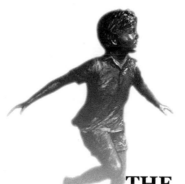

THE
PICU BOOK

A Primer for Medical Students, Residents and
Acute Care Practitioners

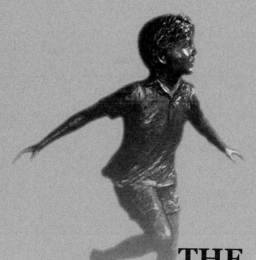

THE
PICU BOOK

A Primer for Medical Students, Residents and
Acute Care Practitioners

editors

Ronald M Perkin • Irma Fiordalisi • William E Novotny

East Carolina University, USA

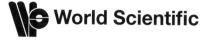

World Scientific

NEW JERSEY • LONDON • SINGAPORE • BEIJING • SHANGHAI • HONG KONG • TAIPEI • CHENNAI

Published by

World Scientific Publishing Co. Pte. Ltd.

5 Toh Tuck Link, Singapore 596224

USA office: 27 Warren Street, Suite 401-402, Hackensack, NJ 07601

UK office: 57 Shelton Street, Covent Garden, London WC2H 9HE

British Library Cataloguing-in-Publication Data
A catalogue record for this book is available from the British Library.

THE PICU BOOK
A Primer for Medical Students, Residents and Acute Care Practitioners

ISBN-13 978-981-4329-60-6
ISBN-10 981-4329-60-6

Typeset by Stallion Press
Email: enquiries@stallionpress.com

Printed in Singapore by World Scientific Printers.

Dedication

We dedicate this work to our PICU team,
whose energy, enthusiasm and desire to excel are inspirational,
and to our colleagues and all health professionals
whose respect and love for children
are a driving force to learn, teach and practice
pediatric critical care medicine.

About the Editors

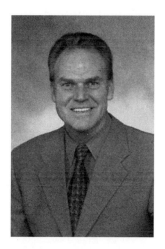

Ronald M. Perkin, MD, MA, FCCM, FAAP

Dr. Perkin is Professor and Chairman, Department of Pediatrics at the Brody School of Medicine, East Carolina University. He also serves as Medical Director, Children's Hospital, University Health Systems of Eastern Carolina and Chief of Pediatrics, Pitt County Memorial Hospital, Greenville, North Carolina.

He obtained his MD degree from the University of South Florida in Tampa, Florida, and completed his internship and residency in Pediatrics at the Children's Hospital in Dallas, Texas. This was followed by a fellowship in Pediatric Critical Care Medicine, also at Children's Hospital in Dallas, Texas. Dr. Perkin is board certified in pediatrics and in pediatric critical care medicine. He is a Fellow of the American Academy of Pediatrics and The American College of Critical Care Medicine.

Dr. Perkin also completed training in Sleep Medicine (1991–1994) at Loma Linda University and is board certified in sleep medicine.

Dr. Perkin completed his MA degree in Biomedical and Clinical Ethics at Loma Linda University's Graduate School in 1997.

Dr. Perkin is a member of many local and national organizations, has received several teaching awards, and has published extensively in the field of pediatric acute and chronic care, and in pediatric sleep medicine.

His military experience was in the US Navy as a pilot.

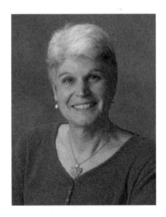

Dr. Fiordalisi

Dr. Fiordalisi is a Professor of Pediatrics, Brody School of Medicine and Director of the Pediatric Intensive Care Unit and Sedation Services at Children's Hospital, University Health Systems of Eastern Carolina in Greenville, North Carolina. She received her MD degree from State University of New York at Brooklyn, Downstate Medical Center and completed pediatric training at Montefiore Hospital and Medical Center-Albert Einstein College of Medicine in the Bronx,

New York. Early experiences in pediatrics included overseas engagements at the International Center for Diarrheal Disease Research in Bangladesh, the Khao-I-Dang Holding Center for Khmer refugees in Thailand and the Department of Community Health at Gondar College of Medical Sciences in Ethiopia. Her interest in pediatric critical care developed after general pediatric and emergency department experience at Kings County Hospital in Brooklyn, New York. She has been board certified in Pediatrics since 1983 and in Pediatric Critical Care Medicine since 1992.

Over the past 25 years, her research interest has been focused on the prevention of brain herniation during treatment of diabetic ketoacidosis. She has many publications in peer reviewed journals and in textbooks regarding the management of this illness.

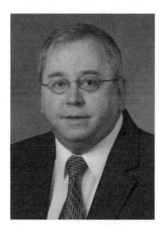

Dr. Novotny

Dr. Novotny is a Professor of Pediatrics at the Brody School of Medicine and serves as Chairman of the Peer Review Committee, Children's Hospital, University Health Systems of Eastern Carolina in Greenville, North Carolina. He earned his MD degree from the Medical College of Ohio at Toledo and completed residency training in pediatrics at Michigan State University. Dr. Novotny completed fellowship training in Pediatric Critical Care Medicine at Children's Hospital, Buffalo, New York. He has been board certified in Pediatrics since 1988 and in Pediatric Critical Care Medicine since 1994. He served in the United States Air Force, during which time he initiated a cardiovascular disease screening program for school-aged children.

Dr. Novotny has special interests in respiratory and cardiovascular pathophysiology and pioneered the use of diagnostic and therapeutic pediatric bronchoscopy in Children's Hospital, Greenville. He has served on the Centers for Disease Control Working Group for investigation and surveillance of acute idiopathic pulmonary hemorrhage in infants and worked on the Task Force for development of clinical practice parameters for the hemodynamic support of pediatric and neonatal patients with septic shock. Dr. Novotny has authored numerous peer-reviewed articles and book chapters relating to his areas of interest.

Contributors

Ira Adler, MD
Clinical Associate Professor
Brody School of Medicine, East Carolina University
Greenville, NC
Chief of Pediatric Imaging
Eastern Radiologists, Inc.
Greenville, NC

Andora Bass, MD
Assistant Professor of Pediatrics
Section of Pediatric Critical Care
Brody School of Medicine at East Carolina University
Greenville, North Carolina

Kathryn D. Bass, MD
Medical Director of Trauma Services
Cook Children's Medical Center
Assistant Professor of Surgery
University of North Texas Health Science Center
Fort Worth, Texas

Cassie A. Billings, BS, Pharm. D.
Clinical Pharmacy Specialist
University Health Systems Pitt County Memorial
    Children's Hospital
Greenville, North Carolina

Catherine Brailer, CPNP-AC
Pediatric Acute Care Nurse Practitioner
University Health Systems, Pitt County Memorial Hospital
  Children's Hospital
Greenville, North Carolina

Alan Branigan, MA, MEd
Director, Educational Support
Eastern Area Health Educational Center
Greenville, North Carolina

Elaine Cabinum-Foeller, MD
Associate Professor
Director of Forensic Pediatrics
Brody School of Medicine at East Carolina University
Greenville, North Carolina

Richard Cartie, MD
Director of Pediatric Critical Care Services
Joseph M. Still Burn Centers, Inc.
Augusta, Georgia

Cathleen Cook, MD
Pediatric Senior Resident
Brody School of Medicine at East Carolina University
Greenville, North Carolina

Charles V. Coren, MD
Chief of Pediatric Surgery
Children's Medical Center
Winthrop University Hospital
Mineola, New York
Assistant Professor of Surgery
State University of New York at Stonybrook
Stonybrook, New York

Christy Denius, BS, CCLS
Certified Child Life Specialist
University Health Systems Pitt County Memorial Hospital
Children's Hospital
Greenville, North Carolina

David Eldridge, MD
Assistant Professor of Pediatrics
Section of General Pediatrics
Brody School of Medicine at East Carolina University
Greenville, North Carolina

David Fairbrother, MD
Assistant Professor of Pediatrics
Section of Pediatric Cardiology
Brody School of Medicine at East Carolina University
Greenville, North Carolina

Irma Fiordalisi, MD
Professor of Pediatrics
Section Head, Pediatric Critical Care
Director, Pediatric Critical Care and Sedation Services
Brody School of Medicine at East Carolina University
Greenville, North Carolina

Susan B. Fox, RN
University Health Systems Pitt County Memorial
Children's Hospital
Greenville, North Carolina

Beng Fuh, MD
Clinical Professor of Pediatrics
Section of Hematology/Oncology
Brody School of Medicine at East Carolina University
Greenville, North Carolina

Melissa Gowans, MD
Assistant Professor of Pediatrics
Section of Pediatric Critical Care
Brody School of Medicine at East Carolina University
Greenville, North Carolina

Roberta S. Gray, MD
Former Clinical Professor of Pediatrics
University of North Carolina School of Medicine and
Director of Nephrology, Carolinas Medical Center
Charlotte, North Carolina

Dynita Haislip, CPNP-AC
Pediatric Acute Care Nurse Practitioner
University Health Systems
Pitt County Memorial Children's Hospital
Greenville, North Carolina

David Hannon, MD
Associate Professor of Pediatrics
Section Head of Pediatric Cardiology
Brody School of Medicine at East Carolina University
Greenville, North Carolina

Glenn D. Harris, MD
Professor of Pediatrics
Section of Pediatric Endocrinology
Brody School of Medicine at East Carolina University
Greenville, North Carolina

Christopher P. Holstege, MD
Chief, Division of Medical Toxicology
Associate Professor, Departments of Emergency
    Medicine & Pediatrics
University of Virginia School of Medicine
Charlottesville, Virginia

Matthew Jordon, Pharm. D.
University Health Systems Pitt County Memorial Hospital
Children's Hospital
Greenville, North Carolina

Karl W Kaminski, RRT-NPS
Respiratory Clinical Specialist
University Health Systems Pitt County Memorial Hospital
Greenville, North Carolina

Cindy Keel, CPNP-AC
Pediatric Acute Care Nurse Practitioner
University Health Systems, Pitt County Memorial Hospital
Children's Hospital
Greenville, North Carolina

Dawn Kendrick, MD
Assistant Professor
Section of Emergency Medicine
Brody School of Medicine at East Carolina University
Greenville, North Carolina

Joseph Lurito, MD
Clinical Associate Professor
Brody School of Medicine, East Carolina University,
Greenville, NC
Senior Neuroradiologist, Central Nervous System Imaging
Eastern Radiologists, Inc.
Greenville, NC

William Novotny, MD
Professor of Pediatrics
Section of Pediatric Critical Care
Brody School of Medicine at East Carolina University
Greenville, North Carolina

Rika O'Malley, MD
Medical Toxicology Fellow
Division of Medical Toxicology
Department of Emergency Medicine
Albert Einstein Medical Center
Philadelphia, Pennsylvania

Tracy Paterson, RN, FNP
Pediatric Sedation Service
University Health Systems, Pitt County Memorial Hospital
Children's Hospital
Greenville, North Carolina

Ronald Perkin, MD, MA
Professor of Pediatrics
Chairman of the Department of Pediatrics
Brody School of Medicine at East Carolina University
Greenville, North Carolina

Melissa Rayburg, MD
Assistant Professor of Pediatrics
Section of Hematology/Oncology
Brody School of Medicine at East Carolina University
Greenville, North Carolina

Timothy Reeder, MD
Associate Professor
Section of Emergency Medicine
Brody School of Medicine at East Carolina University
Greenville, North Carolina

Scot Reeg, MD
Clinical Instructor, Orthopedic Surgery
Brody School of Medicine at East Carolina University
Greenville, North Carolina
Center for Scoliosis and Spinal Surgery
Greenville, North Carolina

Adam K. Rowden, DO
Assistant Professor of Emergency Medicine
Jefferson Medical College
Division Director and Fellowship Program Director
Division of Medical Toxicology
Department of Emergency Medicine
Albert Einstein Medical Center
Major, United States Air Force Reserve
Philadelphia, Pennsylvania

Jose M. Saavedra, MD
Associate Professor of Pediatrics
Division of Gastroenterology and Nutrition
Johns Hopkins University School of Medicine
Baltimore, Maryland

Scott Sagraves, MD, FACS
Associate Professor
Department of Surgery, Trauma Director
Brody School of Medicine at East Carolina University
Greenville, North Carolina

Matthew Salzman, MD
Associate Division Director and Associate Program Director
Division of Medical Toxicology
Director, Clinical Decision Unit
Department of Emergency Medicine
Albert Einstein Medical Center
Philadelphia, Pennsylvania

Charlie Sang, MD
Associate Professor
Section of Hematology/Oncology
Brody School of Medicine at East Carolina University
Greenville, North Carolina

Steven Chad Scarboro, MD
Emergency Medicine Senior Resident
Brody School of Medicine at East Carolina University
Greenville, North Carolina

Jeffrey Schmidt, MD
Clinical Associate Professor of Pediatrics
Section of Pediatric Critical Care
Brody School of Medicine at East Carolina University
Greenville, North Carolina

Jana Sperka, MD
Pediatric Senior Resident
Brody School of Medicine at East Carolina University
Greenville, North Carolina

Robert Dennis Steed, MD
Associate Professor of Pediatrics
Section of Pediatric Cardiology
Brody School of Medicine at East Carolina University
Greenville, North Carolina

Jennifer Sutter, MD
Clinical Assistant Professor
Section Head, Pediatric Endocrinology
Brody School of Medicine at East Carolina University
Greenville, North Carolina

Eric A. Toschlog MD, FACS, FCCM
Associate Professor of Surgery
Director, Surgical Critical Care
Director, Surgical Critical Care Fellowship Program
Brody School of Medicine at East Carolina University
Greenville, North Carolina

Victoria Trapanotto, DO
Clinical Associate Professor of Radiology
Brody School of Medicine, East Carolina University
Greenville, North Carolina
Eastern Radiologists, Inc.
Greenville, North Carolina

Debra Tristram, M.D.
Professor of Pediatrics
Section Head of Pediatric Infectious Disease
Brody School of Medicine at East Carolina University
Greenville, North Carolina

Joel Vanderford, MD
Pediatric Senior Resident
Brody School of Medicine at East Carolina University
Greenville, North Carolina

Alexandra Vasilescu, MD
Fellow, Division of Gastroenterology and Nutrition
Department of Pediatrics
Johns Hopkins University School of Medicine
Baltimore, Maryland

E. Michael Villareal
Medical Student IV
Brody School of Medicine at East Carolina University
Greenville, North Carolina

Jonathan R. Workman, MD, FACS
Clinical Associate Professor of Surgery
Brody School of Medicine at East Carolina University
Greenville, North Carolina
Eastern Carolina Ear, Nose and Throat
Head and Neck Surgery
Greenville, North Carolina

Contents

Complied by C. Keel, I. Fiardalisi and W.E. Novotry

Chapter 1

Introduction

This book is a clinical guide in the practice of pediatric critical care and can serve as a roadmap for an introductory journey through this broadly based and challenging subspecialty. What makes pediatric critical care unique is its scope, which embraces the neonate through the young adult and may encompass any medical and surgical subspecialty during a critical illness. Team leadership, multidisciplinary involvement, clear goals and communication, and patient and family participation are among the essential ingredients for success. It is our hope that this book will provide orientation and inspiration for those privileged to participate in the care of the critically ill pediatric patient.

1.1 How to Use This Book

This handbook is divided into 15 chapters, each of which is subdivided into sections. The Table of Contents will reveal that each chapter encompasses an approach to an organ system or category of problem frequently encountered in a pediatric intensive care unit (PICU). Infectious diseases are addressed within the discussion of specific organ systems and in the *Appendix, part 2*, rather than as a separate chapter. Since critical care is in large part a study of relationships between organs and organ systems, reference to relevant sections within this handbook are commonly made, and recognizable by parentheses with the referenced section in italics. Key points, lists, management considerations and other useful information are often summarized in boxes or figures throughout the text. The boxes and figures are numbered (based on the section of their location) in bolded font so that the text to which they are relevant can be found easily. The editors encourage use of a reliable pediatric drug dose reference, and recommend that drug doses, indications, contraindications, adverse reactions and other considerations always be double checked from a dedicated medication resource before prescribing any medication.

All abbreviations used in this book are alphabetized and identified in the *Appendix, part 1*. The *Appendix, part 2* contains useful reference materials, decision trees, formulae, definitions and guidelines for empiric antibiotic therapies. Familiarity with its contents will serve as a sturdy foundation for stimulating exploration of this exciting field of pediatric medicine.

1.2 General Approach to the Critically Ill Child

Rapid assessment of airway, breathing, circulation and neurologic status are paramount in the evaluation of any ill child, regardless of the underlying disease. Although in practice, the evaluations of these systems occur simultaneously, the ingredients of this primary assessment are discussed in sequence to reflect priorities in interventions. The basics of the metabolic, hematologic and infectious disease aspects of the general assessment are outlined. Critically ill patients are dynamic; electronic monitoring is essential but does not replace frequent bedside reassessments.

Assessment of Airway and Breathing (Box 1.2.1). The airway is the pathway by which gases move in and out of the lungs. Breathing refers to the events of respiration (oxygenation and ventilation). Disease that interferes with the airway or breathing can result in respiratory distress (increased work of breathing) and respiratory failure (inadequate oxygenation and/or ventilation to meet metabolic needs). Respiratory distress can lead to respiratory failure, followed by cardiovascular insufficiency and cardiac arrest if adequate oxygenation and ventilation are not restored. Deterioration of neurologic function during respiratory or cardiovascular compromise indicates respiratory or cardiovascular failure; timely treatment of the underlying disturbance should result in neurologic improvement.

Box 1.2.1

Signs of Respiratory Distress:	Signs of Respiratory Failure:
• Tachypnea • Retractions • Nasal flaring • Positional preference • Difficult inspiration (stridor) • Difficult expiration (wheezing) • Grunting respirations	• Signs of respiratory distress or inadequate respiratory effort • Inadequate aeration • Apnea • Agitation; depressed mental status, decreased muscle tone • Cyanosis, shock, arrhythmias

---

Observation of the pattern of breathing, attention to airway and lung sounds (grossly audible or only heard with a stethoscope), and the response to interventions may help identify the cause of respiratory difficulties.

Assessment and management should proceed simultaneously. Continuous ECG monitoring and pulse oximetry should be instituted on arrival to the PICU if not already in progress. Respiratory failure in a non-intubated patient is typically recognizable based on clinical findings; however, supportive data may be required in individual cases (**Boxes 1.2.2 and 1.2.3**).

Box 1.2.2   Clues to the Origin of Respiratory Distress/Failure

- Upper airway obstruction: inspiratory and/or expiratory stridor, voice change; "sniffing position" preference; drooling; obstructive apnea (chest wall movement without adequate gas movement in the airways)
- Lower airway obstruction: prolonged expiration (wheezing); ↑ expiratory work of breathing
- Parenchymal lung disease: grunting respirations, rales (crackles), ronchi, decreased or asymmetric breath sounds
- Abnormal control of ventilation: abnormal breathing pattern resulting in hypoventilation and hypoxemia; central apnea (no air or chest wall movement)
- R/O cardiac causes: poor perfusion, hyperdynamic precordium, displaced PMI, abnormal heart sounds, jugular venous distension, hepatomegaly and cardiomegaly are suggestive of primary cardiac disease.

> **Box 1.2.3   Causes of Respiratory Distress in the Mechanically Ventilated Patient**
>
> - Dislodged or malpositioned ETT/TT
> - Obstructed or kinked ETT/TT
> - Airway secretions
> - Pneumothorax
> - Pleural effusion
> - Worsening lung disease
> - Worsening heart disease
>
> - Inadequate ventilatory support
> - Patient-ventilator asynchrony
> - Insufficient analgesia
> - Insufficient sedation
> - Altered mental status (delirium)
> - Abdominal distension that compromises ventilation

Tools for the assessment of respiratory distress and failure:

- Determine relevant **historical events**
- Focus on key physical features that characterize the respiratory status:

  ▸ Level of consciousness
  ▸ Color
  ▸ Respiratory rate and rhythm: Observe and count respirations; impedance pneumography may be inaccurate

  ▸ Work of breathing
  ▸ Auscultation: Serial re-assessments are critical to defining direction and response to treatment
  ▸ Feel for crepitus

- Continuous oxygen saturation (SaO_2) by **pulse oximetry** (Pox) and end-tidal CO_2 monitoring (**Boxes 1.2.4, 1.2.6, and Fig. 1.2.1**)
- **Blood gases** to confirm sufficiency or insufficiency of oxygenation and ventilation, provide information regarding acid-base balance, document validity of Pox and non-invasive CO_2 data and responses to interventions. Blood gases are interpreted based on the source of the specimen. Arterial blood is the gold standard for measurement of blood pH and partial pressures of oxygen (PaO_2) and carbon dioxide ($PaCO_2$). Specimens from alternative sources may be useful

Box 1.2.4   Pulse Oximetry: Key Points

- 98% of arterial O_2 is bound to hemoglobin (Hb) at atmospheric pressure.
- SaO_2 measures the percentage of Hb saturated by O_2. The SaO_2 is in equilibrium with the PaO_2, (the partial pressure of O_2 dissolved in blood).
- Changes in pH, temperature and 2,3 DPG influence this equilibrium, resulting in greater or lesser affinity of Hb for O_2 with consequences on O_2 delivery (see *Oxyhemoglobin Dissociation Curve, Appendix, part 2, III*).
- Limitations:
  - ▶ Provides no information regarding ventilation
  - ▶ Motion artifact may distort readings
  - ▶ Readings become inaccurate at lower saturations (<70%)
  - ▶ Often a lag between acute tissue hypoxemia and desaturation by Pox
  - ▶ Does not detect hyperoxia
  - ▶ At pH 7.40, SaO_2 by Pox does not fall below ~90% until PaO_2 <60–70 mmHg
  - ▶ The PaO_2 may decline from a very high value (*e.g.* 200) to ~65 mmHg without a significant decrease in SaO_2 by Pox.
- **Readings may be distorted by:**

▶ Incorrect probe placement	▶ Poor perfusion or severe anemia
▶ Ambient light	▶ Venous congestion
▶ Motion	▶ Abnormal Hb: *e.g.* carboxy
▶ Electromagnetic radiation (MRI, cell phones, electrocautery)	and met-hemoglobin
	▶ Nail polish or very dark skin

- SaO_2 in the presence of Hb F is accurately read by Pox, but the PaO_2 is lower at a given saturation because of ↑ affinity of Hb F for O_2.
- The oxy-Hb dissociation curve is shifted to the right in Hb SS. Although Pox misreadings have been reported, the error is not sufficient to cause misdiagnosis of hypoxemia or normoxemia in sickle cell disease. Therefore, Pox readings are clinically useful during treatment.
- The PaO_2 and calculated O_2 saturation are falsely elevated in the presence of met-Hb and carboxy-Hb. Pox SaO_2 ↓s as met-Hb ↑s, but plateaus at 85%.

Box 1.2.5   Comparison of Capillary and Venous Blood Gas Values with ABG Values

	Sample source	
	Capillary	**Venous**
pH	Similar or ↓	↓
PCO_2	Similar or ↑	↑
PO_2	↓*	↓
Base deficit	Same	Same

* May correlate with $PaCO_2$ in the neonate.

Box 1.2.6   Differential Diagnosis of Flat $ETCO_2$ Waveform

- ETT not in trachea
- ETT obstruction
- Obstruction distal to ETT
- Apnea
- Device malfunction

- Inadequate pulmonary perfusion (*e.g.* pulmonary embolus; no flow during CPA)
- Widespread cell death (no CO_2 production)

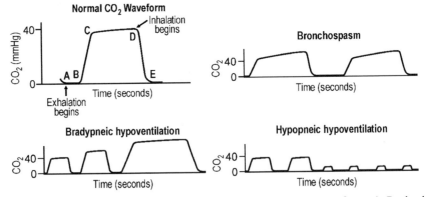

Fig. 1.2.1. $ETCO_2$ Waveform Examples.   Normal CO_2 waveform: A–B, dead space ventilation; B–C, expiration of detectable CO_2; C–D, alveolar emptying plateau; D, end-tidal CO_2; D–E, inspiratory phase. Increased $PaCO_2$ is not necessarily reflected in ↑ $ETCO_2$. Bronchospasm: $ETCO_2$ may be normal, ↑ or ↓ despite a rising $PaCO_2$; Bradypneic hypoventilation: $ETCO_2$ ↑; Hypopneic hypoventilation: $ETCO_2$ ↓.

if obtained from a freely flowing peripheral vein (VBG) or freely flowing warmed capillary bed (CBG) in a well perfused extremity. Use of a tourniquet or squeezing to obtain blood may result in artifactual lowering of the pH and elevation of the PCO_2. Capillary PO_2 may correlate with PaO_2 in a well perfused neonate, but does not reliably reflect oxygenation beyond that age group (**Box 1.2.5**).

- **End-tidal CO_2 ($ETCO_2$) monitoring** detects (qualitatively) or measures (quantitatively, using infra-red light) CO_2 at the end of a tidal breath. The device may be "mainstream" (directly in the airway of an intubated patient; this device may be too bulky and contributes to dead space especially in small patients) or "side-stream" (at the nose, nose and mouth or side port of an ETT adapter; side-stream sampling makes it possible to monitor non-intubated patients; when measured from the distal ETT, sampling error may result in higher $ETCO_2$ readings).

NOTE: $ETCO_2$ depends on: ventilation, lung perfusion and cell metabolism. A colorimetric $ETCO_2$ detector accurately identifies the presence of CO_2 via an ETT and is 100% sensitive in confirming its location in the trachea provided lung perfusion is adequate. If $ETCO_2$ exceeds 15 mmHg, litmus paper in the device changes from purple to yellow. Capnometry provides a digital $ETCO_2$ quantitative measurement. Capnography provides a measurement and a waveform that describes the pattern of CO_2 exhalation over time with each breath. Either method is useful in patients receiving supplemental oxygen since ventilatory failure may not be reflected by oxygen desaturation by Pox until very late. Lack of CO_2 delivery to the lung during cardiac arrest results in a flattened waveform and absent detection of CO_2. Emergence of detectable CO_2 during CPR occurs before return of pulses and is the earliest indicator of return of spontaneous circulation. In viable conditions with normal lung function, the difference between $ETCO_2$ and $PaCO_2$ is $< 5\,mmHg$. Correlation with measured $PaCO_2$ is essential to interpretation of $ETCO_2$. As ventilation to perfusion mismatch increases, the difference between $ETCO_2$ and $PaCO_2$ increases. Monitoring trends and the $ETCO_2$ waveform are useful so long as the limitations of the device are realized (**Fig. 1.2.1 and Box 1.2.6**).

- **Transcutaneous CO_2 (TCO$_2$) monitoring** uses a heated electrode on the skin to measure capillary pH and extrapolates the PCO_2 using the Henderson-Hasselbalch equation; this device has been shown to approximate $PaCO_2$ more accurately than $ETCO_2$ in infants and children less than 40 months with lung disease, but overestimation of PCO_2 due to local heating of the sampling site is a problem. The device requires calibration and site rotation, and is unreliable in the presence of shock, hypothermia and during use of vasoconstrictive medications.
- **CXR** to identify support tube (ETT, NG tube, *etc.*) locations, R/O conditions that may need specific intervention (*e.g.* pneumothorax), characterize lung disease and help provide other clues to diagnosis (*e.g.* rib fractures).
- **Further studies as indicated:** Ultrasound evaluation for fluid, diaphragmatic motion; CT for lung abscess, trauma, congenital malformations, pulmonary embolus (CT angiography); bronchoscopy for possible foreign body, diagnostic culture, removal of secretions, *etc.*

General Approach to Management. Respiratory distress warrants immediate evaluation to determine its cause, prevent progression to respiratory failure and provide therapy specific to the disturbance. If respiratory failure is evident in a non-intubated patient, airway patency and ventilatory support should be ensured (*Bag-Mask Ventilation and Tracheal Intubation 15.2; Non-invasive Ventilatory Support 2.8.2*).

Initial interventions for respiratory distress include:

- 100% oxygen by facemask
- Ensure that the patient's position optimizes airway patency ("head elevation, sniffing position"). For a supine infant, place a small roll under the shoulders; the supine child should have a roll placed under both the neck and the occiput (if the cervical spine is stable). Apply a cervical collar in cases of uncertain cervical spine stability (*Bag-Mask Ventilation and Tracheal Intubation, 15.2, Fig. 15.2.1*).
- Ensure that the upper airway is clear of secretions; suction if necessary (120 mmHg) with a semi-rigid catheter.

- Rule out cardiac causes of respiratory distress.
- If stridor is present, minimize agitation, allow position of comfort; potential therapies include racemic epinephrine, steroids, heliox
- If reactive airway disease is known or suspected, β-agonists and steroids are the mainstay of therapy (*Acute severe asthma 2.3.1*).
- If a tracheostomy tube (TT) is present, ensure its location and patency by auscultation and suctioning via the tube with sterile technique at 40–60 mmHg. If occlusion is suspected, the TT should be replaced (*Tracheostomy 11.2.3*).
- If non-invasive Pox and CO_2 monitoring are performed, periodic correlation with ABG's is recommended.
- Identify actual or potential infection, note quality of respiratory - secretions, culture as indicated and treat with appropriate antibiotics.

Assessment of Circulation. The goal of this assessment is to determine the adequacy of the cardiac output (CO), to identify and reverse shock, and identify compensatory mechanisms that may be relieved by appropriate interventions before decompensated shock (hypotension) occurs. **CO (blood volume circulated/min) = HR (heart rate, beats/min) × SV (stroke volume, volume/beat)**; CO decreases if either HR or SV decreases unless there is a compensatory increase in the other factor. Pediatric patients are more dependent on HR to increase CO to meet metabolic demands than adults. Blood pressure also is related to CO: **CO = MAP (mean arterial blood pressure)/SVR (systemic vascular resistance) or MAP = CO × SVR.** As CO decreases, SVR increases and BP is preserved (**Fig. 1.2.2**). Skin, gastrointestinal and renal perfusion are sacrificed to provide a greater portion of the cardiac output to heart and brain. Examination of skin provides early, readily accessible information regarding physiologic compensatory responses. Skilled clinical assessments are critical, and serially performed examinations form the foundation of circulatory care in all patients.

Tools for the assessment of circulation:

- **Heart rate:** objective; sensitive in response to decreases in CO; non-specific. Inappropriately low HR's during poor perfusion often heralds impending cardiopulmonary arrest or may signal hypothermia.

- **Blood Pressure** (BP): objective and should be readily measurable. Erroneous readings may occur, but should not be attributed to equipment failure unless this is demonstrable. BP is preserved by compensatory increases in HR, SVR and sometimes, SV until decompensation (hypotension) occurs (**Fig. 1.2.2**). BP can be monitored non-invasively (cuff) or invasively (indwelling arterial catheter; "arterial line"). Normal BP varies with gender, size and age. Non-invasive measurement requires an appropriate cuff size: bladder width should be

---

Box 1.2.7   Troubleshooting Sinus Tachycardia

- Dehydration
- Shock
- Fever
- Pain

- Hypoxia; hypercarbia
- Sepsis
- Acidosis
- Anemia

- Drug-related
- Raised ICP
- Anxiety
- Seizures (non-convulsive)

Box 1.2.8   Troubleshooting Bradycardia

• Hypoxia • Hypotension; terminal arrhythmia • Hypothermia • Spinal cord injury • CNS disease • Raised ICP • Hypertension • Conditioning • Sleep • Reflexive	• ↑ Vagal tone (*e.g.* coughing, vomiting, airway instrumentation) • Autonomic dysfunction • Cardiomyopathy; myocarditis; Kawasaki's Disease; SLE • Pulmonary hypertension	• Drug-related (*e.g.* β–blockers, Ca^{++} channel blockers; digoxin) • Sick sinus syndrome • Surgical injury • AV block, congenital or acquired • Toxin-related; *e.g.* organophosphates • Obstructive hyperbilirubinemia

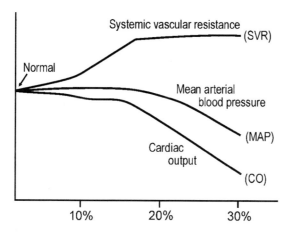

Fig. 1.2.2. Hemodynamic Response to Hemorrhage. The X-Axis shows the percent of blood volume lost. Hypotension is a late event in pediatric shock. Modified from Schwaitzberg, S.D., Bergman, K.S., Harris, B.H. A pediatric trauma model of continuous hemorrhage. *J Pediatr Surg* **23**:605–609, 1988.

~40% of mid-upper-arm circumference; the inflatable cuff should encircle 80–100% of the arm. A cuff that is either too narrow or too short (undercuffing) yields an artificially high BP; a cuff that is too wide or too long may cause an erroneously low BP reading. Auscultation with the use of a mercury sphygmomanometer is the method of choice; all normative data were obtained by this method. Electronic oscillometric devices measure the mean BP; systolic and diastolic pressures are calculated and are less reliable. Indications for placement of an arterial catheter include close monitoring of BP and when vasoactive drugs are used. An indwelling arterial catheter provides the most accurate measurement of BP in a sick patient provided the equipment is functioning well and the users are knowledgeable and skilled. Accuracy depends on:

→ The resonant frequency and damping characteristics of the system; troubleshoot by the "rapid flush test" (**Fig. 1.2.3**)
→ The location of the transducer at the level of the right atrium
→ Correct "zeroing" of the pressure transducer with the atmosphere

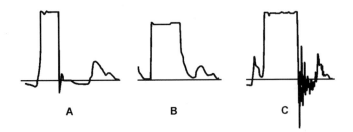

Fig. 1.2.3.   Rapid Flush Test.   Open and close the valve/stopcock quickly while a continuous flush is infusing. A, normal: <3 negative deflections. B, overdamped: seen with air in the system. C, underdamped: multiple deflections around the baseline; seen with excessive tubing length, high CO states. Intra-arterial Pressure Curves, redrawn from Celinski SA, Seneff MG, Arterial line placement and care, in Rippe JM, Irwin RS (eds.), *Intensive Care Medicine*, 6th ed. Lippincott, Williams & Wilkins, Philadelphia, p. 39, 2008.

→ Integrity of tubing and adapter connections

→ Vascular factors (*e.g.* vasospasm) may alter the normal waveform (**Fig. 1.2.4**) and lead to a reading that does not reflect systemic BP.

• **Palpation of peripheral pulse volume**, especially foot pulses: subjective; when compared to central pulse volume, diminished foot pulses signal increased SVR, a lesser difference between systolic and diastolic pressures, and compensation for inadequate CO. Foot pulses are affected before radial pulses. Although not quantifiable, this component of the evaluation is considered indispensible by many experienced examiners.

• **Capillary refill time (CRT):** More reproducible assessment than pulse volume; apply light pressure to a fingernail bed positioned slightly above the level of the heart until blanching occurs, then release. Normal color should return within 2 seconds. Prolongation of CRT occurs with shock, increased SVR, acidemia, hypothermia and environmental cooling.

• **Skin color and temperature:** Nail beds are normally pink. Inadequate skin perfusion causes pallor, mottling and cyanosis, beginning distally and progressing centrally as severity increases.

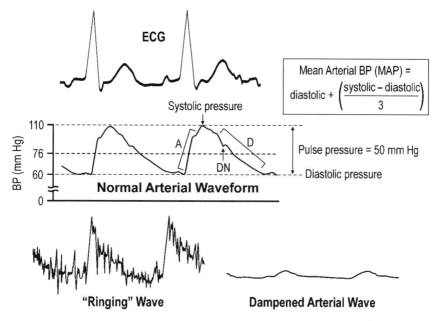

ECG

Systolic pressure

$$\text{Mean Arterial BP (MAP)} = \text{diastolic} + \left(\frac{\text{systolic} - \text{diastolic}}{3}\right)$$

110
76
60
0
BP (mm Hg)

A   D
DN

Normal Arterial Waveform

Pulse pressure = 50 mm Hg

Diastolic pressure

"Ringing" Wave

Dampened Arterial Wave

Fig. 1.2.4. Arterial Waveform. Systolic peak pressure occurs after the QRS complex. The peak of the anacrotic limb (A) is the systolic blood pressure; the dicrotic limb (D) reflects diastole. DN, dicrotic notch, reflects aortic valve closure. The transducer should be positioned at the mid-axillary line (RA level). "Ringing" occurs with rapid movement of the catheter tip, hyperdynamic states, ↑BP, ↑SVR, aortic regurgitation. Damping occurs with ↓SVR, hypovolemia, aortic stenosis. Loss of integrity of the system or malposition of the transducer distorts the waveform and leads to erroneous readings.

Causes other than shock include environmental cooling, hypothermia and severe anemia.

- **Altered mental status:** Consistent with decreased cerebral oxygenation and decompensated shock
- **Measure serial ABG's:** Assess acid-base balance and correlate oxygenation and ventilation with non-invasive devices in use.
- **Measure serum lactic acid:** Elevation of serum lactate is most commonly due to inadequate tissue oxygenation (type A lactic acidosis) as seen in shock. This is attributed to anaerobic metabolism (increased production of lactate) and possibly, hepatic (and

to a lesser extent, renal) hypoperfusion (decreased utilization and excretion of lactate). Lactate is also increased with use of potent vasoconstrictors (*e.g.* epinephrine and β-agonists). Serial measurement of lactic acid is useful in monitoring the progress of resuscitation from shock, and generally decreases within one hour of circulatory improvement, although may transiently increase with "washout".

- **Urine output (UOP):** Reflects renal blood flow. Under conditions of normovolemia, hourly UOP is ~1/3 to 1/2 the hourly maintenance fluid allotment. Oliguria or anuria is consistent with decreased renal perfusion in the absence of intrinsic renal disease or obstruction to outflow. R/O an obstructed bladder catheter as a cause of "poor UOP" in a patient with a urinary catheter.

- **Central venous pressure (CVP):** Assists in assessment of volume status and allows for measurement of O_2 saturation in central venous blood ($ScvO_2$; reflects adequacy of systemic O_2 delivery and extraction). CVP measurement requires a central venous catheter with its tip in a central vein near the right atrium. If the tricuspid valve is normal, CVP reflects right ventricular preload, and is affected by right ventricular compliance, afterload (both pulmonary and systemic) and contractility; CVP is also affected by intrapleural pressures. Trends in CVP and its response to interventions (*e.g.* volume administration, diuresis, vasoactive drugs) are useful in guiding therapy. "Normal" CVP varies, but is usually < 5 mmHg in healthy patients. For patients with evidence of shock, a CVP < 8–10 mmHg may indicate a need for volume administration (*Important Cardiopulmonary Interactions, 3.2*; **Fig. 1.2.5**).

- **12-lead ECG, echocardiogram** to further evaluate for problems such as arrhythmias, ischemic patterns, evidence of electrolyte disturbances or intoxications, voltage abnormalities, cardiomegaly, anatomic abnormalities, pericardial disease, myocardial dysfunction and pulmonary hypertension.

- **CK-MB** and **troponin I** are useful indicators of myocardial necrosis; **brain natriuretic peptide (BNP)** reflects severity of CHF. These may be used to supplement serial monitoring in these conditions.

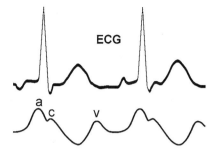

Fig. 1.2.5. Normal CVP Waveform. a, atrial contraction; c, tricuspid valve closure; v, ventricular contraction and atrial filling.

General Approach to Management. Shock requires immediate evaluation to determine its cause, prevent progression to arrest and provide therapy specific to the disturbance so that normal perfusion can be restored.

- Give supplemental O_2 until perfusion is normalized
- Except in cases of congestive heart failure most instances of pediatric shock require fluid resuscitation. Isotonic sodium salt solution such as NaCl 0.9% 10–20 ml/kg has been recommended for initial resuscitation. If signs of congestive heart failure (cardiomegaly, hepatomegaly, jugular venous distension, pulmonary edema) are uncertain, *cautious* administration of NaCl 0.9% 5 ml/kg may be given with close monitoring for the effects of this intervention.
- Patients with septic shock may require ≥ 60 ml/kg of resuscitation fluid during the first hour of treatment.
- Vasoactive drugs are indicated when shock is present despite a CVP ≥ 10 mmHg or as indicated by physical and echocardiographic evaluation.
- Serial examinations of perfusion, monitoring of UOP, blood gases and serum lactate guide progress.

Neurologic Assessment. Serial neurologic evaluations are an integral part of intensive care monitoring and are typically performed at least hourly for patients with instability of any organ system. (*Altered* *in Mental Status 5.1*) Problem management is based on specific findings (*Central Nervous System Disease and Dysfunction, Chapter 5*).

Tools for the assessment of the CNS:

- Determine **relevant historical events**.
- Age-appropriate evaluation of **mental status**; assess cortical and brainstem function; assess **pupillary exam**.
- Evaluate for cervical spine instability by history, physical examination and imaging if necessary. Immobilize the C-spine if injury is suspected.
- **Assess the need for analgesia**; select agents and doses that will not endanger respiratory effort (in non-intubated patients) and circulation.
- When possible, avoid neurotropic drugs when the mental status is not stable until a diagnosis can be made.
- Note seizure activity or movement suspicious for seizure; EEG may be required if non-convulsive status or pseudoseizure is suspected.
- **R/O hypoglycemia** with bedside glucose testing if seizure or other neurologic symptoms are present; consider other metabolic causes of neurologic dysfunction (*Altered Mental Status, 5.1*).
- **Image the brain** (CT) if intracranial abnormality is suspected; serial head CT's may be required to monitor evolution or development of pathology. Brain and/or spine MRI may be needed to identify non-acute blood products, ischemic changes, demyelinating disease, encephalitis, vascular lesions not demonstrable by CT, optimal imaging of the posterior fossa, etc.
- **LP** if CNS infection is suspected and no contraindications are present.
- Measure levels of antiepileptic drugs (AED's) if indicated (*e.g.* during recurrent seizure while receiving AED's or after loading); consider metabolic causes of seizure (*Status Epilepticus, 5.2*).
- Identify and treat raised ICP.

Assessment of Metabolic Status. The extent of this assessment is based on history and physical findings. **Glucose and electrolytes**, including **calcium and magnesium** are measured in most all PICU patients because of the frequency of abnormalities in the critically ill, the diagnostic clues they provide and potential complications such as arrhythmias from uncorrected disturbances. In addition to a review of airway, breathing and circulatory status, elements of this evaluation include:

- **Patient weight:** For over-weight patients, use ideal weight (*Appendix, part 1*) for fluid and electrolyte calculations; establish the drug-specific weight for medication dosing. Serial weights (daily in some cases) should be monitored.
- Correct and monitor for **hypoglycemia** (see *Hypo- and Hyperglycemia, 6.4*).
- Choose i.v. fluids (IVF) based on glucose and electrolyte need; Stress related hyperglycemia is common in PICU patients, and often improves spontaneously during the first several hours of treatment. Glucose-containing i.v. fluid should be withheld during this time to avoid serum glucose in excess of 180 mg/dL for prolonged periods. Administration of insulin may be required to control hyperglycemia to an acceptable range (~80–180 mg/dL). For patients with CNS disease, glucose control should be more strict (e.g. 80–150 mg/dL). If IVF does not contain glucose, blood glucose should be monitored closely so that dextrose can be provided as soon as hyperglycemia resolves. This is particularly important in infants and young children whose glycogen stores are marginal. Hypoglycemia or ketoacidosis may result from inadequate glucose delivery.
- Unanticipated hyperglycemic events should prompt a search for stress such as new infection, seizure, deterioration in ventilation, or inadvertent glucose delivery.
- Provide sodium, at least 75 mEq/L for patients beyond the neonatal age group. For patients with CNS disease, isotonic fluids should be given. Withhold potassium until UOP and renal function are ensured, and K^+ release (*e.g.* rhabdomyolysis, collections of blood, tumor lysis) is not a concern. Electrolytes should be measured at least daily in patients who are receiving i.v. fluids.

- **Monitor UOP, stool, and other losses** incurred from drainage sites such as nasogastric (NG) or other enteric tubes, ventriculostomy (CSF) drainage, chest tubes, wounds and blood, including iatrogenic blood loss. Losses from these sites may generate a "new" deficit if not replaced with fluid of similar composition. In addition to water and salt, proteinaceous losses may occur over time depending on the drainage site and disease. Plasma components should be evaluated for replacement by periodic measurement of total protein, albumin and immunoglobulin in serum.
- **Electrolyte replacement:** See *Electrolyte Disturbances 6.2* for specific interventions.
- **Monitor renal function** biochemically by urea nitrogen (BUN) and creatinine; if these are abnormal, estimate creatinine clearance (Cl_{cr}) and adjust drug doses as indicated for renal insufficiency.
- Evaluate hepatic insufficiency (albumin, bilirubin, PT, PTT, fibrinogen, ammonia) as indicated and adjust medication dosing as appropriate.
- Consider toxicologic evaluations (*Poisonings, Chapter 14*).
- Consider stress ulcer prophylaxis for very sick patients, particularly those who are not receiving gastric feeding.
- Provide nutrition as soon as safe and appropriate (*Nutritional Requirements in the Hospitalized and Critically Ill Child, 8.1*).
- Plan a bowel regimen for patients receiving enteral feeding and narcotics.
- Consider prophylaxis in patients at increased risk for deep vein thrombosis (DVT):

  ‣ Adolescents
  ‣ Patients with inflammatory disease, including active infection
  ‣ Active malignancy
  ‣ Pregnancy
  ‣ History of prior DVT or known thrombogenic disorder
  ‣ Major trauma and/or burns
  ‣ Immobility (>48 hrs)
  ‣ Obesity

Hematologic Assessment. Clinical data dictate the extent of hematologic investigations.

Tools include:

- **CBC:** Identify anemia, thrombocytopenia, neutropenia, marked leukocytosis; R/O drug-related effects such as leukocytosis secondary to steroids, bone marrow suppression due to cytotoxic agents, *etc.* Note cell characteristics such as *toxic granulations* in neutrophils in infection.
- **PT, PTT, INR, Fibrinogen:** important when platelets are decreased or coagulopathy or liver dysfunction is suspected; a breakdown product of fibrin, **D-dimer**, is often elevated in but not specific for DIC, DVT, and pulmonary embolus.
- **Hemoglobin electrophoresis:** important for quantification of hgb S in acute chest syndrome and CNS complications of sickle cell disease.
- Measurement of **carboxyhemoglobin** (R/O carbon monoxide exposure); **methemoglobin** (R/O methemoglobinemia; monitor for methemoglobin toxicity during nitric oxide therapy).

Fever and Infectious Disease. History, physical examination and the above data provide clues to whether or not infection is likely to be present or should be ruled out in the diagnostic process. "Normal" body temperature varies depending on time of day (lower in morning than late afternoon) and site of measurement; the gold standard for core temperature is the temperature in the pulmonary artery (PA);

Box 1.2.9   Causes of Fever

- Infection
- Systemic inflammatory response syndrome (SIRS)
- Seizures
- Trauma
- Drug withdrawal
- Drug induced (antibiotics, intoxications, malignant hyperthermia)
- Transfusion related
- Environmental; heat stroke
- Neoplasm
- Dehydration; anhidrosis
- Collagen vascular disease
- Deep vein thrombosis/ Pulmonary embolus
- Central fever
- Paroxysmal autonomic instability with dystonia ("PAID"; post TBI)

urinary bladder, nasopharyngeal and lower esophageal sites have approximated PA temperatures. The data regarding tympanic temperatures are disparate and evolving. Rectal temperature may lag behind PA core temperature by as much as 2.5 hrs. Axillary temperature correlates poorly with PA temperature, particularly in the presence of fever. There is also evidence that brain temperature in an injured brain is typically higher than temperature measured at other sites, including the PA. Note that abnormal temperature is not uniformly present during infection.

Fever is associated with tachycardia, increases in O_2 consumption, CO and catecholamine release. Fever in infected animals improves survival; its presence in patients with cardiopulmonary disease may profoundly affect their stability *i.e.* further tachycardia may not be tolerated. The need to "treat fever" in PICU patients rests on individual assessment of potential risks and benefits. The differential diagnosis of fever should also be individualized; if infection cannot be ruled out based on historical and physical data, potential sites of infection should be cultured (*e.g.* blood, wound, urine, airway secretions, CSF, stool, *etc.*) or otherwise evaluated [*e.g.* antigen-detection by polymerase chain reaction (PCR), imaging studies, *etc.*] when appropriate; empiric therapy may be indicated based on circumstances. Relevant antibiotic therapies are discussed in sections devoted to specific organ systems.

Communication in the PICU. Clear communication and construction of a unified plan is critical for safe and effective patient care. Breakdown in communication, including breakdown in "hand-offs" in care, continuity of care or care planning were responsible for up to 80% of sentinel events reported to the Joint Commission (JCAHO, 2006).

Qualities of effective hand-offs in patient care include the following:

• Data are current, accurate and complete; use a standardized format with an organ-system approach (**Box 1.2.10**); checklists are helpful.
• Minimize unnecessary interruptions.
• Use direct communication rather than "messengers".

> **Box 1.2.10   Suggested Problem-Oriented Patient Report**
>
> - Neurologic/Psychiatric
>   Pain and sedation management
> - Respiratory
>   Ventilator management
> - Cardiovascular/perfusion
> - Fluids, electrolytes, nutrition
>   (renal/GI)
> - Hematologic
> - Infectious diseases; temperature
>   status; recent or relevant
>   culture data
> - Musculoskeletal and
>   Mobilization issues
>
> - Endocrinologic
> - Skin
> - Scheduled laboratory studies
> - Radiology
> - Consultations
> - Vascular access
> - DVT/peptic ulcer
>   prophylaxis
> - Other
> - Social/family needs;
>   communications
> - Communications with
>   primary care providers

- "SBAR" (Situation, Background, Assessment, Recommendation) format can be helpful for addressing new problems.
- "Readback" of verbal information and telephone orders solidifies understanding between caregivers.

Current physical findings, **medications** and data relevant to the organ-system should be discussed in each category. Plans, anticipated outcomes and alternative care pathways should be identified where relevant and appropriate. A system of "checks and balances" should flow within the team. Patient information, orders, medications, dosages, laboratory data and treatments should be reviewed and checked by care-givers at different levels of care delivery to minimize error.

The PICU environment is one that should promote communication among team members; while making these efforts, it is imperative that patient confidentiality be maintained. The Privacy Rule of the Health Insurance Portability and Accountability Act (HIPAA) of 1996 addresses the use and disclosure of personal health information in an effort to balance the need for sharing information among relevant providers while protecting the privacy of patients. Each health care provider should be familiar with these regulations and ensure that personal health information remains protected.

1.3 Transport of the Critically Ill Child

The pediatric critical care transport team provides mobile pediatric critical care services en route to specialty care centers when local resources are unable to meet patient needs. Early consultation between the referring and accepting centers is essential for optimal outcome for the critically ill child.

The Emergency Medical Treatment and Active Labor Act (EMTALA) of 1986 included three provisions to protect patients from premature or unwarranted transfer to another facility: (1) an appropriate medical screening examination must be provided at the emergency department (ED); (2) the referring hospital must stabilize any emergency condition or transfer the patient and (3) a patient cannot be transferred to another health care facility unless (a) the stabilized patient requires a higher level of care; (b) the patient is not stable but benefits of transfer outweigh risks or (c) the necessary specialty on-call physician fails to appear within a reasonable period and benefits of transfer outweigh risks.

Key steps in the transfer of care process are *preparation, anticipation and transportation.* Preparation involves advanced as well as patient-specific planning. In addition to development and preservation of pediatric critical care skills that permit the team to conduct all the assessments and procedures discussed in the *General Approach to the Critically Ill Child, 1.2,* the transport team must anticipate the spectrum of circumstances posed by a "scene run", the referring facility, the patient(s), families, first responders, bystanders, the identified mode of transport and ability to communicate with the accepting team. This requires pre-determined protocols, maintenance of an appropriate equipment inventory, and specialized training in providing care in transit. A specific plan of action for "the worst case scenario" is continually reviewed and revised as illness, injury and circumstances evolve.

Team composition is part of preparation and anticipation. Transport teams vary in composition to include local EMS personnel, ED or in-patient personnel from the referring hospital, or critical care transport teams (CCTT), some of which may be dedicated to pediatric or neonatal patients. Dimensions of expertise vary with team composition. Pediatric CCTT's are usually composed of a nurse with pediatric critical care expertise and at least one additional provider (*e.g.* a second nurse, paramedic, respiratory therapist, physician or nurse practitioner). Selection of the mode of transport is based on availability, weather conditions and patient needs **(Box 1.3.1)**.

Box 1.3.1 Transport Modes: Advantages and Disadvantages

	Ambulance	Helicopter	Fixed Wing
Advantages	Spacious Operable in most weather conditions Able to stop for procedures	Rapid transport times ↓ Out-of-hospital time	Ideal for long transports Assessments and procedures are easy to perform en route
Disadvantages	↑ Out-of-hospital time Risk of traffic delays	Dependent on weather conditions Lung sounds inaudible; Difficult to assess pulses; Difficult to perform some procedures	Requires advanced planning Long start-up time Surface transport from hospital to aircraft results in delays
Approximate costs for critical care transports (2009)	$2000.00 plus $15.00 per mile	$9–10,000.00 plus $62.00 per nautical mile	$2–3000.00 per flight hr. plus $13.00 per patient-loaded mile

---

Box 1.3.2   Patient Preparation for Transport

- Referring physician discusses the patient with the receiving physician.
- Receiving physician or a designee activates the transport team with knowledge of:

  ▶ The patient's name, weight, medical condition, current vital signs, airway status, circulatory status, mental status, blood glucose, vascular access, need for continuous infusions, therapies rendered and need for blood products.

  ▶ The name of the referring physician, the referring facility, contact telephone number and the patient's location at that facility.

  ▶ The receiving physician communicates patient-specific needs to the CCTT for immediate planning, including needs for isolation; the team is composed based on patient needs.

- The mode of transport is determined based on medical needs, mode availability and weather.
- The referring facility prepares:

  ▶ Signed EMTALA form
  ▶ Signed consent form for transport
  ▶ Complete copy of the medical record

  ▶ All laboratory results, including notation of those still pending
  ▶ Copies of radiologic studies including plain films, CT scans, *etc.*

Typically, critically ill children are transported to tertiary care centers because of the need for a higher level of care and the benefits of transport outweigh the risks. The transporting team should be able to provide *at minimum* the level of care provided by the referring facility, and optimally, be able to provide a level of care approaching that offered by the accepting unit. The referring facility helps prepare the patient for transport to the best of its ability **(Box 1.3.2)**.

Upon arrival at the referring facility, care transitions to the CCTT which becomes the eyes, ears and hands of the PICU team. The patient is assessed and contact with the accepting physician (or the designated physician in charge of the transport) is made. The receiving team is made aware of key information obtained through the CCTT.

Necessary interventions are performed, and a plan of care is developed as anticipatory discussion occurs and orders are formulated.

Airway and perfusion status are re-assessed continually during transport and after any transfer from bed to bed. Emotional support is provided by the transport team to the patient and family members. On arrival to the PICU, the CCTT re-evaluates prior to transferring the patient to the hospital bed; an "SBAR" (Situation, Background, Assessment, Recommendations) report, including all medications given and interventions performed by the CCTT is provided to complete the transition of care to the PICU team.

1.4 Patient and Family Centered Care

Patient and family-centered care (often called "family centered care" or FCC) refers to a partnership in care between and among patients, families, and professional care-givers, and is applicable to care for all age-groups. Unlike family-focused care, which positions the health professional as the expert and designer of the plan of care, FCC emphasizes a collaborative approach to care delivery and decision-making. The composition of "the family" is defined by the patient and/or guardian(s). The partnership is based on trust and a mutual interest in working for the patient's best interests, as defined by those sharing in the partnership. Open communication is paramount in this relationship. Each member brings an essential ingredient and each partner is respected for his/her contribution; the health care experience provides an opportunity to build upon the strengths of the participants, and create a pathway for education and growth at all levels.

FCC in pediatrics is based on the understanding that the family is the child's primary source of strength and support, and that the perspectives of the child and family are important in clinical decision-making. FCC facilitates learning about and participating in one's own healthcare, and eases the transition into adult service systems. Increased family access to PICU patients has led to an increase in parental presence during bedside rounds, invasive procedures and CPR, typically with a favorable impact on patient care and family satisfaction. For these reasons, it is incumbent upon the PICU team to support access of the family to the PICU patient; parental or care-giver participation is particularly essential for the complex and chronically ill, for whom the insights of those who provide daily care are indispensible for the acute care team. Survey data and small observational studies suggest that children have greater coping abilities when a parent or loved one is present; also, an anxious adult may be relieved by the ability to be present to support the child if he/she chooses. Guidelines for implementation of FCC are listed in **Box 1.4.1.**

FCC involves consideration of the needs of the entire family in developing a plan of care, particularly since these needs may ultimately play a role in the patient's future. Complete and successful resolution of the critical illness and the management of poor outcomes are linked to an appropriate use of resources along with family-centered discharge planning.

Box 1.4.1   Guidelines for the Implementation of Family Centered Care

- The family should be given the option of presence whenever possible.
- A "family facilitator" should be present esp. if the situation warrants timely narratives, explanations and support. The facilitator (*e.g.* chaplain, child life specialist, social worker, psychologist, physician, nurse or respiratory therapist) should not be involved in patient care at that time but should be trained in crisis management, and should be capable of providing accurate information. He/she should also be able to assess the emotional stability of the family, identify unstable behaviors and support the family throughout the crisis.
- Policies and procedures as well as educational opportunities should be available for staff as well as family participants. The staff should be familiar with any contraindications to family presence (*e.g.* combative or threatening behavior; suspected drug/alcohol abuse, *etc.*).
- Support for families who choose not to be present for various interventions should be provided.
- A multidisciplinary unit council or similar body should oversee the FCC effort, educate and support participants and new staff, and incorporate the FCC mission as a quality of care and patient safety issue in the PICU.

1.5 Quality and Safety in the PICU

Quality medical care refers to care that is appropriate for the individual patient and his/her illness, is delivered in a timely fashion and is not harmful. Safety refers to the avoidance of preventable errors. Medical errors resulted in approximately 195,000 deaths per year in the early part of the 21st century. Medication errors are the most common cause of adverse events among hospitalized patients of all ages. Slonim *et al.* (2003) reported approximately two to three medical errors per one-hundred hospitalized pediatric patients.

Stevens, Matlow and Laxer illustrate the difference between quality and safety (**Fig. 1.5.1**): "The left side of the graphic represents 10 children who have come to the hospital for treatment, each one experiencing a specific level of care ranging from low to high quality. The middle section depicts the focus of quality improvement, which is to raise the ceiling so that higher levels of care can be

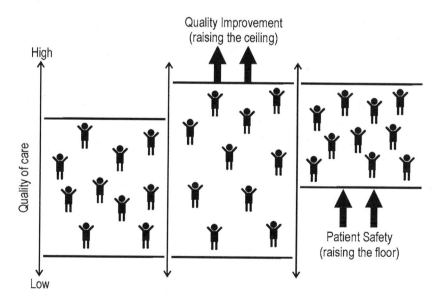

Fig. 1.5.1. Concepts in Quality and Patient Safety. Redrawn with permission; Stevens P, Matlow A, Laxer R, Blueprint for Patient Safety, in Matlow a, Laxer RM (eds.), *Pediatr Clin N Am*, W.B. Saunders, Philadelphia, **53**:1255, 2006.

achieved. The far right section depicts the focus of patient safety, which is to raise the floor so that fewer patients experience poor levels of care or are harmed. Ultimately, quality improvement and ...safety work together..."

Each hospital, service and unit should have a mechanism by which to address input of real or potential adverse events, problems and safety concerns. The environment should be receptive to input from all levels of staff, patients, families and visitors, and have the capacity to evaluate and respond to issues that threaten patient safety and impair the delivery of high quality care. A "high reliability" organization refers to one whose mission is high risk, but which achieves a lower than expected rate of failure. Such industries are highly focused on both near-miss and adverse events, are able to dissect potential or actual problems intensively and glean maximal learning from the event and the evaluation process. There is an emphasis on tailoring the system to meet organizational goals; in health care, these are safe and effective patient-centered care delivered in a timely and cost-effective manner with optimal staff and patient–family satisfaction. This is balanced by an emphasis on personal accountability and a climate that promotes the reporting of real or potential safety concerns by all users with honest discussion of issues.

Human factors engineering, *i.e.* the concept that human performance is to some extent shaped by the environment, especially the systems and technologic environment, is an important component in problem analysis. The multi-disciplinary PICU is unique among intensive care units. The diversity of patient problems, developmental and pharmacologic needs, and unique psychosocial issues can create a stressful environment that poses additional challenges to "raising the floor" of safety. Quality indicators for PICU's have yet to be defined; the following measures have been proposed and are undergoing study:

- Standardized mortality ratio
- Severity-adjusted length of stay
- Unanticipated re-admission to the PICU

- Pain assessments and management
- Medication safety
- Catheter-related infection
- Unplanned extubation

The response must arise from strong leadership and a unified multidisciplinary team if our goals are to be met.

Chapter 2

Care of the Pediatric Airway, Breathing and Respiratory System

2.1 Apnea

Apnea is defined as the cessation of respiratory airflow at the nose and mouth. Apneas may be classified as one of three types: obstructive, mixed, or central (**Fig. 2.1.1**). Obstructive apneas are associated with continued effort to breathe against an occluded upper airway. During central apneas, no effort is made to breathe, and ventilation ceases. Mixed apneas begin with a central component followed by inspiratory effort against an obstructed airway.

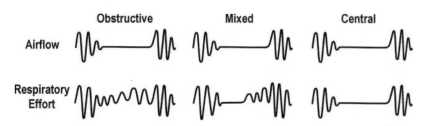

Fig. 2.1.1.   Types of Apnea.

Central sleep apnea (CSA) is characterized by repeated apneic episodes during sleep that result from temporary loss of respiratory effort. Central apneas are considered significant if they last >20 sec. or if they are associated with oxygen desaturation or bradycardia. Brief central apneas not associated with oxygen desaturation to <90% are common during sleep. Recently published data further help define normal values for oxygen saturation (SpO_2) by pluse oximetry during sleep: (1) SpO_2 < 95%, obtained *repeatedly* while an infant is breathing at a regular rate and amplitude is considered abnormal regardless of age; (2) *occasional* falls in SpO_2 by ≥10% may be regarded as normal during the first 6 months of life; (3) falls in SpO_2 decrease with increasing patient age. When symptomatic CSA occurs, several underlying diseases should be considered as potential causes (**Box 2.1.1**).

It is important to remember that premature infants who are < 46 weeks post-conceptional age may develop central apnea, periodic breathing, and bradycardia when exposed to narcotics, sedative and anesthetic drugs. The apnea may occur for up to 18 hours after exposure to the drug.

Obstructive sleep apnea syndrome (OSAS) is the most common form of sleep-disordered breathing in childhood. Obstructive sleep apnea (OSA) is defined as an absence of airflow at the nose and mouth despite continued respiratory effort during sleep. Discrete events that

---

Box 2.1.1   Causes of Central Apnea

- Neurologic: Intracranial hemorrhage, seizures, congenital central alveolar hypoventilation, hydrocephalus, trauma, Arnold-Chiari malformation
- Pulmonary: Chronic hypoxemia from intrinsic lung disease
- Cardiac: Patent ductus arteriosus; congestive heart failure; cardiac arrhythmias
- Gastrointestinal: Vagal stimulation as may occur with feeding (associated with bradycardia); gastroesophageal reflux

- Metabolic: Inborn errors of metabolism, hypoglycemia, electrolyte disorders, placental transfer of sedative drugs
- Hematologic: Anemia
- Infectious: Pertussis, respiratory syncytial virus, botulism, meningitis
- Neuromuscular disorders: Congenital myopathies, infantile myasthenia gravis, diaphragmatic paralysis
- Factitious or induced: Respiratory depressant drugs; Munchausen by proxy

are partial in nature (*i.e.* reduced but not absent airflow) are termed *obstructive hypopneas* and are often accompanied by hypoxemia, hypercapnia, and sleep disruption. The patency of the upper airway during sleep is determined by the bony and soft tissue anatomy of the airway and the upper airway muscle tone. The latter is influenced both by state [wakefulness vs. sleep and rapid eye movement (REM) *vs.* non-REM sleep] and by neural and chemical controls. A number of conditions predispose to OSAS; the most common are listed in **Box 2.1.2**. These etiologies have the features of an anatomically or functionally narrowed upper airway in common. With the onset of the obesity epidemic in children, the landscape of sleep-disordered breathing has changed dramatically, with many children and adolescents now at risk for severe obesity-related OSAS. Complications of OSAS include systemic and pulmonary hypertension, failure to thrive, nocturnal enuresis, and worsening of parasomnias such as sleepwalking. Because neither history nor physical examination is sufficient to firmly establish the diagnosis of OSAS, a polysomnogram (PSG; sleep study) is required to make the diagnosis.

Box 2.1.2   Conditions Predisposing to Obstructive Sleep Apnea Syndrome in Children

- Adenotonsillar hypertrophy
- Obesity
- Craniofacial abnormalities

- Down syndrome
- Sickle cell disease
- Cerebral palsy

Normative PSG values have been established for children and are quite different from those in adults (**Box 2.1.3**). The importance of using age-appropriate normative values is illustrated by the fact that normal children have only 1–2 obstructive apneas or hypopneas per hour of sleep, whereas adults may have as many as 5 obstructive events per hour of sleep and still be considered normal.

Box 2.1.3   Pediatric Polysomnography: Normal Values*

	Normal	Abnormal
Apnea hypopneas index (AHI)**	<1	>1
Maximal end-tidal PCO_2 ($P_{ET}CO_2$; torr)	≤ 53	>54
Duration of hypoventilation		
($P_{ET}CO_2$ >45torr; % of total sleep time)	$\leq 45\%$	$>46\%$
Minimal SpO2 (%)	92%	$<91\%$
Fall in SpO2 (%)	$\leq 8\%$	$>9\%$

* Data for patients 1.1 to 17.4 years from Marcus CL, *et al.* Normal polysomnographic values for children and adolescents. *Am Rev Resp Dis* **146**: 1235, 1992.
** (Number of apneas + Number of hypopneas)/Number of hrs of sleep.

Some patients with OSAS are at increased risk for postoperative complications, particularly those related to anesthesia and sedation. These patients may require a higher level of care, often in the PICU for intensive cardiorespiratory monitoring. Complications of adenotonsillectomy (T&A) include postoperative bleeding, upper airway obstruction secondary to airway edema, pulmonary edema and respiratory failure. Diagnostic groups at the highest risk for postoperative complications are listed (**Box 2.1.4**). A preoperative review of the history and the PSG usually identifies patients who

Box 2.1.4   Conditions Associated with Increased Complication
Risk Following Adenotonsillectomy

- Age <3 yrs
- Severe obstructive sleep apnea syndrome (profound hypoxemia; apnea-hypopnea index >10; significant hypoventilation)
- Morbid obesity
- Neuromuscular disease
- Pulmonary hypertension
- Down syndrome
- Craniofacial anomalies

will require post-operative care in the PICU versus those who can be scheduled for same-day surgery. Unlike the majority of children with OSAS, respiratory control in patients with morbid obesity and OSAS can be altered with resetting of chemoreceptor function, resulting in daytime hypoventilation. In this instance, ventilation may be dependent on hypoxic drive, requiring that oxygen be used judiciously and with close monitoring, both pre- and post-operatively.

Therapy to support children with respiratory compromise following T&A or other airway surgery can include prolonged intubation or a nasopharyngeal airway. The use of non-invasive ventilation, either continuous or bi-level positive airway pressure is attractive, as it avoids intubation and can often be performed in a pediatric unit after the patient is stable (*Non-invasive ventilatory support, 2.8.2*). However, some have questioned the safety of non-invasive positive airway pressure in the immediate postoperative period, with concerns regarding subcutaneous emphysema dissecting at the surgical site, bleeding, or uncomfortable drying of the upper airway.

Most children with OSAS are treated with T&A as first-line therapy, even if other anatomic or functional abnormalities are likely contributing to the upper airway obstruction. However, some will undergo a more extensive procedure, uvulopalatopharyngoplasty, which includes removal not only of the tonsils but the tonsillar pillars and uvula as well. This procedure is most often reserved for patients with cerebral palsy or Down syndrome, who have a high probability for residual obstruction following T&A alone. Mandibular distraction osteogenesis is being used with increasing frequency for infants and children with syndromes that include micrognathia. Pierre Robin syndrome, Treacher-Collins syndrome, and conditions that include hemifacial microsomnia are examples. Treatment of OSAS in patients with Beckwith-Wiedemann (and occasionally Down syndrome) may require tongue reduction surgery. As a whole, children who require complex surgical treatment for OSAS tend to have more severe sleep disordered breathing and other risk factors for post-operative difficulties. Thus, they should be observed in the PICU post-operatively and may require several days of intubation following surgery.

Occasionally, the initial presentation of patients with OSAS will be acute respiratory failure. This is less common in the current era, when the recognition of sleep disordered breathing has increased, and the literature contains little evidence to guide treatment. These patients may be otherwise normal or have one of the risk factors listed in **Box 2.1.4**. Unlike the majority of patients with OSAS, they may have experienced long-term hypercapnia with resultant blunting of their respiratory drive, necessitating extreme caution in the use of supplemental oxygen. Pulmonary hypertension with right heart failure and pulmonary edema are often present, requiring treatment with diuretics and cardiology evaluation. Long-standing upper airway obstruction may have prevented adequate clearance of pulmonary secretions, and treatment with antibiotics may be indicated. Systemic steroids can be administered to acutely decrease the size of adenoidal and tonsillar tissue.

2.1.1 *Apparent life-threatening events*

An apparent life-threatening event (ALTE) is defined as an event that is frightening to the observer, in which the infant is observed to have color change (cyanosis or pallor), change in muscle tone (limpness, rarely stiffness), and apnea, and in which vigorous stimulation, mouth-to-mouth breathing, or cardiopulmonary resuscitation are required to revive the infant. In most cases, observers feared that the infant was in the process of dying. Sometimes, infants appear to respond quickly, and they may appear entirely normal when examined at a later time. Other infants require intensive intervention or resuscitation, and may exhibit signs of a serious hypoxic event several minutes later. It is this latter group who will usually be admitted to a PICU for observation and treatment.

There are multiple identifiable causes of ALTEs; after evaluation approximately 50% of these infants will have a specific diagnosis; the

---

Box 2.1.5   Frequently Identifiable Causes of Acute Life-Threatening Events (ALTE)

- **Infection**: Sepsis; meningitis; respiratory infections such as RSV, pertussis and others; urinary tract infection in neonates
- **Gastrointestinal**: Gastroesophageal reflux disease; pharyngeal incoordination stimulating laryngeal chemoreceptors; malformations
- **Seizure**
- **Breath-holding spells**
- **Other neurologic disorders**: CNS tumors; CNS hemorrhage; hydrocephalus; Arnold-Chiari malformation; neuromuscular disorders
- **Cardiac arrhythmias**
- **Abnormalities of respiratory drive**: Immature respiratory center (*e.g.* apnea of prematurity); respiratory center dysfunction (central hypoventilation syndrome, also called "Ondine's curse"); drug/toxin exposure
- **Obstructive sleep apnea**
- **Metabolic, Endocrinologic, Hematologic**: Hypoglycemia; hypocalcemia; abnormal metabolism of fatty acids; electrolyte disorders; anemia
- **Child Maltreatment**: Non-accidental head trauma; intentional suffocation; Munchausen syndrome by proxy

---

most common of these are related to the gastrointestinal tract or seizures. **Box 2.1.5** outlines the main clinical diagnostic groups. ALTE can be a symptom of many specific disorders including gastroesophageal reflux, infection, seizures, airway abnormalities, hypoglycemia or other metabolic problems, as well as impaired regulation of breathing during sleep and feeding. These episodes can occur during sleep, wakefulness, or feeding; they typically occur in infants beyond 37 weeks gestational age. Clinical management of these infants does not necessarily require exhaustive investigation, but rather a careful and focused clinical assessment beginning with history and physical examination (**Box 2.1.6**) and close observation. For infants with

---

Box 2.1.6   Evaluation of an ALTE

- **Elicit historical details from the person(s) who witnessed the event:**
  - ▶ Color (red, pale, cyanotic)
  - ▶ Tone (flaccid, rigid; seizure activity)
  - ▶ Respiratory effort (apnea, obstructed, irregular)
  - ▶ Sleep state (awake or asleep)
  - ▶ Position (prone, supine, upright)
  - ▶ Noises (stridor, choking)
  - ▶ Eye movements (closed, startled, rolled, fluttering)
  - ▶ Relationship to feeding
  - ▶ Fluid in mouth and/or nose
  - ▶ Duration
  - ▶ Need for intervention
  - ▶ Environmental factors (*e.g.* temperature; smoke)
- **Obtain past medical and family history**
- **Check results of newborn screening tests**

ALTE, an aggressive approach to identifying the cause and instituting appropriate therapy is necessary. The diagnostic evaluation may include, but is not limited to the steps described in **Fig. 2.1.2**. Although not every infant will require all these tests, many are typically performed before the episode is termed "unexplained". The diagnosis of apnea of infancy (AOI) is used when an identifiable cause for the ALTE cannot be found. If a treatable cause for ALTE cannot be found and if the original event was of sufficient severity to be of concern about potential sequelae of subsequent events, most clinicians will manage these patients with home apnea-bradycardia monitoring. Home apnea-bradycardia monitors alert parents and caregivers to prolonged central apneic pauses and/or bradycardia by sounding an alarm (usually 90 dB). Trained caregivers must respond to evaluate the event and revive the infant if necessary.

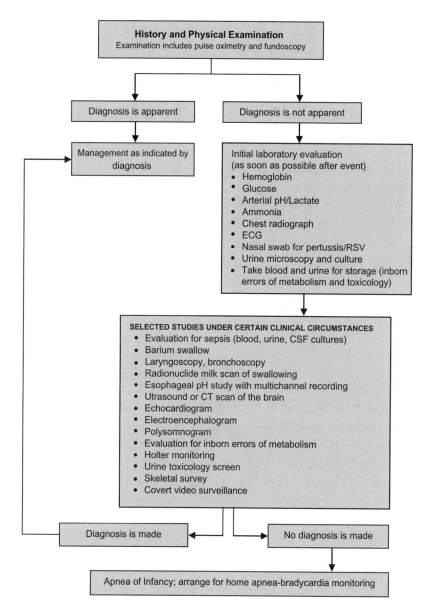

Fig. 2.1.2. Investigation of First ALTE.

2.2 Upper Airway Obstruction (UAO)

The "upper airway" includes the extrathoracic airways beginning at the nose and lips and is variably defined to extend as far as the main-stem bronchi. The narrowest portion of the upper airway in adults and children >10 yrs is at the level of the vocal cords. For children <10 yrs, the narrowest portion of the upper airway is at the cricoid cartilage. The upper airway includes bone and soft tissues of the upper airway and the rigid glottic and subglottic airway which has more cartilaginous support.

Poiseuille's Law states that resistance to laminar flow through a tube (R) is directly related to viscosity (n) of the medium in the tube and the length (L) of the tube, but inversely proportional to the radius (r) to the fourth power (**Fig. 2.2.1**) of the inner diameter of the tube. When air flow is turbulent, resistance is inversely proportional to r raised to the fifth power.

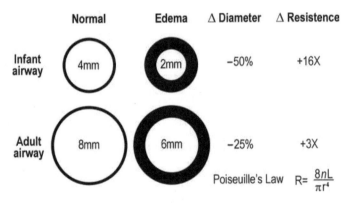

Fig. 2.2.1.   Relationship of Airway Diameter to Airway Resistance.

Abnormal sounds generated within the respiratory tract during breathing are the result of turbulent gas flow. Turbulent flow in the nasopharyx results in snoring; turbulent flow arising from the oro- or hypopharyx results in a low-pitched noise caused by narrowing of the pharyngeal airway. Inspiratory stridor is a high pitched noise produced by obstruction of the extrathoracic airway below the pharyx (*i.e.* the supraglottic, glottic or subglottic space). Expiratory stridor

---

Box 2.2.1   Differential Diagnosis of Airway Obstruction

Congenital (examples):

- Birth trauma
- Calcification of tracheal cartilage
- Laryngeal webs
- Subglottic stenosis
- Tracheal anomalies
- Tumors and cysts
- Vocal-cord paralysis
- Craniofacial dysmorphology (Syndromes such as Pierre Robin, Treacher-Collins, Hallerman-Streiff, Möbius, Delange, Freeman-Shelton)
- Immunologic stridor (hereditary angioedema)
- Laryngomalacia
- Laryngotracheoesophageal cleft
- Metabolic (*laryngysmus stridulosa*)
- Neurogenic stridor (reflex laryngospasm)
- Vascular rings and slings

Congenital (continued)

- Macroglossia (Beckwith-Wiedemann syndrome, congenital hypothyroidism, glycogen storage diseases, Down syndrome, diffuse muscular hypertrophy of the tongue, localized lingual tumors)

Acquired (examples):

- Infectious (epiglottitis, croup, acute spasmodic laryngitis, diphtheria, retropharyngeal abscess)
- Iatrogenic (post-extubation, post-instrumentation, post-surgical)
- Immunologic (juvenile rheumatoid arthritis)
- Neoplasm (laryngeal papillomatosis)
- Trauma (foreign bodies, external trauma, thermal and chemical injury)

Adapted from Maze A, Bloch E. Stridor in Pediatric Patients, *Anesthesiology* **50**: 132–145, 1979.

typically arises from the intrathoracic portion of the upper airway, and stridor present on both inspiration and expiration (biphasic stridor) suggests obstruction between the glottis and subglottis or severe obstruction at any level below the pharynx. Causes of airway obstruction are listed (**Box 2.2.1**).

Transmural pressure (TMP) refers to the gradient between the intraluminal pressure of a tube and the pressure surrounding the outer walls of the tube.

TMP = Pressure inside a tube/Pressure outside a tube

A TMP < 1.0 is considered a "negative TMP" and a TMP >1.0 is considered a "positive TMP". Extrathoracic TMP is the ratio of pressure inside the extrathoracic airway to the surrounding pressure (atmospheric). During inspiration the TMP is < 1, promoting collapse of a (non-stented) airway.

If airway obstruction in this portion of the airway is not fixed, airway narrowing and therefore turbulent gas flow, is exacerbated during inspiration. During expiration, TMP in the extrathoracic airways is positive (>1), and this relative increase in airway diameter may assist in relieving obstruction.

Intrathoracic variable obstruction refers to the relationship between TMP of intrathoracic airways and intrapleural pressure. During inspiration, negative (extraluminal) pleural pressure results in positive TMP (a ratio >1) for the intrathoracic airways leading to relative increases in intrathoracic airway diameter. During exhalation increased positive pleural pressure and lesser intrathoracic airway pressure causes relative airway collapse (TMP < 1). Intrathoracic airway obstruction is more likely to present with wheezing for this reason.

Diagnosis and Assessment. During initial evaluation it is essential to determine the severity and suspected source of the obstruction. History and physical examination help narrow the extensive differential diagnosis of UAO. Infection should be identified as soon as possible. A scoring system may assist in the evaluation of stridor (**Box 2.2.2**).

Imaging of the upper airway with plain films of the neck, chest and/or CT scan may be useful in making a diagnosis. Radiographic investigations are suitable only for stable patients. If instability is even potentially present, the patient should be accompanied by the airway management team at all times. Direct visualization of the airway using nasopharyngoscopy, direct laryngoscopy, or flexible or rigid bronchoscopy may be required for diagnosis and therapy.

Management based on diagnosis. Interventions based on symptoms of UAO may be both therapeutic and diagnostic based on response.

- UAO with any component of edema may be responsive to nebulized epinephrine (NE), which presumably decreases airway

Box 2.2.2   Assessment of Children with Stridor: Severity Score

Score	0	1	2	3
Stridor	None	With agitation	Mild at rest	Severe at rest
Retraction	None	Mild	Moderate	Severe
Air entry	Normal	Normal	Decreased	Severely↓
Color	Normal	Normal	Cyanotic with agitation	Cyanotic at rest
Level of consciousness	Normal	Restless if disturbed	Restless if undisturbed	Lethargic

Total score: <6 = mild severity; 7–8 = moderate severity; > 8 = severe.

Adapted from Rothrock SG, Perkin R. Stridor: A review, update, and current management recommendations. *Pediatr Emerg Med Rep* 1:29–40, 1996.

mucosal edema and increases airway diameter. NE results in symptomatic improvement and decreases the need for tracheal intubation in patients with croup and severe distress. Nebulized racemic epinephrine 2.25% (0.25–0.50 mL in 3 mL saline solution) can be administered every 20 mins if side effects (rebound stridor, tachycardia, hypertension, and myocardial infarction) are not prohibitive. Hereditary angioedema is not usually responsive to NE.

- Corticosteroids decrease inflammation of airway mucosa. In croup this usually occurs within six hours of administration. Dexamethasone (0.6 mg/kg/day; max. dose 10 mg/day PO, IM, IV as single dose or divided every 6 hours) is an effective anti-inflammatory agent and should be considered in any patient requiring NE for relief of UAO or with upper airway edema.
- Helium-Oxygen (heliox; HeO_2): Gas flow is inversely proportional to the square root of the density of the inhaled gas. Helium is a low density gas that improves flow and decreases the work of breathing due to UAO. Heliox may be used as a single or additional therapy in airway obstruction. Helium:oxygen mixtures of 80:20, 70:30, and 60:40 are available; use the highest helium concentration possible that assures adequate oxygenation.

- Endotracheal intubation to secure a critically narrowed airway should be accomplished by the most skillful operator available. The size of the endotracheal tube often may need to be smaller than predicted by age, Broselow scoring or fifth fingernail width (*Bag Mask Ventilation and Tracheal Intubation, 15.2*). Endotracheal intubation may also be *a cause* of airway narrowing particularly in airway burns or trauma, those intubated with an oversized endotracheal tube or those who undergo prolonged periods of intubation. Antimicrobials should be considered if an infectious source is the known or suspected cause of an airway obstruction (**Box 2.2.3**). Vancomycin should be added to these regimens if MRSA is a

---

Box 2.2.3   Empiric Antimicrobial Therapy for Airway Obstruction

Disease	Antibiotic Choices
Peritonsillar abscess	Penicillin +/− metronidazole
Epiglottitis or bacterial tracheitis	Cefuroxime *or* [nafcillin + (cefotaxime or ceftriaxone)]
Parapharyngeal or retropharyngeal abscess	Ampicillin-sulbactam *or* (ceftriaxone or cefotaxime) + (clindamycin *or* ticarcillin-clavulanate *or* piperacillin-tazobactam); metronidazole may be given in place of clindamycin

---

reasonably potential pathogen. Definitive therapy should be guided by antibiotic sensitivity testing.
- Surgical interventions may be indicated to relieve some causes of upper airway obstruction (*e.g.* foreign bodies, retropharyngeal abscess, choanal atresia, intranasal tumors, tongue cysts, severe congenital sublgottic stenosis, severe laryngeal clefts, tracheal stenosis, tracheo-esophageal fistula, vascular rings).
- Vaccines have decreased the occurrence of upper airway obstruction caused by *Corynebacterium diphtheriae* and *Haemophilus influenzae*.

2.3 Lower Airway Obstruction

2.3.1 *Acute severe asthma*

Asthma is the most common hospital admission diagnosis in pediatrics and affects nearly 7% of children in the US. It is a chronic inflammatory disorder with reversible airways obstruction. Acute severe asthma is defined as a peak expiratory flow rate <40% of predicted value or personal best. Some of these patients do not improve with initial emergent interventions (status asthmaticus) and often require admission to a PICU.

Pathophysiology. Acute severe asthma is characterized by airway inflammation, bronchospasm, and mucus hypersecretion with plugging. This combination leads to significant airway obstruction and increased airways resistance. Because of the narrowed and obstructed airways, airflow is impaired during exhalation more so than during inhalation. This leads to air trapping, lung hyperinflation, and increased work of breathing (dynamic hyperinflation). Hypoxemia develops because regional alveolar overdistension causes decreased perfusion to those lung units and gas exchange is impaired (V/Q, mismatch; *Respiratory Failure, 2.7*). In atelectatic lung units, pulmonary blood flow is maintained, but ventilation is impaired also leading to V/Q mismatch and hypoxemia. Hypoxemia causes stimulation of the respiratory centers leading to a respiratory alkalosis. As obstruction and V/Q mismatch worsen, carbon dioxide elimination becomes impaired and respiratory acidosis ensues. As the lungs become more hyperinflated, intrathoracic pressure increases which may impair cardiac output (*Important Cardiopulmonary Interactions, 3.2*). Respiratory failure develops as V/Q mismatch worsens and the respiratory muscles become fatigued.

Clinical presentation. Patients present with variable signs and symptoms depending on the acuity of the exacerbation and their tolerance to chronic poorly controlled asthma. Most patients present with non-productive cough, tachypnea, and wheezing. Patients with status asthmaticus may also have respiratory distress, with inability to speak in full sentences, and diminished breath sounds instead of wheezes due to poor air movement. Severity of asthma and response to therapy are mostly determined by history and physical findings. Laboratory findings may include respiratory alkalosis or acidosis or hypoxemia. Metabolic acidosis may be present due to dehydration (poor intake with increased insensible fluid losses) or lactic acidosis (from excess use of respiratory muscles or stimulated by β_2-agonist therapy). Elevated WBC count may implicate an infectious respiratory agent as the trigger. During treatment, hypokalemia may develop from β_2-agonist therapy. Chest radiograph often shows hyperinflation, flattened diaphragms, and areas of atelectasis. In status asthmaticus, it is also important to evaluate for pneumothorax or pneumomediastinum and pneumonia.

Box 2.3.1	Pharmacotherapy in Status Asthmaticus
1st tier (in ED and initial management in PICU)	• Methylprednisolone load with 2 mg/kg IV followed by 1 mg/kg/dose IV q6hrs • Continuous albuterol 10–20 mg/hr nebulized • Ipratropium bromide 250 mcg/dose (<5 yrs) or 500 mcg/dose (>5 yrs) nebulized q6hrs × 24 hrs • Consider magnesium 25–50 mg/kg IV q 6 hrs
2nd tier	• Heliox *(Other Aids to Support Oxygenation and Ventilation, 2.9)* • Terbutaline load with 10 mcg/kg IV followed by 0.1 mcg/kg/min. May ↑ stepwise to 10 mcg/kg per min (monitor for tachycardia) • Epinephrine 1:1000 concentration 0.01 ml/kg or 0.01 mg/kg (max 0.5 ml or 0.5 mg) subQ q 15–30 min × 2 (non-selective β-agonist therefore more side effects compared to β_2-agonists)
3rd tier	• Aminophylline load with 6 mg/kg IV then start infusion at 1 mg/kg/hr (target levels of 10–20 mcg/ml) • Ketamine 1 mg/kg IV then start infusion at 1 mg/kg/hr. Dissociative anesthetic drug with bronchodilating properties; may be considered in spontaneously breathings patients, but may cause laryngospasm. Preferred in mechanically ventilated patients; often used with benzodiazepines to prevent hallucinations.

Box 2.3.2	Supportive Care in Status Asthmaticus
Humidified O_2 therapy	• Supplemental O_2 may prevent hypoxemia and reduce work of breathing (*Other Aids to Support Oxygenation and Ventilation, 2.9*)
Intravenous fluids	• Provide isotonic fluid (0.9% NaCl or Lactated Ringer's solution) for volume resuscitation • Ongoing fluid therapy should include maintenance fluids (which should account for any ↑ insensible losses) plus supplemental potassium (barring any contraindications); any remaining fluid deficit should be included in the fluid plan; dextrose may not be necessary initially as patients are frequently hyperglycemic from stress and steroids; if hyperglycemia is persistent, treatment with insulin may be appropriate (*Hypo- and Hyperglycemia, 6.4*).
Pulmonary hygiene	• Chest physiotherapy, postural drainage, and repositioning may aid in mucus clearance. • Dornase alfa 2.5 mg/dose q 12 hrs may be nebulized (or instilled in intubated patients) for patients with unresolving atelectasis; avoid acetylcysteine as it may worsen bronchospasm.

Management of acute severe asthma should be aggressive and prompt to avoid progression to respiratory failure and death. Therapies target the underlying mechanisms of airway inflammation, bronchospasm, and mucus plugging (**Box 2.3.1**). Supportive care of fluid status, oxygenation, and comfort are important adjuncts (**Box 2.3.2**).

Non-invasive positive pressure ventilation (NPPV) has not been well established in patients with status asthmaticus but may be an effective temporizing measure as other therapies are optimized and medications reach steady state. In awake patients without vomiting or excessive secretions, NPPV may decrease work of breathing and improve hypoxemia (*Non-invasive ventilatory support, 2.8.2*) without the dangerous airway manipulation required to intubate and mechanically support the patient.

Intubation and mechanical ventilation in patients with status asthmaticus significantly increases the risk of death and morbidity (from barotrauma, cardiac dysfunction, pulmonary edema, worsened bronchospasm from airway manipulation, and myopathy). Only 5–10% of PICU status asthmaticus patients require mechanical ventilation, many of whom are intubated at outlying facilities. The decision to intubate must be approached cautiously and only if other aggressive measures have failed. Hypercarbia alone is not an indication for tracheal intubation. Other factors include refractory hypoxemia, severe work of breathing, altered mental status, and impending respiratory and/or cardiac arrest. Intubation should be done by a clinician experienced in airway management with a cuffed ETT placed. Appropriate drugs to facilitate intubation include ketamine, fentanyl, midazolam, and propofol along with succinylcholine, vecuronium, or rocuronium. The goals during mechanical ventilation should be relief of respiratory muscle work, correction of hypoxemia, and prevention of ventilator-induced lung injury. Permissive hypercapnea (allowing CO_2 to rise by minimizing peak inspiratory pressures tidal volumes and respiratory rate) should be tolerated to minimize barotrauma and volutrauma. A dual control mode of ventilation (*e.g.* adaptive pressure ventilation, pressure-regulated volume control, or auto control +) may be the best mode to use initially. A targeted tidal volume can be set to more closely control minute ventilation, but the pressure to achieve that set volume is minimized and limited (*Invasive mechanical ventilation, 2.8.1*). Positive-end expiratory pressure should be carefully increased to reach the critical airway opening pressure to stent open narrowed airways. Low respiratory rates (6–12/min) should be used to prolong the expiratory time which helps prevent breath stacking and allows for maximum CO_2 elimination. Optimally, patients should be weaned to pressure support ventilation as soon as tolerated to allow patients to set their own inspiratory to expiratory ratio.

Patients who fail standard management for status asthmaticus may benefit from the use of inhalational anesthetics (halothane, sevoflurane) which have bronchodilatory effects. This therapy requires a means of scavenging exhaled gases and the direction of a clinician experienced with their use. Refractory patients may also be considered for ECLS (*Other Aids to Support Oxygenation and Ventilation, 2.9*). Survival rates are 88% for status asthmaticus patients requiring ECLS.

2.3.2 *Bronchiolitis*

Bronchiolitis is an acute obstructive respiratory illness caused by one or more viral pathogens, but most commonly respiratory syncitial virus (RSV; **Box 2.3.3**). It is the most common cause of acute lower respiratory tract infection in children <12 mos and the most common cause of hospitalization in children <6 mos. It is most prevalent in winter but may occur at any time of year.

Box 2.3.3   Viral Causes of Bronchiolitis

- Respiratory syncitial virus
- Human metapneumovirus
- Influenza

- Rhinovirus
- Coronavirus
- Adenovirus
- Parainfluenza

Pathophysiology. Airway obstruction occurs in bronchiolitis from respiratory epithelium necrosis (cellular debris in the airway) and inflammatory mediated edema within and around the airway. RSV also causes loss of epithelial cilia which impairs airway clearance. Some airways become completely plugged while others are only partially obstructed leading to a mixture of over and under-distended alveolar units. Some lung areas are atelectatic while others are hyperinflated. As with acute severe asthma, this heterogeneity leads to V/Q mismatch and hypoxemia (*Acute severe asthma, 2.3.1*).

Clinical presentation. Patients present with a spectrum of signs and symptoms. Findings early in the course of illness are usually rhinorrhea, cough, fever, and poor feeding. As the illness progresses, patients become more tachypneic, irritable, and hypoxic with increased accessory muscle use and nasal flaring. Pulmonary findings include wheezing, crackles, rhonchi, areas of decreased breath sounds, and a prolonged expiratory phase. In the most severe cases, patients become more hypoxic due to worsening V/Q mismatch, have respiratory rates nearing 100/min, become lethargic, and may develop respiratory muscle fatigue. A few patients develop respiratory failure despite aggressive therapy. Risk factors for developing more severe disease include age < 3 mos and history of CHD, neurologic disease, or prematurity.

Laboratory findings may include respiratory alkalosis (in the early phases of illness) or acidosis (as V/Q mismatch worsens or respiratory muscles become fatigued). Many patients also have hypoxemia. Metabolic acidosis may be present due to dehydration (poor intake with increased insensible fluid losses) or lactic acidosis from excess use of respiratory muscles. Elevated white blood cell count may indicate a secondary bacterial infection, such as *Streptococcus or Staphylococcus*. The chest radiograph often shows a mixture of atelectasis and hyperinflation, peribronchial cuffing, and flattened diaphragms. Some patients may also have consolidated infiltrates if a secondary pneumonia is present.

Management of bronchiolitis remains mostly supportive as many proposed therapies have not proven effective in clinical studies. One of the most important measures to improve work of breathing is clearance of secretions from the upper airways by suctioning (because ~60% of airways resistance is in the upper airways and infants predominantly breathe through the nose). Other methods to improve pulmonary hygiene (chest physiotherapy, postural drainage, intermittent percussive ventilation, *etc.*) may also be helpful adjuncts for relieving mucus plugging. Supplemental oxygen is often required in bronchiolitis due to the frequency of hypoxemia. Patients with respiratory destress should not be fed orally because of the risk of aspiration. Infants with GERD are particularly vulnerable to aspiration during illness with bronchiolitis. Other supportive therapies are very similar to those for status asthmaticus (*Acute severe asthma, 2.3.1, Box 2.3.2*). Pharmacologic therapies have been the most controversial topics in bronchiolitis management and are outlined (**Box 2.3.4**).

Box 2.3.4   Pharmacotherapy in Bronchiolitis

β_2-agonists	• Frequently trialed in bronchiolitis patients but no clinical evidence to support its use. • Some patients with anecdotal response to albuterol may actually be benefiting from the humidification effect.
Nebulized racemic epinephrine	• May be superior to pure β_2-agonists due to the α-adrenergic effect of pulmonary bronchiolar arteriolar vasoconstriction which may decrease airway edema.
Corticosteroids	• No conclusive benefit has been found from inhaled or systemic steroids. • May consider trial of steroids in patients with repetitive episodes of wheezing or other signs of atopy.
RSV immuno-globulin	• Immunoglobulin enriched with anti-RSV antibodies. • No clinical evidence to support its use.
Palivizumab	• Monoclonal antibodies against RSV used for prophylaxis in high-risk infants. • Decreased viral load in patients with active RSV infection but no change in clinical course.
Ribavirin	• Antiviral agent with in vitro activity against RSV. • Cochrane database review found no benefit.
Montelukast	• Antileukotriene drug that is being studied for anti-inflammatory benefits in bronchiolitis.
Ipratropium	• Nebulized anticholinergic that has shown no benefit in bronchiolitis patients.
Nebulized NaCl 3%	• May help humidify the airways and assist in mobilization of secretions.

Helium-oxygen mixture (heliox) reduces work of breathing and improves delivery of gas to distal airways in patients with obstructive pulmonary diseases (*Other Aids to Support Oxygenation and Ventilation, 2.9*). Studies of heliox in bronchiolitis have shown some potential benefit but further investigation is needed before it is incorporated into standard care.

Non-invasive positive pressure ventilation (NPPV) may be beneficial for the infant with worsening respiratory distress or apnea. It can be delivered by nasal continuous positive airway pressure (NCPAP) or high-flow nasal cannula. NPPV may stent open obstructed airways reducing work of breathing, improving pulmonary compliance, and improving gas exchange (*Non-invasive ventilatory support, 2.8.2*).

Some patients progress to require invasive conventional mechanical ventilation (CMV) for apnea or respiratory failure. The strategy during CMV should target minimizing barotrauma by allowing permissive hypercapnea and using low respiratory rates to facilitate adequate exhalation time. Patients who fail these strategies (inadequate gas exchange, complications from airleak) may require high frequency ventilation (*Invasive mechanical ventilation, 2.8.1*). Patients who continue to deteriorate or show no improvement from these aggressive measures should be considered for extracorporeal life support (ECLS; *Other Aids to Support Oxygenation and Ventilation, 2.9*).

2.4 Foreign Bodies (FB) in the Airways

FB aspiration can be a dramatic or nearly unrecognized event with high morbidity and mortality. Rescue from upper airway obstruction, recurrent pneumonia or "respiratory failure in search of a cause" requires a high index of suspicion. Children below 3 years are most commonly involved; peanuts, seeds, pieces of food and pieces of toy items are the most frequently aspirated FB's. A careful history leads to the diagnosis in witnessed events. Signs and symptoms are dictated by the location of the FB in the respiratory tree; diagnostic tools are summarized (**Box 2.4.1**).

Management. In an arrested or unresponsive child, grasp tongue with thumb and jaw with index finger, lift and examine for presence of FB. If a FB is visualized, remove it from the pharynx. If unable to ventilate in an infant < 1 year of age, perform 5 back blows and 5 chest thrusts. In an older child, perform a Heimlich maneuver. In event of

Box 2.4.1   Signs, Symptoms and Evaluation of Aspirated Foreign Bodies Based on Location

• Laryngeal: Partial obstruction may cause changes in voice, croupy cough, dyspnea, stridor or hemoptysis. Auscultation of neck and chest may be helpful in localizing the site of obstruction.
• Tracheal FB
  ‣ A "slap" is often heard at the mouth during a cough.
  ‣ A wheeze, often not responsive to β2-agonist therapy may be heard at the mouth.
  ‣ A "thud" may be felt over the chest.
  ‣ A wheeze may migrate from one hemithorax to the other as FB moves.
  ‣ Severe respiratory distress may rapidly develop as FB shifts in airways
• Bronchial: May have persistent cough and/or dyspnea; wheezing (sometimes localized) often not responsive to β2-agonist therapy; there may be a localized decrease in breath sounds. Hemoptysis may occur.
• Plain X-rays detect only 10% of FB's, but may be suggestive of the diagnosis in selected cases. Useful studies include:
  ‣ High quality view of soft tissues of the neck
  ‣ Anterior-posterior end-inspiratory views of chest to detect air trapping or atelectasis distal to point of obstruction.
  ‣ Anterior-posterior end-expiratory view of chest to identify air trapping.
  ‣ Bilateral decubitus chest films to detect air trapping in a child who cannot cooperate for expiratory views. A FB in the dependent lung may create a ball-valve effect and prevent the dependent lung from normal deflation.
• Fluoroscopy of the chest may identify air trapping with movement of the mediastinum away from a bronchus that is obstructed by a FB.
• Computerized tomography of airways with ≥16 detector multi-slice scanner may help identify a non-radio-opaque FB.
• Flexible bronchoscopy (with sedation) or flexible naso-laryngoscopy may be useful in isolated inspiratory stridor. Flexible bronchoscopy may be useful in identification or to "R/O" FB, but rigid bronchoscopy is usually required for FB removal.

complete airway obstruction unresponsive to these interventions, emergency surgical intervention may allow for emergent oxygenation and ventilation, and removal of the FB through a tracheostomy.

In a stable child, perform a diagnostic evaluation as outlined above and consult with the appropriate surgical service (*e.g.* Ear, Nose and Throat Surgery; Pediatric Surgery). Rigid bronchoscopy for FB removal by a surgeon is the management of choice. Flexible bronchoscopy may be useful in removal of a peripheral FB that cannot be seen by the rigid bronchoscope. Tracheal intubation may be required for safety during FB removal.

2.5 Pneumonia and Pleural Fluid

The airways and alveoli are typically sterile and free of inflammation during health. Pneumonia is an inflammatory process in which the airspaces are filled with exudative fluid and lung is solidified (consolidated). Bacteria most frequently enter the respiratory tree through aspiration. If opsonized (*e.g.* coated with IgG or complement) a macrophage will ingest the organism. If not engulfed (esp. with *Streptococcus pnuemoniae*) and if bacterial multiplication continues, a core of vascular congestion and edema forms ("red hepatization"). Eventually phagocytosis of bacteria by neutrophils causes degradation of cell elements ("gray hepatization"). Finally neutrophils phagocytize antibody coated bacteria and monocytes clear debris ("zone of resolution"). If the reticular structure is not injured complete healing of alveolar epithelium occurs.

Community acquired pneumonia (CAP) is a lung infection with air space disease on CXR in an otherwise healthy child who has had limited or no contact with the medical setting. Viruses are the most common cause in all age groups. In neonates, maternal genital tract flora predominate, while in older children and adolescents the cause is most commonly *S. pneumoniae* and agents of atypical pneumonias (*Mycoplasma* and *Chlamydophila*) are more common (**Box 2.5.1**). In children less than 3 yrs of age high fever (>38.5°C) combined with respiratory distress is suggestive of bacterial pneumonia whereas in older children clinical signs are less helpful than simply a history of "difficulty breathing." Newborns with pneumonia may present without cough but with other signs of respiratory distress (*General Approach to the Critically Ill Child 1.2*) including grunting, retracting and nasal flaring; in addition, this age group may present only with signs and symptoms of sepsis. Some common associations with pneumonias and the most common causes by age group are listed (**Boxes 2.5.1 and 2.5.2**).

Close monitoring is indicated if the oxygen requirement exceeds 60%. PICU admission is indicated if positive pressure breathing is necessary, fatigue is present, apnea or irregular respirations occur or hemodynamic compromise is evident (*General Approach to the Critically Ill Child 1.2; Respiratory Failure 2.7*). Initial antibiotic regimens for CAP are listed in **Box 2.5.3**.

Ventilator associated pneumonia (VAP) is currently defined as a pneumonia in mechanically ventilated patients that develops later than or at 48 hours after that patient has been placed on the ventilator. If VAP occurs within 48 to 72 hours after tracheal intubation it is referred to as early-onset pneumonia; it often results from aspiration which complicated the intubation process. Pneumonia that occurs later than 72 hours is called late-onset pneumonia or true VAP. Early onset disease is usually caused by is usually caused by *S. pneumoniae, Hemophilus influenza* or *Moraxella catarrhalis*. True VAP is most often caused by *Pseudomonas aerugenosa (and related species), Enterobacter cloacae, S. aureus* or viruses. Antibiotic coverage often includes ticarcillin-clavulanate, piperacillin-tazobactam *or* meropenem plus vancomycin (if appropriate). Clinically useful signs of VAP are listed (**Box 2.5.4**). CXR changes are required to diagnose VAP. If no underlying cardiac or pulmonary disease is present one CXR with abnormal findings is needed; otherwise two serial CXR's demonstrating new, progressive or persistent infiltrate(s) or new cavitation that develops 48 hrs. after intubation is required. Laboratory diagnosis of VAP is detailed (**Box 2.5.5**).

A **parapneumonic effusion (PPE)** is a pleural effusion (fluid between the visceral and parietal pleura) that forms adjacent to inflammation associated with pneumonia. The fluid is initially sterile but later may be invaded by bacteria. **Empyema** refers to fluid that becomes purulent. *S. pneumoniae* is the most common organism causing PPE but MRSA is being reported with increasing frequency. Organisms associated with empyema are listed and stages of a PPE are

Box 2.5.1	Characteristics of Pneumonia in Infants (Non-Neonates) and Children			
Agent	Age (yrs)	Associated Signs And Symptoms	Auscultatory Findings	CXR
Virus	<5	Preceding URI	Diffuse, bilateral rales or ronchi	Diffuse interstitial air space disease
Bacterial (typical)	All	+/− antecedent URI, fever, cough, malaise, vomiting, chest pain	↓Breath sounds, ↑bronchial sounds	Focal consolidation, pleural fluid, cavitations
Bacterial (atypical)	>5	Malaise, myalgia, headache, conjunctivitis, sore throat, ↑ cough	Possible wheezing	Interstitial infiltrates
Myco-bacterium tuberculosis	All	Low grade fever and cough for 1–2 weeks	↓Local breath sounds with bronchial obstruction	Hilar adenopathy* with small parenchymal focus (subpleural).

* Also occurs with fungal infections.

detailed (**Boxes 2.5.6 and 2.5.7**). Persistent fever for 2 days after starting antibiotics for pneumonia should be investigated for presence of a PPE. Alternatively, a PPE in a child who has no fever or pneumonia (or who has mediastinal masses) should be investigated for malignancy or tuberculosis.

Box 2.5.2   Common Causes of Pneumonia by Age Group

Age Group	Bacterial	Viral	Other
Neonates	Group B *Streptococcus*, *E. coli, Klebsiella, Enterobacter* spp., *Listeria monocytogenes*; other enteric and environmental bacilli	Respiratory syncytial virus (RSV), Enterovirus, Rhinovirus, Adenovirus, Parainfluenza, HSV, Cytomegalovirus (CMV)	*Ureaplasma urealyticum, Chlamydophila (C.) trachomatis*
1 month–6 yrs	*S. pneumoniae*, Group A *Streptococcus*, *Staphylococcus aureus*	RSV, Human metapneumovirus, Parainfluenza (PIV)type III, Adenovirus	*Mycoplasma (M.) pneumoniae* (often >4 yrs old), *C. pneumoniae*
> 6 yrs	*S. pneumoniae*	RSV, Influenza A & B, PIV	*M. pneumoniae, C. pneumoniae*
Immunocompromised host	*Pseudomonas* spp., *Enterobacteriaceae, Legionella pneumophila*, Anaerobic bacteria, *Enterococccus* spp.,	CMV, Varicella zoster, Ebstein Barr virus, *Toxoplasma* spp., Adenovirus	*Nocardia* spp., *Rhodococcus equi, Actinomyces* spp., *Pneumocystis jiroveci*
Animal exposures	*Francisella tularensis* (rabbits); *C. psittaci* (birds); *Coxiella burnetti* (sheep); *Salmonella choleraesuis* (pigs)		

Box 2.5.3   Initial Antibiotic Therapy for Community Acquired Pneumonia

Uncomplicated pneumonia (no parapneumonic effusion or lung abscess)	Cetriaxone, *or* cefotaxime *or* cefuroxime (+ampicillin for *Listeria* in neonates) [+vancomycin or linezolid if suspect methicillin-resistant *S. aureus* (MRSA) or penicillin-resistant *S. pneumoniae*]
Possible atypical bacterial pathogen (afebrile infant or adolescent)	Macrolide (azithromycin *or* erythromycin)
Complicated pneumonia (*i.e.* parapneumonic effusion or lung abscess)	Ceftriaxone *or* cefotaxime *or* cefuroxime + (vancomycin *or* clindamycin *or* linezolid) + macrolide
Aspiration pneumonia	Ampicillin-sulbactam or clindamycin
Pneumonia in immunocompromised host	Broad spectrum Gram positive and Gram negative coverage *plus* vancomycin* (*S. aureus*) or trimethoprim-sulfamethoxazole (TMP/SMX) (*Pneumocystis jirovecii*)

* Note: Vancomycin not needed if TMP/SMX (which also covers MRSA) is given. TMP/SMX may be substituted for vancomycin if *P. jiroveci* is suspected or confirmed by bronchoalveolar lavage or lung biopsy.

Under normal conditions, pleural fluid volume is always in balance since it is filtered by parietal pleura and absorbed by visceral pleura. Transudative effusions are caused by imbalance of systemic factors (*e.g.* heart failure, renal failure, hepatic failure). Local factors (*e.g.* fibropurulent PPE, pulmonary embolism, cancer) more often cause exudates. **Box 2.5.8** lists some of the characteristics of transudates and exudates.

Box 2.5.4   Clinical Signs Useful in Diagnosis of VAP

Age	<12 mos	1–12 yrs	>12 yrs
Criteria	*At least three of "a" criteria must be met*	*At least three of "b" criteria must be met*	*At least one of "c" criteria and two of "d" criteria must be met*
T> 38°C			c
T<37°C or > 38.4°C	a	a	
WBC < 4000/mm³ or > 12,000/mm³			c
WBC < 4000/mm³ or >15,000/mm³		b	
WBC < 4000/mm³ or > 15,000/mm³ with bands > 10%	a		
Worsened gas exchange	necessary	b	d
Cough, dyspnea or ↑RR	a	b	d
Rales or bronchial breath sounds		b	d
Respiratory secretions ↑ or purulent (new)	a	b	d
Apnea, ↑RR or ↑work of breathing	a		
Wheezing, rales or rhonchi	a		
HR <100/min or > 170/min	a		

Adapted from Wright ML, Romano MJ, Ventilator Associated Pneumonia in Children, *Seminars* in *Pediatric Infectious Diseases* **17(2)**:58–64, 2006.

Box 2.5.5   Laboratory Data that Confirm Diagnosis of VAP

At least one of the following must be present:

- Growth from blood culture without other source than lung.
- Growth from pleural fluid culture.
- Growth from bronchoalveolar lavage (BAL)*.
- BAL with ≥ 10,000 colony forming units/ml.
- BAL with >5% of cells with intracellular bacteria.
- Histopathology: abscess or fungal hyphae visualized or growth from lung parenchymal culture.

---

* Note: Growth from a tracheal aspirate has 93% sensitivity but only 41% specificity for bacterial pneumonia.

Box 2.5.6   Bacteria Frequently Associated with Empyema in Children

- MRSA
- *Streptococcus pneumonia*
- Alpha-hemolytic *Streptococcus*
- Coagulase negative *Staphylococcus aureus*
- Group A *Streptococcus*
- *Actinomyces* spp.

Ultrasonography can be useful is identification of PPE, especially when CXR demonstrates an opacified hemothorax ("white out") on the involved side. Also, ultrasonography can demonstrate septations in the fluid and assess for optimal sites for thoracentesis. Chest CT may be helpful if fluid cannot be aspirated or if medical management fails.

The goals of therapy for PPE are evacuation of fluid that will allow re-expansion of lung (especially if cardiorespiratory function is compromised) and sterilization of infected fluid. Beyond these general goals specific management approaches are controversial although surgical drainage [video-assisted throracoscopy ("VATS") or thoracostomy or decortication] is often favored when loculated or organized PPE is present.

Box 2.5.7   Characteristics of Parapneumonic (Pleural) Effusions

	Time into Illness	Fluid Characteristics	CXR Findings
Transudate	Indefinite	Normal glucose and pH; low WBC	Layers out on lateral decubitus CXR
Exudate*	24–72 hrs	Normal glucose and pH; Normal to high WBC	May or may not layers out on lateral decubitus CXR
Fibrino-purulent	7–10 days	Low glucose and pH; PMNs↑ and bacterial invasion present	If "loculated" will not layer out on lateral decubitus CXR
Organized	2–4 weeks	Dry tap from "pleural peel"	"Peel" will not layer out on lateral decubitus CXR

* "Early exudates" may share some characteristics of transudate (see below).

Box 2.5.8   Characteristics of Transudates and Exudates*

Characteristic of PPE	Transudate	Exudate
Specific gravity	< 1.016	> 1.020
Protein (g/L)	< 2	> 2.9
Protein (PPE/serum ratio)	< 0.5	> 0.5
LDH	< 200	> 200
LDH (PPE/serum ratio)	< 0.6	> 0.6
WBC	< 1000/mm^3	> 1000/mm^3
RBC	< 10,000/mm^3	Variable
Glucose	Same as serum	< serum
pH	7.4–7.5	< 7.4

* Not all criteria are required to classify a fluid as "transudate" vs. "exudate".

With free-flowing PPE a simple thoracentesis should not initially exceed drainage of 10 mL/kg; after this fluid is removed the drain should optimally be clamped for one hour to avoid lung re-expansion pulmonary edema. This procedure may improve cardiopulmonary function, and provide specific information regarding the cause of the PPE. If a fibrinopurulent effusion is present, the Gram stain is positive, pus is present, a large free-flowing PPE is present, or there is no clinical improvement after 48 hours of antibiotic therapy alone then a chest tube should be inserted until drainage decreases to 10–15 mL per day. Free-flowing fluid often drains through a "pigtail catheter" whereas large bore drains may be necessary if the PPE is viscous. Fibrinolytic therapy (alteplase or streptokinase) may be instilled into the pleural space to solubilize secretions and improve drainage (especially through small catheters). Air leaks from the lung are contraindications to the use of these agents.

Loculated effusions (especially with pleural thickening and trapped lung), presence of symptoms/signs for over 1 week, lack of response to antibiotics with or without chest tube or bronchopleural fistula with pyopneumothorax are all indications for surgical therapies. VATS earlier than 48 hours into the hospital course has been proposed as an effective therapy with PPE associated with fibrinous septations of pyogenic material. VATS requires only 2 to 3 incision sites. Contraindications to VATS include the lack of ability to create a "pleural window" to access the pleural cavity, or very viscous or fibrinous PPE. A "mini-thoracotomy" or a thoracotomy provides access to the pleural space via incisions along the rib line; these permit evacuation of very viscous or fibrinous PPE.

Decortication is the surgical excision of constricting membrane from the lung and chest wall. Because lung function often returns to baseline in children without this procedure decortications may be often avoided.

Pleurodesis is a procedure where the pleural surfaces are abraded either chemically or mechanically to permanently evacuate the pleural space of air or fluid. This is seldom used in pneumonia with PPE. It has been used for recurrent pneumothoraces in AIDS patients with *Pneumocystis jiroveci* or in cystic fibrosis. This procedure may also be employed for systemic, non-infectious causes of PPE.

2.6 Chronic Lung Disease

Abnormalities in pulmonary function are generally divided into restrictive and obstructive categories. Restrictive disease implies a decrease in lung volumes and is usually accompanied by a proportionate decrease in expiratory and inspiratory flow rates. Examples of restrictive diseases would be decreased air movement from neuromuscular weakness (*Respiratory Failure in Neuromuscular Disease, 2.10*), chest wall deformity (*e.g.* scoliosis), and reduced intrathoracic volume due to tumors, atelectasis, or interstitial deposits. Obstructive diseases have a greater decrease in expiratory flow rate than volume measurements and generally start with narrowing of the airways from numerous causes (**Box 2.6.1**).

This discussion focuses on chronic lung disease of infancy (CLDI), the final common pathway of a heterogeneous group of pulmonary disorders that begin in the neonatal period. Bronchopulmonary dysplasia (BPD) is the most common form of CLDI seen in the PICU. BPD represents a spectrum of CLDI associated with prematurity and surfactant deficiency. Myriad other conditions can also cause airway and parenchymal inflammation that leads to chronic airflow obstruction, increased work of breathing, and airway hyperactivity (**Box 2.6.1**). Usually the inciting factors are not only the underlying disorders, but also the effects of the supportive treatment, including mechanical ventilation, barotrauma, and oxygen toxicity. These early lung disorders have far-reaching consequences that extend into childhood including frequent PICU admissions for exacerbations of airway disease or complicating conditions that are not confined to the respiratory system. BPD is truly a multisystem disorder (**Box 2.6.2**).

Pulmonary function in patients with BPD can be characterized generally by rapid, shallow breathing patterns, increased dead space

Box 2.6.1   Causes of Airway Obstruction/Wheezing Based on Age and Rapidity of Onset

Onset	< 1 Year	> 1 Year
Acute	• Bronchiolitis/Viral pneumonia • Asthma • BPD • Aspiration events • Tracheoesophageal disease • Gastroesophageal reflux	• Asthma • Airway foreign body • Infections: Viral, bacterial, atypical, parasitic • Anaphylaxis • Irritants: cigarette smoke, pollutants, chemical exposures (hydrocarbon ingestion) • Hypersensitivity pneumonitis
Chronic	• Asthma • Cystic fibrosis • Cardiovascular anomalies: Vascular rings and slings, double aortic arch, cardiomegaly with airway compression, pulmonary edema • Defective host defenses: Immotile cilia syndrome; immune deficiencies • Structural anomalies: Tracheal/bronchial stenosis or — malacia, lobar emphysema, pulmonary sequestration, bronchogenic cyst	• Asthma • Cystic fibrosis • Neoplastic diseases: Pulmonary, mediastinal and metastatic tumors • Adenopathy: Neoplasms, tuberculosis, sarcoidosis, autoimmune diseases, lipid storage diseases, pulmonary hemosiderosis, α-1 anti-trypsin deficiency

ventilation, decreased dynamic compliance, maldistribution of ventilation, and abnormal ventilation-perfusion matching. Infants with BPD characteristically have a marked increase in airway resistance. Many mechanisms can be responsible for this elevated airways resistance,

---

Box 2.6.2   Contributors to Acute Respiratory Distress in Infants with CLDI/BPD

- Bronchospasm
- Airway abnormalities
  - ▶ Mucus plugging
  - ▶ Laryngo-, tracheo- or broncho-malacia
  - ▶ Granuloma
  - ▶ Stenosis, caused by prolonged tracheal intubation

- Infection and inflammation
- Aspiration pneumonia
- Pulmonary edema
- Pulmonary hypertensive crisis
- Agitation
- Heart failure

---

including marked metaplasia of the bronchial epithelium with partial luminal obstruction; increased mucous production; inflammation or infection, decreased mucociliary clearance; mucosal edema; reactive bronchoconstriction; small airways closure at low lung volumes; and pulmonary vascular engorgement or edema. Spirometric values reflecting airflow are consistently lower in survivors of BPD at any age than in controls born at term, with substantial airway obstruction and alveolar hyperinflation.

Patients with BPD commonly have reactive or hyper-responsive airways, with as many as 50–60% of adolescents with BPD reportedly affected; they are often erroneously thought to have asthma. Although children with asthma and those with BPD share some clinical characteristics, particularly wheezing, these two obstructive lung diseases do not appear to have the same underlying type of airway inflammation. Inflammation in asthma is associated with eosinophilia of the lung whether or not IgE-mediated inflammation is present; this is not the case in BPD, at least during infancy. Patients with reactive airways (RAD) and history of BPD demonstrate only partial reversal of airflow obstruction in response to beta-2 agonists as compared to patients with asthma. Unlike asthmatics, BPD survivors demonstrate some distortions of normal lung architecture on high resolution CT, and are unlikely to have an atopic history. (See Baraldi E, Filippone M, Chronic lung disease after premature birth, N Engl J Med 357:1946–1955, 2007 for a detailed discussion of this topic.)

In addition to small airway hyperactivity and obstruction, large airway injury can also contribute to acute respiratory exacerbations in patients with BPD. If an infant's respiratory distress is atypical or unresponsive to the usual therapeutic maneuvers, lesions of the trachea and bronchial tree should be considered; flexible bronchoscopy may be diagnostic for problems such as tracheomalacia, bronchomalacia, polyps, granulomas, and inspissated secretions. Early diagnosis of such abnormalities is useful since specific therapies may be warranted.

Pulmonary hypertension contributes significantly to the morbidity and mortality of infants with BPD. The pulmonary circulation is characterized by increased vascular resistance and abnormal vasoreactivity, Infants with BPD have an exaggerated pulmonary vasoconstrictor response to acute hypoxia. Elevated right ventricular afterload leads to cor pulmonale or perhaps LV dysfunction, which adversely affects ventilation-perfusion matching, promotes pulmonary edema, and further decreases oxygenation. Chronic hypoxia, systemic hypertension, chronic adrenergic stimulation from stress or drug therapy, cor pulmonale, or metabolic and nutritional factors are suggested mechanisms for the development of LVH.

Exacerbation of Disease in Children with CLDI/BPD. Infants with BPD admitted to the PICU with acute respiratory symptoms present a difficult diagnostic and therapeutic problem because of the severity and complexity of their cardiorespiratory disease (**Box 2.6.2**). The usual presenting symptoms of increased work of breathing and wheezing are often multifactorial. Diagnosis, monitoring, and therapy must be instituted promptly to interrupt potentially lethal cycles and prevent the need for mechanical ventilation. Monitoring and evaluation are described in **Box 2.6.3**.

Treatment:

Oxygen is the most essential medication. Proper O_2 therapy can decrease the work of breathing, promote growth and reduce

Box 2.6.3   Monitoring and Evaluation of the Patient with CLDI or BPD

- Continuous observation for retractions, flaring, fatigue, and apnea is necessary. The quality of air movement and the presence of wheezing and rales should be recorded. Any acute change should be investigated.
- Initiate continuous pulse oximetry and record inspired O_2 concentration at least every 2–3 hrs; record circumstances of any decrease in O_2 saturation.
- Obtain capillary or arterial blood gases on admission and then as indicated. An acceptable limit for $PaCO_2$ is up to 60 mmHg. In some cases a higher $PaCO_2$ must be accepted depending on each infant's degree of illness, history, and previous blood gas values.
- Obtain a CXR on admission and as needed to evaluate hyperinflation, atelectasis, edema, and heart size. If possible, prior CXRs should be obtained for comparison.
- Perform pulmonary function testing if possible.
- Observe for ↑ in secretions and obtain cultures as indicated.
- Institute a "minimal touch" policy, organizing care and monitoring (nursing, respiratory, laboratory) so the infant is disturbed as little as possible.
- Obtain an ECG and echocardiogram to assess cardiac function and estimate pulmonary arterial pressure.
- Monitor for signs of right heart failure (*e.g.* edema, weight gain, oliguria, tachycardia, tachypnea, and increased O_2 requirements).
- Obtain serum electrolytes initially and as needed, especially in infants receiving diuretics. Assess the nutritional status, liver and renal function.
- Weigh the infant at least daily and investigate excessive weight gains (*i.e.*, > 30 g/day in infants < 12 months of age).

pulmonary vascular resistance. Supplemental O_2 therapy is indicated in infants when the PaO_2 is < 55 mm Hg or the O_2 saturation is < 90% at rest. O_2 therapy does not produce respiratory depression in infants with CLDI. Requirements may vary, depending on illness, agitation, feeding, or sleeping and the FiO_2 should be adjusted accordingly to maintain O_2 saturation >92%. Unrecognized and untreated hypoxemia has been proposed as one mechanism by which chronic pulmonary hypertension develops in patients with advanced lung disease. O_2 therapy may be indicated for several months or even years; provisions for home use of O_2 should be part of discharge planning as indicated. It is important to emphasize that infants and children with BPD may experience frequent episodes of oxygen desaturation during sleep, probably related to hypoventilation and/or upper airway obstruction. If these periods of desaturation are prolonged, central apnea and periodic breathing may result. The provision of supplemental O_2 should decrease the number of these episodes as the average saturation level improves. Eliminating sleep-associated hypoxemia also improves growth in infants with BPD.

Inhaled medications, such as bronchodilators (including β_2-agonists and anticholinergic agents), can improve short-term lung function, but whether they can prevent exacerbations and improve the quality of life remains to be seen. Without reliable evidence, it makes sense to use inhaled bronchodilators only in patients with clinical evidence of reversible airway obstruction and to treat signs of exacerbations. When inhaled drugs are used, the method of administration is important. Metered-dose inhalers, with a spacer and mask, seem to have several advantages over nebulizers.

Corticosteroids suppress inflammation and the release of chemical mediators that may trigger bronchospasm and increase responsiveness to β-adrenergic agonists. Benefits of steroid therapy in non-ventilator-dependent infants with BPD have not been assessed. Short-term steroid use during acute episodes of wheezing and bronchospasm may be useful, just as it is in older children with asthma. Long-term steroid use is discouraged. The use of inhaled corticosteroids for prophylaxis in children with established BPD has neither reduced the incidence of symptoms nor improved the outcome.

Methylxanthines. Infants with BPD have bronchiolar smooth muscle hypertrophy and hyperactive airways, and bronchodilators improve pulmonary function in these infants. Methylxanthines may improve the function of respiratory muscles and central ventilatory drive in addition to relaxing bronchial smooth muscle and stimulating ciliary motility. Worrisome side effects include gastrointestinal irritation, reduced esophageal sphincter pressure, irritability, vomiting, and alteration in sleep patterns. These complications may contribute to nutritional and respiratory problems.

Percussion and postural drainage. In general, infants with BPD have difficulty clearing secretions, and during acute illness when secretions are more copious, they need frequent percussion, postural drainage, and suctioning to prevent mucous plugging and atelectasis. While chest physiotherapy has been shown to be beneficial in infants with BPD by aiding in removal of secretions, it may be detrimental in some infants. Therefore, the overall clinical gain expected from this mode of therapy must be individualized, carefully assessed, and restricted to patients who can be closely monitored.

Fluid management and use of diuretics. Infants with BPD tolerate excessive or even normal amounts of fluid intake poorly and tend to accumulate fluid in the interstitium of the lung. Fluid administration should be limited to the minimum needed to provide necessary calories for the infants' metabolic needs and growth.

When increased lung water persists despite fluid restriction, diuretic therapy may be useful. Furosemide (1–2 mg/kg/dose IV) is associated with improvement in lung compliance and a decrease in airways resistance, but gas exchange is usually unaffected. The beneficial effects of furosemide on lung function appear to be in part non-diuretic in nature and due to non-renal effects whether in the lung or in the systemic circulation. Long-term furosemide use is associated with many complications: electrolyte imbalance, alteration in calcium and phosphate homeostasis, renal stone formation, undesirable effects on bone growth. In addition, furosemide-induced hypochloremia promotes bicarbonate retention, an undesirable effect in patients with chronic hypercarbic respiratory failure. Oral therapy with chlorothiazide (15–40 mg/kg/day) or a combination of chlorothiazide and spironolactone (2–4 mg/kg/day) results in a diuresis equivalent to that from furosemide therapy but may not provide equal improvement in lung function. Overzealous use of diuretics resulting in volume contraction may decrease cardiac output and stimulate neurohormonal systems much like antidiuretic hormone or catecholamines, which may be detrimental.

Vasodilators. Despite O_2 administration, pulmonary hypertension often persists and prevents acceptable cardiac function and interferes with gas exchange. Although vasodilator therapy may be beneficial in decreasing pulmonary arterial blood pressure in selected patients, if cardiac output falls or ventilation-perfusion ratios become more abnormal, the net effect on O_2 delivery may be detrimental (*Important Cardiopulmonary Interactions, 3.2*). Vasodilators which are not selective for the pulmonary circulation can potentially worsen hypoxemia, increase pulmonary edema, and cause systemic hypotension. Sildenafil is a selective phosphodiesterase-type 5 (PDE-5) inhibitor which is well-tolerated, safe and effective for infants with pulmonary hypertension and CLDI or BPD. It acts in pulmonary vascular smooth muscle to inhibit degradation of cyclic GMP, which promotes pulmonary vasodilation. Systemic hypertension may complicate CLDI/BPD and should be evaluated and treated (*Hypertension, 7.2*).

Nutrition. Poor nutritional status can adversely affect cardiopulmonary function by impairing respiratory muscle function, ventilatory drive, and pulmonary defense mechanisms. Inadequate caloric intake is common among patients with CLDI/BPD due to (1) increased caloric requirements (≥ 130–$150 \, kcal/kg/day$) and O_2 consumption, (2) frequent illnesses and (3) interruptions in feeding that often accompany these illnesses. Constant attention to provision of adequate calories for growth is critical. If severe fluid restriction limits caloric intake, judicious use of diuretics may permit larger volumes of feeding. Nutritional supplements can be used to increase caloric density of feeding; however, the increased osmotic load may result in diarrhea or insufficient free water to maintain normal renal function. Attention must also be given to requirements for iron, vitamins, and mineral supplementation.

Parenteral nutrition should be initiated early and at any time oral intake is compromised. Hyperalimentation with high carbohydrate load ($> 8 \, mg/kg/min$) should be avoided if pulmonary function limits the ability to handle increased CO_2 production.

Infants with BPD commonly have feeding difficulties, which are often exacerbated by acute respiratory symptoms. These difficulties may be caused by dysfunctional suck/swallow (bulbar dysfunction), gastroesophageal reflux, prolonged gastric emptying time, or rumination, causing food inhalation on swallowing. Recognition of recurrent aspiration can sometimes lead to a dramatic improvement after institution of appropriate medical or surgical therapy. Infants with aspiration because of bulbar dysfunction may benefit from bypassing the swallowing mechanism temporarily through nasogastric or gastrostomy feedings. Infants with recurrent aspiration caused by gastroesophageal reflux may also benefit from tube feedings along with therapy with metoclopramide (0.1–0.2 mg/kg/dose) or erythromycin. Temporarily, transpyloric feedings may be appropriate if gastroesophageal reflux is severe. Fundoplication occasionally is necessary. The condition of infants with rumination often improves when the same caretaker is allowed to participate consistently in feedings.

Hematologic Considerations. It is important to provide patients in respiratory distress (for whatever reason) with an adequate O_2-carrying capacity. Blood transfusion may be required.

Antimicrobial Therapy. Infants with BPD are at risk for developing respiratory failure with viral or bacterial infections. If pneumonia or bronchitis is suspected, cultures should be obtained and appropriate antibiotics started. During peak RSV season, nasal washings should be obtained for diagnostic testing.

Behavioral and developmental support. Many behavioral, physiologic, and autonomic effects are apparent in infants with BPD. Common characteristics include excessive drops in O_2 saturation secondary to external stimuli, skin mottling, difficulty in temperature regulation, and poor tolerance to any nursing procedure. In the absence of hypoxemia sedative medications may facilitate management. Organize care such that the infant is disturbed as little as possible and facilitate participation in an infant-developmental intervention program as soon as possible.

2.7 Respiratory Failure

Respiratory failure is inadequate oxygenation and/or ventilation to meet metabolic demands. Acute respiratory failure (ARF) refers to onset within a timeframe that causes acute disturbances in tissue oxygenation and/or respiratory acidosis ($PaCO_2 > 45$ mmHg) or acidemia ($pH < 7.35$); respiratory failure is the precipitant for approximately half of all PICU admissions. ARF is distinguished from respiratory distress and is typically recognizable clinically (*General Approach to the Critically Ill Child 1.2*); however, $PaO_2 < 60$ mmHg while breathing room air or $PaCO_2 > 50$ mmHg coupled with respiratory acidosis or acidemia have been arbitrary benchmarks for ARF. Infants and children are at greater risk for ARF than adults based on anatomic and developmental differences related to (1) airway size (*Upper Airway Obstruction, 2.2, Fig. 2.2.1;* Poiseuille's law applies to both upper and lower airways); (2) increased chest wall compliance, with a more horizontal orientation of the ribs resulting in a decreased mechanical advantage when an increase in negative intrathoracic pressure (to accomplish inspiration) is needed; (3) underdeveloped respiratory tract architecture in infants and young children (less cartilaginous support in the airways); absence of the inter-alveolar pores of Kohn (appear during 1–2 yrs of life) and the broncho-alveolar canals of Lambert (appear after 6 yrs of age), both of which provide for "collateral ventilation" during airway obstruction; (4) decreased elastic recoil of the lung, particularly in those < 6 yrs, tends to decrease functional residual capacity (FRC), favoring atelectasis when compliance is decreased. Turi JL, Cheifetz IM. Acute Respiratory Failure. DS Wheeler *et al.* (eds). Resuscitation and Stabilization of the Critically Ill Child, Springer-Verlag, London, 2009).

Normal gas exchange depends upon *all* of the following: airway patency, a normal alveolar-pulmonary capillary interface, adequate cardiac output and pulmonary circulation, and the ability to move gases in and out of the lungs (*i.e.* ability to move the chest wall).* The

---

* A dramatic example of ARF (under controlled circumstances) is the apnea test during evaluation of brain death. Despite witholding mechanical ventilation for periods of ~10 minutes and development of profound respiratory acidemia, Pox saturations and vital signs can remain in an acceptable range with adequate pre-oxygenation. CO_2 moves quickly from blood to alveolus, but removal of CO_2 gas requires chest wall movement (ventilation). Oxygen diffuses more rapidly through the respiratory tree than does CO_2, but eventually, the inability to remove CO_2 would prevent O_2 from reaching the alveoli and hypoxemia would ensue.

latter requires normal CNS respiratory input, normal respiratory muscle strength and function and unimpaired chest excursion. ARF is often characterized as hypoxemic or hypercarbic not because they occur in isolation, but because one or the other disturbance frequently predominates. If the first disturbance is severe and not corrected, the other will follow.

Box 2.7.1   Mechanisms Leading to Hypoxemic Respiratory Failure

- Ventilation/perfusion (V/Q) mismatch: This is the most common cause of ARF in the PICU, and refers to an uneven distribution of oxygenated alveoli with well perfused alveoli.

  Inspired oxygen is normally distributed based on positioning of the lung with respect to the ground (gravity), lung compliance and resistance to gas flow within the lung. In the dependent portions of the lung, gravitational pressure is the greatest and intrapleural pressure is less negative. If intra-alveolar pressure (P_A) remains constant, the alveolar transmural or distending pressure (pressure inside the alveolus minus the pressure outside the alveolus, or P_A minus negative intrapleural pressure) is decreased, resulting in less distension of alveoli in these regions. However, in the spontaneously breathing patient, these alveoli are also more compliant than those in the non-dependent regions. Therefore, increased compliance in dependent lung ultimately results in greater ventilation in these segments. Similarly, normal perfusion is greater in the lung base than in the apical regions, although the increase in perfusion from apex to base is greater than the increase in ventilation from apex to base with relatively greater perfusion than ventilation in dependent lung. Therefore, there is a physiologic imbalance in ventilation as it relates to perfusion, but the gradient is relatively "matched". (*Appendix, part 2, III*)

  During disease, P_A, compliance and resistance are altered by presence of alveolar debris (inflammation, blood, infectious agents, *etc.*) and airway narrowing (bronchospasm, inflammation, foreign body, *etc.*). As intrapleural pressure exceeds P_A transmural forces and

  (Continued)

Box 2.7.1   Mechanisms Leading to Hypoxemic Respiratory Failure (Continued)

decreased lung compliance each favor alveolar collapse, esp. in the dependent portions of the lung. Decreased elastic recoil of the alveoli in infants and young children also contributes to alveolar collapse as compliance decreases. As regional alveolar inflation changes depending on the affected areas of lung, poorly inflated alveoli may continue to be perfused, resulting in return of deoxygenated blood to the circulation. Regional hypoxia ($P_A O_2 < 50$–60 mmHg) often causes local pulmonary vasoconstriction, but this mechanism is insufficient to counter the effect of V/Q mismatching when lung disease is extensive. Alveoli may be completely or partially involved. As the pulmonary capillaries traverse this bed of variably affected alveoli, some areas of pulmonary-to-alveolar contact result in poor-to-no oxygenation. In addition, airway narrowing (*e.g.* asthma) may result in alveolar overdistension; this can result in ↑ pressure on the surrounding capillary bed and ↑ resistance to perfusion of these areas; this would cause an increase in V/Q mismatching. All these disease states result in V/Q mismatch.

- Shunt: This occurs whenever blood returns to the left heart without being oxygenated. Physiologic shunting occurs via veins that drain lung and heart tissue, accounting for a normal shunt fraction < 5% of the total cardiac output. Abnormal shunting most commonly results from circulation of blood to alveoli that are devoid of ventilation; abnormal arterial-venous connections (*e.g.* congenital or acquired collateral vessels in children with congenital heart disease) may also cause intra-pulmonary shunts. (*Appendix, part 2, III*).
- Diffusion abnormality: Usually occurs in combination with V/Q mismatch; associated with thickening of the alveolar-capillary interface, marked reduction in the total surface area of gas exchange, or when hyperdynamic circulation does not allow enough time for oxygenation to occur.
- Hypoventilation: A decrease in the minute ventilation (*Appendix, part 2, III*). In the absence of supplemental oxygen, the ↓ in oxygenation is directly proportional to the ↑ in $PaCO_2$.
- Low FiO_2: *e.g.* Low barometric pressure/high altitude.

Box 2.7.2   Clinical Features of Acute Respiratory Distress
Syndrome

- A severe, acute lung injury, usually occurring 48–72 hrs after an insult such as infection, aspiration, sepsis, trauma or hypotension. The primary insult may or may not involve the lungs.
- Hypoxemia with $PaO_2/FiO_2 \leq 200$ mmHg.
- Bilateral alveolar infiltrates similar to those seen in pulmonary edema, but without signs of venous congestion, cardiomegaly or pleural effusions on CXR (*i.e.* "non-cardiogenic pulmonary edema").
- Normal pulmonary capillary wedge pressure if measured.
- Nearly all patients require mechanical ventilation.

Hypoxemic respiratory failure may result from any disturbance in respiration leading to inadequate oxygenation of blood (**Box 2.7.1**). Focus on these components of oxygenation should not minimize the importance of adequate pulmonary circulation, adequate oxygen carrying capacity, and the ability of tissues to extract and utilize oxygen normally. A disturbance in any of these can lead to respiratory failure since oxygen delivery to the brain and respiratory system would eventually be affected. Features of the prototypic form of acute hypoxemic respiratory failure, the acute respiratory distress syndrome, are described (**Box 2.7.2**). Oxygenation strategies are discussed in *Mechanical Support of Ventilation, 2.8.*

Hypercapneic respiratory failure is caused by insufficient alveolar ventilation, *i.e.* inability to move CO_2 out of the lungs and/or the result of an increase in dead space ventilation (*Appendix, part 2, III and* **Box 2.7.3**).

Box 2.7.3   Mechanisms of Hypercapneic Respiratory Failure

- Decreased minute ventilation (failure to move adequate volume of gas into and out of the lung):
  - ▸ CNS diseases such as infection, TBI, HIE, rasied ICP, tumors, esp involving the brain stem; metabolic encephalopathy; spinal cord injury; respiratory depression from medications (analgesic and sedatives) or intoxications; congenitally disordered breathing including autonomic regulatory disturbances, unresponsiveness to hypercarbia (*e.g.* primary central hypoventilation); Chiari malformations, *et al.*
  - ▸ Neuromuscular disease: These may lead to weakness of the respiratory muscles (*Respiratory Failure in Neuromuscular Disease, 2.10*). Acute causes include Guillain-Barre syndrome, ADEM, infant botulism, tick paralysis, toxins (*Terrorism Agents, 14.3*), drugs (neuromuscular blocking agents; gentamicin, esp. in patients with pre-existing neuromuscular disease), electrolyte imbalance, *viz.* hypokalemia, hypocalcemia and hypophosphatemia. Hypokalemia and hypophosphatemia can cause respiratory muscle failure based on their roles in generating an action potential, energy production, and at the neuromuscular junction. Corticosteroids may cause muscle weakness particularly in the context of critical illness and when given in the presence of other risk factors.
  - ▸ Muscle fatigue: This is hastened by hypoxemia and in children < 2 yrs because of a mechanically disadvantaged diaphragm and highly compliant chest wall.
  - ▸ Distortions or restrictions of the chest wall: These may be congenital or acquired as in severe spasticity with kyphoscoliosis, obstructive lung disease (*e.g.* cystic fibrosis or severe asthma); the ↑ in FRC results in loss of elastic recoil of respiratory muscles at end-expiration with flattening of the diaphragm, leading to ↑ work of breathing to accomplish the next inspiration.
- Increased dead space ventilation (ventilation of non-perfused lung): Physiologic (or total) dead space refers to tidal volume not expected to participate in gas exchange (*e.g.* extra-thoracic and the large intrathoracic airways) plus the volume that ventilates non-perfused alveoli (*Appendix, part 2, III*). Dead space ventilation may be ↑ by artificial airways, excessive length or compliance of mechanical ventilator circuitry and pulmonary embolism.

2.8 Mechanical Support of Ventilation

The goals of mechanical ventilation are to support oxygenation and alveolar ventilation while minimizing work of breathing and iatrogenic lung injury. Currently, positive pressure devices are used almost exclusively. These require the ventilator to generate forces that overcome the elastic and resistive components of the lung, airway, and chest wall in order to displace a volume of gas. Therefore, it is important to recognize and optimize the interplay between the ventilator and the patient. Indications and complications are listed (**Boxes 2.8.1 and 2.8.2**)

Box 2.8.1   Indications for Mechanical Ventilation

- Respiratory failure, actual or impending
- Moderate to severe cardiac dysfunction
- Support of patient intubated for airway protection secondary to CNS dysfunction
- Support of patient intra- and post-operatively
- Optimization of CO_2 (for management of ↑ ICP or pulmonary hypertension)

Box 2.8.2   Complications of Positive Pressure Ventilation

- Ventilator-induced lung injury (barotrauma, volutrauma, atelectotrauma)
- Oxygen toxicity
- Overdistension leading to pneumothorax, V/Q mismatch, ↑ PVR
- Atelectasis
- ↑ Intrathoracic pressure leading to ↓ cardiac output from ↓ venous return
- Ventilator-associated pneumonia
- Sinusitis and otitis media
- Inadvertent extubation
- Trauma (subglottic edema/injury; vocal cord, nasal or nasopharyngeal injury)

2.8.1 *Invasive mechanical ventilation*

Invasive mechanical ventilation refers to ventilation delivered through an artificial airway; the various patterns of gas delivery are characterized as ventilator "modes" which describe ventilator function. The terms used by manufacturers can be confusing as different nomenclature is used for similar modalities. A ventilator mode is defined by the following characteristics which are directly controlled (or set):

(1) the control variable; every mode has a set pressure, volume, or flow (used infrequently in PICU settings) for each mandatory breath (**Box 2.8.3**).
(2) the relationship between mandatory versus spontaneous breaths (*e.g.* CMV, SIMV); **Box 2.8.4**
(3) the phase variables (which determine how a breath is initiated, the size of a breath, and what terminates a breath; **Box 2.8.5**); and
(4) whether or not spontaneous breaths are assisted.

Patient factors influencing ventilation: Support of the respiratory system by invasive mechanical ventilation depends on the interaction between the mode settings and the indirectly controlled patient variables. These variables are determined by the individual patient's anatomy and physiology and include resistance (affected by the resistance of the airways as well as the endotracheal tube) and compliance (affected by the lungs and the chest wall). *Resistance* describes the change in pressure needed to effect a change in flow. *Compliance* describes the change in pressure needed to effect a change in volume. Therefore, in a pressure controlled mode, the delivered tidal volume will change based on the dynamic compliance of the respiratory system (*Appendix, part 2, III*). Conversely, in a volume controlled mode, the pressure required to deliver that tidal volume will change based on the dynamic compliance.

Dual control modes: Since compliance can frequently change, the patient's minute ventilation (TV × RR; *Appendix, part 2, III*) can be highly variable. To achieve more consistent minute ventilation while still limiting the pressure, manufacturers have developed dual control modes [*e.g.* Pressure-regulated volume control (PRVC), Adaptive pressure ventilation (APV), and Auto Control +].

Box 2.8.3   Control Variables in Mechanical Ventilation

	Pressure controlled (PC)	Volume controlled (VC)
Controlled variable	Each breath delivers a set pressure.	Each breath delivers a set tidal volume (TV)
Indirect variable	The TV delivered is variable and determined by the set pressure and the lung/chest wall compliance.	The pressure required to deliver the set TV is variable and is determined by the set TV and the lung/chest wall compliance.
Advantages	Peak inspiratory pressure (PIP) < the PIP in VC ventilation for the same TV. Lung units with variable time constants are recruited more effectively. During air leak, maintains pressure despite volume lost. Higher initial flow may meet patient demands better.	Tighter control over minute ventilation; avoids volutrauma when normal tidal volumes are delivered to healthy lungs with a stable and normal FRC.
Disadvantages	Minute ventilation not guaranteed since compliance changes affect TV.	Constant (invariable) flow may not meet patient demand and lead to asynchrony. PIP > PIP in PC ventilation for the same TV.

Box 2.8.4   Mandatory vs. Spontaneous Breaths: Definitions

- Mandatory breath: Initiated by the ventilator; its characteristics are determined by the set control variable.
- Spontaneous breath: Initiated by the patient; its characteristics are determined by the patient.
- Continuous mandatory ventilation (CMV): All breaths are controlled by the ventilator; no gas flow is delivered for the patient's own breaths making CMV uncomfortable for spontaneously breathing patients
- Intermittent mandatory ventilation (IMV): Spontaneous breaths allowed in between mandatory, controlled breaths; however, patient breaths are not synchronized with the ventilator breaths. Thus, the patient breaths can be interrupted (or "stacked") by a mechanical breath.
- Synchronized IMV (SIMV): Spontaneous breaths are synchronized with the mandatory, controlled breaths, allowing the patient to complete a breath without interruption by a mechanical breath. If no breath is initiated by the patient within a specified time, then a breath is delivered by the ventilator.
- Pressure support ventilation (PSV) and volume support ventilation (VSV): All breaths are spontaneous with frequency, inspiratory time (i-time), and TV controlled by the patient. However, the ventilator can be set to assist these breaths with a pre-set inspiratory pressure or volume (pressure or volume-supported breaths; assisted spontaneous breaths).

Box 2.8.5   Phase Variables, Effects and Mechanical Ventilator Options

Phase Variable	Effect	Options
Trigger variable	Initiates breath	Pressure, volume, flow (most common) or time
Limit variable	Determines size of breath	Pressure, volume, or flow
Cycle variable	Terminates breath	Pressure, volume, flow or time (most common)

A target TV is set and the ventilator uses closed loop, breath-to-breath feedback to adjust the pressure to achieve this target. The lowest pressure necessary is used and a pressure limit is set to prevent barotrauma. Therefore this mode is a pressure controlled mode.

Ventilator settings: The basic settings during conventional mechanical ventilation are the mode of ventilation, set rate (if any), controller variable (PC or VC), positive end-expiratory pressure (PEEP), and set oxygen percentage (FiO_2). PEEP is the lower limit of airway pressure during the breath cycle and is the main determinant of the mean airway pressure. Maintaining alveolar inflation during mechanical ventilation requires setting at least physiologic PEEP (3–4 cm H_2O) and may require increasing levels of PEEP in states of poor compliance (i.e. in acute lung injury or acute respiratory distress syndrome). Pressure control (ΔP) + PEEP = peak inspiratory pressure (PIP; **Fig. 2.8.1**).

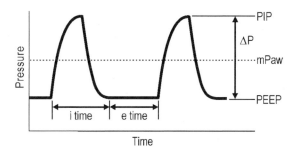

Fig. 2.8.1. Mechanical Ventilator Breaths Displayed on a Pressure vs. Time Graph (i time, inspiratory time; e time, expiratory time; PIP, peak inspiratory pressure; PEEP, positive end expiratory pressure; mPaw, mean airway pressure; ΔP, pressure control or change in pressure).

Other ventilator modes: Adaptive support ventilation (ASV) utilizes closed loop feedback to provide the necessary level of support to the patient. The ventilator adjusts the variables to meet the minute ventilation demands based on the ideal body weight and percent minute volume (set). A paralyzed patient would receive all mandatory breaths (CMV) while an awake patient may only be receiving pressure supported breaths (PSV).

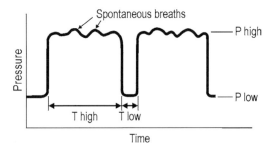

Fig. 2.8.2.   Airway Pressure Release Ventilation (APRV). Breaths are displayed on a pressure vs. time graph. (T high = time spent at p High, T low = time spent at P low, P high = high level of pressure or CPAP used during "inspiratory hold", P low = low level of pressure or PEEP during exhalation).

Airway pressure release ventilation (APRV; also known as Bilevel or Duo-Pap; **Fig. 2.8.2**) is a mode that allows the clinician to provide a higher mean airway pressure while minimizing ventilator induced lung injury. The mandatory breaths are set at a high level of pressure (or CPAP) and the ventilator dumps gas during brief periods of time at a low level of pressure ("P low"). The short time at P low prevents complete exhalation and alveolar collapse. In APRV, patients may also spontaneously breathe with the assistance of pressure support, which augments CO_2 elimination.

Weaning from invasive mechanical ventilation: The risks of prolonged ventilation vs. premature extubation should be balanced. Weaning from support should begin when the underlying process is improving, the oxygen requirement is reasonable (usually < 50%), and the patient can begin spontaneous breathing independently to achieve adequate gas exchange without excess work of breathing. Traditionally, ventilator support is gradually weaned; however, the patient may also begin spontaneous breathing trials.

High Frequency Ventilation (HFV) The high frequency devices deliver very small tidal volumes (less than physiological dead space) at supraphysiologic frequencies (> 60 breaths per min).

High Frequency Oscillatory Ventilation (HFOV) is a type of high frequency mechanical ventilation commonly used as a lung-protective strategy in patients with acute respiratory distress syndrome (ARDS). It is commonly implemented when adequate ventilation and oxygenation can no longer be achieved using lung-protective strategies on conventional mechanical ventilation (CMV). HFOV is unique in that oxygenation and ventilation are more dependent on airway resistance than lung compliance and tidal volumes delivered are less

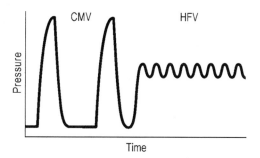

Fig. 2.8.3. Comparison of Conventional Mechanical Ventilation (CMV) and High Frequency Ventilation (HFV). CMV breaths with higher peak pressure and lower PEEP compared to the lower tidal volume, higher frequency breaths during HFV.

than anatomical dead space. The goal of HFOV is to recruit alveolar units without causing overdistention.

Mechanisms of gas exchange. The following are some of the primary physical principles that have been proposed to explain gas exchange with HFOV.

- **Convection:** Lung parenchyma off of proximal primary airways receive direct bulk flow.
- **Diffusion:** Both O_2 and CO_2 molecules diffuse according to the concentration gradients that exist across the alveolocapillary membrane.
- **Dispersion:** Turbulent flow augments the mixing of gases.

- **Pendeluft:** Gas flow is governed by regional variation in airway resistance and compliance.
- Unequal **laminar flow** velocity profiles: over repeated cycles, gas in the center of the airways is directed toward alveoli while gas along the airway wall is directed toward the mouth.

Ventilator and Initial Settings (Box 2.8.6). There are currently two HFOV ventilators marketed by Viasys Healthcare,™ the Sensormedics 3100A (usually for children under 35 kg) and 3100B (for children > 35 kg and adults). These ventilators are driven by an oscillating piston that produces both positive and negative airway pressures across the mean airway pressure (mPaw) at high frequencies.

Box 2.8.6   Initial Settings and Strategies for HFOV

- The initial **mPaw** is usually set 2–8 cm H_2O higher than that used on conventional ventilation and is the primary determinant of **oxygenation**. Initial alveolar recruitment requires higher mPaw than maintenance of recruited alveoli (**Fig. 2.8.4**). If FiO_2 cannot be weaned below 0.6 while maintaining O_2 saturations >90%, mPaw should be increased in increments of 2 cm H_2O. Once FiO_2 is below 0.6, mPaw should be weaned to prevent overdistention.
- **FiO_2** is usually set at 1.0 and weaned as alveolar recruitment improves; goal of $FiO_2 \leq 0.6$.
- **Amplitude** (ΔP) is the peak and trough pressure excursion across the mPaw and is a determinant of **ventilation**. It is the pressure generated by the force of the ventilator piston which is controlled by the power setting. As ΔP increases, tidal volumes and ventilation increase. Initial amplitude can be determined by the lowest ΔP that gives adequate visible "chest wiggle". Initial amplitude has also been estimated by using a ΔP value that is 10–30 cm H_2O > the $PaCO_2$. Changes in ΔP should be made in 5–10 cm H_2O increments.

(Continued)

Box 2.8.6   Initial Settings and Strategies for HFOV (Continued)

- The rate of oscillations or **frequency** is measured in cycles per second (**Hertz or Hz**). Although it is a determinant of **ventilation** it should not be regarded the same as CMV rate. As Hz decrease, tidal volumes increase therefore decreasing Hz increases ventilation. Initial frequency settings are dependent on patient weight and habitus ranging from 12–20 Hz in neonates to 3–5 Hz in adults. ΔP should be maximized prior to decreasing Hz to improve ventilation. Note that decreases in Hz reduce the dampening effect of airway branching and effectively increase the ΔP that reaches the alveoli. Changes in frequency should be made in 1 Hz increments (**Fig. 2.8.5b**).
- See **Fig. 2.8.5** for methods of improving ventilation.
- An **inspiratory time** of 33% of the cycle is most commonly used. It can be increased to 50% to improve CO_2 removal.
- If hypercapnea persists after optimizing ΔP and Hz, allowing a small endotracheal tube cuff leak (by slightly deflating the ETT cuff) may allow improved CO_2 removal. However, this should be used as a "last resort" maneuver.

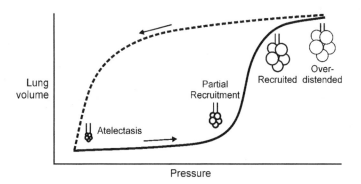

Fig. 2.8.4.   Alveolar Recruitment in HFOV.

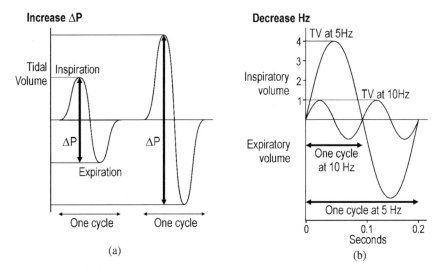

Fig. 2.8.5.   Strategies for Increasing Ventilation in HFOV. TV, tidal volume. A. The effect of changing the power setting (↑Power causes ↑ΔP). Note that an ↑ in ΔP does not change the time for completion of one respiratory cycle. B. The effect of decreasing Hertz. Note that by decreasing Hz from 10 to 5, the TV is increased fourfold, and ventilation is augmented. The time to complete one cycle on 5 Hz is twice as long as the time to complete one cycle on 10 Hz. (These diagrams are for illustrative purposes only and are not necessarily drawn to scale.)

Lung-protective benefits of HFOV:

- Maintains alveolar recruitment without instituting an opening and closing cycle as happens with CMV; this decreases alveolar shear injury.
- ΔP is dampened at each level of airway branching; therefore, the ΔP at the alveolus is significantly reduced, also decreasing shear injury.
- Evidence suggests that HFOV may reduce lung inflammatory responses when compared with CMV.

Transitioning from CMV to HFOV and **Complications of HFOV** are outlined in **Boxes 2.8.7 and 2.8.8**.

Box 2.8.7 Considerations in Transitioning from CMV to HFOV

- Monitoring should include Pox, transcutaneous CO_2 detection (TCOM), ABG's and serial CXR. $PaCO_2$ and PaO_2 may deteriorate rapidly if predetermined ventilator settings are not adequate. In this situation, there may be insufficient time to wait for blood gas results and the clinician is dependent on accurate bedside monitoring. Monitors should be calibrated and reading accurately prior to initiating HFOV. ABG and CXR should be obtained within the first hour of initiating HFOV. Serial ABGs should be frequent until values stabilize. Serial CXR's are necessary to assess appropriate lung inflation (lung expansion 8–10 ribs posteriorly) to avoid overdistention and barotrauma. These may be required with each escalation of settings, or even with de-escalation if the prior film is worrisome or borderline for overinflation (≥ 10 ribs posteriorly).
- A gradual increase in $PaCO_2$ and/or ΔP on a given power setting ("drift") may indicate air trapping and overdistention.
- Intravascular volume should be optimized prior to initiating HFOV. Higher m Paw ↑s intrathoracic pressure and can ↓ preload. Hypotension may occur when initiating HFOV therefore IV fluid for resuscitation (and ionotropic support) should be available at the bedside.
- Analgesia, sedation, and NMB should be started and optimized prior to HFOV. Once the patient and settings have stabilized, NMB may not be required continuously.
- VAP prophylaxis should be continued as with CMV.
- As with CMV continue permissive hypercapnea and hypoxia to allow the least toxic ventilator settings.

High Frequency Jet Ventilation (HFJV) uses a jet injector to deliver gas down the trachea at a high velocity. The high velocity jet pulses may be beneficial for delivering gas past areas of air leak (tracheal trauma, pneumothorax, pulmonary interstitial emphysema). Exhalation occurs continuously and passively (by recoil of the lung) during HFJV and is a potential advantage for patients

---

Box 2.8.8   Potential Complications of HFOV

- Hypotension: The higher mPaw used with HFOV ↑s intrathoracic pressures and ↓s preload which in turn ↓s CO and can result in hypotension. This can be avoided with maintenance of adequate intravascular volume.
- Air leak (pneumothorax, pnemomediastinum, pneumoperitoneum): Can occur secondary to volutrauma or barotrauma. This can result from overdistention of the lungs, often seen as hyperinflation on CXR. The pressure required to open alveoli is higher than the pressure needed to maintain that expansion (**Fig. 2.8.3**). Once alveoli are recruited, mPaw should be weaned and lung inflation monitored closely with serial CXR's. Barotrauma can also result from frequency set too low causing significantly ↑alveolar ΔP. Hz should be set according to "chest wiggle" and should not be decreased until amplitude (ΔP) is maximized.
- Ventilator malfunction: Sudden decompression of the ventilator circuit because of an air leak or circuit disconnect will result in ventilator shut down. Manual bag ventilation with a PEEP valve should always be available at the bedside.
- ETT obstruction: Sudden rise in $PaCO_2$ or increase in ΔP suggests airway or ETT obstruction. Suctioning may not clear the obstruction and bronchoscopy or changing the ETT may be required.

---

with poor carbon dioxide elimination, air-trapping, or bronchospasm (*e.g.* patients with pulmonary hypertension, bronchiolitis, congenital diaphragmatic hernia or obstructive lung disease). If these patients have concurrent acute lung injury, they may benefit from a higher mean airway pressure setting to improve oxygenation as is done routinely with HFOV. The HFJV device by Bunnell is used in infants and small children. Key points are summarized in **Box 2.8.9**.

Box 2.8.9   Key Points in Use of High Frequency Jet Ventilation

- The **inspiratory time** is set at 0.02 sec and is effective in almost every case.
- The **rate** or frequency may be set at 240–660 bpm. Higher rates are generally used in LBW premature infants. Lower rates are used in larger infants and children and are beneficial with pulmonary diseases that cause significant gas trapping. Also, the set rate determines the I:E ratio since i-time is fixed.
- **Peak inspiratory pressure**, which is greatly attenuated down the airways before reaching the alveoli, is the primary determinant of TV and therefore CO_2 elimination. It is also important to remember that as the PEEP is increased, the ΔP is smaller unless PIP is also adjusted.
- The **mPaw** setting, which maintains a constant distending pressure during HFV, requires **a tandem conventional ventilator** be used in-line for the application of PEEP. As with HFOV, clinicians should focus on setting the appropriate mPaw instead of being fearful of increasing the PEEP.
- The in-line CMV can be used to give "sigh breaths" at 5–10 bpm for lung recruitment. To limit iatrogenic lung injury, these breaths should be eliminated as soon as the collapsed alveoli have been reopened and mPaw has been optimized.
- Changes in pulmonary compliance and airway resistance are reflected in the servo pressure, which increases with ↑ compliance and/or ↓ resistance. Note that a pneumothorax, before creating tension, may be reflected as an ↑ in the servo pressure when the lung is very poorly compliant, and suddenly leaks. Hence this change should be viewed in conjunction with all available measures.

2.8.2   Noninvasive ventilation (NIV)

Noninvasive ventilation refers to techniques of augmenting alveolar ventilation without an artificial airway. Due to the complications associated with tracheal intubation (*e.g.* airway injury, aspiration during intubation, barotrauma, hemodynamic instability, nosocomial pneumonia, and increased length of hospital stay) NIV is becoming a popular first alternative, especially in chronic disease processes. There are two types of NIV: positive pressure (NPPV) and negative pressure. Negative pressure ventilation is not commonly used and will be described only briefly.

Negative pressure ventilation is the oldest form of artificial ventilatory assistance. A number of types of negative pressure ventilators are available, and all work by applying intermittent negative pressure to the thorax, causing intrathoracic transpulmonary pressure to become "positive" (pressure inside the airway is > pressure outside the airway; *i.e.* the ratio of pressure inside:outside the airway is > 1). This results in a decrease in pleural pressure, allowing ambient gases to fill the lung. Exhalation is passive; when the negative pressure exerted by the ventilator is realeased, the expanded lung recoils and empties. Negative pressure ventilation simulates normal tidal breathing more closely than positive pressure ventilation and is particularly useful in respiratory insufficiency due to diaphragmatic or respiratory muscle failure.

The three basic types of negative pressure ventilators are tank, jacket, and cuirass ventilators. The advantages of tank ventilators are that they do not need to be fit to the patient, require only one tight seal around the neck, and are the most efficient type of negative pressure ventilators, providing the largest tidal volume for a given pressure change. Jacket ventilators include a rigid internal framework and a suit that must be sealed at the arms, neck, and legs. Good fit is important and often difficult to achieve. These ventilators may be more appropriate for home use. Standard sized cuirass (shell) ventilators are available, but the cuirass is most efficient when individually molded for the patient. When a good fit is achieved, it is easy to care for, and older patients find it easier to apply and remove compared to the jacket ventilator. Cuirass ventilators are useful for home ventilation but need to be remade when the child grows, gains weight, or has other changes in chest shape.

All negative pressure devices have a significant limitation in that they may precipitate upper airway obstruction especially during rapid eye movement (REM) sleep. Another problem is lack of airway protection which may lead to aspiration, especially in patients with bulbar dysfunction.

Noninvasive Positive Pressure Ventilation (NPPV) has been more widely utilized recently because of convenience, portability and its compatibility using with a variety of ventilators. Gas is delivered to the patient through the mouth, nose, or mouth and nose via appropriate patient ventilator interfaces (cannulae with prongs or masks). By definition, this technique is distinguished from those ventilatory techniques that bypass the patient's upper airway with an artificial airway (*e.g.* ETT, laryngeal mask airway, or tracheostomy tube). Because NPPV does not involve an invasive procedure, it may be readily applied and removed, circumventing potential delay in providing respiratory support.

When applied in appropriate circumstances, the shortcomings of NPPV (lack of airway protection and secretion removal) are relatively few in number. NPPV has a role in the management of acute or chronic respiratory failure and in some patients with heart failure. Noninvasive approaches can preserve normal swallowing and speech. Cough, physiologic air warming and humidification are also preserved. Selected patients may be able to feed orally during intervals off NPPV. Tracheal intubation is inherently uncomfortable; deep sedation is often required, further prolonging the weaning process, and sometimes obscuring physical findings of intercurrent problems. Attempts to limit sedation may precipitate discomfort, agitation, patient-ventilator dysynchrony, and sympathetic over-activity. Alert patients often find NIV more comfortable and less frustrating than tracheal intubation.

NPPV may be provided by continuous positive airway pressure (CPAP), high flow nasal cannula (HFNC) or bi-level positive airway pressure (BLPAP). CPAP provides only a single level of airway pressure, which is maintained throughout the respiratory cycle. It does not actively assist with ventilation. In the acute setting, its main uses are for upper airway obstruction and for hypoxemic respiratory failure. It can improve oxygenation by increasing the mean airway pressure, increasing functional residual capacity, and opening under-ventilated and collapsed alveoli, enhancing gas exchange and oxygenation. Work of breathing is decreased through an increase in lung compliance. CPAP is typically delivered by mask or nasal device. The mask fit should not be airtight; a small leak is more comfortable for the patient and is associated with fewer complications. The CPAP flow delivery device should: provide high flows (*i.e.*, exceeding twice the minute ventilation), have an adjustable FiO_2, and maintain constant CPAP levels regardless of the flow through the threshold resistor valves. During mask CPAP, monitor the patient's response, particularly level of comfort, respiratory rate, and oxygen saturation (SpO_2). The patient who is benefiting from mask CPAP usually appears comfortable with an observed decrease in respiratory rate and improvement in aeration. Pulse oximetry is helpful in adjusting the FiO_2.

Nasal CPAP is commonly delivered by single or double (binasal) prongs. These prongs are available in both short (nasal) and long (nasopharyngeal) forms. Nasal masks have been developed that deliver CPAP effectively while causing minimal nasal trauma. Nasal cannulae with an outer diameter of 3 mm and flows up to 2 L/min have been reported to deliver CPAP. Delivery of effective pressures with nasal cannulae can be challenging because low flow rates and leaks between the cannulae and the nasal passages make it difficult to maintain CPAP.

High-flow nasal cannulae (HFNC) systems are an alternative to CPAP, allow greater positive distending pressure and deliver *heated and humidified* gas to the airways. Traditional nasal cannula gas flow in young children is limited to 2–3 L/min because of patient discomfort, mucosal irritation and dryness. The warmth and humidification of the HFNC systems help mitigate these problems. In general, the outer diameter of the nasal prongs should be no greater than half the inner diameter of the nares. Limited studies in preterm infants suggest that HFNC provides airway distending pressure and respiratory support comparable to nasal CPAP.

Bilevel positive airway pressure (BLPAP) provides an inspiratory positive airway pressure for ventilatory assistance and lung recruitment, and an expiratory positive airway pressure to help recruit lung volume and to maintain adequate lung expansion (**Box 2.8.10 and Fig. 2.8.6**). The singular advantage of the addition of a preset inspiratory pressure over CPAP is the capability to augment the patient's tidal volume. The added inspiratory assist theoretically should further reduce the work of breathing.

Box 2.8.10   BLPAP (Bilevel Positive Airway Pressure)

BLPAP systems are machines which can deliver preset adjustable levels of inspiratory positive airway pressure (**IPAP**) and expiratory positive airway pressure (**EPAP**).

- What is EPAP?
  EPAP is the amount of positive pressure maintained in the airway during *Expiration*.
- What does EPAP do?
  EPAP can minimize or eliminate upper airway resistance and small airway collapse which is frequently present.
- What is IPAP?
  IPAP, also known as pressure support ventilation, is the amount of positive pressure delivered to the airway during *Inspiration*.
- What does IPAP do?
  IPAP increases lung volume during inspiration by providing positive pressure. Positive pressure is produced in response to the patient's inspiratory effort. This reduces the work the respiratory muscles must normally do to increase volume.

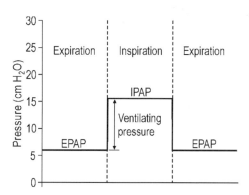

Fig. 2.8.6.   The Difference Between IPAP and EPAP is called "*Ventilating Pressure*".

Published studies in pediatric patients predominantly reflect the use of BLPAP with use of the BiPaP® system (Respironics Corp, Murrysville, PA), a flow triggered, portable device introduced in 1989. BLPAP systems are primarily flow triggered machines. In the spontaneous mode, BLPAP responds to the patient's own flow rates and cycles between higher pressure (inhalation) and lower pressure (exhalation) even if there are air leaks in the patient's circuit. When inspiration is detected, the higher pressure is delivered for a fixed time or until the flow rate falls below a threshold value. An automatic cycle feature can be added for central apnea or poor inspiratory effort. In this spontaneous/timed mode, BLPAP supports any breathing efforts initiated by the patient, along with a minimum set respiratory rate.

Physiologic Effects of NPPV. Numerous studies have confirmed the efficacy of properly-adjusted NPPV in decreasing the work of breathing when the waveform of flow or pressure is appropriately matched for respiratory synchrony. This is reflected in indicators of patient stress (*e.g.* RR, HR, and O_2 consumption). The positive airway pressure applied during inspiration (IPAP) will increase mean airway pressure, an effect accentuated by also maintaining positive pressure during expiration (EPAP). Increasing mean airway pressure tends to improve oxygen transfer across the lung in patients with acute parenchymal diseases, an effect that has been most clearly documented in the older literature pertaining to the use of mask CPAP in pulmonary edema. Improved oxygenation is usually attributed to better recruitment of collapsed lung units, together with beneficial redistribution of lung water and attenuation of the work of breathing. However, excessive increases of mean airway pressure have the potential to decrease venous return, cardiac output, and blood pressure, although this adverse result is much less common during triggered ventilation than during passive inflation. Furthermore, in the presence of a focal consolidation of the lung resistant to recruitment, increased alveolar pressure in the uninvolved lung regions may divert blood flow to the consolidated zones, increasing the pulmonary-shunt fraction.

Application of NPPV in Children. The increase in morbidity and mortality associated with tracheal intubation and mechanical ventilation makes NPPV an attractive alternative. Also, children with chronic respiratory failure are typically managed long term with a tracheostomy and assisted ventilation via volume-regulated ventilators; this approach is fraught with potentially serious complications, both medical and social. Even though few published studies support the use of NPPV as a treatment for chronic pediatric respiratory diseases, application of NPPV in younger patients is keeping pace with its growing use in adults. Although NPPV may be more difficult to initiate in younger children, this therapy can be applied in infants of <1 year of age. For example, recurrent airway occlusions that result in hypoxemia and disturbed sleep can occur in children with Duchenne muscular dystrophy. Such events can be reduced or eliminated by nocturnal NPPV. However, important differences between children and adults in the anatomy and mechanical function of the respiratory system as well as the spectrum of diseases causing respiratory failure bear on the application of NPPV in the pediatric-age patient.

If the nasal mask interface is to be successful in augmenting alveolar ventilation, the resistance of the upper airway must be overcome. Important anatomic and mechanical features of the developing upper airway often require high inspiratory pressure (**Box 2.8.11**).

Box 2.8.11   Factors that Cause Obstruction of the Upper Airway and May Limit the Efficacy of NPPV via Nasal Mask in Pediatric Patients

- The nasal resistance is a relatively higher fraction of the total respiratory resistance in pediatric patients compared to adults.
- Acute nasopharyngeal obstruction with secretions often develops during upper respiratory infections.
- Adenoids and tonsils hypertrophy in response to respiratory infections.
- Congenital anomalies accompanied by maxillary hypoplasia can result in nasopharyngeal airway obstruction.
- The tendency to mouth-breathe in response to naso-pharyngeal obstruction leads to oral leak of nasally or naso-orally delivered flow (see text).

During infancy, resistance of the nasal airway is relatively high, and is a significant fraction of the total pulmonary resistance. In young children, the nasopharyngeal airway is prone to obstruction; the adenoids and tonsils develop naturally between 2 and 7 years and can enlarge in response to recurrent infections and allergies. Adenotonsillar hypertrophy is the most important cause of obstructive sleep apnea in the pediatric population. In addition, thick copious secretions can obstruct the nasopharyngeal airway in children with respiratory tract infections.

The size and shape of the nasopharyngeal airway are determined chiefly by the development of the midfacial bones. Congenital craniofacial anomalies with maxillary hypoplasia (*e.g.* Down syndrome) are often associated with obstructive sleep apnea or, in severe cases, obstructive hypoventilation syndrome. Young infants with choanal atresia or mandibular hypoplasia (*e.g.* Pierre Robin anomaly) can also present with hypoventilation and severe respiratory distress.

Compared to the adult larynx, the immature larynx is positioned relatively anterior and contributes more to upper airway obstructive syndromes. Tonic activation of the laryngeal muscles during the first year of life produces an expiratory "braking mechanism," and thereby preserves lung volume. Infants and young children are more likely than adults to present with laryngeal airway obstruction in association with laryngomalacia, gastroesophageal reflux, and infectious laryngitis. Gastroesophageal reflux can cause laryngeal edema when acid reflux from the stomach reaches the larynx. NPPV may contribute to the tendency to have gastroesophageal reflux when NPPV contributes to gastric insufflation. However, NPPV is not currently contraindicated in pediatric patients with gastroesophageal reflux.

Obstruction of the nasopharyngeal airway necessarily leads to mouth-breathing. This compensatory response may be counterproductive during nasal NPPV, when oral air leak can significantly limit the efficacy of NPPV. Although NPPV devices are flow-triggered by the patient's respiratory effort, the onset of inspiration may be difficult to sense in the presence of large air leaks. In addition, the duration of the inspiratory phase is dependent on the decrease in flow coincident with the attainment of the preset maximum inspiratory pressure; when the oral air leak is significant, patient inspiratory efforts may fail to trigger inspiratory flow. If a backup rate is used, the timer will trigger inspiratory pressure, but inspiratory flow will be prolonged (in an attempt to maintain the inspiratory pressure); if the child attempts to exhale during inflation, patient-ventilator asynchrony results. This is especially common in young children and infants who compensate for respiratory dysfunction by breathing rapidly.

A number of respiratory conditions are amenable to a trial of NPPV in pediatric-age patients (**Box 2.8.12**).

Box 2.8.12   Respiratory Conditions Amenable to a NPPV Trial in Pediatric Patients

- **Impaired Central Respiratory Drive**: Congenital and acquired central alveolar hypoventilation; infectious and metabolic encephalopathies.
- **Acute Hypoxemic Respiratory Failure**: Pneumonia, bronchiolitis; acute chest syndrome in sickle cell disease; atelectasis; pulmonary edema; ARDS.
- **Obstructive Lung Disorders**: Cystic fibrosis; bronchopulmonary dysplasia; status asthmaticus; bronchiolitis obliterans.
- **Restrictive Disorders**: Duchenne's muscular dystrophy; spinal muscular atrophy; myotonic dystrophy; thoracic kyphoscoliosis.
- **Disorders Associated with Obstructive Hypoventilation**:
  - ▶ Morbid Obesity: Prader-Willi syndrome; obesity hypoventilation syndrome.
  - ▶ Cerebral palsy: associated with upper airway obstruction from laryngeal dysfunction and/or malposition of the tongue.
  - ▶ Myelomeningocele with bulbar dysfunction and vocal cord paresis (frequently accompanied by chronic aspiration lung injury).
  - ▶ Craniofacial syndromes with maxillary hypoplasia: Apert's syndrome; Cruzon's syndrome; Treacher-Collins syndrome; Carpenter's syndrome; Down syndrome.
  - ▶ Severe primary laryngo- and tracheo-malacia (often associated with GERD).
  - ▶ Severe obstructive sleep apnea syndrome.

NPPV in Acute Hypoxemic Respiratory Failure. In children, the reported use of NPPV has primarily been in patients with chronic respiratory failure secondary to neuromuscular disease or chronic lung disease. Favorable experience with NPPV in pediatric patients with acute respiratory failure is accumulating. The most common diagnosis in a reported case series was pneumonia, and a significant number of children with neurodevelopmental disabilities were managed effectively with this method.

Recent reports suggest that NPPV may have a role in treating children with acute asthma exacerbation; however, in the emergency room or ICU, a trial of NPPV should be considered in children with severe lower airway obstruction refractory to standard medical therapy, who do not have apnea, mental status changes, or other contraindications. NPPV also deserves consideration in disorders

---

Box 2.8.13   Patient and Equipment Monitoring Requirements for NPPV in Pediatric Patients as a Life-support Therapy*

- ABG's
- End-tidal or transcutaneous CO_2 (when correlated with ABG's) may be helpful.
- Continuous pulse oximetry
- Respiratory waveform
- ECG
- Blood pressure
- Gastric distension

- Degree of respiratory distress:
  - ▸ Respiratory rate
  - ▸ Nasal flaring
  - ▸ Use of accessory muscles
  - ▸ Location and severity of retractions
- Breath sounds
- Subcutaneous emphysema
- CXR

Monitoring of the NPPV System and Mask Interface:

- Airway pressures, including high and low pressures and disconnect alarms
- FiO_2

- Inspiratory gas temperature
- Charting of serial ventilator settings

---

* Removal from NPPV may result in imminent death.

predominated by alveolar hypoxia, including pneumonia, acute pulmonary edema, and acute respiratory distress syndrome.

Utilization of NPPV in these acute respiratory disorders should not be attempted outside the emergency room, recovery room, or ICU. The appropriate setting should also be one that routinely handles unstable children and has practitioners skilled in the application of NPPV. Children treated with NPPV in acute respiratory conditions must be closely monitored **(Box 2.8.13)**. Contraindications to the use of NPPV as a life support therapy in children are similar to those that apply to adults; guidelines for patient selection are listed in **Box 2.8.14**.

NPPV in Chronic Respiratory Conditions. Use of NPPV is dramatically increasing as is the range of chronic diseases in which it is utilized. In pediatric patients, studies of NPPV include children with acute and chronic upper airway obstruction, OSA, cystic fibrosis (CF), muscular dystrophy and other forms of congenital myopathy, chronic lung disease and central hypoventilation.

Box 2.8.14 Selection Guidelines for NPPV Use in Pediatric Patients

- Progressive respiratory failure or insufficiency in the absence of apnea or impending cardiorespiratory collapse with the following:
  ▶ Acute respiratory acidosis
  ▶ Respiratory distress
  ▶ Use of accessory muscles or paradoxical abdominal movement
- Failure of NPPV would not produce immediate morbidity or mortality
- Hemodynamic stability
- Absence of on-going emesis
- Absence of excessive secretions
- Intact upper airway protective reflexes
- Absence of acute facial trauma
- Intact consciousness (appropriate sedation is *not* contraindicated)
- Adequate mask-fit achievable and tolerated

The Patient-Device Interface. Selection of a well fitting interface is important because inappropriate selections may cause excessive air leakage, patient discomfort, and skin breakdown. Proper fit of the mask or nasal prongs should be optimized to achieve effective support and maintain comfort. If the nasal mask, is not well tolerated, application of nasal pillows might be helpful. Sinusitis or deviation of the nasal passages can contribute to increased resistance and may be more amenable to use of a full face mask.

Recommended Settings for Initiation of NPPV (Box 2.8.15 and Fig. 2.8.7). Children with central hypoventilation syndromes and depressed ventilatory drive must have an NPPV unit with a backup rate that will cycle in the absence of spontaneous respiratory effort. Relatively high IPAP levels may be necessary to improve gas exchange in children with obesity hypoventilation syndrome and other conditions

---

Box 2.8.15   Steps in Initiating NPPV

- Determine patient suitability (**Box 2.8.14**)
- Explain the process to the patient and family as appropriate
- Select and fit a mask
- Select and set a ventilator (**Fig. 2.8.7**)
- Start ventilation at low pressure (inspiratory, 8–10 cm H_2O; expiratory 4–6 cm H_2O), with the patient holding the mask in place.
- Typically, in most types of chronic hypercarbic respiratory failure in children, the $PaCO_2$ gradually decreases even at relatively low inspiratory pressures (*i.e.* 10–12 cm H_2O).
- Adjust pressures for patient comfort.
- Titrate the O_2 flow rate or FiO_2 to maintain desired O_2 saturation.
- Check for air leaks and readjust mask as needed.
- Check patient frequently; offer reassurance; coach breathing pattern.
- Increase inspiratory pressure gradually to relieve respiratory distress.
- For patients with persistent hypoxemia despite high flow supplemental O_2, the expiratory pressure can be adjusted upward in 2 cm H_2O increments until the SaO_2 is consistently >90%. If an expiratory pressure >8 cm H_2O is required, use of a ventilator with an O_2 blender that delivers accurate, high FiO_2 is recommended before further increasing the expiratory pressure.

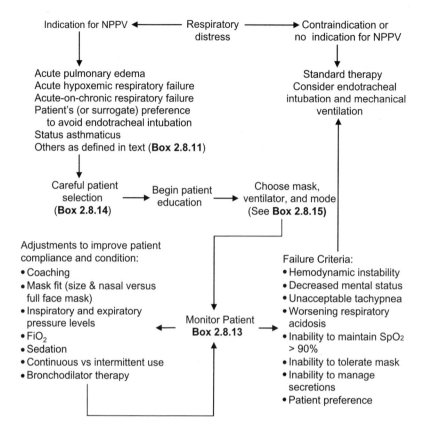

Fig. 2.8.7.   Institution of Non-invasive Ventilation.

that reduce respiratory system compliance or increase inspiratory airway resistance. In children with severe status asthmaticus and hypoxemia, NPPV at inspiratory pressures < 20 cm H_2O may improve oxygenation, but does not consistently reverse hypercarbia.

NPPV via a bilevel ventilator may not reduce a child's $PaCO_2$ when exhaled CO_2 does not clear the in-line exhalation valve or when the dead space of the nasal mask is large. The problem with CO_2 rebreathing may be eliminated by raising the PEEP above 4 cm H_2O or substituting an isolated one-way exhalation valve in the ventilator circuit. Higher EPAP settings are also often necessary if patients have atelectasis, hypoventilation associated with ventilation/perfusion mismatch, or a component of OSA.

With NPPV ventilation, the FiO_2 can be raised by connecting oxygen tubing to a port on the mask or a T-connection in the ventilator circuit; the problem with this method is that FiO_2 delivery is not precise. Alternatively, oxygen can be blended into the circuit by diverting the connection tubing between the pressure-targeted unit and nasal mask through a conventional heater/humidifier/oxygen source. This method has the advantages of conditioning the inspired gas and allowing some estimate of the FiO_2 via an oxygen sensor electrode in the circuit.

Patients with profound hypoxemia may be better oxygenated using a "critical care" ventilator with an oxygen blender. In most applications, the patient's $PaCO_2$ decreases coincident with a reduction in respiratory distress, but the change in $PaCO_2$ may be delayed, especially in very obese children or in cases of severe status asthmaticus.

Obstacles to Successful Uses of NPPV. Absolute contraindications to NPPV are uncommon in children. In general for NPPV to be successful a patient should posses the following characteristics: (1) capable of spontaneous ventilation; (2) cooperative and fully conscious; (3) able to protect his/her airway (adequate cough and minimal sputum retention) and (4) is hemodynamically stable.

Excessive secretions may be hazardous in children with depressed sensorium or impaired bulbar function and are relative contraindications to NNPV. Adequate expiratory muscle function is critical for clearing airway secretions and mucus plugs, particularly during respiratory tract infections. Patients utilizing NPPV must be able to generate adequate peak cough expiratory flows either unassisted or by assisted means. Techniques of manual assisted coughing include use of an applied abdominal thrust; alternatively, a mechanical insufflation-exsufflation device may be helpful in selected patients.

Complications of NPPV. Minor complications related to the "interface" between patient and device are the most common and include local skin irritation, drying of the nasal and pharyngeal mucosa, nasal congestion, and eye irritation. Skin irritation may be reduced by the use of special adhesives or by replacing the mask with nasal pillows. Mucosal drying can be reduced by adding a humidifier to the inspiratory circuit. Major complications of NPPV have not been reported frequently. Isolated case reports include pneumocephalus, bacterial meningitis, conjunctivitis, massive epistaxis, and atrial arrhythmia. Potential complications include pneumothorax, pneumopericardium, and aspiration from gastric distention.

2.9 Other Aids to Support Oxygenation and Ventilation

Airway patency is essential for adequate oxygenation and ventilation. Simple but effective interventions such as application of nasal cannula oxygen for hypoxemia can be thwarted by nasal obstruction due to secretions, particularly in the young infant. The importance of clearing of upper airway secretions by atraumatic techniques (*e.g.* a well lubricated suction catheter via each nare) cannot be over-emphasized. See **pulmonary hygiene** below.

A nasopharyngeal (NP) airway may also facilitate spontaneous breathing in a patient with NP obstruction and should be considered in patients with mouth-breathing or patients with large adenoids and/or tonsils with upper airway obstruction, especially during sleep.

Oxygen therapy is the most common intervention used for support during respiratory illnesses. The variety of oxygen delivery systems are categorized as either low-flow or high-flow systems (**Box 2.9.1**). Low-flow systems deliver gas flow which may not be adequate to meet total patient inspiratory requirements but these devices are more economical and more comfortable for the patient. High-flow systems deliver gas flow which meets all patient inspiratory requirements, deliver FiO_2 more accurately, and allow the control of temperature and humidity.

Potential risks associated with oxygen therapy include combustion, cellular toxicity, physiological changes associated with hyperoxia, pulmonary vasodilation, respiratory insufficiency in patients with some chronic pulmonary diseases, and retinal damage in premature infants.

Box 2.9.1   Oxygen Delivery Systems (Continued)

Device	Characteristics	FiO$_2$ Delivery	Flow (L/min)
Nasal cannulae	Comfortable and inexpensive; FiO$_2$ is dependent on amount of entrained air.	24–50%	Low (<6)
High flow nasal cannulae	Accommodate higher flow rates (vary by device); may be heated and humidified. Use O$_2$ blender to achieve desired FiO$_2$.	21–100%	High (4–60)
Simple face mask	FiO$_2$ dependent on amount of entrained air and liters of flow.	35–55%	Low (6–10)
Venturi mask	Oxygen-to-air entrainment ratios provide fixed FiO$_2$ when recommended flow rates are set.	24–50%	High (variable)
Non-rebreather face mask	Face mask with an added reservoir bag; fresh gas infusion via an inflow system allows FiO$_2$ to approach 100%. Unidirectional valve between face mask and reservoir prevents rebreathing CO$_2$.	~100%	Low (15)
Partial rebreathing face mask	Face mask with an added reservoir bag; no unidirectional valve.	<60%	Low (15)
Oxygen hood	Provides oxygen enriched environment; covers head of neonate or infant; higher FiO$_2$ requires a good seal; allows O$_2$ analyzer to be close to the patient.	<90%	High (>9)
Oxygen tent	Covers the entire infant or toddler	<50%	High

Helium is a biologically inert gas that is one-seventh the density of air or oxygen and can be administered clinically as a helium-oxygen mixture (**Heliox**). The low density of heliox facilitates improved gas flow through high resistance airways. Also, carbon dioxide diffuses more rapidly in heliox than in air or oxygen alone. It is commercially available in premixed ratios of 80:20 (20% O_2), 70:30, and 60:40. The higher the percentage of helium, the greater the therapeutic benefit achieved; however the patient's oxygen requirement must be taken into consideration. Note that because gas may be more effectively delivered to the distal airways, the patient's oxygenation may improve while on Heliox therapy.

Heliox can also be used as the driving gas for aerosolized medications (*e.g.* albuterol) or delivered through a conventional mechanical ventilator. It is clinically useful for improving gas flow in upper airway obstruction seen in croup and post-extubation stridor, and in lower airway obstruction associated with asthma, bronchiolitis and chronic obstructive lung disease.

Inhaled Nitric Oxide (iNO). In 1987–88, endothelium-derived relaxing factor (EDRF) was identified as nitric oxide (NO). NO is a gaseous compound endogenously produced by many cells of the body. It is synthesized from the reaction of L-arginine and oxygen by one of three nitric oxide synthase (NOS) isoenzymes. NO produces vascular smooth muscle relaxation by binding the heme moiety of cytosolic guanylate cyclase, increasing intracellular levels of cyclic guanosine 3′, 5′-monophosphate (cGMP) which in turn elicits intracellular signaling leading to vasodilation. NO is also a second messenger gas that plays a mediator role in neurotransmission and inflammatory responses. Inhaled exogenous NO (iNO) has been investigated since 1988 and some therapeutic effects and key points regarding clinical use are listed in **Boxes 2.9.2 and 2.9.3**.

Surfactant acts to optimize surface tension on the alveolar surface which reduces work of breathing, prevents collapse and overdistension, and decreases transudate of fluid. Similar to neonatal

> **Box 2.9.2   Therapeutic Effects of Inhaled NO**
>
> - Reversal of pulmonary hypoxic vasoconstriction and reduction of pulmonary hypertension with improvement of oxygenation.
> - Vasodilation of lung regions ventilated by iNO with improved ventilation/perfusion matching resulting in increased oxygenation.
> - Improved cardiac output from decreased RV afterload.
> - iNO rapidly binds to hemoglobin and is metabolized to methemoglobin and nitrate; these inactive molecules are released into the systemic circulation, preventing iNO from causing systemic vasodilation.
> - iNO may affect vascular endothelium by inhibiting platelet aggregation and decreases adhesion molecule expression (and other anti-inflammatory effects).

respiratory distress syndrome (RDS), acute lung injury (ALI) in other populations includes a component of surfactant dysfunction, making its potential role in therapy attractive. However, adult studies overall have not been favorable; benefit has been shown in a limited number of animal and pediatric ALI/ARDS studies. Few negative effects were seen other than its expense. However, the use of exogenous surfactant has not become widely accepted because more studies are needed to answer questions regarding optimal preparation, safety, and efficacy.

Corticosteroids have also been evaluated in the treatment of ALI/ARDS because a significant portion of the organ damage is due to dysregulated inflammation. Therefore, blunting this response with steroids has been theorized to benefit patients with ALI/ARDS, but early studies showed no consistent benefit. More recent studies have focused on patients with refractory (or unresolving) ARDS and have used longer courses of steroids than in previous studies. Further investigation will determine the potential benefit of this strategy.

Positioning strategies, such as prone positioning, have been practiced in pediatric patients with respiratory illnesses for many years.

Box 2.9.3   Clinical Use of iNO: Key Points

- The FDA approved use of iNO in 1999 for persistent pulmonary hypertension of the newborn.
- "Off label" uses without evidence-based clinical benefit may include: pediatric ARDS, post-operative cardiac patients with pulmonary hypertension/decreased right heart function; acute chest syndrome (sickle cell disease); pulmonary leukostasis (leukemia). Off-label use requires consent after explanation of risks and benefits.
- The NO product, *INOmax*® and its delivery system, the Datex-Ohmeda *INOvent* (Datex-Ohmeda, Madison, WI) are currently marketed as a combined package by INO Therapeutics (Clinton, NJ).
- iNO is usually delivered through a ventilator circuit but can be administered via non-invasive ventilation or a nasal cannula.
- The recommended starting concentration is 20 parts per million (ppm); concentrations above 40 ppm (up to 80 ppm) have not shown any significant increase in response and significantly increase the potential for toxicity. Toxic levels of iNO are uncommon with administration of iNO at < 40 ppm.
- iNO dose should be titrated downward according to clinical response; iNO should be weaned cautiously because sudden withdrawal can result in hypoxemia or cardiovascular collapse.
- Methemoglobin (met-Hb) levels should be monitored and should remain < 5%; patients with decreased methemoglobin reductase activity are at risk for higher met-Hb levels.

Prone positioning may improve ventilation/perfusion (V/Q) matching (*Respiratory Failure, 2.7*). In injured lungs, dependent portions of the lungs become atelectatic. These collapsed, poorly ventilated lung units continue to be perfused and deoxygenated blood is returned to the circulation. The non-dependent lung units often become overdistended during CMV which causes local pulmonary vasoconstriction. Blood is diverted away from these areas and gas exchange is impaired. V/Q mismatch results in physiologic shunt and hypoxemia which may be improved by prone positioning. A second potential benefit from prone positioning is an improvement in pulmonary mechanics from reduced chest wall compliance (which may be particularly beneficial in patients with neuromuscular disease). However, studies of prone positioning in ALI/ARDS patients have demonstrated no improvement in mortality or ventilator-free days. Therefore, prone positioning is not considered a part of standard care in ALI/ARDS.

Patients with obstructive airway disease may benefit from upright positioning. This strategy has been shown to decrease airway resistance. Decubitus positioning may benefit patients with unilateral lung disease when placing the injured lung in the non-dependent (upward) position, thus improving V/Q matching. With any of these strategies, care must be taken to prevent pressure injury to the skin. Standard repositioning to relieve pressure points is imperative.

Pulmonary hygiene refers to mechanisms to assist in secretion clearance and resolution of atelectasis. Options include coughing, deep breathing exercises (incentive spirometry), changes in body position (postural drainage), suctioning of the upper airway, suctioning of the trachea, and chest physiotherapy. Devices which assist with pulmonary hygiene are listed in **Box 2.9.4**.

Bronchoscopy is also used as an adjunct to improve oxygenation and ventilation. It can be therapeutic or diagnostic (**Box 2.9.5;** *Foreign Bodies in the Airways, 2.4*).

Extracorporeal life support (ECLS), or extracorporeal membrane oxygenation (**ECMO**), is the use of cardiopulmonary bypass principles to achieve adequate gas exchange in refractory cardiac or respiratory failure. The goal is to improve oxygen delivery while resting the heart and/or lungs. For respiratory failure, the oxygen index (OI) correlates with risk of mortality and is used to guide the initiation of ECLS. OI is calculated by $(mPaw \times FiO_2 \times 100)/ PaO_2$. OI of 25–40 is associated with a 50% mortality rate and OI > 40 correlates with an 80–100% mortality rate without ECLS. For patients with cardiac failure, ECLS is used for severe but reversible cardiac dysfunction (**Boxes 2.9.6 and 2.9.7**).

Box 2.9.4   Devices that Assist Pulmonary Hygiene

Device	Characteristics
Intrapulmonary percussive ventilator (IPV)	High flow jets of air delivered to the airways at 100–300 cycles/min; may be used during spontaneous or mechanical breathing.
Mechanical insufflator-exsufflator (CoughAssist)	Simulates cough; alternately applies a positive and negative pressure to the airway. Used in patients with neuromuscular disease and impaired cough.
Positive expiratory pressure devices (PEP)	Exhaling through the device causes "fluttering" of the airway pressures; loosens secretions; marketed as FLUTTER and Acapella® devices.
Intermittent positive-pressure breathing (IPPB)	Spontaneous breaths are augmented by pressure from the device which passively fills the lungs.
High frequency chest wall oscillation devices (ABI vest®)	High-frequency chest physiotherapy device; uses an insufflated vest or wrap which percusses patient's chest.

Box 2.9.5   Bronchoscopy in the PICU

Diagnostic
- Vocal cord dysfunction
- Subglottic or tracheal stenosis
- Airway malacia
- Foreign body
- Airway compression
- Bronchoalveolar lavage
- Airway inflammation or edema
- Anatomic variations
- Pulmonary hemorrhage
- Endobronchial mass
- Gastroesophageal reflux disease

Therapeutic
- Tracheal intubation
- Foreign body removal
- Mucous plug clearance
- Instillation of medications

Box 2.9.6   Conditions Potentially Managed with ECLS

Neonatal respiratory-related diseases	**Cardiac diseases**
• Meconium aspiration syndrome	• Myocarditis
• Respiratory distress syndrome	• Cardiomyopathy
• Sepsis	• Cardiogenic shock
• Pneumonia	• Refractory, life-threatening arrhythmia
• Congenital diaphragmatic hernia	• Post-operative support after cardiac surgery
• Persistent pulmonary hypertension	
• Air leak syndrome	• Support after cardiac arrest (rapid deployment ECLS)
Pediatric respiratory-related diseases	
• Pneumonia (bacterial, viral, or aspiration)	• Post-transplant support
• ARDS	
• Severe acute asthma	

Box 2.9.7   General Guidelines for Patient Selection for ECLS

• Failure to respond to conventional management
• Reversible disease process
• Gestational age > 32 wks and weight > 2 kg
• No immunosuppression
• No intraventricular hemorrhage
• No severe neurologic dysfunction
• No non-survivable comorbidity

Venoarterial (VA) ECLS provides near-complete support for both heart and lungs. Venous blood is drained by a central venous cannula to the extracorporeal circuit where it is anti-coagulated then circulated by a pump through the artificial lung (often referred to as the membrane oxygenator). Oxygen and carbon dioxide gas exchange occur in the artificial lung by passive pressure gradients. The blood is then pumped through the heat exchanger and back to the patient through the arterial cannula. The cannulae may be placed percutaneously (most commonly right internal jugular vein and carotid artery) or directly into the right atrium and aorta via sternotomy. Venovenous (VV) ECLS uses a percutaneously placed double-lumen cannula (one for drainage and one for reinfusion) or two separate central venous cannulae (IJ and femoral). Cardiac function must be adequate to pump the venous blood, part of which has been through the artificial lung, into the lungs and out to the systemic circulation. However, many patients on VV ECMO show improvement in cardiac function because of improved oxygen delivery and decreased intrathoracic pressure (*Important Cardiopulmonary Interactions, 3.2*).

2.10 Respiratory Failure in Neuromuscular Disorders (NMD)

Respiratory muscle weakness is the inevitable consequence of many childhood NMDs (**Box 2.10.1**). The leading causes of morbidity and mortality in children with NMD are (1) inspiratory muscle weakness, which results in atelectasis and V/Q mismatch and (2) expiratory muscle weakness which results in an ineffective cough with decreased clearance of secretions and foreign material from the lungs, both of which increase the incidence and severity of pneumonia. Frequent or severe pneumonias in a child with NMD indicate that ventilatory muscle weakness is significant.

Respiratory muscles will fatigue when the energy supply is no longer adequate to meet the demand, whether because of increased resistive forces (*i.e.* airway obstruction), increased elastic loads (*i.e.* edema), or decreased energy supply. Blood flow to the diaphragm and other inspiratory muscles is determined by cardiac output, perfusion pressure, oxygen-carrying capacity of the blood, and the ability to increase perfusion of the respiratory muscles in response to increased demand of oxygen delivery. Decreased blood flow to these muscles will decrease substrate delivery. With increased activity, the diaphragm requires approximately 10 to 20 times greater

Box 2.10.1   Neuromuscular Diseases which Influence Respiratory Function

Level of Involvement	Disease
Central: Upper motor neuron	Cerebral palsy
Brainstem	Arnold-Chiari Malformations Types I & II
Spinal Cord	Spinal cord injuries, including myelitis: C1–C6
Motor Neuron	Spinal muscle atrophy; Poliomyelitis
Peripheral Nerve	Guillian-Barré; Polyneuropathy; Leukodystrophies; Phrenic nerve injury; Hereditary sensory autonomic neuropathy (Riley-Day); Hereditary sensory motor Neuropathies (Charcot-Marie-Tooth); sustained use of neuromuscular blocking agents
Neuromuscular Junction	Congenital myasthenia; Tetanus; Myasthenia gravis; Botulism
Muscular Dystrophies and Myopathies:	
Dystrophinopathies	Duchenne; Becker
Nondystrophinopathies	Emery-Dreifuss; Limb-girdle; Autosomal recessive; Fukuyama type; Merosin-deficient; Merosin-positive
Myotonic Dystrophy	Congenital myotonic dystrophy
Congenital Myopathies	Nemaline; Central core; Centronuclear; Multicore; Minicore; Myotubular
Metabolic Myopathies	Acid maltase deficiency
Mitochondrial Myopathies	Pyruvate dehydrogenase deficiency; Respiratory Complex I; Respiratory Complex IV
Inflammatory Myopathies	Systemic lupus erythematosis; Polymyositis; Rhabdomyolysis

oxygen delivery to meet its metabolic demands. Factors that impair oxygen delivery to the muscles (*e.g.* hypoxemia, anemia, decreased CO), can hasten the onset of fatigue. Ventilatory muscle function can likewise be affected by metabolic disturbances. Decreased serum concentrations and total body stores of potassium, phosphorus, magnesium, or calcium can result in decreased muscle strength. Similarly, malnutrition can markedly reduce the strength and endurance of respiratory muscles. A number of drugs can adversely influence respiratory muscle function. These include corticosteroids that promote atrophy and aminoglycosides and calcium channel blockers that can interfere with neuromuscular transmission.

Patients with progressive neuromuscular weakness will eventually develop sleep-disordered breathing. Most commonly, hypoventilation occurs because of their weakness and low tidal volume breathing; this problem is often accentuated during REM sleep, when intercostals and accessory muscles do not contribute to ventilatory effort. Patients with upper airway muscular weakness or bulbar dysfunction can also demonstrate obstructive apneas during REM sleep. Both hypoxemia and hypercapnia result from these breathing derangements during sleep. These disturbances cause frequent arousal from sleep, reduced sleep efficiency, and eventual sleep deprivation. Once nocturnal hypercapnia is present, diurnal hypercapnia will inevitably follow if ventilator support is not introduced. Diaphragmatic insufficiency may be present in the setting of neuromuscular disease with hypoventilation and prominent desaturations and arousal in REM sleep. In severe cases REM sleep will be absent, and in extreme cases the life of the individual will be at risk. The identification of REM sleep hypoventilation requires polysomnography. This test should be considered for patients with a known NMD who complain of excessive daytime sleepiness with multiple awakenings at night. In severe cases patients will develop orthopnea, nocturnal and early morning headaches, vomiting, and cyanosis, particularly when sleeping supine, all in the context of signs of progressive cardiopulmonary morbidity. Unexplained failure to wean from a respirator may be the presenting manifestation of diaphragmatic weakness in patients with undiagnosed motor neuron disease or myopathies.

Although patients are on occasion admitted to the PICU because of an NMD that has or is at risk of producing respiratory failure, a much more common scenario is the development of weakness in the course of treatment of acute illness syndromes such as sepsis and/or respiratory failure. As a complication of critical illness, weakness frequently slows and even dominates the course of recovery from critical illness (**Box 2.10.2**).

Pulmonary function testing in patients with NMD helps to evaluate the respiratory status of patients at the time of diagnosis, monitor their progress and course, evaluate them for surgery or sedation, indicate the need for mechanical ventilation and, in some instances, assess prognosis. Clinically useful tests and measurement are listed in **Box 2.10.3** and illustrated in **Fig. 2.10.1**. Serial monitoring of lung function is mandated for all children with NMD when it is able to be performed (usually after the age of 5 yrs) and

---

Box 2.10.2   Causes of Intensive Care Unit-Acquired Muscle Weakness

Risk Factors:
- Severity of illness
- Medications: corticosteroids, aminoglycosides, prolonged use of neuromuscular blocking agents
- Poor glycemic control
- Hypocalcemia
- Hypermagnesemia
- Immobility
- Prolonged controlled mechanical ventilation
- Sepsis/ SIRS

Prevention and Treatment:
- Minimize exposure to corticosteroids, aminoglycosides and neuromuscular blocking agents
- Glycemic control
- Correct hypocalcemia and hypermagnesemia as indicated
- Nutritional support
- Avoid excessive sedation and analgesia
- Early, targeted physiotherapy

Box 2.10.3   Clinically Useful Measures of Respiratory Sufficiency in Patients with Neuromuscular Disorders

- Lung Volumes:
  ▶ Total lung capacity (TLC)
  ▶ Residual volume (RV)

- Spirometry
  ▶ Peak flow rate (PFR)
  ▶ Cough peak flow rate (CPF)
  ▶ Vital capacity (VC)
  ▶ Forced VC in 1 second (FVC$_1$)

- Respiratory muscle strength:
  ▶ Maximal expiratory pressure (MEP)
  ▶ Maximal inspiratory pressure (MIP)

- Other tests:
  ▶ Pulse oximetry
  ▶ Capnography
  ▶ Blood gases (arterial, capillary, venous)
  ▶ Polysomnography

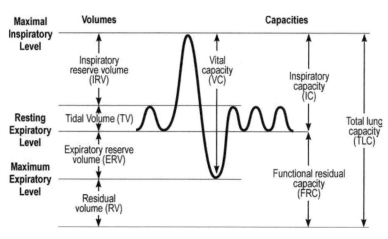

Fig. 2.10.1.   Lung Volumes and Capacities.

may be limited by technique, facial weakness, alterations in mental status and inconsistent effort. Normal vital capacity (VC) is usually > 50 ml/kg body weight. Vital capacity ≥ 60% of its predicted value represents a low risk for nocturnal hypoventilation, whereas a VC < 40% is a good predictor of nocturnal hypoventilation in children with NMDs of varying etiologies. When VC is reduced to 30 ml/kg, cough becomes poor and secretions begin to accumulate. Further reduction in VC to < 20 ml/kg results in atelectasis that may not be visible on CXR, hypoventilation and respiratory failure.

The tests most widely used to assess respiratory strength are the maximum inspiratory pressure (MIP) and maximum expiratory pressure (MEP). After the first year of life, normal values for MIP range between 80 and 120 cm H_2O. When MIP becomes < 50 cm H_2O, the patient requires assistance in secretion removal and is noted to have weak tongue movements. Further reductions of MIP to < 30 cm H_2O are associated with aspiration and ventilatory failure. Similarly, MEP of less than 45 cm H_2O is seen in patients with ineffective cough, possible atelectasis, pneumonia and respiratory failure.

The maximum flow generated during a voluntary cough maneuver can be used to assess the strength of the respiratory muscles. Cough peak flows (CPF) correlate with the ability to clear secretions from the respiratory tract. The normal value for CPF in adults is 360 L/min, and values below 160 L/min are associated with inadequate airway clearance. Baseline CPF values of 160 L/min are insufficient for patients with muscular dystrophy as these patients can experience decreased muscle function during respiratory illnesses. Thus, at CPF less than 270 L/min, assisted cough techniques are recommended. The target CPF of 270 L/min may not be appropriate for children because those younger than 13 yrs. often are not able to generate values of 270 L/min. CPFs < 270 L/min are more likely when VC is < 2.1 L in children with muscular dystrophy.

Daytime $PaCO_2$ levels greater than 45 mmHg have been used to predict sleep disordered breathing and eventual ventilatory failure. In infants with severe NMD, infant lung function testing is technically demanding and untested in the clinical setting, but monitoring with polysomnography or with oximetry if polysomnography is not available, particularly during sleep, is extremely helpful in assessing respiratory muscle weakness and resultant hypoventilation. Serial monitoring of lung function is mandated for all children old enough to cooperate. Spirometric evaluation, MIP, MEP, and CPF are usually obtained after 5 yrs of age.

Management of children with NMD must focus on improving the performance of respiratory muscles in general by providing assistance to the expiratory muscles to ensure adequate airway clearance and assistance to the inspiratory muscles to correct impairments in ventilation. Medications such as the methylxanthines, particularly aminophylline, can improve contractile properties of the diaphragm and render the diaphragm less susceptible to fatigue. This is a therapeutic option during acute exacerbations of disease and should constitute a trial limited to 1–2 weeks.

Cough assist. Coughing works by helping to clear airway secretions from the lungs. These secretions act as a protective layer covering the bronchi and bronchioles. They trap environmental particulate matter as well as bacteria and viruses that are inhaled during respiration. Cilia protruding from bronchial epithelial cells move this protective layer in a proximal direction. Coughing augments the ciliary clearance of these secretions.

Coughing consists of three components: An inspiratory phase, a contraction phase; and an expiratory phase. During the inspiratory phase, the patient inhales, usually to 60% to 90% of total lung capacity. In the contraction phase, the patients' glottis closes and the expiratory muscles begin to contract; allowing intrathoracic pressure to increase. The final, expiratory phase of a cough occurs when the glottis opens and there is a sudden expiratory rush of airway. During this phase, large shearing forces are generated, clearing off parts of the secretory lining and carrying with them the trapped foreign material. During this expiratory phase flow rates usually exceed 360 L/min. In children with NMD both the inspiratory and expiratory muscles are weak and limit the effectiveness of the cough. The expiratory muscles, in particular, can have a dramatic influence on the quality of a cough. Two tests that greatly predict the adequacy of a patient's cough are the CPF and MEP. In general, a CPF < 270 L/min and/or MEP < 45 cm H_2O require cough assisting techniques. There are a wide variety of techniques available to assist a patient's cough ranging from manual techniques to mechanically assisted maneuvers.

Any method used requires a combination of improved insufflation of the lungs to achieve sufficient lung volumes for an effective cough (phase 1) in conjunction with adequate forced expiration techniques to augment the patient's natural, but weakened cough (phase 3). Ideally the patient should be able to (briefly) hold his or her breath before exhaling to maximize the pre-cough lung volumes and help generate sufficient intrathoracic pressures (phase 2).

Mechanical equipment is available to help inflate the lungs. Patients who require the use of volume-cycle ventilator for treatment of respiratory insufficiency can use the ventilator in assist mode to breath stack. The Cough Assist® machine (the mechanical insufflator-exsufflator; Respironics Corp, Millersville, PA) has proven to be a boon to airway clearance in patients with neuromuscular weakness. It provides both an inspiratory phase (to inflate the lungs) and an expiratory phase (for the actual cough). Manual and automatic modes can be used and are effective for children and adults with muscle weakness of varied causes. With this device, the duration of treatment and pressures used can be preset to maximize the efficacy of the cough and the patient's comfort. There is no increase in the risk of complications such as pneumothorax, gastroesophageal reflux, or pulmonary hemorrhage. It also can be used through various interfaces such as the mouth, a full face mask, or an endotracheal or tracheostomy tube.

The use of chest physiotherapy in patients with NMD is controversial. Although manual chest physiotherapy, intrapulmonary percussive ventilation, and high-frequency chest wall oscillation are effective at aiding clearance in conditions of highly viscous secretions (*i.e.* cystic fibrosis), the underlying problem in NMD is primarily inability to clear *normal* secretions and/or an increased volume of secretions associated with infection. However, these techniques are useful in NMD with focal atelectasis from mucous plugging.

Ventilatory support. Respiratory failure relates directly to the loss of inspiratory muscle force and VC and shows characteristic evolution from normal ventilation during daytime and sleep- induced hypopneas at mild degrees of inspiratory muscle weakness, to rapid eye movement (REM) and non-REM sleep hypoventilation in more severe respiratory muscle impairment. Continuous nocturnal hypoventilation, common at VC < 40% of predicted, precedes daytime hypercapnia. Daytime ventilatory failure is present with VC < 20% predicted and represents an indication for supportive ventilation, usually non-invasive positive-pressure ventilation (*Noninvasive ventilation, 2.8.2*). NPPV applied intermittently and preferably during sleep, relieves respiratory muscles for the work of breathing and augments alveolar ventilation. A tracheostomy and PPV may be necessary if NPPV is not well tolerated or if ventilatory support is required for 24 hrs/day.

Chapter 3

Care of the Circulation

Resuscitation and maintenance of circulation requires an understanding of its components, knowledge of available tools, potential therapies and bedside vigilance. Maintenance of adequate circulation means adequate delivery and extraction of oxygen to permit normal cell metabolism. Metabolic demands change with age, activity and disease. The essence of circulatory care requires an understanding of cardiac output, oxygen carrying capacity, cardiopulmonary interactions and disturbances in oxygen consumption. Knowledge of equations used for calculation of hemodynamic variables aids in understanding these relationships.

3.1 Determinants of Cardiac Output (CO) and Oxygen Delivery (DO_2)

Cardiac output is the volume of blood ejected from the heart into the systemic circulation in one minute:

CO (L/min) = Stroke volume (SV, volume/beat) × Heart rate (HR, beats/min); when indexed for body surface area, cardiac index (CI) = $L/min/m^2$.

CO may be measured directly by thermodilution or dye dilution; these techniques involve administration of an injectate (iced saline or dye) into a central vein and measuring the change in either temperature or dye concentration in the pulmonary artery (PA). Thermodilution remains the bedside gold standard for measurement of CO, but non-invasive methods (*e.g.* cardiac ultrasonography) are increasingly sought because of reproducibility of results and risks of complications associated with PA catheters.

Critical illness is associated with an increase in demand for oxygen, acutely answered by an increase in CO. CO in infants and young children is heart rate-dependent (**Fig. 3.1.1**); SV can be augmented only minimally because the immature myocardium is less compliant, generates less force and shortens more slowly than the adult myocardium, given the same load. For infants, tachycardia is an important mechanism by which CO may be increased; failure to generate an effective tachycardia in face of increased demand often precedes circulatory failure and cardiac arrest.

Stroke volume depends on preload, afterload, muscular synergy, myocardial contractility (systolic function) and diastolic function.

Preload: Ventricular end diastolic volume (VEDV); the greater the VEDV, the greater the stretch of myocardial muscle. This results in greater force of the subsequent contraction and a larger SV, until a physiologic limit is reached (Starling's law; *Important Cardiopulmonary Interactions, 3.2*; *Fig. 3.2.3*). Since volume/pressure (V/P) relationships are well correlated in a normal heart, right VEDV

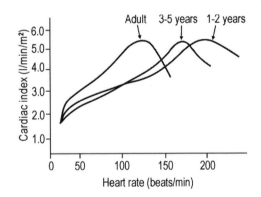

Fig. 3.1.1. The Relationship Between CO (or CI) and HR. Note that the ability to increase CO by raising the HR is limited as age increases. While medications that prevent increases in HR may be necessary for certain patients, they also have potential to limit appropriate increases in CO during times of illness.

is reflected by right atrial (RA) or central venous pressure (CVP) and left VEDV is reflected by pulmonary capillary wedge pressure (PCWP) or diastolic pressure in the PA. The preload (or *diastolic filling volume*) necessary for optimal SV depends on ventricular compliance:

$$\text{Compliance (C)} = \Delta\text{Volume}/\Delta\text{Pressure}$$

Compared to a normally compliant ventricle, the more rigid ventricle is less compliant and requires a greater filling pressure to achieve the same EDV.

Afterload: The "load" against which the heart must eject blood. Afterload is related to ventricular wall stress, which can be estimated by echocardiography. If P_v is ventricular pressure and r is the radius of the ventricular chamber:

$$\text{Ventricular wall stress} = (P_v \times r) \div 2(\text{wall thickness})$$

Resistance (R) offered by the circulatory system contributes to afterload and is difficult to measure but can be inferred. Resistance to blood flow through a vascular bed is determined by length and diameter of the "tube" and viscosity of the circulating medium. Resistance to laminar flow through a vessel is inversely proportional to the radius of the vessel raised to the fourth power; a 50% decrease in vessel diameter (vasoconstriction) results in a 16 fold increase in resistance to flow. LV afterload is determined by resistance of the aorta and systemic circulation; RV afterload is determined by resistance in the PA and the pulmonary circulation. An increase in afterload above normal leads to a decrease in SV, increased myocardial work and therefore increased myocardial O_2 consumption (VO_2), a consequence to be avoided, particularly when O_2 demands rival supplies in critical illness. (**Boxes 3.1.1 and 3.1.2**)

R across the systemic circulation (systemic vascular resistance index, SVRI) in dyne sec/cm^5/m^2 can be calculated by:

$$\frac{[\text{Mean arterial pressure (MAP)} - \text{CVP}]}{\text{CI}} \times 80$$

Normal SVRI = 800–1600 dyne sec/cm^5/m^2

Box 3.1.1 Factors Influencing Systemic Vascular Resistance	
Increased SVR	**Decreased SVR**
Findings may include: • Tachycardia • Cool, mottled skin • Prolonged capillary refill time • Decreased pulses • Narrowed pulse pressure	**Findings may include:** • Tachycardia • Warm, flushed skin • "Flash" capillary refill time • Bounding pulses • Widened pulse pressure
Common causes: • Hypovolemic, cardiogenic and late ("cold") septic shock • Hypothermia • High stress states ($\uparrow$ catecholamine output) • Cardiac tamponade	**Common causes:** • Early ("warm") septic shock; anaphylaxis; spinal shock • Vasodilator therapy • Cirrhosis • Anemia

R across the pulmonary circulation (pulmonary vascular resistance index, PVRI) in dyne sec/cm^5/m^2 can be calculated by:

$$\frac{(\text{Mean PAP} - \text{PCWP})}{\text{CI}} \times 80$$

Normal PVRI = 80–240 dyne sec/cm^5/m^2

- **Muscular synergy:** Synchronous myocardial contraction; dysrhythmia, tumors, contusions or areas of ischemia may impair SV.
- **Contractility:** The ability of heart muscle to contract independently of preload and afterload; contractility is assessed clinically by echocardiogram using direct measures of SV, shortening fraction, ejection fraction, and systolic time intervals.
- **Diastolic function:** Ability of heart muscle to relax and distend with blood; myocardial relaxation is an active process. Diastolic dysfunction is diagnosed by Doppler echocardiography or cardiac catheterization.

Box 3.1.2   Factors Influencing Pulmonary Vascular Resistance (PVR)

Increased PVR	Factors that Decrease PVR
Findings may include: • Hypoxemia • Right heart strain or failure • Tricuspid regurgitation • RV diastolic dysfunction **Causes:** • ARDS • Hypoxemia and hypercapnea • Under- or over-inflation of lungs • Acidemia • Sepsis • Hypothermia • Pulmonary edema • Pulmonary emboli • Systemic to pulmonary shunts • Valvular heart disease • Idiopathic pulmonary hypertension	• Respiratory and metabolic alkalosis • Optimizing oxygen delivery (DO_2): Correction of hypoxemia; allowing hyperoxia; optimizing hemoglobin; augmentation of CO when indicated • Avoiding increased intrathoracic pressure and establishing normal lung volumes • Sedation; muscle relaxation • Vasodilator therapy: Phosphodiesterase inhibitors (milrinone, sildenafil) Nitroglycerin Inhaled nitric oxide Inhaled (or IV) prostacyclin Endothelin receptor antagonist (bosentan)

Adequate *oxygen delivery* (*DO_2;* **calculated in ml/min/m^2**) requires adequate CO and adequate oxygen content in arterial blood (CaO_2): CaO_2 = the amount of O_2 bound to hemoglobin (Hb) + the amount of O_2 dissolved in blood, or

$$CaO_2 \text{ in ml } O_2/L \text{ blood}$$
$$= Hb \text{ in g/L} \times 1.34 \text{ ml } O_2/g \text{ Hb} \times (SaO_2/100)$$
$$+ (PaO_2 \text{ in mmHg} \times 0.003 \text{ ml})$$

NB: If Hb is expressed in g/dL, then multiply g/dL by 10 to convert to g/L.

Normal CaO_2 = 17–20 ml/100 ml of blood. SaO_2 is the percent O_2 saturation of arterial blood and PaO_2 is the partial pressure of oxygen in arterial blood.

The amount of oxygen in venous blood (CvO_2 in ml/min) can be calculated using the same equation, with O_2 saturations and partial pressure of O_2 from mixed venous blood (blood from the pulmonary artery):

$$CvO_2 \text{ (ml } O_2/L \text{ blood)} = Hb \text{ (g/L)} \times 1.34 \text{ ml} \times (SvO_2 /100)$$
$$+ (PvO_2 \text{ mmHg} \times 0.003 \text{ ml})$$

Normal CvO_2 = 12–15 ml/100 ml. Normal mixed venous SvO_2 is 75–80%. If mixed venous blood is not accessible, SvO_2 and PO_2 from superior vena cava (SVC) blood may be substituted. Normal SvO_2 from SVC blood is 70%.

DO_2 is the rate at which oxygen is made available to tissues; this is a function of cardiac output (or cardiac index) and the content of oxygen in arterial blood:

$$DO_2 \text{ in ml/min} = CO \text{ in L/min} \times CaO_2 \text{ in ml } O_2/L \text{ blood} \quad \textbf{or}$$
$$DO_2 \text{ in ml/min/m}^2 = CI \times CaO_2$$

Normal DO_2 = 400–600 ml/min/m^2; O_2 delivery decreases if CO falls or oxygen content of arterial blood is decreased. DO_2 can be augmented by (1) increasing CO by volume administration or vasoactive drugs and/or (2) increasing hemoglobin by blood transfusion and/or (3) improving oxygen saturation. The PaO_2 contributes little to arterial oxygen content, unless marked anemia is present. In that setting, a maximal amount of inspired oxygen should be provided since dissolved oxygen is the main source of O_2 until hemoglobin can be increased.

Oxygen consumption (VO_2) describes the rate of removal of O_2 from arterial blood:

$$VO_2 \text{ in ml/min} = CO \times (CaO_2 - CvO_2) \quad \textbf{or}$$
$$VO_2 \text{ in ml/min/m}^2 = CI \text{ } (CaO_2 - CVO_2)$$

Normal VO_2 = 140–160 ml/min/m². VO_2 remains relatively constant over a wide range of variations in DO_2. Oxygen consumption increases when metabolic demands increase. When DO_2 and O_2 extraction can keep pace with needs, tissues remain well oxygenated and lactic acid production is curtailed. In critically ill patients with evidence of tissue hypoxia, augmentation of DO_2 may improve oxygen extraction.

The oxygen extraction ratio (O_2ER) describes the relationship between O_2 consumption and delivery:

$$O_2\,ER = VO_2/DO_2, \text{ or } (CaO_2 - CvO_2)/CaO_2$$

Normal $O_2\,ER$ = 22–30%; an $O_2ER > 35\%$ indicates a marked increase in O_2 consumption or decrease in O_2 delivery, or both. If an increase in O_2 extraction is not sufficient to meet metabolic demands, and DO_2 is already maximal, the VO_2 falls and anaerobic metabolism ensues. Relationships between DO_2, VO_2, O_2ER and serum lactate under varying clinical conditions are shown in **Fig. 3.1.2.**

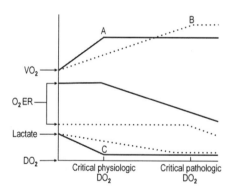

Fig. 3.1.2.   Relationships Between Physiologic (Solid Line) and Pathologic (Dotted Line) O_2 Supply (DO_2), Consumption (VO_2), and Lactate Under normal physiologic circumstances, a maximal ↑ in VO_2 at point A is met by a maximal ↑ in DO_2 with a nearly unchanging oxygen extraction ratio (O_2ER). Serum lactate falls as DO_2 increases (point C). Under pathologic conditions of O_2 utilization, DO_2 must ↑ greatly before VO_2 plateaus (point B). This is associated with a marked ↓ in O_2ER compared to the physiologic condition. The lower the DO_2 the greater the lactate production.

3.2 Cardiopulmonary Interactions

Oxygen delivery (DO_2) is dependent on coordination between the pulmonary and cardiovascular systems. Understanding basic principles of heart and lung interaction helps the bedside clinician to treat cardiopulmonary imbalances that impair or threaten oxygen delivery. Fundamentals of cardiopulmonary physiology with clinical applications are presented.

"Venous pressure curves" are curves that can be generated in an arrested animal with a pump that replaces the heart (**Fig. 3.2.1**). Mean circulatory filling pressure (MCFP) is the pressure present when blood flow is stopped; this pressure is generated by blood volume and compliance of the blood vessels. An individual venous return curve can be plotted for a given MCFP (x, y, and z) with values of right atrial pressure (RAP) ≤ MCFP. Blood flows from the MCFP (maximum upstream driving pressure) to the (lower) RAP. The greater the RAP (the closer the MCFP is to the RAP), the greater the back pressure preventing blood return to the heart; as RAP approaches MCFP blood flow through the circulatory system slows to a stop.

In the living animal (under circumstances where blood volume is constant), if RAP rises, the nervous system can trigger vascular compliance to decrease (and MCFP to increase); thus blood flow can be maintained. In contrast, in a critically ill child, if venous compliance is increased by nitroglycerin, furosemide, or the vasomotor paresis of sepsis, the MCFP is decreased; if RAP remains constant the blood flow to the RA slows. The venous pressure curve can be altered by changing the intravascular volume (**Fig. 3.2.1**). An overly distended heart is relieved by an increase in venous compliance. In contrast, the decreased CO of sepsis is at least partially corrected by raising the MCFP by volume resuscitation.

During spontaneous (negative pressure) breathing intrathoracic pressure (ITP) and RAP become sub-atmospheric (far to the left on the x axis of **Fig. 3.2.1**) and blood flow increases inversely to negative RAP but then plateaus. Extra-thoracic blood vessels are exposed to atmospheric pressure and collapse under negative "transmural pressure" (Tmp). Tmp is the pressure difference between two sides of a wall and equals pressure inside a cavity minus pressure outside a

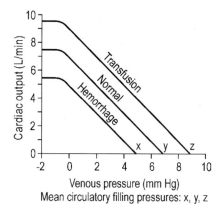

Venous pressure (mm Hg)
Mean circulatory filling pressures: x, y, z

Fig. 3.2.1. Venous Flow Curves During Hypovolemia, Normovolemia and Hypervolemia. Right atrial pressure and mean circulatory filling pressures are plotted on the *x* axis. During hypervolemia (*e.g.* transfusion) the venous flow curve shifts right/upward (y to z). During hypovolemia (*e.g.* hemorrhage) the venous flow curve shifts left/downward (y to x).

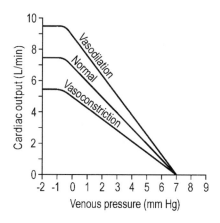

Venous pressure (mm Hg)

Fig. 3.2.2. Venous Flow Curves During Arteriolar Vasodilatation and Vasoconstriction. Arteriolar vasodilatation or vasoconstriction causes the venous pressure curve to pivot on the mean circulatory pressure to the right or left respectively. Increased arteriolar tone traps blood on the arterial side of the circulation during vasoconstriction and allows relatively less blood to flow to the RA for a given MCFP-RA difference; during vasodilatation blood is released to the venous side of circulation and more blood flows to the RA for a given MCFP-RA difference.

cavity. (A "positive" Tmp distends a cavity and a "negative" Tmp collapses a cavity.) In contrast, in heart failure and pericardial tamponade RAP is elevated. Tmp remains positive and extrathoracic vessels do not collapse with inspiration. Blood flow may continue to increase with inspiration and decreasing RAPs (An explanation of TMP is discussed further in *Upper Airway Obstruction, 2.2*).

"CO curves" can also be generated by rapidly transfusing sympathectomized animals and measuring CO at different RAP's (**Fig. 3.2.3**). Starling's law states that increases in end diastolic volume (EDV) increase CO until a physiologic limit is reached. The clinically useful indicators of EDV are CVP or pulmonary arterial wedge pressure (PAWP). At a certain maximum EDV further increases result in no further increases of CO (**Fig**. 3.2.3). CO curves vary depending on myocardial function. Myocardial contractility is augmented when for a given EDV, the stroke volume and CO become greater than at a lesser degree of myocardial contractility. At equilibrium, a point is defined where blood flow on the venous return curve equals blood flow on the cardiac output curve.

Respiratory activity has profound influence on blood flow in the vena cava. Usually, during spontaneous inspiration, ITP decreases and

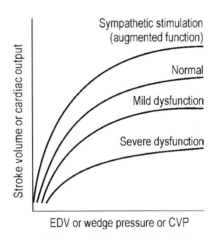

Fig. 3.2.3.   Cardiac Output Curves (Starling Curves):   A series of curves upon which the ventricle functions. The curves demonstrate the ability of the ventricle to change its force of contraction and therefore the stroke volume in response to changes in end-diastolic volume (EDV).

the Tmp of the RA increases, favoring venous return into the distended RA. Also, during inspiration the diaphragm compresses intra-abdominal capacitance vessels and MCFP increases, further augmenting blood flow into the RA. In contrast, if high positive airway pressure is applied (as occurs during positive pressure ventilation), the diaphragm may compress the subdiaphragmatic surface of the liver and decrease inferior vena cava blood flow into the RA. If positive airway pressure is (partially) transmitted to the intrapleural space (which at rest has a negative pressure), then both ITP and RAP increase during positive pressure ventilation (PPV). As the ITP becomes less negative, the RA Tmp and RA size decrease and venous return as well as CO decrease. The effect of PPV on venous return, and CO is, however, ultimately dependent on several factors:

- Location of the ventricle on the CO curve (**Fig. 3.2.3**).
- Adequacy of circulatory reflexes controlling venous capacitance changes that can in turn influence MCFP (See above).
- The extent to which positive airway pressure is transmitted to heart chamber walls. This depends on both lung compliance and airway resistance.

Blood flow through the lung is dependent on three interrelated pressures: pulmonary arterial (Ppa), alveolar (Palv) and pulmonary venous (Pven). If Palv exceeds Ppa blood flow stops; this may occur in lung exposed to excessive positive airway pressure (overdistension); these conditions are called "zone 1." PA blood flow under these conditions is shunted to lung regions where Palv is lower than Pap. If pulmonary hypertension is present (Ppa > Palv), zone 1 conditions are unlikely to occur. In "zone 2", where Ppa > Palv > Pven, blood flow is primarily determined by Ppa minus Palv (the blood vessel is partially compressed by Palv as it traverses the alveolus) and resistance to flow is increased. In "zone 3," Ppa > Pven > Palv and the vessel is completely open throughout its trans-alveolar course; flow is determined by the difference between Ppa and Pven.

Pulmonary vascular resistance (PVR) is affected when lung volume deviates from functional residual capacity (FRC; lung volume

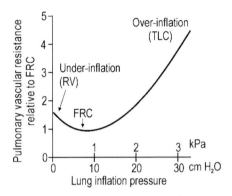

Fig. 3.2.4.   Lung Volume and Pulmonary Vascular Resistance.   RV, residual lung volume; TLC, total lung capacity; FRC, functional residual capacity.

at end exhalation during tidal breathing; **Fig. 3.2.4**). When under-inflated (near residual volume, or air remaining in the lungs at the end of maximal expiration), lung vessel resistance increases as result of hypoxic vasoconstriction related to alveolar collapse as well as collapse of extra-alveolar vessels. When lung is overinflated (either by a positive pressure breath, spontaneous inhalation or air-trapping as in asthma), mechanical obstruction of blood vessels develops (near total lung capacity). During spontaneous tidal inspiration the venous capacity of the lungs increases; during expiration (return to FRC), venous capacitance decreases and blood return to the heart is augmented resulting in increased CO and systemic blood pressure.

Ventricular interdependence: During spontaneous inspiration (see above) blood return to the right side of the heart increases. As the right ventricle fills, the interventricular septum bows toward the left ventricle (LV) at end diastole (**Fig. 3.2.5**). As LV volume decreases ("diastolic ventricular interdependence") so does LV stroke volume, CO and systemic blood pressure.

Under conditions of increased PVR the interventricular septum also deviates from right to left during systole; the RV enlarges because of its inability to empty into a high pressure circuit. LV pressure assistance to the RV decreases ("systolic ventricular inter-dependence")

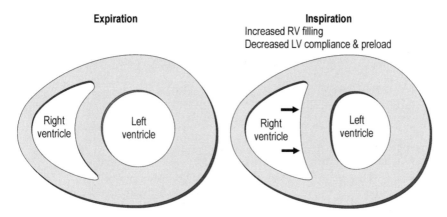

Expiration

Inspiration
Increased RV filling
Decreased LV compliance & preload

Fig. 3.2.5.   Diastolic Interventricular Dependence.

because the LV is now restricted by an enlarged RV and the LV cannot contract effectively and support ejection of the RV. Decreased CO from the LV can cause RV ischemia and failure. Clinically, episodes of hypotension can accompany periods of pulmonary hypertension in post-operative congenital heart disease patients as a consequence in part of ventricular interdependence.

During spontaneous inspiration (decreased ITP) distending pressure is exerted on the outer LV wall and ventricular ejection is hampered ("increased afterload"). In contrast, during expiration the LV wall has extramural force compressing the LV ("decreased afterload"). This effect is exaggerated during grunting respirations or a positive pressure breath. Therefore, if LV failure is present, PEEP or PPV improves LV function. The RA, RV and pulmonary vasculature are all exposed to the same ITP and therefore ITP changes do not affect right sided pressure relationships.

As a result of (1) changing LV filling during spontaneous lung inflation (increased pulmonary venous capacitance during inspiration), (2) interventricular dependence during the respiratory cycle and (3) changes in transmural stresses related to the phases of the respiratory cycle, normal fluctuations in systolic blood pressure (SBP) occur during the respiratory cycle. In a healthy individual this SBP

Box 3.2.1   Cardiac Disease, Heart Function and Ventilation

Problem	Intervention	Effects
LV *systolic* heart failure		
• ↓ Ventricular volume		↑ Intrathoracic pressure (ITP)
• ↓ Stroke volume	Positive pressure	↓ LV afterload
• ↓ CO	Ventilation (PPV)	↓ Myocardial VO_2
		↓ Respiratory muscle VO_2
***Diastolic* heart failure**		
• ↓ Ventricular filling volume		NPV may ↑ ventricular Tmp
• ↓ Stroke volume	Negative pressure	PPV ↑s ITP and ↓s
• ↓ CO	ventilation (NPV)	ventricular filling; these worsen diastolic
	PPV	dysfunction
Cavopulmonary anastomosis (Fontan procedure)		
• ↓ Ventricular filling	Promote ↑	Negative ITP
• ↓ CO	venous return	enhances ventricular
• ↓ PVR	by promoting	filling. PPV is
• Ventricular diastolic dysfunction	negative pressure breathing or minimizing positive ITP by minimizing the mean airway pressure and PEEP.	associated with ↑ ITP and ↓ venous return. ↑ PEEP from 0 to 12 cm H2O causes ↓ CO by 25%

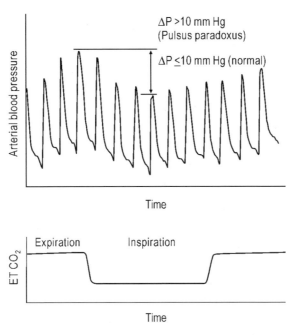

Fig. 3.2.6.   Changes in Systolic Blood Pressure During Spontaneous Breathing.

variation is ≤ 10 mmHg. Pulsus paradoxus is a SBP decrease > 20 mmHg associated with breathing (**Fig. 3.2.6**). During mechanical ventilation the pattern of changes is reversed (SBP is higher during inspiration). Conditions that may contribute to pulsus paradoxus include asthma, cardiac tamponade, restrictive cardiomyopathy, RV infarction, hypovolemic shock, and CHF (**Box 3.2.1**).

3.3   Cardiopulmonary Resuscitation (CPR) in Infants and Children

CPR is an attempt to restore spontaneous, effective ventilation and circulation. Effective CPR provides adequate coronary and cerebral blood flow (approximately 25% to 33% of normal CO) until return of spontaneous circulation (ROSC) occurs (**Box 3.3.1**). Respiratory arrest is the most likely cause of cardiopulmonary arrest (CPA) in

---

Box 3.3.1   Principles of Basic CPR

- Chest compression time should equal relaxation time; relaxation time should permit full chest recoil. The lower sternum is compressed to a depth of 1/3 the anterior-posterior chest diameter.
- Compressions in infants:

  1 person CPR: use "2-finger sternum compression" (index and middle fingers)
  2 person CPR: use "2-thumbs sternum compression" (hands encircling the chest)
- Compression: rescue breath ratio:

  1 person CPR: 30:2 (each breath delivered over 1 to 1.5 sec).
  2 person CPR: 15:2.
- Interrupt chest compressions with each positive pressure breath until an artificial airway is established then uninterrupted compressions can be delivered.
- "In-hospital" CPR should deliver 100 compressions/min. After each 2 min period, perform a 10 sec pulse assessment, then switch rescuer positions.
- Ventilation in adults to achieve ETCO2 > 10 mmHg has been associated with improved ROSC and hospital survival. Over-ventilation may cause ↓ CO and ↓ ROSC.

---

children. Asystole (most common), bradycardia and pulseless electrical activity (PEA) are often presenting rhythms. Pulseless ventricular tachycardia (VT) or ventricular fibrillation (VF) occurs in approximately 15% of children with out-of-hospital, usually sudden, cardiac arrest, especially in the setting of underlying heart disease or toxic ingestion.

Priorities for Initial CPR. In the setting of asphyxial CPA or prolonged VF both artificial ventilation and chest compressions should be initiated immediately. During the first minutes after sudden onset VF (no preceding hypoxia) chest compressions take precedence over

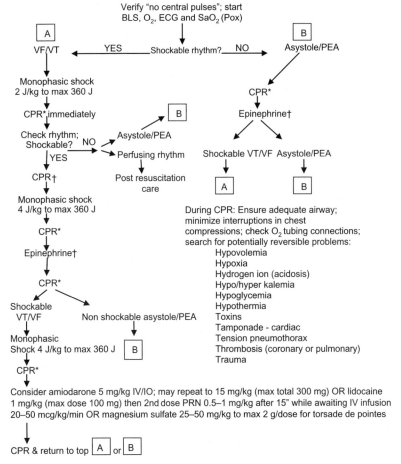

Fig. 3.3.1. Pulseless Arrest Algorithm.

ventilations. If VF is present, defibrillate as soon as possible since the likelihood of ROSC decreases after 3 to 4 min of VF (**Fig. 3.3.1**). Treatment of "shock resistant rhythms" includes epinephrine administration and CPR (for 30 to 60 sec) before re-attempting electrical therapy. Algorithms for management of VT, SVT and bradycardia with poor perfusion are noted in **Figs. 3.3.2 and 3.3.3**.

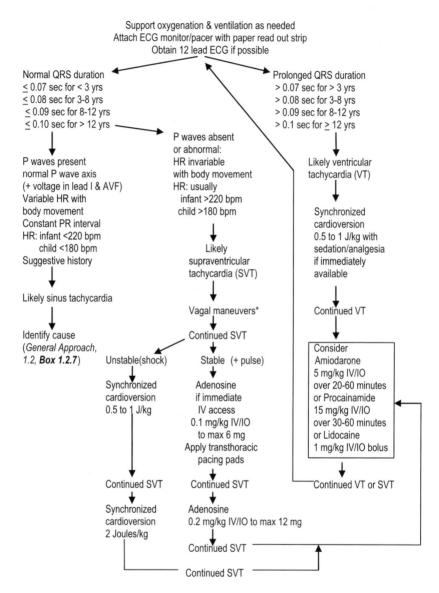

Fig. 3.3.2.   **Tachycardia with Poor Perfusion.**

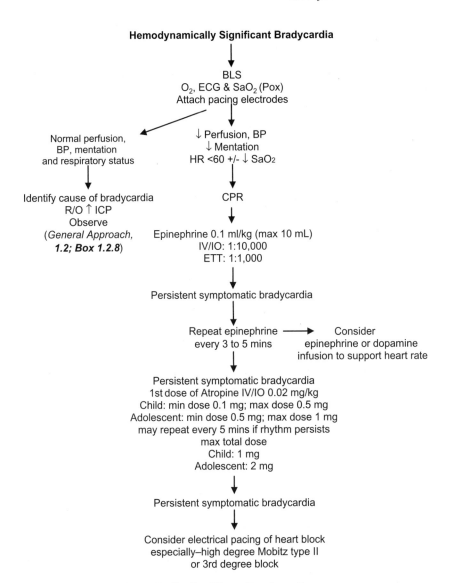

Fig. 3.3.3. Hemodynamically Significant Bradycardia.

Key points about rhythm algorithms (Figs. 3.3.1–3.3.3 and Box 3.3.2):

- *Medications* given by peripheral IV should be followed by saline flush and elevation of extremity used for injection. Epinephrine, atropine, lidocaine, naloxone and vasopressin are absorbed via tracheal administration. Deliver endotracheal medications via a tubing that reaches beyond the ETT tip.
- Do not give *procainamide* and *amiodarone* simultaneously.
- For *narrow complex sinus tachycardia* identify and treat the cause (*General Approach to the Critically Ill Child, 1.2; Box 1.2.7*).

Box 3.3.2   Mechanisms of Blood Flow During CPR

Cardiac pump mechanism	The heart is directly compressed between sternum and vertebrae causing mitral and tricuspid valve closure; blood is propelled antegrade from the ventricles. During the relaxation phase the ventricle fills with blood. (This mechanism would not be operative with compression delivered in any other direction *e.g.* laterally).
Thoracic pump mechanism	During compression of chest from *any direction,* intrathoracic pressure exceeds extrathoracic venous and arterial pressure. The tricuspid and peripheral venous valves (especially in the internal jugular veins) close and prevent retrograde blood flow. The mitral valve remains open and the heart beyond the tricuspid valve acts as a passive conduit for blood flow. Blood in the thoracic pump is vented by arteries leaving the thorax which are relatively resistant to collapse leading to areas of lower extrathoracic pressure. During relaxation of compression blood returns to the heart from the veins.

- *Electrical therapy* for *un*-witnessed pulseless VT (PVT) or VF: Give two minutes of CPR before delivering a shock. For witnessed PVT/VF arrest, defibrillate as soon as possible. Resume CPR immediately (for 5 cycles) and only then recheck rhythm. Pediatric sized paddles are recommended for children <15 kg. Positioning of paddles or electrodes should be to the right of the sternum just beneath the clavicle and the second paddle/electrode lateral to the left nipple in the anterior axillary line. Alternative placement of defibrillator pads is just to the left of the sternum overlying the heart and over the left side of back.
- *Vagal maneuvers for SVT:* e.g. apply ice over the eyes and forehead, or ask the patient to blow through a straw. If hemodynamic instability is present, cardiovert unless adenosine can be administered quickly through a reliable vascular access site (Fig. 3.3.2).
- Hemodynamically significant *bradycardia* should be treated with basic CPR. (**Fig. 3.3.3**; *General Approach to the Critically Ill Child, 1.2*; *Box 1.2.8*). Atropine is effective for vagally-induced bradyarrhythmias or in suspected AV block. Electrical pacing for heart block or sinus node dysfunction can be accomplished transcutaneously or transvenously. Bradycardia associated with hypoxic heart damage or respiratory failure requires correction of hypoxemia and should not be paced. When indicated, demand pacing avoids induction of ventricular arrhythmia. Use adult sized pacer pads for children >15 kg. Skeletal muscle contraction can be minimized by using large electrodes, a 40 msec. pulse duration and the smallest amplitude needed for QRS capture.
- Key points to consider during resuscitative efforts are summarized in the mnemonic "PAGE TOBE" (**Box 3.3.3**). Potentially reversible causes of CPA should be addressed in each arrested patient. An emergency CXR and echocardiogram may reveal mechanical causes of arrest (tension pneumothorax; pericardial tamponade). An alternative mnemonic to "PAGE TOBE" is "H (6) T (5)" as noted in pulseless arrest algorithm (**Fig. 3.3.1**).
- **Box 3.3.4** outlines the main issues in post-resuscitative care.

**Box 3.3.3   What Should be Checked During a "Code"?
            Remember to "PAGE TOBE"**

P   Potassium

A   ABG

G   Glucose

E   Electrolytes (calcium*, magnesium) *Calcium use during CPR
     is usually restricted to hypocalcemia (DiGeorge, loop diuretic
     usage, renal failure, pancreatitis, severe hyperventilation,
     massive infusion of blood products), hyperkalemia,
     hypermagnesemia and calcium channel blocker overdose. Treat
     with calcium chloride or calcium gluconate if any of the above
     are expected.

T   T(4) Temperature, Tamponade, Tension pneumothorax,
     Thrombosis (coronary or pulmonary)

O   Overdose of drug

B   B(2) Breath sounds (reassess oxygenation and ventilation);
     consider systemic Bicarbonate treatment to improve
     myocardial response to catecholamines.

E   E(2) Echocardiogram and candidacy for ECLS (ECMO)

Box 3.3.4   Summary of Post-resuscitation Care

- Optimize cardiopulmonary function; identify the cause and prevent
  recurrence of arrest.
- Temperature: Avoid both hyper and marked hypothermia (*HIE, 5.3*).
- Respiratory: Check tracheal/gastric tube position on CXR.
  Avoid hypoxia, hypocapnea, autoPEEP.
- Cardiac: Maintain normal to slightly elevated BP.
  Echocardiogram within 24 hours may help optimize fluid and
  vasoactive drug therapy.
- CNS: Identify and treat seizures aggressively
- Glucose: Keep in an acceptable range (usually, 80–150 mg/dL)
- Monitor need for blood products.
- Identify and treat infection.
- Provide family support by updates from medical and nursing staff,
  social services, pastoral support, *etc.*

3.4 Arrhythmias

Disturbances in the conduction system, or dysrhythmias, can have a significant impact on a patient's circulatory status. Broadly defined, these fall into two main classifications: **tachyarrhythmias**, which are typically due to either a reentrant circuit or an ectopic focus and **bradyarrhythmias**, which are usually due to a disruption in the conduction of the cardiac electrical impulse through the atrioventricular (AV) node or an abnormally low intrinsic heart rate. In all these cases, the most important keys to the management of these patients are recognition, accurate diagnosis, and an understanding of the underlying pathophysiology. As in all cases where there is clinical concern, the first steps of management include Airway and Breathing, before Circulation. It cannot be over emphasized that an ECG (12 lead tracing if possible) is essential in addressing any arrhythmia. This documentation is critical at all stages: during the arrhythmia, initiating treatment, and after conversion to sinus rhythm. In all aspects of dysrhythmia management, the **pediatric cardiologist should be consulted**. In all aspects of dysrhythmia care, PALS algorithms should be initiated if the patient is clinically unstable (*Cardiopulmonary Resuscitation, 3.3,* **Figs. 3.3.1 to 3.3.3**).

Tachyarrhythmias are those dysrhythmias with an abnormally fast heart rate, beyond that which is expected for a child's age. While "normal rates" vary with age, a dysrhythmia is not just an abnormal rate, but more importantly, an abnormal conduction mechanism. In identifying the mechanism, it is often helpful to classify the tachycardia according to the QRS morphology and whether or not it is narrow or wide. Ninety percent of all tachycardias in the pediatric population fall under the category of **narrow complex** tachycardias. These include supraventricular tachycardia (SVT), atrial flutter, and atrial tachycardia. Sinus tachycardia (*General Approach to the Critically Ill Child, 1.2; Box 1.2.7*) should be distinguished from the narrow complex tachyarrhythmias based on rate (<220/min), presence of a normal P wave before each QRS complex and variation of rate, rather than the fixed rate associated with the tachyarrhythmias.

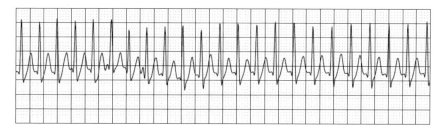

Fig. 3.4.1.   Narrow Complex Tachycardia.

Wide complex tachycardias (QRS duration > 140 msec) include ventricular tachycardia (VT), SVT with aberrancy, or SVT with antegrade conduction down an accessory pathway.

Diagnosis. For illustrative purposes, two rhythm strips will be used to demonstrate the two classes of tachyarrhythmias.

Narrow complex tachycardias. The most common type in this classification is **supraventricular tachycardia (SVT)**. It is an abnormally fast cardiac rhythm that begins above the level of the ventricles. Among the SVTs, the most common types are "reentry" in nature, activating the ventricles through the normal His/Purkinje system and then "reentering" the atrium through another route, either an accessory pathway or the AV node itself. In childhood SVT, more often than not, there is an abnormal electrical connection called an accessory pathway with conduction properties that allow the electrical circuit to conduct from the ventricles back up to the atrium and then down the AV node. This is known as **atrioventricular reentry tachycardia (AVRT)**. A second type of reentry SVT involves a reentry circuit within the AV node itself. These individuals have both a slow conducting and fast conducting part of the AV node, known as the slow and fast pathways; they allow the reentry circuit to revolve within these two components of the AV node. The resulting rhythm is known as **atrioventricular node reentry tachycardia (AVNRT)**. Other diagnoses within the category of narrow complex tachycardia include **sinus tachycardia, ectopic atrial tachycardia (EAT), atrial flutter, atrial fibrillation**, and **junctional ectopic tachycardia (JET)**. While rarely an unstable rhythm, sinus tachycardia is usually a sign of another problem such as sepsis, pericardial effusion, hyperthyroidism, or ingestion. EAT results from an automatic focus within either of the atria and is often seen in patients with a history of congenital heart surgery. Likewise, atrial flutter is due to a large reentry circuit involving both slow conducting and fast conducting tissue within the atrium. Atrial fibrillation is an uncommon tachyarrhythmia in children. It can occur spontaneously, in patients who have a history of congenital heart disease with dilated atrial tissue, or in patients who have been in "traditional SVT" for a significant period of time. Lastly, JET is an unusual rhythm that involves an automatic focus within the AV node. Although it can occur in patients with structurally normal hearts, it most typically occurs patients with CHD in the acute postoperative period due to swelling or injury involving the AV node as a result of the surgery.

Acute Management. In general, most narrow complex tachycardias, with the exception of JET, are usually well tolerated with minimal hemodynamic compromise. As a result, they allow a systematic approach for both diagnosis and treatment (**Box 3.4.1**).

Wide complex tachycardias (**Fig. 3.4.2**) are assumed to be due to **ventricular tachycardia (VT)** until proven otherwise. Since this dysrhythmia can quickly become hemodynamically unstable and degenerate into ventricular fibrillation (VF), rapid intervention is indicated. The differential diagnosis should also include **SVT with aberrancy**, as some rapidly conducting reentry rhythms, typically AVRT, can result in wide complex bundle branch block morphology of the QRS complex. If the patient has Wolff-Parkinson-White (WPW) syndrome, antegrade conduction down the accessory pathway, known as **antedromic reciprocating tachycardia (ART)**, will create a widened QRS. In the post-operative patient with bundle branch block at baseline, sinus tachycardia is also a consideration.

Acute Management (Box 3.4.2). Aggressive management is indicated, as wide complex tachycardias can be associated with hemodynamic instability and poor cardiac function. Laboratory evaluation should include electrolytes (specifically, potassium, calcium and magnesium), arterial blood gases; urine toxicology screen should be considered.

Box 3.4.1   Acute Management of Hemodynamically Stable Narrow Complex Tachycardia*

- **Vagal maneuvers:** Infants: Plastic bag filled with slurry of ice and water and held on the face for 5–10 sec. Older children: Valsalva maneuver by "bearing down" or holding a deep breath for as long as possible before slowly exhaling. Carotid sinus massage may also be used.
- **Adenosine:** Should be given by rapid IV push in a large bore IV, as close to a central vein as possible. Result will be brief period of asystole and AV node block. This is useful in terminating reentry rhythms. If atrial flutter is present, adenosine administration is diagnostic, as the AV node will be blocked, slowing conduction to the ventricles, and an ECG will demonstrate multiple P waves at a regular rate (i.e. saw-tooth pattern). Atrial fibrillation will not be terminated and minimal P wave activity will be demonstrated. JET will terminate briefly, followed by re-initiation and may show AV dissociation.
- **Calcium channel blockers:** This is useful if the tachycardia does not terminate with escalating doses of adenosine and is thought to be AVNRT. Calcium channel blockers should only be used with close monitoring and not given to infants < 1 yr of age.
- **Procainamide:** For patients with recalcitrant SVT secondary to an accessory pathway (AVRT), a loading dose followed by an infusion has a direct action on the accessory pathway.
- **Esmolol:** May be used in patients in whom rate control is desired and who have a stable blood pressure.
- **Amiodarone:** A slowly administered loading dose followed by a continuous infusion can be used for tachycardias that are resistant to other medical therapies. Additionally, it is the drug of choice in the management of JET. Care must be taken, as hypotension, varying degrees of AV block, and ventricular tachyarrhythmias can be induced.

(Continued)

Box 3.4.1   Acute Management of Hemodynamically Stable
Narrow Complex Tachycardia* (Continued)

- **Electrical therapy:** When medications fail to terminate the dysrhythmia, **transesophageal pacing** may be useful for patients with a reentry SVT or atrial flutter. Alternatively, and particularly if the dysrhythmia is atrial fibrillation, **synchronized direct current (DC) cardioversion** may be used. Should the patient become unstable, **defibrillation** is indicated. In the specific case of JET, **atrial overdrive pacing** can be used to provide synchrony and improve cardiac output until JET resolves.
- **Maintenance therapy:** Medication type and duration will vary, depending on the etiology of the dysrhythmia, as well as the age of the patient. Additionally, an electrophysiology (EP) study and ablation may be necessary to eliminate the arrhythmia substrate.

* If hemodynamic instability (shock) is present, follow the algorithm for tachycardia with poor perfusion (*Cardiopulmonary Resuscitation, 3.3, Fig. 3.3.2*).

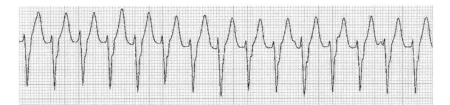

Fig. 3.4.2.   Wide Complex Tachycardia.

Bradyarrhythmias include the dysrhythmias characterized by a heart rate less than typically expected for age. The conducting pathway may not be necessarily abnormal. Typical bradyarrhythmias include varying degrees of **AV block** (typically 2nd or 3rd degree) or an abnormally slow sinus bradycardia *(General Approach to the Critically Ill Child, 1.2, Box 1.2.8)*.

Diagnosis: Obtaining an ECG is imperative.

Acute management: For patients with hemodynamically stable bradyarrhythmias, close monitoring may be all that is necessary until the

---

**Box 3.4.2   Acute Management of Hemodynamically Stable
Wide Complex Tachycardia**

- **Lidocaine:** A loading dose (1 mg/kg; max 100 mg) followed by continuous infusion (20–50 mcg/kg/min) is "first line" for stable monomorphic VT. Patients with shock, heart failure or liver disease may require lower doses.
- **Procainamide:** Second line therapy if lidocaine fails to terminate the dysrhythmia.
- **Amiodarone:** A slowly administered loading dose (5 mg/kg) followed by a continuous infusion (7 mcg/kg/min) can be used for resistant tachycardia. Close monitoring is necessary, as hypotension, varying degrees of AV block, and ventricular tachyarrhythmias can be induced.
- **Electrical therapy: Synchronized DC cardioversion** can be used to terminate recalcitrant dysrhythmias. Should hemodynamic instability occur at any point, **defibrillation** is indicated.
- **Maintenance therapy:** As with narrow complex tachycardia, medication type and duration will vary, depending on the etiology of the dysrhythmia, as well as the age of the patient. Additionally, an electrophysiology (EP) study and ablation may be necessary to eliminate the arrhythmia substrate.

---

dysrhythmia resolves. For patients with 2nd and 3rd degree AV block, a transvenous pacing catheter can be placed for ventricular pacing to increase cardiac output. In the postoperative cardiac patient with epicardial pacing wires, AV sequential pacing is particularly beneficial.

Isoproterenol infusion may be necessary for patients with bradycardia secondary to sick sinus syndrome. Close monitoring is necessary, as hypotension may be a consequence.

Maintenance therapy: Permanent pacemaker placement may be necessary if the bradyarrythmia persists beyond the acute setting. If significant AV node dysfunction persists in the postoperative cardiac surgery patient 7–10 days after surgery, permanent pacemaker placement is indicated. Pacemaker therapy is also useful for patients who have sick sinus syndrome and in whom both bradycardia and tachycardia may be an ongoing issue.

3.5 Shock

Disrupted oxygen delivery and/or oxygen utilization results in shock. During shock, physiologic compensatory mechanisms are overwhelmed, and vital organ system failure can result unless the process is reversed. **Shock is characterized by inadequate peripheral perfusion with preservation of blood pressure** (compensated shock) **or hypotension** (decompensated shock; *General Approach to the Critically Ill Child, 1.2*) The strategy for its reversal is dependent upon its cause, which is often identifiable by history and physical examination. Laboratory data, invasive measurements and echocardiograms may be required for diagnosis. Note that one type of shock (*e.g.* anaphylaxis) may share features with another (*e.g.* hypovolemic shock), leading to similarities in findings and initial management. It is important to define its cause in each case so that definitive therapy can proceed. Reassessment after each intervention is critical to identification of the correct diagnosis and therapy.

Hypovolemic Shock: Circulating volume insufficient to meet metabolic demands leads to hypovolemic shock. This is the most common cause of shock in the pediatric population. Treatment is directed at replacing that component of the circulation that has been lost. The reversal of hypovolemic shock should occur quickly; this phase of treatment does not address the remainder of the rehydration process which should follow (*Dehydration, 6.1*), typically at a more gradual pace.

Fluid and electrolyte losses: Causes include: vomiting, diarrhea, enteric drainage, abnormal renal losses (*e.g.* polyuric renal failure, diabetes insipidus, diuretics), high fever, inadequate intake. (See *Fluids, Electrolytes and Metabolism, Chapter 6*).

Treatment: NaCl 0.9%, Lactated Ringer's Solution (LR) or 5% albumin IV 20 ml/kg aliquots; repeat until shock is corrected; 20–50 ml/kg is often required in the first hour.

Hemorrhage (Box 3.5.1): Causes include: fractures, hepatic/splenic injuries, GI bleeding, peri-operative blood loss, intracranial bleeding or scalp laceration in the infant.

Box 3.5.1 Hemorrhagic Shock: Clues and Treatment:		
% Blood Loss	**Signs**	**Treatment**
<15%	↑HR	Maintenance fluids; monitor vital signs, mental status, UOP
15–30%	↑HR, ↑RR, ↑CRT, ↓Pulse pressure, Anxiety	NaCl 0.9% or LR 20 ml/kg; Repeat as needed and monitor as above
30–40%	↓Systolic BP, altered mental status, ↓UOP	NaCl 0.9% or LR 20–40 ml/kg and/or PRBC (cross-matched) 10 ml/kg
>40%	Coma; no UOP	NaCl 0.9% or LR 20–40 ml/kg and/or PRBC (cross-matched or O negative) 10–20 ml/kg

HR, heart rate; RR, respiratory rate; CRT, capillary refill time; UOP, urine output

Plasma losses: Causes include: sepsis, burns, nephrotic syndrome, hypoproteinemia, acute hemorrhagic pancreatitis, peritonitis, chest tubes, intra-abdominal and other compartment drains; massive hemorrhage.

Treatment:

• Burns: NaCl 0.9% or LR during the first 24 hrs; albumin 5% may be appropriate thereafter.
• Nephrotic syndrome: NaCl 0.9%; avoid use of albumin; consider steroid supplementation if receiving chronic steroid therapy.
• Pancreatitis and peritonitis: Albumin 5% is useful in the early phase of shock resuscitation.
• Post-operative albumin loss via external drain or into the interstitium: Albumin 5% may be superior to crystalloid solutions in maintenance of post-operative lung function.
• If massive transfusion of PRBC is required, plasma should also be replaced using fresh frozen plasma.

Cardiogenic Shock (Boxes 3.5.2 and 3.5.3): Myocardial dysfunction sufficiently severe that cardiac output cannot meet metabolic demands results in cardiogenic shock. Cardiogenic shock may be readily recognizable, especially in patients with known heart disease, but may require differentiation from other causes by:

- History: often, subtle dyspnea with exertion or feeding; respiratory distress; abdominal pain, vomiting
- Physical examination: tachycardia, tachypnea and cyanosis (nonspecific, but may be out of proportion to the perfusion abnormality); jugular venous distension; abnormal breath sounds (rales or "crackles"); abnormal heart sounds (gallop and/or murmur); hepatomegaly
- ECG, which may be diagnostic for cause of shock (*e.g.* arrhythmia).
- May worsen after fluid is given.

Box 3.5.2   Causes of Cardiogenic Shock with Examples

- Arrhythmias
- Congenital heart disease
- Hypoxic ischemic: Cardiac arrest, anomalous coronary artery, high output failure causing cardiac ischemia, MI
- Cardiac trauma
- Infectious or post-infectious: Viral myocarditis; bacterial, fungal, Rickettsial, protozoal, helminthic
- Metabolic: Hypothermia; hypoglycemia, hypocalcemia, hypophosphatemia, acidosis; hypo-or hyper-thyroidiism; inborn metabolic errors (see *IEM*, 6.3); pheochromocytoma; nutritional deficiencies
- Post-bypass
- Toxins: Carbon monoxide; heavy metals; alchohol
- Drugs: Antibiotics (hypersensitivity myocarditis); doxorubicin; cyclophosphamide, cocaine
- Radiation toxicity
- Collagen vascular diseases: SLE; JRA; Kawasaki's disease
- Neuromuscular disorders: Muscular dystrophies, spinal muscular atrophy, Friedrich's ataxia
- Familial dilated cardiomyopathy

Box 3.5.3   General Approach to Treatment of Cardiogenic Shock

- Provide supplemental oxygen or mechanically assist breathing as indicated; establish adequate oxygenation to both the systemic and coronary circulations.
- Minimize metabolic demands by treating hyperthermia and pain. Small doses of narcotics may be safer than standard dosing. Avoid agents that lower blood pressure.
- Correct anemia
- Treat arrhythmias
- Optimize preload with NaCl 0.9% **2 to 5 ml/kg IV, or administer a diuretic if indicated.**
- Consider LV afterload reduction with sodium nitroprusside or milrinone and RV afterload reduction with milrinone
- Consider inotropic support with dopamine or dobutamine 5–10 mcg/kg/min or epinephrine starting at 0.01 mcg/kg/min. Milrinone or continuous infusion of calcium may be helpful.
- Correct metabolic disturbances such as hypoglycemia, acidosis (ventilation or base administration), hypocalcemia or hypophoshatemia.

- Cardiomegaly is seen frequently on CXR.
- Central venous pressure is increased.
- Myocardial function is abnormal on echocardiogram.

Specific therapies for specific conditions are dictated by echocardiographic findings and cardiologic evaluation:

Myocarditis: Angiotensin converting enzyme inhibitors, digitalis, diuretics and beta-blockers. Immunosuppressive therapy with IVIG may be useful.

Kawasaki syndrome: IVIG 2 grams/kg over 12 hrs; start aspirin 80–100 mg/kg/day divided every 6 hrs until the 14th day of illness.

Cardiomyopathies:

- Hypertrophic forms have narrowed outflow tracts (may narrow further with use of inotropic agents or diuretics)
- Dilated forms: Diuretics and inotropes may be useful

Box 3.5.4   Obstructive Shock: Causes, Clues and Treatment

Pericardial effusion: Dyspnea, orthopnea, cough, chest pain; jugular venous distension, muffled heart sounds, pulsus paradoxus (>10 mmHg), S–T segment elevation on EKG; ECHO is diagnostic.

Pneumothorax: Tracheal deviation, decreased breath sounds on the affected side, hyper-resonance to percussion; diagnosis should be made at the bedside; CXR is diagnostic.

Treatment includes supplemental oxygen, volume support and definitive relief of obstruction with pericardiocentesis or thoracentesis (*Chest Tube Placement and Removal, 15.4*).

Obstructive shock results from external compression of a ventricle sufficient to impair cardiac output (**Box 3.5.4**). *Distributive shock* results from vasomotor instability and maldistribution of blood flow (**Box 3.5.5**).

Box 3.5.5   Distributive Shock: Causes, Clues and Treatment

- **Anaphylaxis:** IgE-mediated; commonly, ingested food.
- **Spinal cord injury** above T-2: reduced sympathetic outflow results in unopposed vagal tone
- **Anaphylactoid reaction:** Non-IgE-mediated; commonly opioids, hyper-osmolar agents, radiocontrast agents, complement activation
  - ▶ **Clues:** Sudden onset after exposure; stridor, drooling, perioral and lingual edema; respiratory distress and altered mental status
  - ▶ **Treatment:** Tracheal intubation as indicated; **Epinephrine** for bronchospasm and urticaria: 1:1000 solution, 0.01 ml/kg subQ to max. 0.5 ml. For angio- and laryngeal edema, hypotension: 1:10,000 solution 0.1 ml/kg IV, IO or IM to max. 10 ml. **For circulatory collapse**: NaCl 0.9% 20 ml/kg; repeat as needed PLUS continuous infusion of epinephrine or dopamine for hypotension that is refractory to fluid resuscitation.

(Continued)

> **Box 3.5.5   Distributive Shock: Causes, Clues and Treatment (Continued)**
>
> ‣ **Treatment:** NaCl 0.9% 20–30 ml/kg; Consider PA catheter; Atropine may be needed for bradycardia.
>
> ▪ **Methylprednisolone** 2 mg/kg followed by 0.5 mg/kg IV every 6 hrs; PLUS Diphenhydramine or hydroxyzine PLUS ranitidine or cimetadine
>
> ‣ **Clues:** Spinal shock is frequently associated with bradycardia
>
> • **Adrenal insufficiency:** cortisol and aldosterone deficiency (salt wasting forms) may present with shock.
>
> ‣ **Clues:** Hypovolemic shock; hypoglycemia; hyponatremia with hyperkalemia
>
> ‣ **Treatment:** D_5 0.9% NaCl 20 ml/kg IV; If there are EKG changes from hyperkalemia, treat with Na^+–K^+ exchange resin (Kayexalate)
>
> ‣ **Give Hydrocortisone:** Infuse the following dose over several minutes then give the same dose by continuous IV infusion over 24 hrs: < 3 yrs, 25 mg; 3–12 yrs, 50 mg; > 12 yrs, 100 mg. Fludrocortisone: as recommended by consulting endocrinologist
>
> • **Septic shock:** See *Septic Shock, 3.6*

3.6 Septic Shock and Multiple Organ Dysfunction Syndrome (MODS)

Septic shock is a form of distributive shock characterized by both inadequate oxygen delivery and oxygen utilization, but commonly has components of cardiogenic and hypovolemic shock (*Shock 3.5*) as well. It is triggered by invasion of a microbial pathogen that elicits characteristic systemic inflammatory and anti-inflammatory responses that variably affect cellular respiration. Improved survival has been in large part the result of early recognition, early administration of antibiotics, and early reversal of perfusion abnormalities.

Pediatric septic shock accounts for close to 50,000 hospitalizations with estimated health care costs approaching $2 billion annually. Overall mortality is near 13% but approaches 40% in very high-risk patients [oncology patients S/P bone marrow transplant; Kutco MC *et al.* Mortality rates in pediatric septic shock with and without multiple organ system failure, *Pediatr Crit Care Med* 4(3): 333–337, 2003]. In 2002, The American College of Critical Care Medicine (ACCM) published evidence-based clinical practice parameters for hemodynamic support in pediatric and neonatal septic shock. These were reviewed and updated in 2007 and published in 2009; studies that implemented the 2002 guidelines reported mortality rates approaching 0–5% in previously healthy pediatric patients and 5–10% for chronically ill pediatric patients.

It is primarily the response of the host's immune system rather than the direct damage caused by the invading organism that is responsible for the morbidity and mortality associated with sepsis. Resulting pathologies and clinical responses vary and reflect perturbations in proinflammatory vs. anti-inflammatory homeostasis. The end result is disruption of cellular respiration and end-organ dysfunction.

Immune response

- Microbial organisms produce or contain a number of molecules [lipopolysacchride (LPS), peptidoglycan, bacterial cell wall components] that are known to bind to receptors of the host's immune responsive cells (macrophages, dendritic cells, neutrophils, endothelial cells, *etc.*).
- Binding of extracellular receptors initiates intracellular signaling that results in gene expression of numerous proinflammatory molecules [interferon (IF)-γ, tumor necrosis factor (TNF)-α, interleukins (IL)-1, 2, 6].
  This sets in motion multiple simultaneous signaling cascades that produce the symptoms of clinical inflammation.
- Antigen presentation to T-lymphocytes by innate immune cells in the presence of proinflammatory mediators escalates the proinflammatory response which is collectively referred to as the Th-1 response.

- In the presence of anti-inflammatory mediators, T-lymphocytes promote a counter-regulatory response. This is referred to as the Th-2 response.
- The balance between proinflammatory and counter-regulatory responses is necessary for the host to survive sepsis. It is now recognized that persistent uncontrolled hyper- or, possibly more common, hypo-immune responses are associated with increased morbidity and mortality. This may explain why numerous clinical trials targeting proinflammatory mediators have failed to improve outcomes.

Endothelial activation and microvascular dysfunction:

- Endothelial injury and activation result in the release of additional mediators such as nitric oxide (NO) and adhesion molecules.
- Coagulation homeostasis becomes disrupted resulting in microvascular thrombosis and disseminated intravascular coagulopathy (DIC).
- Expression of inducible nitric oxide synthase (iNOS or NOS-2) may increase 1000-fold during septic shock with marked production of NO.
- Direct effects of NO on the vasculature cause the inappropriate vasodilation and capillary leak characteristic of "warm shock".
- NO is in part responsible for alterations in cellular respiration (see mitochondrial dysfunction below).
- NO also plays a counter-regulatory role by way of inhibition of platelet aggregation and adhesion molecule expression.

Mitochondrial dysfunction:

- Abnormalities of cellular respiration and mitochondrial dysfunction are hallmarks of septic shock. Anaerobic metabolism predominates leading to lactic acidosis.
- Initially, the perfusion abnormalities of septic shock resulting in inadequate **oxygen delivery** are in part responsible for anaerobic conditions. However, mitochondrial dysfunction and anaerobic metabolism persist after restoration of perfusion, oxygen delivery, and intracellular oxygen content. The problem shifts to failure of cellular **oxygen utilization**.

- This phenomenon has led to the creation of such terms as "cytopathic hypoxia," "cytopathic cytotoxicity," and "cell hibernation." Some have hypothesized that this may be an immediate protective response to limit cellular metabolic demand in the face of compromised substrate delivery. However, over time this contributes to end-organ dysfunction (see below). Potential mechanisms explaining the alterations in cellular oxygen utilization include: (1) Nitric oxide (NO) reversibly inhibits mitochondrial respiratory chain enzymes; (2) NO production of peroxynitrite intermediates which irreversibly inhibit mitochondrial respiratory chain enzymes; (3) Inhibition of pyruvate delivery into the tricarboxylic acid (TCA) cycle with increased pyruvate reduced to lactic acid; (4) Activation of poly(ADP-ribose) polymerase resulting in depletion of NAD+/NADH stores.

Definitions and Clinical Presentation. In 1992, The American College of Chest Physicians and Society of Critical Care Medicine (ACCP/SCCM) established clinical consensus criteria for the purpose of unifying the definition of Systemic Inflammatory Response syndrome (SIRS) and Sepsis for research purposes in adults (**Box 3.6.1**). Pediatric-specific definitions were later formulated and are listed in **Boxes 3.6.2 and 3.6.4**. These definitions serve not only to provide more accurate comparisons between patient populations in clinical research but also to aid in early clinical recognition and management.

ACCM practice guidelines (2002, 2009) for hemodynamic support of pediatric and neonatal septic shock define septic shock by clinical, hemodynamic, and oxygen utilization variables. The recognition of the following triad of clinical signs is emphasized for the diagnosis of septic shock before hypotension occurs:

- Abnormal core body temperature; hypothermia *or* hyperthermia.
- Altered mental status (confusion, lethargy, obtundation, seizures).
- Abnormal perfusion: inappropriate peripheral vasodilation with brisk capillary refill, bounding pulses, warm skin (**warm shock**) *or* vasoconstriction with capillary refill time (CRT) >2 seconds, diminished pulses and mottled, cool extremities (**cold shock**).

Box 3.6.1   ACCP/SCCM Definitions of SIRS and Sepsis in Adults*

- **Infection:** Microbial phenomenon characterized by an inflammatory response to the presence of microorganisms or the invasion of normally sterile host tissue by those organisms.
- **Systemic Inflammatory Response Syndrome (SIRS):** The systemic inflammatory response to a variety of severe clinical insults. The response is manifested by two or more of the following conditions:

  ‣ Temperature > 38°C or < 36°C.
  ‣ Heart rate > 90 beats/min.
  ‣ Respiratory rate > 20 breaths/min or $PaCO_2$ < 32 mmHg
  ‣ WBC >12,000 cells/mm^3, < 4000 cells/mm^3, or > 10% immature (band) forms

- **Sepsis:** The systemic response to infection manifested by ≥ 2 of the above SIRS conditions.
- **Severe Sepsis:** Sepsis associated with organ dysfunction, hypoperfusion, or hypotension. Hypoperfusion and perfusion abnormalities may include, but are not limited to, lactic acidosis, oliguria, or an acute alteration in mental status.
- **Septic Shock:** Sepsis with hypotension, despite adequate fluid resuscitation, along with the presence of perfusion abnormalities that may include, but are not limited to, lactic acidosis, oliguria, or an acute alteration in mental status. Patients who are on inotropic or vasopressor agents may not be hypotensive at the time that perfusion abnormalities are measured.
- **Multiple Organ Dysfunction Syndrome:** Presence of altered organ function in an acutely ill patient such that homeostasis cannot be maintained without intervention.

* From The American College of Chest Physicians/Society of Critical Care Medicine Consensus Conference: Definitions for sepsis and organ failure and guidelines for the use of innovative therapies in sepsis. *Crit Care Med* 1992; **20**:864–874.

Box 3.6.2   International Consensus Conference on Pediatric Sepsis Definitions*

- **Infection:** A suspected or proven (by positive cultures, tissue stain, or polymerase chain reaction test) infection caused by any pathogen *or* a clinical syndrome associated with a high probability of infection. Evidence of infection includes positive findings on clinical examination, imaging, or laboratory tests (*e.g.*, WBC in a normally sterile body fluid; perforated viscus; pneumonia on CXR; petechial or purpuric rash; purpura fulminans).
- **Systemic Inflammatory Response Syndrome (Diagnosed when two or more of the following criteria are present):**
  - ▸ Core temperature of > 38.5°C or < 36°C.
  - ▸ Tachycardia defined as a mean HR > 2 SD above normal for age in the absence of external stimulus, chronic drugs, or painful stimuli *or* otherwise unexplained persistent ↑ in HR over a 0.5–4 hr time period *or* for children < 1 yr: bradycardia, defined as a mean heart rate < 10th percentile for age in the absence of external vagal stimulus, β-blocker drugs, or congenital heart disease *or* otherwise unexplained persistent ↓ in HR over a 0.5 hr time period.
  - ▸ Mean RR > 2 SD above normal for age or mechanical ventilation for an acute process not related to underlying neuromuscular disease or the receipt of general anesthesia.
  - ▸ Leukocyte count elevated or depressed for age (not secondary to chemotherapy-induced leukopenia) or > 10% immature neutrophils.
- **Sepsis:** SIRS in the presence of, or as a result of, suspected or proven infection
- **Severe Sepsis:** Sepsis plus one of the following: cardiovascular organ dysfunction or acute respiratory distress syndrome or 2 or more other organ dysfunctions (**See Box 3.6.4**).
- **Septic Shock:** Sepsis and cardiovascular organ dysfunction.

* From Goldstein B, Giroir B, Randolph A. International Consensus Conference on Pediatric Sepsis. International pediatric sepsis consensus conference: definitions for sepsis and organ dysfunction in pediatrics. *Pediatr Crit Care Med*; 6:2–8, 2005.

Box 3.6.3   Signs and Symptoms of End-Organ Dysfunction in Septic Shock

- Pulmonary: Pulmonary edema, respiratory failure, ARDS.
- GI/Hepatic: Vomiting, diarrhea, ascites, ↑transaminases, ↑bilirubin.
- Electrolytes and acid-base balance: ↓Calcium, ↓phosphorus, ↑magnesium, acidosis. Lactic acid may predominate intracellularly and consume body buffer stores; therefore, metabolic acidosis caused by lactic acidosis may be present without lactic acidemia.
- Renal: ↓Urine output, ↑BUN, ↑creatinine.
- Endocrine: Hypo- or hyper-glycemia, hypothyroidism, sick euthyroid syndrome, adrenal insufficiency.
- Hematologic: leukocytosis, leukopenia, thrombocytopenia, anemia, coagulopathy, DIC.
- Infectious disease: Elevated markers of inflammation and acute phase reactants.

Warm shock:

- More common in adults than infants and children.
- Marked by "luxurious" peripheral perfusion with vasodilation, brisk capillary refill, and bounding pulses.
- Often associated with diastolic hypotension and widened pulse pressure.
- Vasodilation in the setting of altered mental status, hypotension, acidosis, hypovolemia, or any end organ dysfunction is *inappropriate* and is evidence of a perfusion abnormality characteristic of septic shock.
- Central venous oxygen saturation ($ScvO_2$ or SvO_2) is usually elevated (normal ~ 70%) secondary to impaired oxygen utilization.

Cold shock:

- More common in infants and children than in adults.
- Vasoconstriction with CRT > 2 sec; peripheral pulses often diminished.

Box 3.6.4   Pediatric Organ Dysfunction Criteria*

- *Cardiovascular*: Despite administration of isotonic intravenous fluid bolus ≥ 40 ml/kg in 1 hour:
  - ▶ Decrease in BP (hypotension) < 5th percentile for age or systolic BP > 2 SD below normal for age *OR*
  - ▶ Need for vasoactive drug to maintain BP in normal range (dopamine >5 mcg/kg/min or dobutamine, epinephrine, or norepinephrine at any dose) *OR*
  - ▶ Two of the following:
    - ▪ Unexplained metabolic acidosis: base deficit > 5.0 mEq/L
    - ▪ Increased arterial lactate > 2 times upper limits of normal
    - ▪ Oliguria: urine output < 0.5 mL/kg/hr
    - ▪ Prolonged capillary refill: > 5 secs
    - ▪ Core to peripheral temperature gap > 3°C.
- *Respiratory*:
  - ▶ PaO_2/FiO_2 < 300 in absence of cyanotic heart disease or preexisting lung disease *OR*
  - ▶ $PaCO_2$ > 65 mmHg *or* 20 mmHg over baseline $PaCO_2$ *OR*
  - ▶ Proven need for > 0.50 FiO_2 to maintain SaO_2 ≥ 92% *OR*
  - ▶ Need for non-elective invasive or noninvasive mechanical ventilation
- *Neurologic*:
  - ▶ Glasgow Coma Score (GCS) ≤ 11 *OR*
  - ▶ Acute change in mental status with a ↓in GCS ≥ 3 points from abnormal baseline
- *Hematologic*:
  - ▶ Platelet count < 80,000/mm³ or a decline of 50% in platelet count form highest value recorded over the past 3 days (for chronic hematology/oncology patients) *OR*
  - ▶ International normalized ratio (INR) > 2
- *Renal*:
  - ▶ Serum creatinine ≥ 2 times upper limit of normal for age or 2-fold ↑ in baseline creatinine
- *Hepatic*:
  - ▶ Total bilirubin ≥ 4 mg/dL (not applicable to the newborn) *OR*
  - ▶ ALT twice the upper limit of normal for age

* From Goldstein B, Giroir B, Randolph A. International Consensus Conference on Pediatric Sepsis. International pediatric sepsis consensus conference: definitions for sepsis and organ dysfunction in pediatrics. *Pediatr Crit Care Med.* 2005; 6:2–8.

- Usually normotensive until late in presentation. Contrary to adults, children are more likely to have elevated systemic vascular resistance (SVR) and decreased cardiac output (CO) on presentation (the combination of vasoconstriction with hypotension has been associated with higher mortality).
- $Scvo_2$ usually decreased ($< 70\%$) secondary to poor CO.

In addition to altered mental status and cardiovascular dysfunction, patients with septic shock commonly present with additional **organ system dysfunction.** Signs and symptoms of other **end organ-dysfunction** are summarized in **Box 3.6.3**; **Box 3.6.4** lists criteria that define organ dysfunction.

Management. Early recognition of septic shock with the early goal-directed reversal of perfusion abnormalities and early institution of appropriate antibiotics continue to be the primary therapeutic influences on improved survival of pediatric septic shock. The 2007 ACCM evidence-based update of the clinical practice parameters for hemodynamic support of pediatric and neonatal septic shock are summarized in **Boxes 3.6.5, 3.6.6 and Fig. 3.6.1**.

Multiple Organ Dysfunction Syndrome (MODS; Boxes 3.6.4, 3.6.6 and 3.6.7)

The progression from sepsis to MODS is poorly understood, and likely multifactorial. Some evidence suggests that end-organ dysfunction secondary to initial hypoperfusion and shock is more common among pediatric patients than adults, and that early reversal of perfusion abnormalities may reverse early-onset organ dysfunction. Sepsis-associated MODS increases mortality, with a 7% and 53% death rate associated with one and ≥ 4 organ failures, respectively. Clinical end-organ dysfunction is often more profound than the end-organ injury present at autopsy, and apoptosis rather than hypoxic-ischemic injury is the predominant finding. The mainstay of therapy remains prevention, with early restoration of end-organ perfusion and support of end-organ function as described (**Box 3.6.6**).

Box 3.6.5   Key Points in the Management of Pediatric Septic Shock

- **Key Goals: (Fig 3.6.1)**
  - ▶ First hour fluid resuscitation and inotropic therapy directed to age-specific goals of threshold heart rates, normal blood pressure, and CRT ≤ 2 sec.
  - ▶ Subsequent hemodynamic support directed to goals of $ScvO_2 >$ 70% and cardiac index 3.4 –5.9 L/min/m^2.
- Support airway, breathing (*Bag-Mask Ventilation and Tracheal Intubation, 15.2*) and establish vascular access as indicated.
- Early institution of inotrope via 2nd PIV until CVC is placed.
- Ketamine with or without atropine is recommended for invasive procedures if indicated; etomidate is not recommended due to reports of adrenal suppression.
- Monitor ECG, BP, MAP, temperature, UOP (*General Approach to the Critically Ill Child, 1.2*).
- Apply age-adjusted hemodynamic goals.
- Measure CO by Doppler echocardiography, pulse index contour cardiac catheter, or femoral artery thermodilution catheter in addition to pulmonary artery catheter.
- Enoximone and levosimendan are potential new potential rescue therapy agents for recalcitrant cardiogenic shock.
- Once resuscitated, diuretics, peritoneal dialysis or hemofiltration (CRRT) should be considered in patients who remain hypervolemic.
- Children are more likely than adults to have absolute adrenal insufficiency defined by basal and peak ACTH-stimulated cortisol levels < 18 mcg/dL. For persistent catecholamine resistant shock and the presence of absolute adrenal insufficiency, give hydrocortisone 1–2 to 50 mg/kg/day dosed intermittently or as a continuous infusion and titrated to reversal of shock.
- Laboratory assessment:
  - ▶ Appropriate cultures to identify infectious source, pathogen and antibiotic sensitivity data to guide therapy.

(Continued)

Box 3.6.5   Key Points in the Management of Pediatric Septic Shock (Continued)

▶ Blood samples for the following help assess for immediate and end-organ injury and function; serial measurements are important in guiding therapy and in helping assess the response to therapy:

- Blood gases
- CBC with differential
- Electrolytes, ionized Ca^{++} and Mg^{++}
- Liver enzymes and function tests
- PT, PTT, INR, Fibrinogen and D-dimer

- Lactic acid
- C-reactive protein (non-specific; may be useful in assessing response to therapy)
- Cortisol (basal and peak value in response to cosyntropin stimulation)
- TSH and free T4

Box 3.6.6   Maintenance PICU Care for the Patient with Septic Shock

- Support beyond the first hour focuses on achieving and maintaining the same clinical, hemodynamic, and oxygen utilization endpoints as desired in the initial therapy.
- Support of end-organ dysfunction should be optimized:
  ▶ Maintain normal perfusion (CRT ≤ 2 sec.; normal peripheral pulses)
  ▶ Maintain age-appropriate HR and perfusion pressure.
  ▶ Maintain CVP 5–10 mmHg; CVP < 8 mmHg at 12 hours of treatment in adults with septic shock may be associated with lower mortatity.
  ▶ Maintain $ScvO_2$ > 70% and cardiac index > 3.3 and < 6.0 L/min/m².

(Continued)

Box 3.6.6   Maintenance PICU Care for the Patient with Septic Shock (Continued)

▶ Low CI, normal BP, high SVR: consider nitroprusside, nitroglycerin, milrinone, inamrinone.

▶ Low CI, low BP, low SVR: consider dobutamine, enoximone.

▶ High CI, low BP, low SVR: consider vasopressin, angiotensin, and terlipressin.

▶ Maintain hemoglobin >10 gm/dL.

▶ Provide coagulation factors as need for bleeding.

▶ Narrow antibiotic coverage based on culture results and sensitivities.

▶ Glycemic control: isotonic IVF containing D10W to provide adequate substrate and keep serum glucose ≥80 mg/dL and insulin infusion to keep serum glucose ≤180 mg/dL (*Hypo- and Hyperglycemia, 6.4*). For CNS disease, goal glucose is 80–150 mg/dL.

▶ Provide adequate sedation and analgesia (*Analgesia, Sedation and Neuromuscular Blockade, 13.2*).

▶ Decompress the stomach; give an H-2 blocker or proton-pump inhibitor for ulcer prophylaxis.

▶ Decompress the bladder; monitor fluid balance.

▶ Provide nutrition.

▶ Provide age-appropriate DVT prophylaxis when indicated.

▶ Follow ventilator associated pneumonia (VAP) prophylaxis guidelines (*Mechanical Support of Ventilation, 2.8*).

▶ Use lung protective mechanical ventilation strategies (*Mechanical Support of Ventilation, 2.8*).

▶ CRRT (*Acute Kidney Injury and Renal Replacement Therapies, 7.1*).

▶ ECMO should be considered for refractory shock.

▶ Experimental therapies: Activated Protein C (adults only); vagal stimulation.

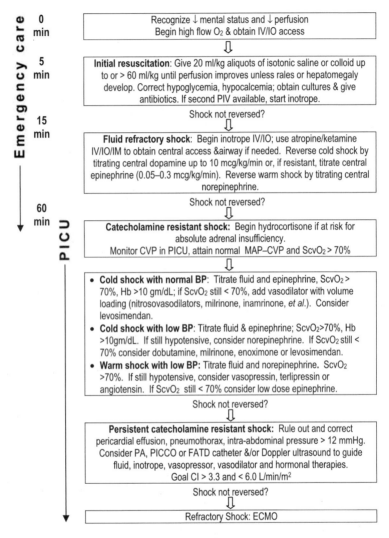

Fig. 3.6.1.   Management Guidelines for Treatment of Septic Shock: "Goal-directed therapy". PA, pulmonary artery; PICCO, pulse contour cardiac output; FATD, femoral arterial thermodilution. From Brierly J *et al.*, Clinical practice parameters for hemodynamic support of pediatric and neonatal septic shock: 2007 update from the American College of Critical Care Medicine, *Crit Care Med*, 37(2): 666–688, 2009.

Box 3.6.7   Management Principles for Patients with Multiple Organ System Dysfunction

- **Protect the lungs** (*Respiratory Failure, 2.7*). Early institution of mechanical ventilation decreases oxygen consumption; use lung protective strategies and allow hypercapnea providing there are no contraindications such as brain swelling (goal blood pH > 7.25).
- **Support the heart** (*Shock, 3.5; Septic Shock, 3.6*). Abnormal hemodynamic variables should be addressed and appropriate interventions implemented before further deterioration is irretrievable. Acceptable variabilities should be discussed. The assistance of near infra-red spectroscopy and serial echocardiograms may augment and refine the therapeutic vasoactive approach.
- **Monitor the CNS** (*Altered Mental Status, 5.1*). Avoid medications that may impact negatively on hemodynamic instability. Adjust dosing regimens for renal or hepatic insufficiency or failure. Seizures should be treated aggressively. Consider EEG and CNS imaging for any change in mental status or neurologic findings of uncertain cause.
- **Support fluid and electrolyte balance** (*Dehydration 6.1 and Electrolyte Disturbances, 6.2*). Focus on intravascular volume resuscitation until capillary leak injury subsides. Avoid unnecessary volume expansion, and use blood products if these are indicated to provide necessary volume as well as RBC and coagulation factors. Monitor electrolytes with particular attention to potassium, calcium, and magnesium, and supplement these as necessary. Optimization of these, particularly calcium, may have a positive effect on cardiac function.
- **Support nutrition** (*Nutritional Requirements in Hospitalized and Critically Ill Children, 8.1*). Sepsis is a hypermetabolic state; nutrition should begin early in the course (usually by day 3) and enteral is preferred over parenteral nutrition.
- **Control glucose.** Maintain serum glucose in a safe range (*Hypo- and Hyperglycemia, 6.4*).

(Continued)

Box 3.6.7   Management Principles for Patients with Multiple Organ System Dysfunction (Continued)

- **Correct marked anemia and coagulopathy associated with bleeding.** Patients with evidence of hypoperfusion, hypoxemia, and/or high FiO_2 requirement need higher hemoglobin (*e.g.* 10 gm/dL) than more stable patients with more satisfactory indicators of oxygenation. Coagulation abnormalities should be addressed in the context of presence or absence of bleeding and individual risk factors.
- **Ensure appropriate, broad-spectrum antibiotic coverage pending identification of the offending organism(s).** Culture all potential sites, including peripheral blood, blood from all access devices, urine, wounds, airway, fluid collections such as pleural effusions, ascites, *etc.* Consider sites such as the oral cavity and sinuses particularly in the immunocompromised. Ensure that drug doses and levels are appropriate based on individual drug characteristics in the presence of organ dysfunction (*e.g.* dosing adjustments in renal or hepatic impairment). Consider the possibility of secondary superinfection if deterioration occurs after initial improvement. Consider the immune status and possible need for supplementation with immune globulin in hypogammaglobulinemic patients and WBC transfusion in severely neutropenic patients (*Appendix, part 2, XI and XII*).

Chapter 4

Heart Disease, Cardiac Surgery and Peri-Operative Care

4.1 Acquired Heart Disease

4.1.1 *Myocarditis*

Myocarditis is an inflammatory process involving the myocardium that can lead to significant cardiac dysfunction, arrhythmias, and even cardiac failure. The diagnosis can be elusive and requires a high index of suspicion. The incidence of clinically significant cases is ~0.10–6% in the general pediatric population with the majority occurring in the first year of life and during adolescence.

Causes. The most common cause of myocarditis is a viral illness (**Box 4.1.1**). These viruses may cause direct myocardial injury, lead to a dysregulated immune response, and sometimes produce toxins. Other etiologies include bacteria, fungi, rickettsiae, protozoa, medications (*e.g.* doxorubicin, daunorubicin, syrup of ipecac), autoimmune diseases, Kawasaki disease and hypersensitivity reactions.

Box 4.1.1   Common Viral Causes of Myocarditis

- Adenovirus (55–60% of cases)
- Parvovirus B19
- Varicella-zoster virus
- Human immunodeficiency virus
- Respiratory syncitial virus
- Coxsackie viruses (30–35% of cases)
- Influenza
- Epstein-Barr virus
- Herpes simplex virus
- Cytomegalovirus

169

Clinical Presentation. The signs and symptoms of myocarditis are highly variable; some patients present with only mild tachycardia and others with cardiovascular collapse. Careful history and thorough physical examination are imperative. There may be history of a viral prodrome, syncope, chest pain, poor feeding, dyspnea, or irritability. Gastrointestinal (GI) symptoms on presentation (abdominal pain, diarrhea, vomiting) are common. Since vague GI symptoms may be the only complaint, incorrect diagnoses of viral gastroenteritis, colic, or psychogenic disorder may be made. Tachycardia (out of proportion to degree of fever or not resolving with conventional measures) is common; distal perfusion, liver size, and blood pressure should be carefully evaluated. The classification system of myocarditis, based on clinical features, histology on myocardial biopsy, and outcomes, portrays the spectrum of disease (**Box 4.1.2**).

Box 4.1.2   Classification of Myocarditis

Type	Characteristics
Fulminant myocarditis	• Heart size on CXR often normal; may present with cardiogenic shock, arrhythmia, or sudden death; ↓ systolic performance • Lymphocyte infiltration with myocyte necrosis • Prognosis highly variable; some patients return to normal premorbid function, others have significant morbidity and/or mortality
Subacute myocarditis	• Cardiomegaly on CXR; may present with subclinical heart failure symptoms; ↓ systolic performance • Lymphocyte infiltration with or without myocyte necrosis • May develop cardiomyopathy
Dilated cardiomyopathy	• Cardiomegaly on CXR, symptoms of heart failure, ↓ systolic performance with dilated LV • Myocyte hypertrophy, interstitial fibrosis, may have no inflammation • May require transplantation

---

Box 4.1.3   Diagnosis of Myocarditis

Study	Findings
Chest radiograph	• Heart size may be normal. • Cardiomegaly, pulmonary edema, or pleural effusion may be present.
Electrocardiogram	• Most commonly shows sinus tachycardia, low-voltage QRS, and/or flattening or inversion of T waves. • Acute dysrhythmias (SVT, atrial ectopic tachycardia, premature beats, VT) occur due to myocardial irritability.
Echocardiogram	• Ventriculomegaly, reduced shortening or ejection fraction, AV valve regurgitation. • Less commonly shows pulmonary hypertension due to ↑ left atrial pressure or intracardiac thrombi.
Cardiac troponin	• Concentration > 0.052 ng/ml is more consistent with acute viral myocarditis than with dilated cardiomyopathy.
Viral studies	• Viral cultures, polymerase chain reaction studies, antibody assays, and viral titers may reveal a viral pathogen.
Endomyocardial biopsy	• Gold standard for histological diagnosis but not routinely performed on every patient.

Diagnosis (**Box 4.1.3**). **Management** is primarily supportive with the goals of optimizing oxygen delivery and minimizing oxygen consumption (**Box 4.1.4**).

4.1.2 *Pericarditis*

The pericardium is a double-layered fibrous sac that surrounds the cardiac chambers and extends to the great vessels, including the systemic and pulmonary veins. The pericardium prevents acute

Box 4.1.4   Management of Patients with Myocarditis

Inotropic support	• β-adrenergic agents (dopamine, dobutamine, and epinephrine) are often warranted but may be arrhythmogenic or ↑ myocardial oxygen consumption. • Milrinone improves left ventricular relaxation (lusitropy) as well as reduces afterload; may cause hypotension.
Diuresis	• Treatment with diuretics should be initiated early.
Antiarrhythmics	• Often initiated if ventricular ectopy or more serious dysrhythmia is present; not given empirically.
Respiratory support	• Beneficial to patients with low cardiac output state. • Goals: Target decreasing oxygen consumption and improving cardiac output (*Important Cardiopulmonary Interactions, 3.2*) • Medications that cause depression of myocardial function should be avoided. Tracheal intubation is a particularly hazardous process in these patients and should be undertaken by the most experienced practitioner available.
Immunomodulation	• High-dose IVIG (2 gm/kg over 24 hrs) • Immunosuppression sometimes considered but less well studied (steroids, infliximab)
Mechanical support	• Extracorporeal life support (*Other Aids to Support Oxygenation and Ventilation, 2.9*) may be necessary for refractory cardiac dysfunction or cardiac failure. • May also consider ventricular assist devices.
Transplantation	• Up to 10% of cardiac transplantations are undertaken for myocarditis. • Post-transplant survival reaches about 70%.

over-distension of the heart, protects the heart from infections and adhesions, maintains the heart in a fixed position in the chest, and regulates the stroke volumes of the two ventricles. Pericarditis is an inflammatory reaction of the pericardium. It occurs in 1 per 850 pediatric hospital admissions. In children less than 2 years, 90% of cases are purulent (infectious) pericarditis.

Pericarditis results from idiopathic, infectious, and non-infectious causes (**Box 4.1.5**). Infectious pericarditis typically results from direct or hematogenous spread to the pericardium from a primary site. Treatment of the primary cause will ultimately result in resolution of pericarditis, although pericardiocentesis may still be required if there is hemodynamic compromise during the acute phase of illness. Post-pericardiotomy syndrome is discussed below.

Box 4.1.5   Causes of Pericarditis

- **Idiopathic**
  - ▶ Benign
  - ▶ Recurrent
- **Infectious Agents**
  - ▶ Purulent: bacteria,
    M. tuberculosis, fungi
  - ▶ Viruses
  - ▶ Mycoplasma
  - ▶ Parasites
  - ▶ Spirochetes
  - ▶ Chlamydia
  - ▶ Protozoa

- **Noninfectious**
  - ▶ Postpericardiotomy syndrome
  - ▶ Rheumatic fever
  - ▶ Connective tissue disorders
    (*e.g.* SLE)
  - ▶ Trauma: blunt or penetrating
  - ▶ Metabolic: uremia, myxedema
  - ▶ Cor pulmonale (as may occur in
    chronic upper airway obstruction)
  - ▶ Hypersensitivity
  - ▶ Neoplasm
  - ▶ Post-irradiation

Pericarditis from any cause begins with fibrin deposition adjacent to the great vessels causing the pericardium to lose its smoothness and translucency. The intruding agent or source of inflammation spreads from direct extension from lung/pleura or the bloodstream. Fluid accumulates in the pericardial space increasing intrapericardial pressure; the rate of accumulation determines the clinical presentation.

Slow accumulation of fluid allows accommodation of large volumes due to gradual expansion of the pericardium. Venous, atrial and ventricular pressures of the heart rise equally. The resultant decrease in venous return due to cardiac compression results in decreased cardiac output (*Important Cardiopulmonary Interactions, 3.2*). Reflex tachycardia and peripheral vasoconstriction are activated to maintain cardiac output (*Determinants of Cardiac Output and Oxygen Delivery, 3.1*; *Box 3.1.1*). Pulsus paradoxus, a greater than 10 mmHg drop in systolic pressure during inspiration, occurs because of decreased inflow to the cardiac chambers (*Shock, 3.5*; *Box 3.5.4*). "Kussmaul sign" is a paradoxical rise in jugular venous pressure during inspiration due to the limitation of blood return to the right atrium from diastolic atrial compression caused by the tense pericardial sac. Symptoms and signs are described in **Box 4.1.6**; useful laboratory data are listed in **Box 4.1.7**.

Box 4.1.6   Symptoms and Signs of Pericarditis

- Symptoms include:
  ▸ Most common: fever, dyspnea
  ▸ Abdominal pain: may be seen in 15–80% of patients
  ▸ Symptoms of upper respiratory infection (10–14 days prior to presentation) may be present in patients with viral pericarditis.
  ▸ Signs and symptoms of other systemic diseases may be present.
- Physical findings include:
  ▸ Tachycardia
  ▸ Tachypnea
  ▸ Jugular venous distension
  ▸ Muffled heart tones
  ▸ Pericardial friction rub (best heard in the leaning forward or kneeling position with the diaphragm of the stethoscope pressed against the chest to amplify the opposing visceral and parietal pericardium); may be absent if there is sufficient pericardial fluid to prevent apposition of the pericardium to the outer myocardial surface.
  ▸ ↓ Peripheral pulses and ↑ capillary refill time may be present in early cardiac tamponade.

Box 4.1.7   Laboratory Data Recommended in Patients with Pericarditis

- CBC, ESR and C-reactive protein
- Chest X-ray: Cardiothoracic ratio may be increased; a large heart with diminished pulmonary vascular markings is classic for pericardial effusion.
- Evaluate for infection: Culture blood and urine for bacteria; culture nasopharynx, stool/rectum for virus. Culture pericardial fluid if indicated.
- Evaluate further as indicated by history and physical findings (*e.g.* ANA, *etc.*)
- Pericardial fluid: Cell count with differential, Gram stain, culture (bacterial and Mycobacterial as indicated), protein, glucose; consider triglycerides, LDH, cytology
- 12-lead ECG: ST elevation in numerous leads with upright T-waves
  Some patients demonstrate the following sequence (Spodick Stages):

  1) ST segment elevation and PR depression
  2) Normalization of ST and PR segments
  3) Diffuse T-wave inversion
  4) Normalization of T waves

- Echocardiogram: Reveals an abnormal fluid collection in the pericardial sac. Cardiac tamponade is present when diastolic collapse of the RA and RV is demonstrated.

Management and Prognosis (Box 4.1.8)

Patients who present with cardiac tamponade and hemodynamic instability require emergent pericardiocentesis. Drainage of the pericardial fluid using echocardiogram guidance is life saving. Purulent pericarditis often requires open surgical drainage with a pericardial drainage tube since the viscous fluid will not drain from smaller tubes. Intravenous antibiotic therapy, based on culture results, is required for 3–4 weeks. The most common offending bacteria are *Staphylococcus aureus* and *Hemophilus influenzae*.

Box 4.1.8   Pericarditis Pearls

- Diuretics given in the setting of pericarditis with pericardial fluid may create hemodynamic instability by decreasing filling pressures resulting in cardiac tamponade physiology.
- Patients may require volume resuscitation prior to or while extracting pericardial fluid to improve preload.
- Sedation and analgesia provided during pericardiocentesis should be accomplished with drugs that avoid or minimize the risk of hypotension.
- A complication of pericardiocentesis includes laceration of coronary arteries and perforation of the heart. If the patient does not improve during pericardiocentesis, ensure that the needle or catheter is in the pericardial space and not the ventricular cavity.
- Typically pericardial fluid will not clot and the hematocrit of the fluid is less than that of venous blood.

Viral pericarditis may resolve spontaneously over 3–4 weeks. Non-steroidal anti-inflammatory therapy (NSAID) with aspirin (80–100 mg/kg/day divided every 6 hrs) or ibuprofen (30–50 mg/kg/day divided every 6–8 hrs) constitutes immediate initial therapy in most cases. If there is poor response to NSAID therapy after 48 hrs, prednisone (2 mg/kg/day divided every 12 hrs) has been recommended in cases where the pericardial fluid continues to accumulate.

Treatment of underlying non-infectious causes typically results in resolution of pericarditis. Patients with hypothyroidism, renal failure, and systemic lupus erythematosus can experience dramatic recovery with treatment of the underlying disease. Rare cases of recurrence not responsive to medical management have required a surgical pericardial window for long-term drainage.

Purulent pericarditis has a mortality rate of 25–75%. A late complication of purulent pericarditis is constrictive pericarditis. A thick, fibrotic, and occasionally calcified pericardium develops which restricts diastolic filling. Surgical resection of the pericardium is curative. The recurrence rate for viral pericarditis is 15–30%. Patients may have associated viral myocarditis requiring therapy even after the pericarditis has resolved.

Postpericardiotomy syndrome is the most common postoperative inflammatory complication in patients who have undergone heart surgery with pericardial invasion. Typically, extensive muscle resection/trauma has been performed; however, cases have been reported with ASD and PDA closure. An autoimmune response with production of antisarcolemmal and antifibrillary antibodies is a potential etiology.

Affected patients develop fever 1–2 weeks post-operatively with malaise, decreased appetite, irritability, and nonspecific chest pain. Physical findings include tachycardia, pericardial rub, and hepatomegaly. Cardiac tamponade is rare. Complete blood count may show a predominance of band forms. The ESR may be elevated. Chest X-ray demonstrates enlargement of the cardiac silhouette and sometimes, a left pleural effusion; the echocardiogram confirms the presence of pericardial fluid.

Anti-inflammatory therapy with NSAID's (aspirin, ibuprofen, indomethacin), or prednisone will typically aid in resolving the inflammatory process. Frequent cardiac ultrasound follow-up is required to document resolution and rule out enlargement of the fluid collection. Pericardiocentesis or surgical drainage/window has been required in cases not responsive to medical management.

4.2 Heart Failure

Heart failure can be defined as cardiac dysfunction from a variety of causes that results in an inability to maintain cardiac output (CO) sufficient to meet metabolic demands. Therapy, therefore, can be directed not only at improving cardiac function, but also at reducing the workload placed upon the heart. Poor CO can result from excessive cardiac work (followed by deterioration of cardiac function, or "high output failure") in addition to disorders that primarily result in low output heart failure. Key points in the clinical assessment are:

- The single best indicator of the adequacy of the patient's cardiovascular system is the strength and quality of the peripheral pulses.
- Capillary refill time is typically prolonged in heart failure.
- Heart rate: Is the heart rate appropriate? Inappropriate tachycardia may be an indication of an attempt to compensate for poor ejection performance.
- Hypotension, particularly with narrowed pulse pressure, is indicative of an inability to generate an adequate stroke volume. Experienced clinicians rarely trust one data point in isolation, particularly when it is inconsistent with other findings. An easily palpable peripheral pulse in a child correlates with a pulse pressure >20 mmHg. If the pulses are 2+ and the blood pressure is 65/50 the blood pressure is probably artifactual.
- Respiratory rate: This is typically increased in CHF; an increase in the work of breathing may be apparent, since the metabolic rate is increased and pulmonary edema may be present due to left heart dysfunction.
- Temperature: Fever presents increased demand on CO because of the systemic demand for more metabolic energy; febrile patients with heart failure should be appropriately cooled, and consideration should be given to fever itself as a cause of heart failure (*e.g.* thyrotoxicosis). Note that skin temperature may be cool while the body temperature may be abnormally increased.
- Evidence of fluid overload and venous congestion: pulmonary edema, hepatomegaly, peripheral edema, jugular venous distension.
- Palpation of the precordium: Apical activity may be displaced and possibly more diffuse (*e.g.* in cardiomyopathy).

- Auscultation: The findings are obviously lesion-specific when there is structural heart disease (*Congenital Heart Disease, 4.4*). In the setting of normal anatomy the presence of an S3 gallop reflects a dilated and perhaps thin walled left ventricle. The presence of an S4 gallop reflects decreased ventricular compliance. Accentuated sound of pulmonary valve closure is indicative of pulmonary hypertension.
- CXR usually reveals cardiomegaly; evidence of pulmonary edema may be present. Pulmonary blood flow may be increased depending on the lesion.
- ECG: Lesion-specific. ST elevation or depression may be present in the setting of a cardiomyopathy/myocarditis.
- High output failure (as seen in left to right shunts, aortic incompetence, A-V malformations, thyrotoxicosis, catecholamine excess, and severe anemia) may be distinguished by history and bounding but poorly sustained pulses (Ninja pulses: "Strike fast and fade away") and a hyperdynamic left ventricular impulse with or without displacement.

Clinical suspicion should prompt a formal pediatric cardiology evaluation to include a complete history and physical examination and echocardiography which helps define anatomic abnormalities, ventricular function (including ejection performance and diastolic function), "loading conditions," *i.e.* systemic and pulmonary vascular resistance, and an assessment of preload (intravascular volume).

Venticular wall stress is the primary determinant of myocardial oxygen consumption. In the treatment of a failing ventricle, the goals of minimizing the ventricular radius, minimizing intraventricular pressure and maximizing ventricular wall thickness all help to decrease wall stress.

$$\text{Wall stress} = (\text{Intracavitary pressure} \times \text{Intracavitary radius}) \div 2 \times (\text{ventricular wall thickness})$$

Management should be individualized with the help of a pediatric cardiologist; helpful interventions are summarized (**Box 4.2.1**); key steps and substitutions in the transition to oral therapy are outlined (**Box 4.2.2**).

Box 4.2.1   Management of Heart Failure

- Minimize factors that contribute to wall stress, or the tension on the ventricular wall. These include:
  - ▸ Optimization of filling pressures with avoidance of excessive volume resuscitation. This is critically important in a dilated, relatively thin-walled ventricle, *e.g.* dilated cardiomyopathy.
  - ▸ Decrease intracavitary pressure; avoid excessive systemic/pulmonary vasoconstriction and minimize systemic/pulmonary afterload as much as tolerated.
  - ▸ Optimize ventricular wall thickness: a gradual increase in ventricular wall thickness can be seen with the judicious use of inotropic agents and diuretics and can improve intrinsic ventricular ejection performance as wall stress decreases. This is more operative in children than in adults since children can increase coronary blood flow in response to the increase in ventricular mass.
- Treatment of decreased ejection performance of the systemic ventricle:
  - ▸ Parenteral inotropic agents:
    - ▪ Dopamine (typical dosage range: 2–20 mcg/kg/min); typically the "first line" inotropic agent. Doses as low as 2 mcg/kg/min have been reported to be effective, but 5 mcg/kg/min is the recommended starting dose with advancement to 10 mcg/kg/min without reservation or concerns regarding augmentation of afterload. It is important to ensure that the patient's volume status is adequate before advancing the dose further. (An increase in heart rate without a reasonable blood pressure response may suggest inadequate intravascular volume or excessive vasodilatation as in sepsis/septic shock). Larger doses may be needed in pre-term infants or when receptor down regulation might have occurred such as in chronic illness, longstanding cardiomyopathy or obstructive sleep apnea. Increased afterload will occur to a mild degree at doses of 10–15 mcg/kg/min and more significantly at higher doses.
    - ▪ Epinephrine (typical dose: 0.1–1 mcg/kg/min); an unequivocally more potent inotrope than dopamine. Epinephrine carries a greater potential for negative side effects, including the risk of significant systemic vasoconstriction at higher doses

(Continued)

Box 4.2.1   Management of Heart Failure (Continued)

and greater increases in myocardial oxygen consumption as compared to dopamine; typically added to the regimen only when dopamine has been maximized. Addition of epinephrine usually permits weaning of dopamine to dopaminergic doses (<10 mcg/kg/min; effective renal stimulation of DA_1 receptors occurs at ≤ 3 mcg/kg/min) in an effort to maintain optimal renal perfusion.

■ Dobutamine (typical dose: 2–15 mcg/kg/min) is a weaker inotrope than epinephrine or dopamine; results in net afterload reduction, which made it somewhat appealing in combination with other inotropes prior to the availability of milrinone. Dobutamine can result in stimulation of beta 2- and beta 1- adrenergic receptors in healthy coronary arteries which can result in coronary vasodilation.

▶ Parenteral vasodilators:

■ Milrinone: (typical dosage range: 0.25–0.75 mcg/kg/min; a 50 mcg/kg load over 15 mins may be given). A selective inhibitor of peak III cyclic AMP phosphodiesterase isozyme in cardiac and vascular muscle, resulting in ↑ contractile force in cardiac muscle and relaxation in vascular muscle, vasodilating both systemic and pulmonary vascular beds. Results in positive synergism of inotropic effect when combined with traditional parenteral inotropic agents. Essential in the treatment armamentarium for heart failure. Optimal dosage should result in improved pulse pressure, pulse quality, and perfusion without a significant decline in blood pressure.

■ Nitroprusside: (initial dose 0.25–0.3 mcg/kg/min; usual dose: 3 mcg/kg/min; range 1–10 mcg/kg/min but doses >4 mcg/kg/min are rarely required); a mainstay of vasodilator therapy prior to the availability of milrinone. Limited indications in the setting of cardiac dysfunction in children.

• Treatment of excessive preload and/or symptoms and sequelae of pulmonary and systemic venous congestion with parenteral diuretics:

▶ Furosemide (typical dose 1–4 mg/kg/day divided every 8–24 hrs). Monitor for hypokalemia, metabolic alkalosis, hypercalciuria and hypocalcemia.

Box 4.2.2   Transition to Oral Therapy

• If there is persistent ventricular dysfunction and therefore a need for outpatient anticongestive therapy, some oral therapy is initiated as IV therapy (particularly milrinone) is weaned.

• The two mainstays of oral anticongestive therapy are the ACE inhibitors and carvedilol.

▸ ACE inhibitors: captopril, enalapril, and lisinopril are all commonly used agents which provide afterload reduction in addition to positive effects on cardiac remodeling. Captopril may serve better as an initial transition agent because its shorter half-life allows for more frequent and relatively small doses making it easily adjustable based on response. None of the oral ACE inhibitors are commercially available in liquid form, and prescriptions have to be compounded. Captopril can be prepared in a 1 mg/mL suspension.

▸ Carvedilol (typical starting dose ≤0.1 mg/kg per dose; advance as tolerated). A beta 1- and beta 2-blocker as well as an alpha 1-blocker which has proven to be effective in the setting of dilated cardiomyopathy. Particularly effective when there is an element of diastolic dysfunction. Can result in ↑stroke volume and stroke work index along with a ↓ in heart rate and ventricular size. Carvedilol has also been shown to ↓ pulmonary mean and wedge pressures and ↑ peripheral vasodilatation. Frequent dosing (q 6 hrs in neonates and infants while hospitalized and q 8 hrs in older children) is necessary because of its short half-life, therefore frequent dosing may be necessary q 6 hr dosing for neonates and infants while inpatient and q 8 hr dosing in older children.

• Diuretics:

▸ Furosemide (typical starting dose 1–2 mg/kg/day divided BID. Note that the parenteral route is ~twice as potent as the enteral route.

(Continued)

> **Box 4.2.2   Transition to Oral Therapy (Continued)**
>
> ▸ Spironolactone should be considered for patients requiring >1 mg/kg/day of furosemide. In the absence of an ACE inhibitor in the regimen, spironolactone is added for its potassium-sparing effects as well as its theoretical beneficial effects on cardiac remodeling. In our practice, we have found that a 2:1 to 2.5:1 dose ratio of oral furosemide to spironolactone will maintain normal potassium balance in most all patients.
>
> ▸ Metolazone is an extremely potent thiazide diuretic which is strongly synergistic with furosemide, esp. if the latter is given ~2 hrs after metolazone is given. Marked potassium loss may occur. Metolazone is not typically utilized unless an ACE inhibitor is already part of the regimen. Metolazone is rarely given on a daily basis.
>
> • Digoxin:
>   Digoxin still appears to have some benefit in the treatment of heart failure when there is ventricular systolic dysfunction. Whether this is purely an inotropic effect or whether additional mechanisms are present is unclear. The dosage required for inotropic therapy (typically 8 mcg/kg per day divided bid) is less than the dosage for antiarrhythmic therapy.

4.3 Pulmonary Hypertension

Pulmonary hypertension (PHTN) occurs when there is an abnormal elevation of pulmonary vascular resistance. After the neonatal period, PHTN is quantified as a mean pulmonary artery pressure 25 mmHg or more at rest and 30 mmHg or more with exercise. Although the initial site of injury is the pulmonary vascular anatomy, there can be significant "end organ" damage as it relates to cardiac anatomy and function. PHTN can be either primary or secondary. Clearly identifying the etiology has significant prognostic and therapeutic implications.

Changes in the pulmonary vascular architecture leading to the development of PHTN are complex and incompletely understood. Key points in the development of this disease involve abnormal interactions between the pulmonary arteriolar vascular smooth muscle cells and the associated endothelium. This typically begins with hypertrophic changes in the vascular medial muscular ring, and subsequent development of intimal fibrosis due to proliferation of the intimal cells. Over time, there is resultant pulmonary artery dilatation and further pulmonary artery occlusion due to worsening intimal fibrosis. This vascular remodeling results in fibrinoid necrosis, *i.e.* the formation of bands of scar tissue which form layers within the wall of the smaller pulmonary arteries, causing significant luminal narrowing. At the same time, injury to the blood vessel lining affects two endothelial products: **nitric oxide (NO)** and **endothelin (ET)**. NO is a vasodilator, while ET is a vasoconstrictor. With endothelial injury, the production and release of ET is increased and the production of NO is decreased. Within the smooth muscle cell, calcium and thromboxane (TXA) are also at work. Once Ca^{++} enters the smooth muscle cell, it initiates smooth muscle contraction leading to vasoconstriction. TXA also causes vasoconstriction and platelet aggregation. In normal individuals, TXA would be opposed by prostacyclin (also called prostaglandin I2 or PGI2), which inhibits platelet aggregation and is a vasodilator. However, in patients with severe PHTN, there is a reduction in the activity of the enzyme that helps synthesize PGI2, creating an imbalance between PGI2 and TXA. Over time, the entire process frequently becomes irreversible and can lead to RV failure.

Etiology. Primary (idiopathic) PHTN occurs in 2 per 1,000,000 children, affecting females more than males. Familial PHTN accounts for ~5% of primary PHTN.

Secondary PHTN. Vascular injury due to increased pulmonary blood flow from congenital heart lesions with chronic left to right shunting may result in the development of PHTN. Additionally, "downstream" obstruction from left-sided heart lesions, including left sided heart failure with high LV end-diastolic pressures or impaired/obstructed pulmonary venous return leads to an "upstream" increase in pulmonary artery pressures and potentially initiation of the vascular injury cascade. Other causes of secondary PHTN include disease processes associated with chronic pulmonary emboli causing occlusion of pulmonary blood vessels, such as sickle cell disease. There is also an association with high altitudes and cocaine abuse. PHTN can also be caused by pulmonary disease associated with hypoventilation. Encompassed in this category are chronic airway obstruction, chronic lung disease (*e.g.* BPD) and other disorders associated with hypoventilation. This can lead to the development **cor pulmonale** *i.e.* heart disease due to a pulmonary etiology which puts increased pressure-related demand on the right heart due to increased resistance in the pulmonary vasculature.

Diagnosis. The child may be asymptomatic before diagnosis or may have vague symptoms such as fatigue, exercise intolerance, chest pain, dyspnea, shortness of breath, dizziness, and syncope. Although the progression of the disease can occur quickly, there may be no correlation between severity of the PHTN and severity of presenting symptoms. Multiple tools can aid in making the diagnosis of PHTN (**Box 4.3.1**).

Box 4.3.1   Tools Helpful in Diagnosing Pulmonary Hypertension

- **ECG**: If cor pulmonale has not developed, this may be normal. Voltages may indicate RVH with RA enlargement and right axis deviation. Abnormal changes may be indicative of right sided heart failure and RVH due to strain on the right ventricle contracting against increased pulmonary artery pressure.
- **CXR:** There is varying correlation, depending on the extent of PHTN and underlying pulmonary parenchymal disease. Cardiomegaly may be present due to RVH. Additionally, the pulmonary artery may appear enlarged and the pulmonary parenchyma may appear underperfused, with "pruning" of the pulmonary vessels.
- **ABG:** This is helpful both with diagnosis as well as monitoring therapeutic efficacy. Hypoventilation can be assessed by the $PaCO_2$ and/or the presence of a base excess; oxygenation is quantified by the PaO_2.
- **Cardiac catheterization:** Measurement of pulmonary artery pressure by right heart catheterization is the gold standard for diagnosing PHTN. This also allows for the inclusion or exclusion of secondary PHTN due to cardiac causes. An important role for catheterization is evaluating the potential for the reversibility of PHTN by measuring pressures before and after vasodilator therapies.

(Continued)

Box 4.3.1   Tools Helpful in Diagnosing Pulmonary Hypertension (Continued)

- **Echocardiogram:** ECHO is becoming the noninvasive mainstay for making the diagnosis of PHTN. Findings associated with PHTN include ↑ pulmonary artery pressure, tricuspid regurgitation (allowing relative quantification of pulmonary artery pressure), pulmonary regurgitation, RVH, pulmonary artery dilatation, and right to left shunting across a patent foramen ovale. Additionally, it can help rule in or rule out cardiac causes with increased pulmonary blood flow from left to right shunting, LV failure, or pulmonary vein obstruction. An ECHO may also demonstrate **Eisenmenger syndrome** *i.e.* irreversible cyanotic PHTN due to chronic pulmonary overcirculation from shunting lesions. Similar to cardiac catheterization, an ECHO can be used to monitor therapy and assess the reversibility of PHTN as treatment progresses.

Treatment. Just as the pathophysiology of PHTN is multifactorial, so is the treatment (**Box 4.3.2**). Consultation with a pulmonologist, in conjunction with a cardiologist, is recommended; this will allow the tailoring of treatment to a patient's individual need. In general, treatment of primary PHTN is life-long. Maximizing

---

Box 4.3.2   Therapeutic Tools in the Management of Pulmonary Hypertension

- **Oxygen:** The primary benefit of O_2 therapy results from its vasodilatory properties in relaxing the pulmonary vasculature. Additionally, ↑ing the patient's FiO_2 maximizes the amount of O_2 available for exchange.
- **Mechanical ventilation:** For patients who are critically ill, this allows tight control of both oxygenation and ventilation. In addition to conventional positive pressure ventilation, various strategies such as high frequency ventilation may be employed to maximize alveolar recruitment and insure ideal gas exchange.

(Continued)

Box 4.3.2   Therapeutic Tools in the Management of Pulmonary Hypertension (Continued)

- **Calcium channel blockers:** Calcium channel blockade plays an important role in pulmonary vasodilatation. Demonstration of a reactive pulmonary vascular bed during catheterization suggests that a positive response to calcium channel blocker therapy may occur.
- **Anticoagulation:** ↑ platelet aggregation, coupled with narrowed pulmonary vasculature requires that anticoagulation be considered. If an embolic component is present, this is mandatory. Hematology consultation may be useful in determining the appropriate anticoagulant and dosing regimen.
- **Nitric oxide:** Delivery of iNO to relax the vascular smooth muscle is an important therapeutic modality for the critically ill patient. It also serves a diagnostic role in helping predict which patients may benefit from oral vasodilators due to a responsive pulmonary vascular bed. Close monitoring is required (*Other Aids to Support Oxygenation and Ventilation, 2.9*). Additionally, cautious weaning is necessary, as rebound PHTN can occur after iNO is withdrawn.
- **Phosphodiesterase inhibitors (*e.g.* Sildenafil):** These drugs result in dilatation of pulmonary circulation and allow for increased oxygenation. Additionally, it can be used in the role of tempering NO withdrawal and preventing rebound pulmonary hypertension.
- **Prostaglandin (*e.g.* Epoprostenol):** The primary role is pulmonary vasodilatation. In long term therapy, it has been shown to improve quality of life, ↑ survival, ↑ exercise capacity, and ↓ pulmonary pressures.
- **Endothelin receptor antagonists (*e.g.* Bosentan):** These medications address the actions of endothelin, which include vasoconstriction and ↓ NO production. Bosentan has been shown to improve exercise capacity.
- **Organ transplantation:** Transplantation may also be an option for patients with end stage disease who do not respond to medical management. Lung transplantation may be a consideration for patients with primary PHTN and preserved cardiac function. In patients with severe LV dysfunction or severe shunting lesions in association with PHTN, a combined heart-lung transplant may be their only option, although it is associated with significant mortality and morbidity.

management has been shown to improve both quality of life as well as survival. The mainstay therapies for primary PHTN often involve an anticoagulant to combat the effects of platelet aggregation and clot formation in the small diameter pulmonary vessels, supplemental oxygen, a calcium channel blocker, and an oral vasodilator. Conversely, goals of therapy for secondary PHTN are directed at correcting its cause. These may include eliminating pulmonary over-circulation by reparing a shunting defect and improving pulmonary venous hypertension by treating LV failure. Likewise, treating the pulmonary arterial obstruction with vasodilators improves RV function. Current therapy involves treating the specific components of the process that lead to and maintain PHTN.

4.4   Congenital Heart Disease and Peri-Operative Care

Left to Right Shunt Lesions. Significant left to right intracardiac shunting from a ventricular septal defect (VSD) or patent ductus arteriosus (PDA) results in left ventricular (LV) volume overload during diastole in addition to increased pulmonary blood flow. A very large VSD or PDA causes pulmonary hypertension that is reversible after surgical or catheter closure of the defect. Left to right shunting from an atrial septal defect (ASD) results in right ventricular (RV) diastolic volume overload without pulmonary hypertension, and usually presents without symptoms in children. Catheter or surgical closure of an ASD is performed electively to prevent RV failure later in life. Complete atrio-ventricular septal defect (AVSD), also called endocardial cushion defect or AV canal, is often seen in infants with trisomy 21. Both RV and LV volume overload may be present as well as pulmonary hypertension. A regurgitant common atrio-ventricular (av) valve, especially the mitral component, may contribute to heart failure (HF, H*eart Failure*, 4.2). Symptoms of HF in infants include poor feeding, failure to thrive, tachypnea and sweating. Signs include tachycardia, tachypnea, hepatomegaly and rarely, edema. Cardiac findings include abnormal precordial lift, systolic murmurs that may be low pitched or subtle if RV hypertension is present, a loud S-2 or a gallop, or the low pitched diastolic flow murmur of excess venous return across the mitral valve. PDA causes a continuous murmur through systole into early diastole unless there is very severe pulmonary hypertension.

Pre-operative Considerations in Left to Right Shunts. Congestive heart failure (CHF) from a VSD or PDA is associated with pulmonary vascular congestion clinically and on radiograph and with LV enlargement and preserved systolic ventricular performance on echocardiogram (ECHO). Admission to PICU preoperatively is needed only for severe decompensation. Lower respiratory infections may precipitate CHF in these infants adding to cardiogenic pulmonary edema and increased work of breathing; respiratory support with mechanical ventilation may be needed. Additional PEEP may improve pulmonary venous congestion and edema. Maintaining a PaO_2 greater than normal with supplemental oxygen should be avoided because this decreases pulmonary vascular resistance leading to increased left to right shunting, pulmonary vascular congestion and decreased systemic arterial perfusion (*Important Cardiopulmonary Interactions, 3.2*).

Pre-operative diuretics may be given IV when appropriate. ACE inhibitors that improve the systemic to pulmonary blood flow ratio can be continued enterally. In very ill infants, milrinone can be substituted or added to promote systemic arterial flow over pulmonary blood flow as well as for inotropic effect.

Cautious volume resuscitation should be given for dehydration with hypovolemia when indicated.

Postoperative Considerations. Catheter closure of a large PDA or large ASD may not require PICU admission. Surgical repair of VSD and AVSD usually requires post operative mechanical ventilator support and low dose inotropic support with milrinone, dopamine or dobutamine. Epicardial temporary cardiac pacing is needed rarely. Regularly scheduled furosemide IV promotes mobilization of tissue edema after cardiopulmonary bypass. Central venous pressure (CVP) monitoring allows for appropriate volume replacement especially if there is increasing heart rate and decreased blood pressure with a low CVP (*General Approach to the Critically Ill Child, 1.2*). A rapid rise in CVP with increasing heart rate and falling blood pressure may signal cardiac tamponade. Continuous near infrared spectroscopy (NIRS) noninvasively monitors central venous O_2 saturation and can detect decreasing cardiac output as a sign of early tamponade or low output syndrome. Infants with Down syndrome may be more likely to experience transient but serious pulmonary hypertension post operatively, which may manifest as a sudden decline in SaO_2 with bradycardia, increasing tachycardia, decreased $ETCO_2$, increased CVP, or with hypotension. This may respond to improved ventilation and increased FiO_2. ECHO evaluation can confirm pulmonary hypertension if a PA catheter is not in use. Nitric oxide therapy (*Other Aids to Support Oxygenation and Ventilation, 2.9*) may be needed until pulmonary hypertensive spells subside. ECHO also can assess ventricular systolic performance and residual shunts or the development of significant AV valve regurgitation especially following repair of AV septal defect.

At the time of transfer from the PICU, transition to enteral therapy is usually underway (*Heart Failure, 4.2*). Infants who have had very large left to right shunts may have relative sinus bradycardia noted post -surgery; this resolves as cardiac adrenergic receptors up-regulate following correction of the shunt with normalization of the pre-operative hyperadrenergic state associated with HF.

Post Discharge Care and Follow-Up. Palivizumab is administered to infants < 24 mos during RSV season since the protective effect of previously administered palivizumab is lost during cardiopulmonary bypass. Endocarditis prophylaxis with antibiotics one hour prior to oral procedures is recommended for six months post-operatively until the surgical patch or suture lines endothelialize. Post-pericardiotomy syndrome may cause large sterile pericardial effusions during the first month after open-heart surgery in children (*Pericarditis, 4.1.2*).

Obstructive Lesions

Coarctation of the aorta, if severe, presents in the first three weeks of life with shock and profound metabolic acidosis following late ductal closure. The clinical presentation may be similar to neonatal sepsis so empiric antibiotic therapy is given until the diagnosis is established. After volume resuscitation, palpable right brachial and carotid pulses with absent femoral pulses (or systolic BP in the lower extremities <systolic BP in the upper extremities) may be a helpful clue that sepsis is not the primary diagnosis. Failure to resolve shock in a neonate with suspected sepsis despite effective volume replacement and inotropic and ventilatory support should prompt consideration for treatment with alprostadil (prostaglandin E1; PGE-1) infusion. PGE-1 results in opening of the ductus arteriosus and re-establishes systemic blood flow from the RV even before ECHO confirmation of the diagnosis. Interrupted aortic arch type B and hypoplastic left heart with aortic atresia present in the same manner as neonatal critical coarctation, but will have absent pulses in all four extremities.

After initiation of PGE-1 infusion (0.05–0.1 mcg/kg/min) reducing the FiO_2 to 0.21 and avoiding hyperventilation and hypocarbia avoids deleterious low pulmonary vascular resistance which can impair adequate ductal flow to the systemic circulation (*Important Cardiopulmonary Interactions, 3.2*). Establishment of urine output and resolution of metabolic acidosis indicate adequate systemic perfusion.

Surgical repair of neonatal aortic coarctation is performed via left thoractomy unless concomitant VSD repair is required. The arterial pressure in the left arm may be lower than the right even after a successful coarctation repair; right radial arterial pressure monitoring is therefore preferable. Repair of interrupted aortic arch often is performed with repair of a large VSD and requires cardiopulmonary bypass and sternotomy. Post-operative considerations are similar to those described with VSD or AVSD. Post-operative management of hypoplastic left heart syndrome is more complex and is discussed below *(***Single-ventricle lesions***).* Infants with aortic arch abnormalities should be given only irradiated blood to avoid potential graft versus host disease in infants with T cell deficiency or thymic hypoplasia with chromosome 22q11 deletion syndromes. In many institutions all infant blood transfusions are irradiated.

Aortic valve stenosis is often treated with balloon catheter dilation. Rarely, severe aortic valve regurgitation may necessitate surgical treatment. Clinically significant vascular perforations or dissections are rare after balloon dilatation, even in small infants, but unexplained post-catheterization hypotension and tachycardia should prompt evaluation including imaging for retroperitoneal hematoma from iliac vessel perforation. Longer term surveillance for recurrence of aortic stenosis or for increasing LV size from catheter-induced valve regurgitation is needed since most affected infants will eventually require aortic valve replacement.

The Ross operation replaces a severely stenotic or regurgitant aortic valve with autotransplantation of the child's pulmonary valve into the aortic position. It is performed with placement of a valved tissue conduit (often human homograft valve) from the RV to the PA. Although the coronary arteries are reimplanted into the new aortic root, ischemic events rarely occur. Late issues usually relate to stenosis or incompetency of the pulmonary valved conduit or to dilatation of the neoaortic root with aortic valve regurgitation.

Congenital mitral stenosis is usually seen in infants or children with other lesions (*e.g.* VSD, coarctation). The rumbling diastolic murmur of flow across the stenotic valve can be subtle. Surgical valvuloplasty can ameliorate symptoms of pulmonary edema but post-operative pulmonary hypertension can be an issue. Pulmonary vasodilators may not be helpful if there is fixed downstream obstruction at the mitral valve but cautious use may be necessary if there is severe reactive pulmonary hypertension. Follow-up for recurrence of stenosis and pulmonary hypertension is needed.

Pulmonary valve stenosis, if critically severe, is associated with cyanosis and right to left atrial shunting in neonates. It requires urgent balloon catheter valve dilation. Rarely, cyanosis worsens during the post-catheterization period. ECHO may show severe subvalvular obstruction from a hypercontractile right ventricular infundibulum after relief of valve stenosis. Volume resuscitation may be sufficient to improve this, but prudent use of beta blockade (*e.g.* esmolol) may be needed. More rarely, cyanosis may occur due to reactive pulmonary hypertension after successful pulmonary valve dilation. This diagnosis can be confirmed by ECHO and lead to specific treatment (*e.g.* nitric oxide).

Cyanotic Heart Lesions

Cyanotic congenital heart disease can be thought of as either separate transposed circulations (*e.g.* transposition of the great arteries), lesions with pulmonary atresia or critically low pulmonary blood flow (*e.g.* severe tetralogy of Fallot), or lesions in which the oxygenated pulmonary venous return mixes completely with the deoxygenated systemic venous return in a common chamber. Complete mixing of the venous returns can occur at the atrial level (*i.e.* total anomalous pulmonary venous connection), the ventricle (*e.g.* any so-called single ventricle lesion such as tricuspid atresia or hypoplastic left ventricle), or at the arterial level (*i.e.* truncus arteriosus).

Transposition of the great arteries (TGA) presents with severe cyanosis in the first day or days of life. Oximetry in the 60–70 % range with normal pulmonary blood flow on CXR is typical. Normal pulmonary blood flow is not delivered to the systemic circulation. Treatment with PGE-1 allows mixing of the separate red (oxygenated) and blue (deoxygenated) circulations. A Rashkind balloon atrial septostomy (BAS) with a catheter through the umbilical or femoral vein allows vigorous interchange of the two circulations with a rise in oximetry to the 80–90% range. Arterial switch operation (ASO) is performed in the first two weeks of life.

Pre-operative concerns in TGA. Some infants with TGA have severe pulmonary hypertension with persistent severe cyanosis even after BAS and require aggressive ventilator management before ASO. Alternatively, attempts to promote a normal O_2 saturation (~100%) with supplemental oxygen while on PGE-1 after BAS can "steal" flow to the pulmonary circulation manifesting as poor perfusion and poor pulses with metabolic acidosis.

Post-operative concerns in TGA. Monitoring and basic management are described (*General Approach to the Critically Ill Child, 1.2*) but additional concerns apply. Implanting the coronary arteries into the neoaortic root can compromise coronary flow especially if coronary anatomy is atypical or there is an intramural coronary artery coursing through the wall of the aortic root. Low output syndrome or episodes of ventricular tachycardia may signal ischemia. A murmur over the PA is common with mild stenosis, but severe pulmonic stenosis is rare.

Late post-operative concerns in TGA. Neoaortic root dilatation can be marked in a few patients but reoperation for severe aortic regurgitation is rare. Angiographic studies indicate that late coronary artery stenosis or occlusion of the transplanted coronary arteries can be found in 2–5% of children or young adults. Symptoms may be absent if there is a well-developed collateral circulation bypassing the obstructed coronary artery. This makes strict recommendations for diagnosis and management of this complication difficult to establish.

Tetralogy of Fallot and Pulmonary Atresia. Infants with tetralogy of Fallot (TOF) have a large VSD with aortic override, pulmonary valve stenosis often with pulmonary artery hypoplasia and RV hypertrophy with hypertrophy and stenosis of the infundibulum of the RV outflow tract (RVOT). Oximetry may be normal at birth if pulmonic stenosis is only moderate. Cyanosis gradually develops over months as RVOT obstruction progresses. If pulmonary atresia is present, then severe cyanosis in the first days of life may occur as the ductus closes if there is no other source of pulmonary blood flow. Some infants with TOF and pulmonary atresia have large collateral arteries arising from the descending aorta that supply adequate pulmonary flow after ductal closure and present with continuous murmurs (heard over the back) but no cyanosis. TOF most commonly presents as an acyanotic infant with a loud systolic murmur of obstruction in the RVOT radiating to the lung fields. The classic boot-shaped heart on CXR may not be apparent in the young infant. A right aortic arch is present in ~25% of cases.

Hypercyanotic spells can occur suddenly in infants with TOF who have no or mild cyanosis. Clinical signs are intense cyanosis and rapid very deep respirations with head bobbing (hyperpnea). Oximetry saturations can be 40% or lower. Although calming or sedating the infant is considered standard treatment, some may present with obtundation already or have lost consciousness. The murmur becomes almost inaudible as there is virtually no systolic flow to the pulmonary arteries due to systolic hyperdynamic contraction of the

RVOT infundibular muscle and nearly complete right to left shunt of systemic venous return to the overriding aorta. Treatment consists of administration of oxygen, calming the infant if agitated, and placing the infant in the knee chest position which increases aortic afterload and venous return to the RV. Judicious administration of morphine is recommended. A vigorous "volume push" of NaCl 0.9% often reverses cyanosis with concomitant return of the murmur. However, if these maneuvers do not result in sustained improvement in oximetry, a continuous infusion of phenylephrine may resolve the spell. Another approach is administration of esmolol to decrease infundibular hypercontractility by continuous beta blockade. Preceding this with continuous infusion of phyenylephrine may prevent esmolol-related systemic hypotension.

Cyanotic Lesions with Complete Mixing of Venous Return

Total anomalous pulmonary venous connection (TAPVC) allows complete mixing of pulmonary and systemic venous return at the level of the right atrium. If the confluence of the pulmonary veins behind the heart returns via a left vertical vein to the innominate vein or to the coronary sinus there may be no obstruction to pulmonary venous return and cyanosis may be minimal with room air Pox saturations of 85–95%. Some cases are misdiagnosed as transient tachypnea of the newborn until worsening pulmonary over-circulation leads to symptoms of poor feeding and respiratory distress. In infra-cardiac TAPVC the pulmonary vein confluence returns to the right atrium via a descending vein through the intra-hepatic venous circulation causing obstruction and more severe neonatal respiratory distress. In some cases there is severe cyanosis from pulmonary hypertension. Pulmonary venous congestion may be seen on CXR unless pulmonary blood flow is reduced by pulmonary hypertension.

Truncus arteriosus causes complete mixing of pulmonary and systemic venous returns at the arterial level. Since the truncal valve and common arterial trunk override a VSD, LV and RV outputs combine before leaving the ascending aorta and the pulmonary arteries that arise from the common arterial trunk. Pulmonary artery flow is abnormally high, pulmonary venous return is excessive, and Pox saturations are 85–95% in most cases. A loud single second heart sound, right ventricular lift and diastolic filling sound or gallop are typical findings. Presentations as late as several months of life with failure to thrive and tachypnea are not rare. Chest radiograph shows a right aortic arch in 1/3 of cases in addition to pulmonary over-circulation.

Single ventricle lesions include hypoplastic left heart syndrome with aortic atresia, hypoplastic right heart syndrome with pulmonary atresia, tricuspid valve atresia, and other complex single ventricle lesions sometimes associated with heterotaxy (asplenia or polysplenia syndromes). If there is pulmonary atresia the clinical presentation is neonatal cyanosis. If there is no pulmonary stenosis the presentation will be pulmonary over-circulation without clinical cyanosis. If there is coexisting aortic coarctation or hypoplasia, shock may occur when the ductus closes. Alprostadil (PGE-1) is needed to maintain ductal patency if there is either pulmonary atresia or severe corctatation or aortic atresia. Avoiding pulmonary overcirculation as described above (under **Coarctation of the Aorta**) is important in cases with aortic atresia or hypoplasia preoperatively. Balloon atrial septostomy may be required preoperatively in cases with mitral atresia or hypoplastic left heart syndrome if an intact atrial septum causes obstruction to pulmonary venous return.

Postoperative considerations: TAPVC and truncus arteriosus undergo complete primary repair when the diagnosis is made after medical treatment of symptomatic HF. Postoperative management is not different from other neonatal cardiac repairs.

Single ventricle lesions with pulmonary atresia are treated with PGE-1 to maintain ductal patency until an aorto-pulmonary shunt (modified Blalock-Taussig shunt) is performed. Single ventricle lesions with unrestricted pulmonary blood flow may need coarctation repair if present; PA banding may be needed to prevent pulmonary hypertension.

If there is coexisting subaortic valve obstruction then anastomosis of the main PA with the ascending aorta (referred to as a

Damus-Kaye-Stansel procedure) is performed to secure unobstructed systemic flow. An aorto-pulmonary shunt provides pulmonary blood flow.

Infants with hypoplastic left heart syndrome with aortic atresia undergo a Norwood procedure. The ascending aorta is augmented using the main PA to create a neoaorta. An aorta to pulmonary artery shunt or RV to PA shunt (Sano shunt) provides pulmonary blood flow. Post-operative support of the systemic single right ventricle after this operation requires avoiding pulmonary over-circulation. Arterial PaO_2 ~40 mmHg is usually ideal. Hypocarbia ($PaCO_2$ <35–40) should be avoided. Destination treatment for all single ventricle patients is the modified Fontan operation (total caval pulmonary connection). A superior vena caval to PA anastomosis (bidirectional Glenn shunt or hemi-Fontan operation) is performed at 4–12 mos. of life. The Fontan is completed between 18 mos to 3 yrs of age when the IVC is routed to the pulmonary arteries with a conduit. A conduit fenestration allowing some venous blood to pass into the atrium may be created to prevent excessive venous pressures.

After bi-directional Glenn shunting, cyanosis may worsen with any elevation in pulmonary vascular resistance. However, in post-Glenn shunt physiology, hyperventilation with hypocarbia reduces pulmonary flow. Therefore, permissive hypercarbia ($PaCO_2$ 45–50 mmHg) may actually enhance pulmonary flow. Another complication of the altered physiology after a bi-directional Glenn shunt is development of veno-venous collateral veins in response to elevated CVP. This occurs when venous channels, formed to decompress the SVC, drain into the pulmonary artery, left atrium or IVC. This causes marked cyanosis. Diagnosis of veno-venous collaterals can be suspected if ECHO imaging shows appearance of significant echo-contrast in the heart during injection of agitated saline into an upper extremity or jugular venous catheter.

Pleural or pericardial effusions can occur during early convalescence after either superior caval-pulmonary shunting or the total cavo-pulmonary connection if venous pressure elevation leads to lymphatic pressure elevation. If venous pressure elevation is transmitted to the thoracic duct these effusions may be chylous. Pleural or pericardial drainage may be needed. Venous pressure elevations may be treatable with increased diuresis, and medical optimization of systolic and diastolic ventricular function. A fat free diet or one containing only medium-chain triglycerides may prevent chylous effusion reaccumulation.

Late Follow Up. Truncus arteriosus patients may require re-operation or interventional catheterization for truncal valve or pulmonary valved conduit regurgitation or stenosis. Repaired TAPVC patients can develop late stenosis of one or more pulmonary veins causing pulmonary hypertension. Atrial tachyarrhythmias can occur years later. If incessant, this may cause secondary dilated cardiomyopathy. Patients with single ventricle lesions may also develop atrial tachyarrhythmias. Declining systolic performance of single ventricle hearts has required cardiac transplantation in some late post-Fontan patients. Failing ventricular performance in these patients may be signaled by edema, pleural effusions or ascites. In some cases a protein losing enteropathy with intestinal lymphangiectasia develops due to venous pressure elevation. All of the above late occurring problems will be managed at some point in the PICU setting.

Chapter 5

Central Nervous System (CNS)

5.1 Altered Mental Status (AMS)

AMS refers to a disturbance of consciousness that extends from the awake and alert state to coma. Causes of AMS are broadly divided between toxic/metabolic disturbances (~75% of cases) and structural CNS lesions. History is the most important factor in identifying the cause of AMS (**Box 5.1.1**).

Spectrum of Disturbance: Normal consciousness requires the integrity of at least one cerebral hemisphere *and* the reticular activating system.

- Alert wakefulness: age-appropriate awareness
- Lethargy: reduced wakefulness, but arousable
- Confusion
- Delirium: fluctuating course of impaired cognition and memory; disorientation; hallucinations may be present
- Obtundation: severely blunted, slowed responses
- Stupor: arousable only with vigorous stimulation; returns to sleep once stimulus withdrawn
- Coma: unarousable unresponsiveness

Evaluation and management should proceed simultaneously. Critical assessment of vital signs, airway, breathing and circulation are essential. If the cause is uncertain or trauma cannot be ruled out, immobilize the cervical spine and image the brain (head CT).

Box 5.1.1   Causes of AMS with Examples

- **Respiratory Failure:** Primary (pneumonia) or secondary (Arnold Chiari malformation with hypoventilation); toxic/metabolic causes of respiratory depression (severe metabolic alkalosis; severe hypophosphatemia); neuromuscular disease; sleep apnea
- **Cardiovascular:** Hypo-or hyper-tension; arrhythmias; right-to-left intracardiac shunting leading to hypoxia or cerebral emboli; cerebral thrombosis; vascular malformations; migraine
- **Primary Neurologic:** Seizure; post-ictal state; non-convulsive status epilepticus; ↑ ICP; traumatic brain injury; hydrocephalus; ventricular shunt malfunction; tumor; blood; abscess; post-infectious encephalomyelitis (ADEM)
- **Metabolic:** Electrolyte disturbances (esp. hyponatremia); hypo- or hyper-glycemia; hyperosmolality; DKA; adrenal insufficiency; hypothyroidism; thyrotoxicosis; liver failure; renal failure; hypo- or hyper-thermia; inborn errors of metabolism; altitude sickness; drug withdrawal; vitamin deficiencies
- **Toxic or Drug-Related:** Drug ingestion or environmental exposures (carbon monoxide, lead, heavy metal poisoning); vitamin intoxication (hypervitaminosis A); steroid psychosis; cyclosporine-induced
- **Infectious:** Meningitis; encephalitis; HIV; hemolytic uremic syndrome
- **Immunologic:** CNS vasculitis (lupus cerebritis); thrombotic thrombocytopenic purpura
- **Acute Abdominal:** Intussusception, volvulus, malrotation, NEC, pyloric stenosis
- **Hematologic:** Anemia; polycythemia; hyperleukocytosis
- **Traumatic:** Intracranial hemorrhage; stroke/ischemia due to vascular injury
- **Psychiatric:** Depression and conversion reactions; Munchausen's syndrome +/− by proxy; psychogenic hyperventilation; ICU or other psychosis

Box 5.1.2   General Approach to the Patient with AMS

- Assess airway, breathing: Give oxygen; treat respiratory failure with tracheal intubation as indicated.
- Ensure circulatory adequacy: treat hypotension. If BP is high, first R/O ↑ ICP as a cause of hypertension (*Raised Intracranial Pressure*, 5.5). Treat hypertension that may be causing AMS.
- Identify and treat hypoglycemia.
- Identify and treat seizure activity.
- Normalize body temperature.
- Identify other potentially reversible, life-threatening causes (*e.g.* epidural or subdural hematoma; raised ICP) by early brain imaging.
- Obtain CSF if there is no contraindication and infection is suspected. Contraindications to LP include: raised ICP, coagulopathy, infection of overlying skin at the LP site. If CSF examination is essential in these situations, neurosurgical consultation should be considered. If the patient is unstable, LP should be postponed and antibiotic therapy should be given empirically.

Imaging should not delay securing the airway, resuscitation of circulation or treatment of hypoglycemia when indicated. Laboratory studies are guided by the history and physical findings.

Key findings and interventions. Historical and physical clues guide laboratory and radiologic evaluation and treatment priorities (**Boxes 5.1.2, 5.1.7 and 5.1.10**).

Evaluate cortical function: The Glasgow Coma Scale (GCS; modified from Teasdale and Jennet; **Box 5.1.3**):

- The GCS was created to categorize arousal in TBI in adults
- The best score achievable at a given time is the designated score.
- Scores ≤ 8 indicate coma and the need for tracheal intubation.
- Simple and reproducible.
- Important alterations (*e.g.* lethargy) are not reflected in the score.
- Separate scores for each category may enhance usefulness (*e.g.* E3, V4, M5 = 12); if an ETT interferes with verbal assessment, the score is modified: E3, V1T, M5 = 9T.

Box 5.1.3   Glasgow Coma Score

Activity	Score	6 mos to 2 yrs	>2 yrs
Eye opening	4	Spontaneous	Spontaneous
	3	To speech/sound	To speech
	2	To pain	To pain
	1	None	None
Best Auditory/ Verbal Response	5	Smiles, listens, follows (interacts)	Oriented
	4	Cries but consolable	Confused
	3	Inappropriate, persistent cry	Inappropriate words
	2	Agitated; restless	Incomprehensible words
	1	None	None
Best Motor Response	6	—	Obeys commands
	5	Localizes pain	Localizes pain
	4	Withdraws from pain	Withdraws from pain
	3	Abnormal flexion	Abnormal flexion
	2	Abnormal extension	Abnormal extension
	1	None	None
Best Total score		14	15

- Alternatively, the descriptive "**AVPU**" (alert, responds to voice, responsive to pain, unresponsive) assessment may be used.

Note: Flexion withdrawal mediated by spinal and brainstem reflexes (*e.g.* stereotypic "triple flexion" at the hip, knee and ankle with toe pinch) should not be confused with purposeful withdrawal. Other alterations in muscle tone are characteristically evoked at various levels of brain function (**Boxes 5.1.4**). The sensory examination may be

Box 5.1.4   Clinical Significance of Disturbances of Muscle Tone

- **Decorticate posturing:** Cortical or diencephalic dysfunction
- **Decerebrate posturing:** Midbrain or pontine dysfunction
- **Hypertonicity:** Corticospinal dysfunction
- **Flaccidity or hypotonicity:** Pontine, medullary or spinal cord dysfunction

limited to the response to tactile stimuli, including observed changes in HR, BP and pupillary size.

Evaluate the Brainstem. Pupillary reactivity to light (CN II, III, the retina and autonomic fibers to intrinsic pupillary muscles): Asymmetry or lack of reactivity should prompt urgent evaluation. A unilateral fixed, dilated pupil indicates ipsilateral CN III paralysis consistent with uncal herniation (*Raised Intracranial Pressure, 5.5*). Anisocoria may also result from seizures, congenital anomalies, ocular trauma, surgery and exposure to certain medications (*e.g.* tropicamide; contamination from a scopolamine patch).

Pupils fixed in mid-position are seen in midbrain lesions. Loss of reactivity can also be seen in intoxications, hypothermia ($\leq 29°C$), anticholinergic exposure (*e.g.* atropine). Fundoscopy: Assess for hemorrhage, venous pulsations, papilledema, and exudates.

Extraocular movements: Note the ability to track. For comatose patients without c-spine injury, assess the doll's eyes maneuver (CN III, IV, VI); If the neck cannot be rotated, or there is no response to the doll's eyes maneuver, the oculovestibular reflex (ice water calorics; CN III, IV, VI, VIII) should be assessed if the tympanic membrane is visibly intact and there is no CSF leak: instill ice water (60 mL) into an unobstructed external auditory canal; the head and upper body should be elevated 30° from the horizontal (**Boxes 5.1.5 and 5.1.6**).

Corneal reflex (CN V,VII): Absence of a bilateral blink response indicates impairment of these CN's and the brainstem between their nuclei. Impairment or absence of the gag reflex (CN IX, X), cough

---

Box 5.1.5   Interpretation of Response to Ice Water Calorics

Ipsilateral tonic eye deviation ("toward ice") *with* contralateral nystagmus (fast component away from ice)	Normal response in awake patient
Ipsilateral tonic eye deviation ("eyes toward ice") *without* nystagmus	Cortical dysfunction (not awake) with intact brainstem
None	Brainstem not intact

Box 5.1.6   Eye Findings Useful in Diagnosis of AMS

Conjugate horizontal nystagmus; Transient or vertical dysconjugate gaze; Ocular bobbing	Metabolic encephalopathies; Neuroblastoma
Fixed dysconjugate gaze; Rotary nystagmus	Structural lesions; focal dysfunction
Bilateral downward gaze ("setting sun sign")	Raised ICP
Transient conjugate gaze	Seizure, usually
Fixed conjugate gaze	Contralateral pontine lesion

Box 5.1.7   Suggested Initial Laboratory Evaluation of Patients with AMS of Unknown Cause

- ABG, carboxyhemoglobin
- Glucose
- Electrolytes, urea nitrogen, creatinine
- Calcium, Mg, phosphorus
- CBC, PT, PTT, fibrinogen
- Liver enzymes, liver function tests, ammonia
- EEG

- 12-lead ECG
- Urine drug screen; consider gastric aspirate for drug screen
- Acetaminophen, aspirin and ethanol levels
- Head CT
- Lumbar puncture
- Chest and abdominal plain films
- Additional metabolic studies to R/O inborn metabolic errors if indicated

---

reflex (CN X), and shoulder shrug (CN XI) indicate progressively lower brainstem dysfunction. Swallowing is impaired with bilateral CN XII dysfunction. Formal apnea testing is indicated when brain death is suspected (*Brain Death, 5.7*).

Delirium is acute brain dysfunction characterized by wakefulness with abnormal fluctuation in the content of thought, manifested by impaired cognition and memory. While this disturbance may occur as

---

Box 5.1.8   Delirium: Three Clinical Types

- **Hypoactive delirium:** Apathy; ↓ responsiveness, social withdrawal, psychomotor retardation; may be difficult to recognize. This may be the most common type.
- **Hyperactive delirium:** Agitation, hallucinations, restlessness, emotional lability; this type is the least common but usually most readily recognized.
- **Mixed delirium:** Hypo- and hyper-active features
- **Common features:** Inability to focus, shift or maintain attention; disorientation; inappropriate speech; disturbed sleep

---

Box 5.1.9   Management of Delirium in Pediatric Patients

- Treat underlying medical risk factors.
- Age-appropriate cognitive stimulation.
- Consistent non-pharmacologic sleep.
- Restoration of circadian rhythm with light and noise control.
- Family presence; pictures of familiar people and objects.
- Provide familiar music and objects.
- Exercise and early mobilization.
- Removal of medical devices as soon as appropriate.
- Provide baseline sensory support devices such as eye glasses and hearing aids.
- Minimize unnecessary exposure to neurotropic agents.
- Consult a clinical psychiatrist if pharmacologic therapy is necessary.
- Minimize doses of anti-psychotic agents if these are warranted.

---

a presenting problem (*e.g.* after medication or toxin exposure), it demands attention most frequently because of its occurrence among critically ill ICU patients. When delirium develops in the latter setting, the term "ICU psychosis" has been used. Current data are derived primarily from its common occurrence among adult ICU patients (40–80%), in whom it is associated with increased morbidity

---

Box 5.1.10   Pearls

- Remember the causes of AMS: "VITAMINS-P": Vascular, Infectious, Toxins, Accidents, Metabolic, Intussusception, Neoplasm, Seizure, Psychiatric.
- Consider empiric treatment for infectious causes in each case, including administration of acyclovir for possible Herpes simplex encephalitis.
- Avoid use of drugs that further alter the mental status.
- Consider prophylactic anticonvulsant drugs when appropriate.
- R/O raised ICP as a cause of hypertension.
- Hypertension may occur secondary to seizures, but may also be the cause of seizures or AMS.
- Post-ictal impairment of consciousness for >1 hr should prompt investigation for a cause other than primary seizure (*e.g.* meningitis, head trauma). Also consider non-convulsive status epilepticus, the effects of sedative drugs (*e.g.* benzodiazepines, barbiturates) or behavioral problems (*e.g.* pseudo-seizures).
- Drooling may be a sign of inability to protect the airway and may signal the need for tracheal intubation.
- Consider pediatric neurology consultation.
- Psychiatric disease in children with AMS is typically a diagnosis of exclusion.
- Treatment of delirium in pediatric ICU patients includes treatment of the underlying illness and restoration of a more physiologic physical as well as neurochemical environment. Consultation with individuals trained in the use of pediatric psychotropic medications should be considered.

---

and mortality. Delirium is suspected to be common among children as well. Lack of validation of age-appropriate tools for diagnosis of delirium by the non-psychiatrically trained has challenged progress in its recognition and treatment. However, study in this area is underway (The Pediatric Confusion Assessment Method for the ICU; Smith ABH *et al.*, Delirium: An emerging frontier in the management of critically ill children, *Crit Care Clin* **25**:593–614, 2009). See **Boxes 5.1.8, 5.1.9 and 5.1.10**.

In addition to environmental factors, neurotransmitter (NT) imbalance generated by a primary illness or medications has been implicated as the cause of delirium. Key points include:

• Hypoactive or mixed delirium: possibly attributable to dopamine deficiency; in adults, this has been treated with atypical antipsychotic agents (first choice agents; *e.g.* risperidone); acetylcholinesterase inhibitors (*e.g.* donepazil) and serotonin antagonists (*e.g.* ondansetron) are alternatives.

• Hyperactive delirium: attributed to hyper-stimulation of central dopamine receptors; in adults, dopaminergic blockade (*e.g.* haloperidol, risperidone, olanzipine, ziprazidone) is recommended. A baseline ECG is important to monitor for QT_c prolongation prior to or during treatment.

• Gamma-aminobutyric acid (inhibitory NT) may lead to unpredictable neurotransmission. Benzodiazepines and propofol (GABA agonists) have been implicated as causes of delirium in the ICU.

• Anticholinergic agents (anti-cholinergic excess and acetylcholine deficiency) are associated with delirium.

• Additional biochemical factors include inflammatory mediators, hypoxia, shock and electrolyte imbalance.

• Iatrogenic factors include sleep deprivation, lorezepam and midazolam exposure, and social alienation.

Among adults, delirium is associated with prolonged mechanical ventilation and hospital stay, inadvertent removal of tubes/catheters, failed extubation, increased hospital cost and mortality rate. Long-term cognitive impairment and post-traumatic stress disorder may be linked to delirium during an ICU stay.

5.2 Status Epilepticus (SE)

Generalized motor or convulsive SE is the presence of recurrent or enduring abnormal neuronal discharges in the brain lasting greater than 10 mins in a child under 5 yrs, or greater than 5 mins in a child over 5 yrs of age. Predominant causes vary with age group (**Box 5.2.1**). Generalized repeated seizures of all motor types (**Box 5.2.2**) are most

---

Box 5.2.1   Common Causes of Convulsive SE in Different Age Groups

Neonatal	Hypoxemia/ischemia, low birth weight, intracranial hemorrhage, metabolic imbalances, cerebral anomalies, central nervous system infections
<1 yr	Fever greater than 38.4°C and acute symptomatic seizure (CNS disease or systemic imbalance predisposing to seizure)
1–2 yrs	Prolonged febrile seizures
>4 yrs	Remote symptomatic seizure (prior CNS abnormality that predisposes to seizure) or cryptogenic seizure (no abnormalities that predispose to seizure)
Considerations in all ages	Infection, trauma, acute intracranial event (*e.g.* hemorrhage), metabolic disturbance (*e.g.* hypoglycemia, hyponatremia, hypocalcemia, hypomagnesemia), hypertension, remote or progressive CNS disease, inadequate ACD levels or ACD intoxication; poisoning or drug overdose.

Box 5.2.2   Primary Generalized Motor Seizure Types Leading to SE

- Tonic-clonic (**Fig. 5.2.1.** EEG of Generalized Motor SE; compare to **Fig. 5.2.2**, Normal EEG)
  - ▸ Tonic phase: 10–30 secs of flexion of neck/trunk/extremities then extension of trunk/extremities
  - ▸ Clonic phase: 30–50 secs of rhythmic jerks
- Clonic: one to several minutes of motor jerks
- Myoclonic: very brief, very rapid jerks of trunk or extremities (on EEG ≅ 350 msec discharges/contractions)
- Tonic: prolonged extension of trunk/neck
- Atonic: sudden loss of tone

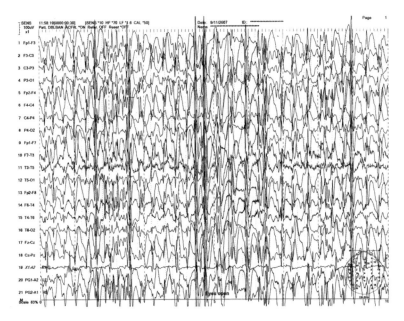

Fig. 5.2.1.   EEG Showing Generalized Status Epilepticus.

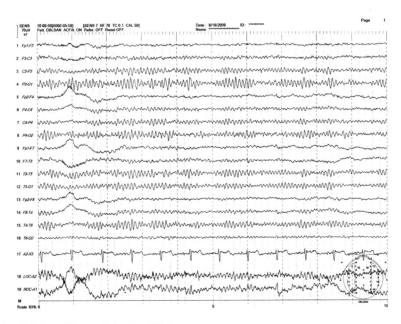

Fig. 5.2.2.   Normal Awake EEG.

Box 5.2.3   Systemic Effects of Convulsive SE

- Secretions accumulate in upper airway and coordination of glottis with ventilatory efforts may be impaired.
- Central control of breathing is variable; hypoxemia may occur in up to 2/3 of patients and $PaCO_2$ may increase to ≥ 60 mmHg range during SE.
- Hormonal release from adrenal glands result in hypertension during initial 30 mins of GCSE but thereafter blood pressure may fall.
- Cerebral autoregulation is impaired during SE.
- Fever in excess of 102°F may be generated during SE.
- Brain glucose utilization may increase by a multiple of six in first hour of SE.

---

likely to result in hippocampal injury; this is associated with abnormalities in memory, learning and behavior. Convulsive SE is often accompanied by several systemic effects (**Box 5.2.3**).

Seizures are characterized as either "complex" (associated with loss of consciousness) or "simple" (preserved consciousness). Seizure activity originating from one cerebral hemisphere is characterized as a "partial" or "focal" seizure; a seizure that involves both cerebral hemispheres is "generalized". Seizures may begin as focal and generalize secondarily.

Overall mortality in pediatric SE is approximately 3% but rises to 20% in acute symptomatic disease with refractory SE (*i.e.* persistent seizures despite at least two drugs administered in adequate doses). Mortality in both adults and children appears to be less when SE lasts < 30 mins *vs.* > 30 mins (2.6 *vs.* 19% mortality). Following non-febrile convulsive SE 34–43% may develop epilepsy and 10–34% may exhibit neuro-developmental deterioration.

Nonconvulsive SE (NCSE) is a cognitive or behavioral change without a motor component lasting for at least 30 mins. Seizure activity should be suspected whenever unexplained motor activity, change in vital signs or alteration in awareness/responsiveness occurs. Outcome depends upon NCSE seizure type (**Box 5.2.4**).

Box 5.2.4   Types of Nonconvulsive Seizures Leading to NCSE

- Absence SE (ASE): blank stare and blinking then return to previous activity; EEG discharges at 3 Hz; this form NCSE is likely to be benign.
- Atypical ASE is frequently occurs in Lennox– Gastaut or myocloinc epilepsy and associated with neurodevelopmental deterioration afterward.
- Partial-complex: aura, behavioral arrest or lateralization of eyes followed by cycles of altered awareness and myoclonic jerks. Automatic motor movements: grimacing, blinking, laughing, crying, bicycling of legs is especially prevalent in older age groups; typically associated with brain malformations or following HIE; EEG shows focal discharges frequently in temporal lobes before generalization. This form of NCSE may affect memory, cognitive ability and may be associated with recurrence of seizures.
- NCSE in critically ill children: coma and unresponsiveness are primary indications for continuous EEG (cEEG) which is diagnostic in detecting subclinical seizures. In adults this form of NCSE is associated with 30–90% mortality.
- NCSE in children with learning difficulties includes electrical SE during sleep, atypical ASE and tonic SE.
- Autonomic SE presents with ictal emesis, pallor or flushing or cyanosis, pupillary changes, thermoregulatory alterations, brief apnea or brief cardiac asystole.

Anticonvulsant drug (ACD) therapy is indicated for all patients with SE. Most episodes of SE are readily identifiable; a high index of suspicion is necessary to distinguish NCSE from a post-ictal state (**Box 5.2.5**). EEG is indicated if NCSE is suspected.

Seizures during the **neonatal period** (usually defined up to 30 days) are often subtle. Typically they cannot be provoked by external stimuli or suppressed by gentle restraint. Frequently neonatal seizures fall into one of several catagories: focal clonic, focal tonic, generalized tonic, myoclonic, spasms or automatisms. Movements that can be provoked by external stimuli or suppressed by gentle restraint that

Box 5.2.5   Anticipated Duration of Post-Ictal State Based on Type of Seizure

Seizure	Median Recovery Time (hrs)	Upper Range of Time to Full Recovery (hrs)
Febrile	0.3	9.0
Idiopathic	1.35	13.2
Remote Symptomatic	1.25	12.1
Acute Symptomatic	4.6	17.0
Treated with benzodiazepine	3.5	14.3
No benzodiazepine	0.5	17.0

Box 5.2.6   Key Points in Searching for Cause of Neonatal Seizures

History: Identify risk factors

- Hypoxemia/ischemia: when hypoxemia/ischemia is moderately severe, muscle tone, Moro, suck and grasp reflexes may be decreased and apnea occurs; seizures often occur within the first 24 hrs of life.
- Infections: meningitis, encephalitis, sepsis from group B streptococcus, Escherichia coli, Herpes, Toxoplasmosis, Cytomegalovirus, Syphilis, Rubella
- Hypoglycemia, hypocalcemia, inborn error of metabolism
- Drug withdrawal or intoxication
- Intracranial hemorrhage
- Genetic/congenital/neurodegenerative disorders
- Benign neonatal or familial neonatal convulsions

Physical examination

- Heart rate changes or apnea make it more likely seizure is ongoing
- Assessment of tone, reflex symmetry (tonic neck, Moro, root, suck), and search for muscle twitching that may be palpable but not visible.
- Fontanelle (bulging with ↑ICP), fundi (look for retinal hemorrhages) and lens (note cataracts)
- Skin: Sturge-Weber, neurofibromatosis, tuberous sclerosis, herpes vesicles, incontinentia pigmenti
- Cranial bruit (AVM)
- Odors: See *Inborn Errors of Metabolism, 6.5; Box 6.5.5.*

Box 5.2.7   Bedside Approach to Treatment of Neonatal Seizure Activity*

A–B–C–D's

- Airway: clear secretions, foreign bodies and vomitus; rotate head/body to side if emesis occurs; position, secure airway as needed.
- Breathing: apply supplemental O_2; during first 1–3 mins of SE hypopnea may occur and supplemental O_2 may be all that is needed; keep Pox >95%.
- Circulation: hypotension may occur after first 30 min of seizure but always search for other causes of hypotension
- Dextrose: beside glucose <50 mg/dL: D10 W 2 ml/kg IV/IO (*Hypo- and Hyperglycemia, 6.4*)

Rapid History for:

- Prior seizure activity or ACD therapy, baseline motor function and consciousness, pertinent perinatal issues, past adverse drug reactions
- Ongoing event described along with history of current illness, medications or trauma

Interventions for Seizure Activity:

- Obtain vascular access, electrolytes, BUN, creatinine, liver function tests, calcium, magnesium, phosphate, complete blood count, arterial blood gas, toxicology panel, ACD levels and cultures as indicated.
- Begin anticonvulsant (and antibiotic and antipyretic) therapies as indicated.
- Traditional ACD therapy:
  - ▶ 1st tier: Phenobarbital loading: 20 mg/kg IV/IO and pyridoxine 100 mg IV push
  - ▶ 2nd tier: Phenytoin loading: 20 mg/kg IV/IO or fosphenytoin (phenytoin equivalents) 20 mg/kg IV/IO/IM.
  - ▶ IM loading of phenobartital or fosphenytoin is for non-emergent loading only.
  - ▶ 3rd tier: Diazepam: 0.25 mg/kg IV/IO or 0.5 mg/kg PR

*Adapted from Novotny WE, Perkin RM. Tremors vs. Seizures: Recognizing and Managing Seizures in Children. *Pediatr Emerg Med Reports* 8:112–122, 2003.

Box 5.2.8   Bedside Approach to Pediatric Generalized Convulsive Status Epilepticus (SE)*

A–B–C–D's

- Airway: suction/position/secure as needed
- Breathing: supplemental oxygen to achieve Pox >95%
- Circulation: ECG monitor, perfusion assessment and blood pressure evaluation
- Dextrose: if low (<60 mg/dL) treat with 2 ml/kg of 25% dextrose to maximum of 25 gm. Maintain glucose in 80–150 mg/dl range.
- Seizures: record awareness, responsiveness, motor activity and vital signs
- Rapid bedside history

    ▶ Prior seizures or ACD, baseline neurocognitive function, allergies or adverse reactions to medications

    ▶ Chief complaint: describe event, acute illness, trauma, medications.

- Interventions for status epilepticus

    ▶ Obtain vascular access and send electrolytes, BUN, creatinine, liver function tests, calcium, magnesium, phosphate, complete blood count, arterial blood gas, toxicology panel, ACD levels and cultures as indicated.

    ▶ Begin anticonvulsant (and antibiotic and antipyretic) therapies as indicated

    ▶ ACD for generalized tonic-clonic SE

        ▪ Prehospital therapy:

        Diazepam PR: 2–5 yrs, 0.5 mg/kg; 6–11 yrs 0.3 mg/kg; >12 yrs 0.2 mg/kg **or**
        Midazolam intranasal: <50 kg 0.2 mg/kg to max 5 mg; >50 kg 0.2 mg/kg to max 10 mg

        ▪ 1st tier therapy: Lorazepam (0.1 mg/kg to max 4 mg IV/IO)
        ▪ 2nd tier therapy: Phenytoin (20–30 mg/kg) or fosphenytoin (20–30 mg/kg phenytoin equivalents) IV/IO. Note that IM use is for non-emergent loading only.

(Continued)

Box 5.2.8   Bedside Approach to Pediatric Generalized Convulsive Status Epilepticus SE* (Continued)

- Seizure >10 mins after phenytoin or fosphenytoin: give levetiracetam 20–30 mg/kg IV at 5 mg/kg/min up to max of 3 gm or valproic acid 20 mg/kg at 5 mg/kg/min
- Seizure >5 mins after levetiracetam or valproic acid give phenobarbital 30 mg/kg IV/IO (may need to secure airway)
- Seizure >10 mins after phenobarbital: give midazolam (0.2 mg per kg up to max 10 mg bolus then 1–18 mcg/kg/min continuous IV) or pentobarbital load of 5 mg/kg followed by 1–3 mg/kg/hr with goal of "burst suppression" (50% burst/50% suppression) for 24 hrs before weaning; monitor EEG continuously or at least 3 times/day (**Fig. 5.2.3**, Burst Suppression).
- Other considerations: Topiramate, ketamine, ACTH and rarely pyridoxine

* Adapted from Novotny WE, Perkin RM. Tremors vs. Seizures: Recognizing and Managing Seizures in Children. *Pediatr Emerg Med Reports* **8**: 112–122, 2003.

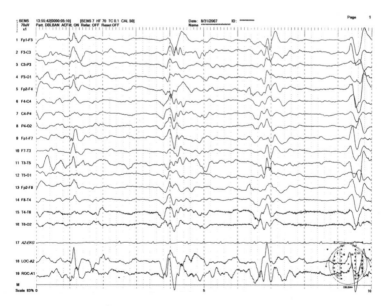

Fig. 5.2.3.   Burst Suppression EEG.

Box 5.2.9   Treatment of Non-Convulsive Status Epilepticus (NCSE)*

Absence SE (ASE)	Clobazam (po), benzodiazepine, valproic acid (IV)
Atypical ASE	Benzodiazepine, acetazolamide, or valproate (IV)
Complex partial SE	Benzodiazepine followed by phenytoin or valproate (IV)
NCSE in children with learning disabilities	Clobazam (po), steroids (po), surgery (multiple subpial transections)
NCSE in coma	Treat as for generalized tonic-clonic SE
Myoclonic SE	Benzodiazepine (IV)

---

* Adapted from Novotny WE, Perkin RM. Tremors vs. Seizures: Recognizing and Managing Seizures in children. *Pediatr Emerg Med Reports* **8**:112–122, 2003.

may be epileptic include generalized tonic movements or automatisms. An EEG may be helpful to distinguish seizure from non-seizure. Key points in identifying the cause of neonatal seizures (**Box 5.2.6**) and the approach to treatment are summarized (**Box 5.2.7**). The approaches to treatment of pediatric SE (**Box 5.2.8**) and NCSE (**Box 5.2.9**) are summarized.

5.3   Hypoxic-Ischemic Encephalopathy (HIE)

HIE refers to brain injury resulting from inadequate oxygen delivery to the brain. Ischemic injury occurs when normal cerebral blood flow (CBF; 50–75 mL/100 g brain tissue/min) falls to less than approximately 18 mL/100g/min causing energy failure. The extent of injury depends upon the severity and duration of ischemia, and whether the insult is global or focal. The most common cause of HIE in post-natal pediatric patients is respiratory failure from any cause leading to cardiopulmonary arrest (CPA). The chief cause of CPA in adults is ventricular fibrillation; by contrast, children are more likely to arrest from asphyxia, after insults from hypoxemia, hypercarbia, acidosis and hypotension have already disrupted the metabolic environment. Post-arrest outcomes are worse among pediatric patients as compared to adults; however, the response of the immature brain to hypoxic-ischemic injury may be more amenable to modification than the adult brain.

During asphyxia (**Fig. 5.3.1**), neuronal O_2 stores are depleted within 30 secs, and ATP and glucose are depleted within 5 mins. However, ischemia up to 10–15 mins may be followed by restoration of ATP during reperfusion. Selected areas of increased vulnerability to hypoxia change with age:

• Infant: diencephalon, hippocampus, midbrain
• Older child and adults: cerebral cortex, hippocampus, Purkinje layer of the cerebellum

During arrest, CBF may be absent or relatively preserved (low flow) by effective chest compressions. Post-arrest CBF is phasic, and varies among brain regions:

• Multifocal no re-flow
• Global hyperemia (transient)
• Delayed hypoperfusion (may last hours to days)
• Restoration of normal flow

During periods of hyperemia and delayed hypoperfusion (secondary injury) biochemical cascades set in motion by inadequate cerebral perfusion advance the primary injury and may lead to either apoptosis ("programmed cell death": requires energy; associated with minimal inflammation) or necrosis (results from more immediate energy failure; associated with marked inflammation). The evolution of secondary injury may occur over as long as 7 days (**Fig. 5.3.1**). Early imaging (head CT) may be normal despite severe hypoxic-ischemic insult, but should be obtained to identify confounding problems.

Minimizing injury during this secondary phase by optimizing CBF and O_2 delivery, minimizing factors that would exacerbate

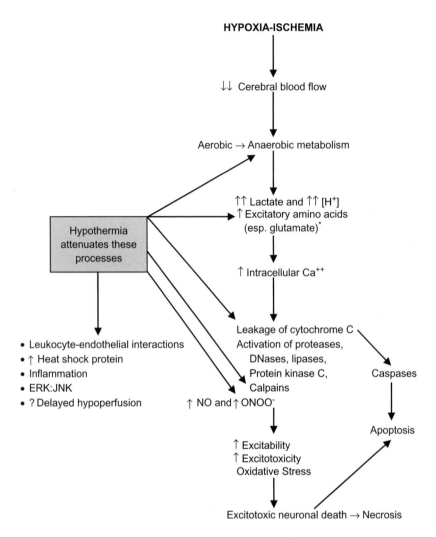

Fig. 5.3.1   Schematic of Pathophysiology in Global Hypoxic-ischemic Encephalopathy.   *Via N-methyl-D-aspartate (NMDA), and alpha-amino-3-hydroxy-5-methyl-4-isoxazole-proprionate, which activate Kainate receptors. ERK, extracellular signal-regulating kinases; JNK, c-JUN NH2 terminal kinases; NO, nitric oxide; ONOO⁻, peroxynitrite.

Box 5.3.1 Therapeutic Goals in HIE

- Maintain normal oxygenation and $PaCO_2$ (35–40 torr). Avoid hyperventilation (causes cerebral vasoconstriction and may promote decreased CBF); avoid hypoventilation (causes cerebral vasodilatation and may lead to increased ICP).
- Maintain BP in the upper range of normal for age.
- Maintain glucose in the 80–150 mg/dL range; hyperglycemia accentuates brain injury.
- Avoid temperatures above normal; cerebral metabolic rate ↑s by 6–7% per degree Celsius. Consider controlled hypothermia in appropriate patients (see text below).
- Treat seizures aggressively if they occur.
- Maintain normal electrolyte balance; avoid hyponatremia, which may exacerbate brain swelling.
- Correct acid-base disturbances.
- Correct clinically significant anemia and coagulopathy.
- Identify and treat infection.
- Provide nutritional support as soon as appropriate.
- Characterize prognosis when possible.

---

increases in ICP, and creating a healthy metabolic environment is the focus of critical supportive care (**Box 5.3.1**). This phase also offers opportunity for future therapeutic interventions.

Prediction of Outcome in HIE (Box 5.3.2). Characterization of prognosis in patients with HIE is among the most common reasons for pediatric neurology consultation in the PICU, and is important for decision-making for physicians and families, and appropriate resource allocation. Data interpretation is confounded since definitions of "good" or "poor" neurologic prognosis vary among studies. A combination of historical data (duration of insult), physical findings, neurologic testing and imaging are used to help assess prognosis. No absolute outcome predictions can be made based on data currently available. See **Box 5.3.3**.

Box 5.3.2   Factors Associated with a High Positive Predictive Value (%) for Poor Neurologic Outcome in Pediatric HIE

- CPR >10–15 mins (90–100)
- Data at ≥24 hrs after insult:

  ▸ GCS <3–5 (90–100)
  ▸ Absence of brainstem reflexes and motor response to painful stimuli (90–100)
  ▸ Bilateral absence of somatosensory evoked potential (EP) at the primary sensory cortical location (N20) not attributable to peripheral or brainstem signal disruption (90–100)
  ▸ Discontinuous, silent or nonreactive EEG (50–100)
  ▸ Brain diffusion weighted MRI revealing watershed and basal ganglia or brainstem injury (80–100 and 100, respectively)

Limitations in the application of these data include small sample sizes and the need for study interpretation. Accuracy is improved as the time interval between hypoxic-ischemic injury and testing is increased (*e.g.* several days).

Box 5.3.3   Pearls

- Hypoxia without ischemia is better tolerated than hypoxia associated with hypotension or reduced perfusion.
- Post hypoxic-ischemic seizures do not contribute to prognosis.
- Hypoxia may lead to dysfunction of other organs which may influence neurologic performance (*e.g.* hepatic dysfunction may prolong the effects of sedative medications).
- The difference between a good outcome and a poor outcome may vary among families, patients and care-givers; these perceptions may change over time.

Therapeutic Hypothermia (Fig. 5.3.1). The International Liaison Committee on Resuscitation recommends that therapeutic hypothermia (32–34°C) be provided for adults who remain comatose after out-of-hospital non-traumatic ventricular arrhythmia-induced CPA. Hypothermia in the range of 33–34°C has been used with success in asphyxiated newborns, particularly those with mild to moderate rather than severe injury. Therapeutic hypothermia may be of benefit in pediatric patients with HIE with the following considerations:

- The optimal timing, depth, duration and method of cooling are not known.
- Overcooling (<32°C) is associated with potentially fatal arrhythmias and requires expertise to be prevented.
- Coagulopathy (mild) and immune suppression may occur; pancreatic, renal, metabolic and endocrinologic abnormalities also have been reported.
- Cooling may be accompanied by an increase in persistent vegetative state among survivors.

5.4 CNS Infections and Acute Disseminated Encephalomyelitis (ADEM)

This group of diseases involves invasion of the CNS by bacteria, viruses, fungi or parasites associated with an inflammatory response. Entry of an infectious agent into the CNS occurs either directly from a contiguous site or via the bloodstream. Meningitis is the inflammation of the pia-arachnoid and CSF, and is characterized by CSF pleocytosis. In the absence of obstruction to CSF flow, the entire cerebrospinal axis is involved. Viral encephalitis refers to virus-mediated inflammation of brain parenchyma causing brain dysfunction without meningeal involvement; meningoencephalitis involves the meninges as well. Cerebritis denotes brain parenchymal involvement caused by bacteria, fungus or parasites. In post-infectious encephalitis (ADEM) a response to a systemic infection (usually viral) or rarely, a vaccine, presents with acute demyelinating inflammation involving the brain and spinal cord.

Box 5.4.1   Key Clinical Findings in Meningitis and Encephalitis

- Fever (not always present)
- Irritability
- Poor feeding; vomiting
- Altered mental status
- Meningeal signs in meningitis: stiff neck, Kernig and Brudzinski signs

- Photophobia
- Headache
- Focal neurologic findings
- Apnea (esp. neonates)
- Seizures (more common in encephalitis than in meningitis)

CNS infections in an immunocompromised host may be devoid of the clinical signs of inflammation, significantly altering the presentation and CSF findings. Also, inflammation without infection may occur (*e.g.* vasculitis involving the CNS or drug-related meningeal inflammation).

Diagnosis of meningitis and encephalitis/meningoencephalitis is made by clinical presentation (**Box 5.4.1**) and CSF analysis (**Box 5.4.2**); brain imaging may be helpful, particularly in encephalitis when CSF may be normal. Optimally, blood and CSF cultures should be obtained before antibiotic therapy is given. If there is difficulty obtaining these promptly, or if imaging is required prior to lumbar puncture (*Lumbar Puncture, 15.5*), administration of empiric antibiotic therapy takes precedence over obtaining CSF for culture. Except for *N. meningitidis*, bacteria in the CSF are usually recoverable for several hours after the first dose of antibiotics. CSF cell counts, glucose and protein usually remain abnormal for days. See **Box 5.4.3** for recommendations for re-evalution of CSF during treatment. See **Box 5.4.7** for "pearls".

Common causative agents and empiric antibiotic therapies in bacterial meningitis:

Neonates (<4 weeks): *Streptococcus agalactiae* (GBS), *E. coli, Listeria monocytogenes, Klebsiella sp.*: ampicillin + cefotaxime or ampicillin + gentamicin (or other aminoglycoside)

Infants (1–23 mos): *Streptococcus pneumoniae, Neisseria meningitides,* GBS, *H. influenza, E. coli*: vancomycin + (cefotaxime or ceftriaxone)

Box 5.4.2   Typical CSF Findings in Selected CNS Infections* and ADEM

	WBC/mm³ (Predominant cells)	Glucose	Protein
Bacterial meningitis*	>100 (Neutrophils)	↓↓	↑↑
Viral meningitis/ meningoencephalitis	N to <100 (Lymphocytes)	N to Slightly ↓	N to Slightly ↑
Herpes simplex encephalitis or meningoencephalitis**	N to ↑ (Lymphocytes)	N to ↓	N to ↑
M. tuberculosis meningitis[†]	>100 (Lymphocytes)	↓↓	↑
Rocky Mountain Spotted Fever with encephalitis	N to <100 (Neutrophils *or* Lymphocytes)	N	N to ↑
ADEM[‡]	N to ↑	N	N to ↑

* Gram stain is positive in 80–90% of untreated cases of bacterial meningitis.
** Red blood cells are increased in ~50% of patients with HSV CNS infection.
[†] Thick enhancement of the brain base is characteristic on head CT.
[‡] RBC's may be present. N, Normal; ↑, increased; ↑↑, very increased; ↓, decreased; ↓↓, very decreased; ADEM, acute disseminated encephalomyelitis.

Box 5.4.3   Recommendations for Repeating Lumbar Puncture in 24–48 hrs After Initiation of Therapy

- If there is failure to improve clinically.
- When there is infection with resistant pneumococci or Gram negative organisms.
- Some experts include "all neonates" with meningitis because delayed sterilization is common and clinical progress may be difficult to assess in this age group.

Children (>2 yrs): *N. meningitides, S. pneumonia*: vancomycin + (cefotaxime or ceftriaxone)

Patients with **VP or VA Shunts**: *Staphylococcus sp.*; Gram negative organisms: vancomycin + (cefepime or ceftazidime or meropenem)

Patients with **basilar skull fracture**: Gram positive and Gram negative organisms: vancomycin + (ceftriaxone or cefotaxime)

Chemoprophylaxis is indicated for close contacts of patients with invasive meningococcal disease and unimmunized household, daycare and nursery contacts of patients with *H. influenza type b* (Hib) invasive disease.

Dexamethasone decreases hearing loss in patients with Hib meningitis, and is recommended for patients >6 weeks of age with Hib meningitis and should be considered for patients >6 weeks with pneumococcal meningitis. Dexamethasone is most effective if given 15–20 mins before or simultaneously with the first dose of antibiotic. The risks of steroid administration should be weighed against its benefits when the cause of the infection is not yet known. Human immunoglobulin should be considered in neonates and others in whom the immune response may be blunted.

Aseptic Meningitis/Meningoencephalitis. This refers to CSF pleocytosis with or without encephalitis and absence of a pathogen from routine bacterial culture of CSF prior to treatment with antibiotics. The causative agents are usually viral; enteroviruses are the most common, followed by herpes simplex and adenovirus. Enteroviral and herpesvirus infections can be diagnosed by polymerase chain reaction (PCR) in CSF; adenovirus is diagnosed by culture or serology. Arboviruses tend to occur in late summer or early fall in the United States, but may occur throughout the year in the south; these are typically diagnosed serologically. Other causes of aseptic meningitis or meningoencephalitis should be considered since specific therapy may be indicated (**Box 5.4.4**). Empiric treatment with acyclovir along with appropriate antibacterial agents is indicated in all cases of encephalitis and meningoencephalitis until these most common and treatable pathogens can be ruled out.

Herpes Simplex Virus (HSV) Encephalitis. Herpes simplex viruses are the most common and most lethal of the viral encephalitides, and

Box 5.4.4   Causes of Aseptic Meningitis Requiring Specific Anti-microbial Therapy

Agents/Diseases	Suggested Treatment
Bacteria	
• *B. henselae* (Cat scratch disease)	Azithromycin or Doxycycline + Rifampin
• *Borrelia burgdorferi* (Lyme disease)	Ceftriaxone
• Brucellosis	Doxycycline + Rifampin + TMP-SMX
• *C. trachomatis*	Doxycycline or Erythromycin
• Ehrlichiosis	Doxycycline
• Leptospirosis	Penicillin; Doxycycline; Ceftriaxone
• *M. tuberculosis*	Usual phase I drugs: Isoniazid + Rifampin + Pyrazinamide + Streptomycin or Ethambutol
• *Mycoplasma*	Erythromucin; Azithromycin; Clarithromycin
• *Rickettsia* (RMSF)	Doxycycline
• *Treponema pallidum* (Syphilis)	Penicillin G; Ceftriaxone
Fungi	
• *Aspergillus*	Voriconazole
• *Blastomyces*	Liposomal Amphotericin B followed by an azole
• *Candida* spp.	Liposomal Amphotericin B + Flucytosine
• *Cryptococcus neoformans*	Amphotericin B
• *Coccidioides immitis*	Amphotericin B
• Histoplasmosis	Liposomal Amphotericin B followed by itraconazole

(Continued)

Box 5.4.4   Causes of Aseptic Meningitis Requiring Specific Anti-microbial Therapy (Continued)

Agents	Suggested Treatment
Parasites	
• Toxoplasmosis	Pyrimethamine + Sulfadiazine or TMP-SMX
• *Entamoeba histolytica*	Metronidazole
• *Trichinella*	Mebendazole + Steroids
• *Naegleria fowlerii*	Amphotericin B + Rifampin
Viruses	
• Adenovirus	Cidofovir (may be indicated)
• Herpesviruses	Acyclovir
• *Influenza*	Oseltamivir*, Zanamivir* +/− Rimantadine** (may be indicated)
• Cytomegalovirus	Ganciclovir; valganciclovir; foscarnet; cidovir may be indicated
• Rabies	Investigative protocol available, Children's Hospital of Wisconsisn

* Active against *Influenza* A and B
** Used in the past for treatment of *Influenza* A

may occur at any age. Mortality among neonates with isolated encephalitis (usually type 2) is 4–15% despite treatment; this increases to 30–50% with disseminated disease with or without encephalitis (**Box 5.4.5**).

Acute disseminated encephalomyelitis (ADEM) appears to be a cell-mediated delayed hypersensitivity reaction to myelin leading to demyelination and sometimes, axonal transection. There are ~3–6 cases per year in regional medical centers, with a history of antecedent viral or bacterial infection within the prior 3 months in ~75% of cases. Fewer than 5% of cases are vaccine associated (most commonly measles vaccine).

Typical clinical findings of ADEM are similar to those of infectious meningoencephalitis, and may include multifocal neurologic deficits, pyramidal and spinal cord signs, cerebellar ataxia and optic neuritis. Brain and spine MRI are essential in making the diagnosis.

> **Box 5.4.5   Key Points in HSV Encephalitis**
>
> - 1–2% of febrile neonates have HSV encephalitis.
> - Concurrent skin lesions are present in fewer than 50% of cases.
> - For neonates, maternal history may be negative for HSV infection.
> - The clinical presentation is often indistinguishable from other causes of CNS infection and empiric treatment with acyclovir is indicated in all cases of encephalitis pending confirmatory data.
> - Diagnosis is confirmed by identification of HSV in CSF by PCR. HSV PCR remains positive up to 7 days after treatment is started.
> - If CSF is not obtainable, the diagnosis may be inferred by positive eye, nasopharyngeal, or rectal culture, or supported by clinical findings and diffusion weighted MRI. Neonates (findings are less specific than in older patients): reduced diffusion (hypointensity on apparent diffusion coefficient images); subtle hyperintensity on concurrent T-2 weighted images may be seen. In children and adults: increased signal on T-2 weighted images in the temporal and frontal lobes, insular cortex and cyngulate gyrus.
> - Head CT may be normal, especially early in the disease.

Initial therapy often includes antibiotics until the diagnosis can be confirmed.

- Most patients have multiple deep and subcortical white matter lesions seen best on T-2 weighted and FLAIR sequences.
- Lesions are often bilateral.
- Brainstem and spinal cord lesions are common; thalamic and basal ganglia lesions may be present.
- The differential diagnosis of ADEM includes: CNS infections, transverse myelitis, multiple sclerosis, optic neuritis, and *neuromyelitis optica* (Devic's disease).

Management summary:

- Stabilization of airway, breathing and circulation. If tracheal intubation is required, use neuroprotective techniques.
- Neurologic evaluation: Note any focal signs; R/O raised ICP; treat seizures.

- Identify potential sources of infection outside the CNS to help guide antibiotic therapy; obtain chest X-ray.
- Obtain blood, urine and other appropriate cultures.
- Obtain CBC, electrolytes, liver chemistries, ammonia, PT, PTT.
- Perform LP if no contraindications are present (*Lumbar Puncture, 15.5*). Head CT should be obtained prior to LP if there is evidence of raised ICP, focal signs, possible head trauma or mass lesion.
- CSF studies: cell count, glucose, protein, Gram stain and culture; PCR for HSV and enterovirus if appropriate; obtain CSF stains for fungi and acid-fast bacilli if the host is immunocompromised; consider exposure history.
- Obtain viral cultures from nasopahrynx and stool if viral agent is suspected.
- Give antibiotics based on age and most likely cause(s). Include acyclovir until HSV infection can be ruled out. Antibiotic administration is a priority, even prior to LP if obtaining CSF is delayed.
- Metabolic care: monitor serum glucose (goal 80–150 mg/dl) and electrolytes, especially serum Na$^+$ concentrations. Salt depletion as well as ↑ADH effect may lead to hyponatremia; this should be prevented (or corrected) to avoid exacerbation of brain swelling and raised ICP.
- Monitor for other complications (**Box 5.4.6**)
- **Specific therapy for ADEM:** Methylprednisolone 20–30 mg/ kg/day, usually for 3–5 days followed by oral steroid taper over

---

Box 5.4.6   Complications of CNS Infections

Bacterial Meningitis and Meningo-encephalitis:	Bacterial Meningitis:
• Brain swelling; ↑ ICP	• Cerebritis
• Respiratory failure	• Brain abscess
• Hemodynamic instability	• Hydrocephalus
• Hyponatremia; SIADH	• Sensorineural hearing loss
• Seizures	• Subdural effusions (rarely need evacuation)
• Brain infarcts	
• CNS hemorrhage; DIC	

Box 5.4.7   Pearls

- Fever is not uniformly present during CNS infection; temperature may be normal or low.
- Infants <1 yr often present with non-specific symptoms, and without signs of meningeal irritation.
- Patients exposed to antibiotics prior to diagnosis of bacterial meningitis may have non-specific symptoms and equivocal CSF findings ("partially treated meningitis").
- A normal head CT does not R/O raised ICP, but does R/O mass lesions, mass effect and primary CNS contraindications to LP. An opening pressure should be obtained if raised ICP is suspected despite a normal head CT.
- Antibiotics against likely bacteria along with acyclovir are generally indicated so long as treatable CNS infection remains a consideration.
- Brain imaging (or re-imaging) should be considered in any patient with CNS complications.
- If there is obstruction to CSF circulation (*e.g.* as may occur with infection of shunt hardware), lumbar CSF may not be representative of ventricular CSF.
- Neurosurgical consultation should be sought for a patient with a CNS shunt and suspicion of shunt infection.

3–6 weeks. Alternatives in selected patients with ADEM include plasmapheresis and immunoglobulin therapy (IVIG).

5.5   Raised Intracranial Pressure (ICP) and Cerebral Resuscitation

Intracranial pressure normally results from the volumetric summation of three non-compressible components in a rigid intracranial vault. These are: brain (80%), blood (10%), and CSF (10%) by volume. Normal ICP is typically in the range of 5–10 mmHg (7–14 cm H_2O) with considerable but transient changes under assorted physiologic circumstances. Severely elevated ICP is the final

---

Box 5.5.1   Etiologies of Increased ICP

- Traumatic brain injury
- Hypoxic-ischemic injury
- Intracranial infections (*e.g.* meningitis, encephalitis, abscess)
- Cerebral venous thrombosis
- Rapid decline in serum osmolality

- Tumors, cysts
- Hydrocephalus
- Encephalopathies (*e.g.* hepatic, Reyes syndrome)
- DKA
- Intracranial hemorrhage
- Hypo-osmolality (*e.g.* water intoxication)

Box 5.5.2   Key Clinical Findings in Increased ICP*

- Headache
- Vomiting
- Altered level of consciousness
- Elevated BP (increased SBP, decreased DBP) with decreased HR (Cushing's triad); sometimes systolic BP is decreased
- Hyper- or hypo-osmolality due to disturbances in antidiuretic hormone release
- Abnormal breathing patterns
- Abnormal muscle tone
- Cranial nerve abnormalities (*e.g.* anisocoria; sixth cranial nerve palsy)

---

* See a more extensive list in *Hydrocephalus and CSF diversion, 11.2.2; Box 11.2.5.*

common pathway to neurologic injury and mortality from a variety of insults. Early identification of patients at risk for development of increased ICP (**Boxes 5.5.1 and 5.5.2**) and timely intervention are keys to optimal care and outcome.

Principle of Compensation

Volume expansion of any one of the intracranial components (*i.e.* brain tissue, blood or CSF) must be accompanied by a decrease in volume of another component; otherwise, ICP will increase

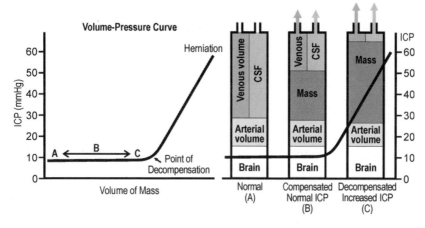

Fig. 5.5.1. **Intracranial Pressure Volume Curve Showing Compensatory Mechanisms for an Expanding Mass.** Modified with permission from Poss BW, Brockmeyer DL, Clay B, Dean JM, Pathophysiology and management of the intracranial vault, in Rogers MC (ed.), *Textbook of Pediatric Intensive Care*, Williams & Wilkins, Baltimore, p. 646, 1996.

(**Fig. 5.5.1**). Physiologic compensation includes extrusion of venous blood and CSF from the intracranial vault as brain or any other substance increases in volume (**Fig. 5.5.1, B**). After compensatory mechanisms are exhausted, ICP rises exponentially (**Fig. 5.5.1, C**).

Open cranial fontanels may help decompress increased ICP. A fontanel may be convex (bulging), flat (normal) or concave (sunken). The bony borders of an open, normal fontanel should be readily appreciable on palpation.

Cerebral Oxygenation is a consequence of three interrelated factors (**Box 5.5.3**); ICP is but one component of this relationship.

Cerebral autoregulation refers to the ability of the brain to maintain stable blood flow despite fluctuations in CPP from 50 to 150 mmHg (**Fig. 5.5.2**). This is accomplished by vasodilatation or vasoconstriction in response to changes in blood pressure. See **Figs. 5.5.3** and **5.5.4** for relationships between cerebral blood flow and metabolic rate, CPP, $PaCO_2$ and PaO_2.

Box 5.5.3   Factors Responsible for Cerebral Oxygenation

- **Cerebral blood flow:** Controlled by cerebral perfusion pressure (MAP–ICP), blood viscosity, diameter of intracranial arteries and arterioles (not easily measured; measured by xenon radiotracer injection)
- **Arterial oxygen content** (CaO_2)
- **Cerebral metabolic rate:** Indexed by jugular venous bulb oxygen saturation (usual goal 60–80%) or by non-invasive cerebral oximetry (typical range 60–80%)

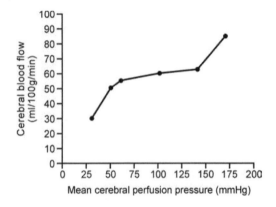

Fig. 5.5.2.   Cerebral Autoregulation: Cerebral blood flow remains relatively constant over a wide variation in CPP. Modified from Hernendez MJ, Brennan RW, Bowman GS, Cerebral blood flow autoregulation in the rat, *Stroke*, 9(2):152, 1978.

Box 5.5.4   Factors that Contribute to Cerebral Autoregulation

- Metabolic: Blood flow is linearly correlated with cerebral metabolic rate.
- Myogenic: Intrinsic constriction or relaxation of blood vessels in response to ↑ or ↓ of BP, respectively
- Chemical: As PaO_2 falls below 50 mm Hg, CBF ↑ hyperbolically. As $PaCO_2$ ↑ within the physiologic range, CBF ↑.
- Neural: Sympathetic nervous control may shift the autoregulation curve rightward in traumatic brain injury (TBI).
- Endothelium dependent mechanisms: Nitric oxide mediates dilation of arteries and arterioles.

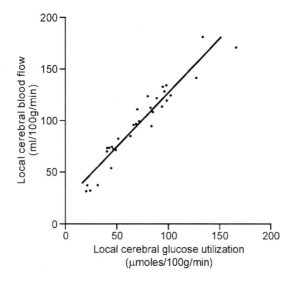

Fig. 5.5.3. Cerebral Blood Flow and Metabolic Rate: With permission from Kuschinsky W, Cerebral blood flow and glucose metabolism in a rat model, *J Basic Clin Physiol Pharmacol* 1:195, 1990.

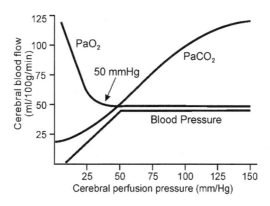

Fig. 5.5.4. Changes in Cerebral Blood Flow as CPP, $PaCO_2$ and PaO_2 Change. Redrawn from Rogers MC, Traystman RJ, An overview of the intracranial vault: physiology and philosophy, *Crit Care Clin* 1:199, 1985.

Types of Brain Herniation and Associated Findings. The brain may herniate through compartments of the skull in several different directions; these are described in **Fig. 5.5.5**.

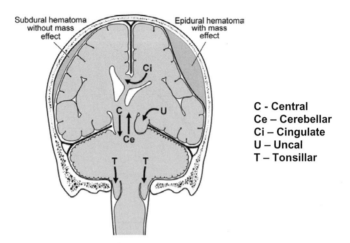

Fig. 5.5.5. Herniation Syndromes:

- **Cingulate (Subfalcine):** Ventromedial portion of the frontal lobe herniates beneath the falx cerebri (**Ci**); headache followed by contralateral leg weakness
- **Uncal (Transtentorial):** Medial temporal lobe herniates through tentorial notch (**U**) causing CN III paresis, contralateral hemiparesis and sometimes, ipsilateral hemiparesis
- **Central:** Temporal lobes and diencephalon herniate through tentorial notch; clinical findings of bilateral uncal herniation (**C**)
- **Cerebellar:** Cerebellum herniates upward through the tentorial notch (**Ce**); hydrocephalus (lateral and third ventricles) with rapid onset of coma and death.
- **Tonsillar:** Cerebellar tonsil(s) herniate downward through the foramen magnum (**T or TT**); "Lhermittes's phenomenon" *i.e.* dysesthesia in arms and legs with forward bending of head until obtundation occurs.

Emergency Management is directed at avoiding secondary brain injury (**Box 5.5.5**; also, *General Approach to the Critically Ill Child, 1.2 and Appendix, part 2, X*).

Patient selection for ICP monitoring is based on degree of risk for development or progression of raised ICP, ability to monitor the compartment with increased ICP, ability to monitor the physical examination, availability of imaging and prognosis. Intraventricular catheters are the "gold standard" for ICP monitoring. They are placed through a burr hole into the frontal or occipital ventricles of the (typically) non-dominant hemisphere; zero pressure is maintained at the Foramen of Monro (typically chosen landmarks are just above

---

Box 5.5.5   Emergency Management of Increased ICP*

- Attend to "ABC's": Give supplemental oxygen; goal for $PaCO_2$ initially 30–35 mmHg until stabilized, then goal of 35–40 mmHg. Volume resuscitate as indicated with 0.9% saline; provide isotonic fluid to avoid ↓ in serum sodium which might precipitate brain swelling.
- Radiologic imaging: Rule out neurosurgically treatable lesions (head CT) as soon as possible.
- Maximize cerebral venous drainage: Elevate head of bed 30°; keep head midline; avoid neck vein compression.
- Analgesia/sedation: Provide as indicated. Caution: may interfere with clinical findings.
- Avoid hyperthermia: May use antipyretics or cooling blanket; avoid shivering which may increase ICP; R/O infection as needed.
- Glucose goal: 80–150 mg/dL.
- Treat seizures: May need EEG in setting with sudden swings in vital signs and ICP.
- Pharmacologic muscle relaxation: If ICP monitor placed and airway secured.
- Osmotherapy: Mannitol [the "gold standard" (see text)].
- Barbiturate coma: Pentobarbital (see text).
- Decompressive craniectomy or lobectomy (non-dominant frontal or temporal lobe): Controversial.

---

* See *Appendix, part 2*, X.

or at the external auditory canal). This type of catheter may be difficult to place under conditions of brain swelling and small ventricles. The associated risk of infection is ≥5%. Alternatively, intraparenchymal monitors are placed through a burr hole and inserted into the brain parenchyma. This device measures surrounding pressure by strain gauge or fiberoptic methods. It is easily positioned but cannot be re-zeroed, and the reading may "drift" over several days. The risk of infection is less than that of the intraventricular catheter.

Mannitol (0.25–1 gm/kg IV over 20 mins) has been the osmotic agent of choice for treatment of increased ICP. It decreases blood viscosity, increases CBF and decreases cerebral blood volume at the time of infusion. Within 20–30 mins, increased blood osmolality draws fluid from the extravascular and intracellular compartments to the intravascular space across an intact blood brain barrier. Administration is followed by osmotic diuresis; hypovolemia and hypotension may follow. Avoid osmolality greater than 320 mOsm/kg H_2O to minimize the risk of acute renal failure.

Hypertonic saline: NaCl 3% (0.1–1 ml/kg/hr *via* CVL; loading doses of 5–10 ml/kg have been used). Hypertonic saline infusions accomplish volume expansion with increased cardiac output and accompanying cerebral vasoconstriction as well as create an osmotic gradient between intravascular and extravascular/intracellular spaces. Serum osmolality as high as 365 mOsm/kg H_2O appears to be well tolerated when induced by hypertonic saline. Too rapid an increase of serum sodium has been associated with a central demyelinating syndrome (*Electrolyte Disturbances, Hyponatremia, 6.2.1*).

Pentobarbital induced coma is a therapeutic option once other interventions including sedation, analgesia, muscle relaxation, osmotherapy and surgical care (*e.g.* evacuation of blood) have been addressed. This intervention decreases cerebral metabolism and therefore decreases cerebral blood flow and ICP. The dose is adjusted to achieve burst suppression on EEG (*Status Epilepticus, 5.2, Fig. 5.2.1*). Elimination is by zero order kinetics; accumulation in muscle, skin and fat results in prolonged effects after drug discontinuation. Complications include hypotension, bronchoconstriction, hypokalemia, ileus, oliguria and anuria.

5.6 Brain Death and Organ Procurement

Historically, death has been associated with cessation of heart beat and/or breathing. Subsequent introduction of cardiac and respiratory resuscitative maneuvers demonstrated that "death could sometimes be reversed". However, along with life-sustaining technology came the recognition that loss of all brain function, despite intact cardiopulmonary function, eventually leads to somatic death; the association of loss of all brain function became recognized as brain death (BD). Recognition of BD not only helps identify potential organ donors but also avoids futile, expensive care. Criteria for BD have been established for adults and for children (**Box 5.6.1**). The clinician should be familiar with state-specific guidelines regarding brain death.

Box 5.6.1   Key Points in Determination of Brain Death in Infants and Children*

- The absence of all brain function, including the brainstem, must persist over time and be irreversible.
- The physical examination is paramount in making the diagnosis of BD. Ancillary testing may be supportive when components of the physical examination are inconclusive or cannot be completed.
- All disturbances or factors that may influence the neurologic examination must be treated, corrected or eliminated. These include:
  ▶ Hypotension, hypothermia (T < 35°C), or severe electrolyte or glycemic abnormalities
  ▶ Severe hepatic or renal dysfunction
  ▶ Metabolic errors causing potentially reversible brain dysfunction
  ▶ The presence of neurotropic agents such as sedatives, NMBs, anticonvulsants, CNS intoxicating drugs. The influence of such drugs should be assessed by drug levels and/or known pharmacokinetics to ensure that they play no role in the neurologic assessment. If the role of a drug in unclear, the diagnosis of BD should be postponed; consideration may be given to ancillary testing.
- The neurologic examination following cardiac arrest or other severe brain injury may not be representative of neurologic potential. Evaluation for BD should be postponed for ≥24–48 hr after the event or until there is clinical certainty.
- Two examinations, including apnea testing, should be performed. Two different attending physicians should complete these examinations; however, apnea testing may be done by the same physician. If apnea testing cannot be performed, anciallary testing should be done.
- The recommended period of observation between the two examinations is 24 hr for neonates from 37 weeks to 30 days and 12 hr for infants and children 31 days to 18 yr.
- Ancillary testing (EEG, radionuclide cerebral blood flow study) does not replace the neurologic examination. These studies are used to support the presence or absence of BD if 1) the physical examination cannot be completed, 2) findingd are uncertain, 3) an interfering drug precludes clinical certainly, 4) it is desirable to shorten the observation period. See **Fig. 5.6.1** for EEG showing electrocerebral silence.

* Nakagawa TA, Ashwal S, Mathur M, Mysore M, Guidlines for the Determination of Brain Death in Infants and Children: an Update of the 1987 Task Force Recommendations, *Pediatrics* **128**:e720–e740, 2011.

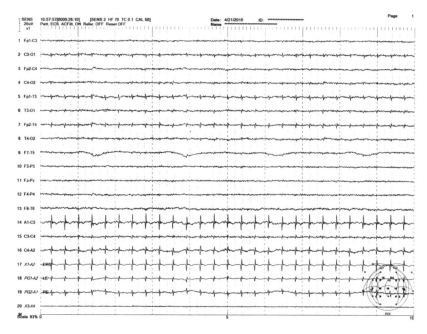

Fig. 5.6.1.   Electrocerebral Silence (ECS) with ECG Artifact.

Box 5.6.2   Physiology of Progression of Brain Injury to BD

• Autonomic nervous system changes:

▶ Sympathetic discharge results in hypertension, bradycardia and hydrostatic pulmonary edema.

▶ Eventual lack of simultaneous sympathetic and parasympathetic discharges results in HR and BP which do not vary; ultimately, asystole occurs.

▶ Eventual loss of sympathetic discharge results in vasodilatation and decreased cardiac inotropy.

• Hypothalamic-pituitary dysfunction:

▶ Compression of the pituitary stalk by herniation of the hypothalamus causes diabetes insipidus in 95% of patients.

Several physiologic changes can be anticipated as brain injury progresses to BD (**Box 5.6.2**). The process of evaluating for BD should be organized; key points are listed (**Box 5.6.3**).

Box 5.6.3   Testing for Brain Death

- Prerequisites: The cause for coma must be known and the cause must be **irreversible**.
  Exclude reversible causes of coma such as hypothermia (T core $\leq 32°C$), circulatory shock, metabolic imbalance, intoxication, presence of neurotropic drugs which could alter findings.
- Ensure the presence of unarousable unresponsiveness to noise or pain (*e.g.* pressure to supraorbital, temporal-mandibular or nail bed regions).
- Evaluate the brainstem (*Altered Mental Status, 5.1*)
- Pupils are in midposition or dilated without direct or consensual response to light in BD. Retinal hemorrhages blocking light from reaching retina or recently administered mydriatic agents or systemically administered anticholinergics (*e.g.* atropine) may invalidate the findings.
- Ocular movements
  ▶ Oculocephalic: Afferent limb involves CN VIII, the labyrinth and neck propriocpetors; efferent are CNs III, IV and VI. Perform only if neck injury is not suspected: rapidly turn head laterally 90° from midline. If ocular hemispheric neural control is damaged but brainstem control is intact then tonic deviation of eyes in the direction opposite to that of head movement will occur; in BD no extraocular movement of the eyes occurs (eyes look forward).
  ▶ Oculovestibular: CN VIII is afferent; CN VI is efferent (*Altered Mental Status, 5.1; Box 5.1.5*) No eye movement response occurs in BD. Eyelid edema may obscure eye movements. Basilar skull fracture may prevent eye deviation on the side of fracture due to CN injury; this invalidates the finding.
- Facial movements
  ▶ Corneal reflex is absent in BD. Eye trauma may interfere with this reflex. CN V is afferent and CN VII is efferent.
  ▶ Grimacing occurs normally with pressure on supraorbital ridge or temporal mandibular joint. This response is absent in BD. CN V is afferent and CN VII is efferent.
  ▶ Jaw reflex normally occurs in response to a tap on the chin with the mouth slightly open; the mouth should close. This reflex is absent in BD. CN V is afferent and efferent.
- Cough is tested by inserting a suction catheter tip into the trachea and applying suction. In BD no cough is elicited. CNs V, X, XI, and the phrenic nerves are afferent. Vagus and phrenic are efferent. The gag reflex is absent in BD. CN X is both afferent and efferent.

(Continued)

Box 5.6.3   Testing for Brain Death (Continued)

- Apnea test: This is a controlled hypercarbic challenge to determine if the patient has any respiratory effort in response to a ≥ 20 mmHg increase in $PaCO_2$ and a $PaCO_2 > 60$ mmHg. The patient is oxygenated, but not ventilated (mechanical breaths are temporarily suspended) during this test. Evidence of hemodynamic instability or oxygen desaturation may result in abortion of the test.
  - ▶ To eliminate nitrogen stores, pre-oxygenate with FiO_2 1.0. During the apnea test ensure delivery of 100% O_2 either by T-piece or place a catheter with 100% oxygen at 6 L/min in the tracheal tube or apply CPAP if needed (*e.g.* pulmonary disease).
  - ▶ An initial ABG should document $PaCO_2$ ~40 mmHg; once this is confirmed, mechanical breathing is withheld and O_2 is passively instilled. $PaCO_2$ usually rises by ~3 mmHg per minute. A POSITIVE test is present when no respiratory effort is present when target $PaCO_2$ is reached (usually within 7–10 mins). Monitor carefully for any chest wall movement (respiratory effort) the entire test.

Box 5.6.4   Movements Compatible with Brain Death

- Spinal reflexes are **elicited** movements. They are characterized by:
  - ▶ Stereotypical movements elicited after a specific trigger
  - ▶ Have constant period of latency and duration
  - ▶ Habituates only with frequent triggers
  - ▶ Includes responses to cutaneous stimulation of extremities or to movement of the head on the neck
- Automatisms are **spontaneous** movements. Examples include:
  - ▶ Lazarus sign: arms move above the chest then at sides of torso; it is known to occur during apnea testing, ↓BP, painful stimuli, passive flexion of head on neck
  - ▶ Finger jerks or undulating toes
  - ▶ Decerebrate movements

A brain dead child may exhibit movements that may be categorized as either spinal reflexes or automatisms (**Box 5.6.4**). Consultation with a neurologist may help to correctly categorize these movements.

Organ procurement from brain dead donors and after cardiac death. After brain death is confirmed the family is notified. If the family is interested in organ donation, care is transitioned to the state organ procurement organization (OPO). The OPO can be initially contacted before death is declared on mechanically ventilated patients with little neurological function (GCS ≤5). Several disease states preclude organ donation (**Box 5.6.5**).

The OPO coordinator and the PICU team often work together in the management of the BD donor to maintain hemodynamic, pulmonary and fluid/electrolyte balance (**Box 5.6.6**).

Box 5.6.5 Contraindications to Organ Donation

- HIV
- Measles
- Rabies
- Parvovirus
- Adenovirus

- Prion-related disease
- Overwhelming infection (not bacteremia)
- Herpetic meningoencephalitis
- Human T-cell leukemia/lymphoma
- Active malignancy

Box 5.6.6 Pretransplant Care of the Brain Dead Child

- **Hemodynamic:** Maintain mean BP of ≥60 mmHg by using dobutamine and/or dopamine at <10 mcg/kg/min with adequate urine output and left ventricular ejection fraction ≥45%. Where indicated give diuretic or IV fluid to maintain CVP 6–8 mmHg or PCWP 8–12 mmHg. Goals: CI >2.5 L/min/m² and SVR >800 dyne-sec/cm⁵/m². If epinephrine and/or norepinephrine are needed in doses >0.05 mcg/kg/min consider steroid or thyroid hormone supplementation. Maintain hemotocrit > 30%.
- **Pulmonary:** Normalize tidal volumes (5–7 cc/kg IBW) to avoid atelectasis or baro/volutrauma. Avoid fluid overload that promotes lung dysfunction following transplantation.
- **Fluid balance:** For diabetes insipidus infuse aqueous vasopressin (usually, 0.5–10 mUnit/kg/hr) to achieve UOP of 2 ml/kg/hr. Replace excessive UO with D2.5% + NaCl 25 mEq/L + K-acetate 35 mEq/L. If an osmotic dieresis occurs from hyperglycemia infuse insulin 0.025 to 1 Unit/kg/hr with hourly glucose goal of 120–150 mg/dL.

Box 5.6.7   Key Points in Donation After Cardiac Death

- Decision is made by patient care team and next of kin that injury is non-recoverable and rapid death is likely if mechanical support is withdrawn.
- Next of kin consents to heparin administration and placement of vascular access (femoral catheters) before withdrawal of support (for organ preservation).
- After surgical "time out" ventilatory and pharmacologic supports are withdrawn; any needed IV analgesia/sedation is provided. No member of the transplant team may declare death or be a member of the palliative care team.
- Once no central pulse can be palpated or no heart beat is auscultated the child can be moved to the operating room for preparation.
- Death is defined as no auscultated heart beat or palpated central pulses or respiratory effort continuously for 5 mins (or up to 10 mins per the Maastricht protocol). After this waiting period, death may be diagnosed and surgery for organ procurement may begin.

Donation after cardiac death is another option for organ donation in the child who is not BD. While not BD, these children typically have non-recoverable severe brain, respiratory or high spinal cord injury which will likely lead to rapid death if mechanical support is withdrawn. Under these circumstances the family may wish to discontinue life support but proceed with organ donation after cardiac arrest. Cardiac death should be assessed as likely to occur within 30 min for a liver donation and within 60 min for kidneys and/or pancreas donation. The heart is almost never recovered. Steps of DCA are listed (**Box 5.6.7**).

Chapter 6

Fluids, Electrolytes and Metabolism

6.1 Dehydration

In times of health, water and salt needs are met through a normal thirst mechanism, adequate intake of salt and water, and kidneys normally responsive to hormonal control mechanisms. "Maintenance fluid" is that volume of fluid required to replace insensible losses that normally occur through skin, respiratory and gastrointestinal tracts, and provide sufficient water for formation of urine. Dehydration denotes a state in which a deficit has accrued. A fluid deficit accrues if (1) maintenance needs are not met and/or (2) abnormal losses occur through skin (*e.g.* excessive sweating, high fever), respiratory tract (*e.g.* hyperventilation, tachypnea), gastrointestinal tract (*e.g.* diarrheal disease, vomiting), urinary tract (*e.g.* polyuric renal failure, diabetes insipidus, adrenal insufficiency, diuretics) or (3) fluids normally "recycled" are externally drained (*e.g.* intestinal drainage, diverted CSF, pleural or intra-abdominal drains). It is important to identify the cause of dehydration in all cases. See **Box 6.1.1**.

The nature of the fluids lost determines the resultant type of dehydration (isotonic, hypotonic or hypertonic). If losses are isotonic to plasma (*i.e.* contain ~135–150 mEq/L Na$^+$), salt is lost in physiologic proportion to water and dehydration is isotonic. Most losses in gastroenteritis, except for secretory diarrhea, are hypotonic, and would result in hypernatremia were it not for thirst followed by intake of hypotonic fluids (water, juice, electrolyte solutions, "sports drinks"). ADH release leads to water conservation, and

Box 6.1.1 Distribution of Total Body Water			
Age	Water as % Lean Body Mass (LBM)	ICF % LBM	ECF % LBM
Newborn	75–80		
< 6 mos	70	45	25
> 6 mos–adulthood	55–60	45–50	20–25

ICF, Intracellular fluid; ECF, Extracellular fluid; Ideal body weight is the "normal" or non-obese weight; Lean body mass is the weight minus all fat.

The ICF and ECF compartments are separated by a semi-permeable membrane that allows free movement of water between compartments; this movement is driven by osmotic forces which determine the volume of each compartment (**Box 6.1.2**). Fluid in the urinary bladder and colon are not available for exchange and are considered physiologically "outside" the body.

hypernatremia is averted. If vomiting or lack of access to oral intake ensues, or if insensible water loss is enhanced (*e.g.* high fever), hypernatremia develops. If net losses are more nearly isotonic (*e.g.* secretory diarrhea, cystic fibrosis, drainage of pancreatic fluids) and partially replaced with hypotonic fluid, the patient will present with hyponatremic dehydration.

Each fluid plan should address the following needs:

- What are the patient's maintenance water needs? These are based on caloric expenditure or body surface area (**Box 6.1.3**).
- Is the patient dehydrated? Physical and biochemical data assist with the answer. Acute losses are more likely to be clinically apparent by physical examination (**Box 6.1.4**). Deficit volumes accrued gradually (many days to weeks) may be associated with normal peripheral perfusion despite severe dehydration; serum

Box 6.1.2 Osmolality

- "Osmolality" is the number of milliosmoles (mOsm) measured per kilogram of water. Normal osmolality (275–295 mOsm/kg H_2O) is dependent on intake, a well perfused, normal kidney, sympathetic output, aldosterone, atrial natriuretic factor, vasopressin and dopamine.
- Non-diffusible proteins, complex phosphates, sulfates, Mg^{++} and K^+ help form the intracellular electro-chemical skeleton; sodium is actively extruded from cells by a Na^+-ATPase driven pump. Interstitial fluid resembles plasma, but is lower in protein.
- The osmotic activity of sodium, its anions, and glucose (especially when increased) are largely responsible for maintenance of ECF volume. These osmoles define the *effective osmolality* (E_{osm}): 2[Na in mEq/L] + [glucose in mg/dL]/18.
- Because water moves freely across cell membranes, intracellular and extracellular osmolalities must equalize. Urea nitrogen moves across membranes along its own concentration gradient and therefore is not an effective osmole.
- Calculated osmolarity (C_{osm}) approximates measured osmolality by +/− 10 mOsm/kg H_2O unless additional (unmeasured) osmoles (*e.g.* alcohol, mannitol) are present:

C_{osm} in mOsm/L solution

$$= 2[\text{Na in mEq/L}] + [\text{BUN in mg/dL}]/2.8 + [\text{glucose in mg/dL}]/18.$$

The difference between calculated osmolarity and measured osmolality is the "osmolar gap".

chemistries, especially BUN and *acute* changes in weight (*i.e.* those that occur over ~24 hrs) provide clues.

- Are there abnormal on-going losses that should be replaced? (*e.g.* diarrheal stools, gastric drainage, fluids from surgically placed drains, *etc.*) If such losses are sufficiently large and not replaced, a deficit volume will accrue.
- What should the electrolyte composition of the fluids be? This is based on maintenance needs, serum electrolytes and solute content of ongoing losses.

Box 6.1.3   Maintenance Water Requirements Based on Basal Caloric Expenditure* Per Day

Age	Weight (kg)	BSA (M²)‡	Calories Expended (kcal)/kg/day
1 week**–6 mos	3–8	0.2–0.35	65–70
6–12 mos	8–12	0.35–0.45	50–60
1–2 yrs	10–15	0.45–0.55	45–50
2–5 yrs	15–20	0.6–0.7	45
5–10 yrs	20–35	0.7–1.1	40–45
10–16 yrs†	35–60	1.5–1.7	25–40
>16 yrs	70	1.75	15–20

* When 1 kcal is expended, 1 ml of water is lost; therefore, the number of kcals/kg/day expended is numerically equal to the mL/kg/day needed to maintain normal water balance.

Half the basal requirement is lost insensibly and half provides water for urine formation. **The usual maintenance water requirement is 1.5 times the basal requirement.** Under conditions of increased energy expenditure (hyperventilation, shivering, fever), the maintenance requirement may increase to twice or three times the basal allotment. For each degree C over basal temperature (~37°), caloric expenditure increases by 13%.

** For term infants <1 week, maintenance requirements begin at 50 mL/kg/day on the first day of life and increase by 10 mL/kg/day until reaching ~100–110 mL/kg/day by the end of the first week. Use of a radiant warmer and/or prematurity will increase the maintenance fluid requirement.

† Note that the older the child, the fewer the kcals/kg/day required; the 16 yrs old needs ~25 kcal/kg/day while the 10 yrs old needs ~40 kcals/kg/day.

‡ Based on body surface area, maintenance volume for patients >10 kg = 1500 mL/M²/day.

Box 6.1.4   Estimating the Volume of Deficit ("Degree or Percent Dehydration") in Normally Nourished Patients*

	Mild	Moderate	Severe
Infants <2 yrs	5% (50 mL/kg)	10% (100 mL/kg)	≥15% (150 mL/kg)
Children ≥2 yrs	3% (30 mL/kg)	6% (60 mL/kg)	≥9% (90 mL/kg)
Heart rate	N**	↑	↑↑↑
Mucous membranes	Sticky	Dry	Dry
Skin temperature	N	Cool to cold distally	Cold; clammy
Capillary refill time‡	N (<2 sec)	↑ (2–3 sec)	↑↑(>3 sec)
Foot pulses‡‡	N	↓ to absent	Absent
Blood pressure	Preserved	Preserved	Low

* For obese patients use the ideal body weight for fluid and electrolyte calculations. Guidelines assume acute losses and isotonic dehydration (*i.e.* normal serum sodium concentration); signs of severe dehydration may be masked by compensatory mechanisms when losses occur gradually or when dehydration is hypertonic (Na^+ >150 mEq/L and/or marked hyperglycemia is present). Additional signs of dehydration include sunken fontanel, sunken eyes, loss of skin elasticity and decreased or absent urine output.

** N = Normal.

† Tachycardia persists until O_2 delivery to the heart fails; bradycardia followed by arrest ensues.

‡ Capillary refill time may be influenced by environmental and body temperatures.

‡‡ Although not quantifiable, foot pulses are often decreased to absent in moderate and severe degrees of dehydration. The qualitative volume of foot pulses is used clinically in assessing, monitoring and re-assessing perfusion during treatment.

- Monitoring of physical findings, urine output, abnormal ongoing losses and serial chemistries during treatment is essential for safety and success.

Content of "Maintenance Fluids":

- Generally, these should provide Na^+ 2–4 mEq/100 kcal expended per day, K^+ 2 mEq/100 kcals expended per day and sufficient dextrose to maintain normoglycemia and to prevent ketosis and catabolism.
- Although these needs are usually satisfied by a solution containing 5% dextrose with NaCl ~40 mEq/L and K^+ ~20 mEq/L, use of this hypotonic fluid has been associated with hyponatremia in sick, hospitalized patients. "Maintenance" fluid for sick patients usually provides $\geq Na^+$ 77 mEq/L.
- If provision of dextrose is not desirable (*e.g.* during stress-related hyperglycemia) the minimum sodium concentration in maintenance fluids is ~77 mEq/L (0.45% NaCl). Very hypotonic fluids should be avoided.
- If acid-base balance is normal, K^+ may be added as acetate to maintain physiologic anion ratios (~1/4 the anion as base).
- On the first day of life, the newborn does not require electrolyte; this is the only instance in which 5–10% dextrose in water without electrolyte is appropriate as maintenance fluid.

Deficit Replacement:

- If hypovolemic shock is present, give isotonic fluid (*e.g.* 0.9% NaCl) 10–20 mL/kg followed by reassessment; this should be repeated until signs of shock are reversed (*Shock, 3.5*). Assign as estimated volume of deficit based on physical findings (**Box 6.1.4**) and "refine" this assessment based on biochemical findings once these are available: *e.g.* if findings are consistent with moderate dehydration, but the BUN is 50 mg/dL, this suggests chronicity, likely with a greater degree of dehydration.

- Identify and treat accompanying hypoglycemia (*Hypo- and Hyperglycemia, 6.4*).
- The remainder of the deficit (deficit volume minus resuscitation fluid volume) is replaced more gradually, depending on whether dehydration is isotonic, hypotonic or hypertonic.

Isotonic dehydration: serum [Na^+] = 135–150 meq/L with evidence of dehydration; *net* losses are isotonic to plasma, *i.e.* for purposes of calculation, the losses *net* ~150 meq/L. Rehydration is planned over 24 hrs, usually half the deficit given in the first 8 hours and the remainder over the next 16 hrs.

Example: For a 1 year old, 10 kg infant, with diarrheal disease and "10% dehydration" (100 mL/kg *or* 1000 mL volume of deficit) and serum Na^+ 138:

- If 0.9% NaCl 30 mL/kg has been given for resuscitation of shock, the remaining deficit volume to be replaced is 70 mL/kg.
- The sodium deficit is ~150 meq (because the patient has lost ~1000 mL); 46 meq of Na^+ have been given during resuscitation, leaving 104 meq to be given during the remainder of the rehydration.
- The maintenance water allotment for this 12 mos old is ~75 mL/kg or 750 mL/day (for 750 kcals expended); maintenance Na^+ requirement is 2–4 meq/100 kcals expended, or ~22 meq/day. This Na^+ requirement is small compared to the deficit of sodium and may be safely omitted for one day.
- Add the remaining deficit of 700 mL to the maintenance water requirement for a total of 1450 mL; total Na^+ owed is 104 meq or ~71 meq/L Na^+.
- If the patient is euglycemic, the IVF would likely contain 5% dextrose in 0.45% NaCl (~77 meq/L NaCl); a greater or lesser concentration of dextrose may be required depending on the patient's glycemic status. If urine is being reliably produced, providing potassium (as the acetate instead of the chloride salt to balance the anion load) is usually appropriate.

- If a significant base deficit is present, some or all of the sodium in the rehydration solution may be given as sodium bicarbonate or sodium acetate.
- The infusion rate would be 75 mL/hr × 8 hrs and 53 mL/hr × 16 hrs.

Hypotonic (hyponatremic) dehydration. For clinical purposes, this is defined as serum [Na$^+$] <130 mEq/L **with evidence of hypovolemia**; sodium has been lost in excess of water. Signs of extracellular deficit (circulatory insufficiency) predominate, especially when the loss is acute, because extracellular water has shifted to the intracellular compartment. Rule out pseudo-hyponatremia by correcting the measured [Na$^+$] for hyperglycemia, identifying severe hyperlipidemia, and comparing measured osmolality *vs.* calculated osmolarity (*Hyponatremia*, **Box 6.2.1**). If renal function is normal, urine sodium is low (usually <20 mEq/L). Hyponatremic hypovolemia with an increased urine Na$^+$ (*e.g.* >20 mEq/L) and increased serum potassium is typical in adrenal insufficiency (*Adrenal Insufficiency, 6.8*)

Assess the degree dehydration and calculate the volume of deficit and the Na$^+$ deficit as for isotonic dehydration. Add to this, the "excess" Na$^+$ deficit leading to hyponatremia by multiplying the difference between measured and desired Na$^+$ by total body water. This is the additional amount of sodium to be delivered to achieve isonatremia (**See Example** below).

When sodium loss is *acute* and severe, circulatory collapse not responsive to isotonic fluids or refractory seizures may require treatment with 3% NaCl. In these settings, the amount of 3% NaCl required to raise the serum Na$^+$ to 125 mEq/L is calculated as follows:

$$(125 - \text{measured Na}^+) \times 0.6 \times \text{weight in kg} = \text{mEq Na}^+ \text{ to be given.}$$

The rate of infusion depends upon severity of symptoms; too rapid an increase in serum sodium caused by overly aggressive therapy is associated with osmotic demyelination syndrome (*Electrolyte Disturbances, 6.2*).

Example: For a 3 month old, 5 kg infant with severe diarrhea for 24–36 hrs with signs of 150 mL/kg deficit or 750 mL ("$>$15% dehydration") and serum Na^+ = 117 mEq/L:

- This infant received 0.9% NaCl 50 mL/kg (250 mL) to resuscitate blood pressure and regain peripheral perfusion.
- To estimate the initial sodium deficit, first calculate what the deficit would be if dehydration were isotonic: ~150 mEq/L in Na^+ losses means ~113 mEq Na^+ lost in 750 mL. Add to this the amount of Na^+ required to increase the measured Na^+ to 135 mEq/L: (135–117) × 0.6 × 5 kg = 54 mEq; Total sodium deficit is 113 + 54 = 167 mEq Na^+.
- During resuscitation, the patient received NaCl 0.9%, 250 mL, containing ~36 mEq Na^+. This salt and volume are "contributions" to deficit replacement. If these are subtracted from the initial deficit, we owe: 500 mL of water and (167–36) or 131 mEq Na^+.
- Maintenance water allotment: 525 mL/day; maintenance Na^+ = 15 mEq/day.
- Total volume to be given in one day: Deficit volume (500 mL) + maintenance volume (525 mL) = 1025 mL; total Na^+ owed: 131 mEq (maintenance Na^+ may be omitted for one day). This results in a solution containing Na^+ approximately 127 mEq/L. The rehydration solution should also contain appropriate amounts of dextrose (depending on glycemic status), potassium (depending on renal status, UOP, *etc.*) and base (depending on acid-base status). Since Lactated Ringer's is a stock solution containing Na^+ 130 mEq/L, it could serve as a rehydration solution with appropriate additives. Once perfusion has been restored during emergency resuscitation, the remainder of rehydration may proceed evenly over 24 hrs (43 mL/hr).
- Replace any abnormal on-going losses such as diarrheal stools, stoma drainage, *etc.* with a fluid similar in content to that being lost.
- In addition to frequent physical examinations, monitor glucose, BUN and electrolytes carefully, including Na^+, K^+, Mg^{++}, Ca^{++} and phosphorus serially; supplement electrolytes as needed.

Hypertonic dehydration results from the presence of salt or other extracellular osmoles (*e.g.* glucose) in physiologic excess of water. Hypernatremia ([Na$^+$] > 150 mEq/L; *Electrolyte Disturbances, 6.2*) and other forms of hyperosmolality (*e.g.* severe hyperglycemia with insulin resistance or deficiency) ultimately result in dehydration which is largely intracellular (water is drawn from cells into the ECF space by sodium and its anion or another osmotically active substance). Extracellular volume, initially preserved, decreases as dehydration becomes more profound. Circulation is spared until late in the course, and neurologic symptoms predominate: quiet when undisturbed, highly irritable with stimulation, high pitched cry, hypertonicity, hyperreflexia, intracranial hemorrhage, seizures and cerebral venous thrombosis. A doughy, velvety-feel to the skin is characteristic. Hypocalcemia and hyperglycemia are frequent associated findings.

Brain cells adapt to hypertonic conditions such as hypernatremia by generation of intracellular osmoles (taurine, myoinositol, glutamate, glutamine betaine, choline compounds) to prevent loss of brain cell water, particularly when hypertonicity develops over a few hours rather than suddenly. In the presence of an osmotically adapted brain, rapid correction of the hypertonic state leads to swelling of brain cells and potentially, seizures, raised ICP, and brain herniation. For this reason, hypernatremia is corrected gradually by lowering serum Na$^+$ 10–15 mEq/L/24 hrs *evenly* or ~1 mEq/L every 2 hrs. See example below.

See **Box 6.2.5** for causes of hypernatremia. DKA and hyperosmolar hyperglycemic syndrome also cause hypertonic dehydration and the management principles of gradual rehydration to effect a gradual decline in osmolality apply to these disorders as well.

Example: A 5 month old 6 kg infant with a 2 day history of diarrhea, vomiting, fever, poor intake and physical signs of 10% dehydration; she is hyper-irritable; serum Na$^+$ = 168 mEq/L BUN = 30 mg/dL. Signs of dehydration are masked by the hypertonic state; the volume of deficit is likely > 100 mL/kg and closer to 150 mL/kg or 900 mL. To decrease the sodium by a total ~ 20 mEq, plan to rehydrate over at least 48 hrs with a goal [Na$^+$] of ~145 mEq/L.

- NaCl 0.9% 10 mL/kg (60 mL) is sufficient to restore perfusion. Remaining deficit is 840 mL.
- Estimate the free water deficit (FWD): for Na^+ <170, this is ~4 mL/kg for each 1 mEq per L Na^+ increase above normal: $4 \times 6\,kg \times (168–145) = 552\,mL$. (For Na^+ >170, use 3 mL/kg for each mEq Na^+ above normal since water losses are not linear if hypernatremia becomes extreme.) Plan to replace this FWD (226 mL) evenly over 48 hrs.
- Solute fluid deficit (SFD) = Remaining deficit (*i.e.* the deficit remaining after volume resuscitation or 840 mL) minus the FWD (which is 552 mL) = 288 mL = 0.288 L
- Solute Na^+ deficit (SND) = SFD (or 0.288 L) × total body water (or 0.6/kg) × [desired Na] or 145 mEq/L = 25 mEq Na^+.
- Maintenance volume = 6 kg × 70 mL/kg × 1.5 = 630 mL/day; maintenance Na^+ = 24 mEq.
- First 24 hrs: Give maintenance water (630 mL) plus half the FWD (276 mL) or 906 mL. To this volume, add the entire SND (25 mEq Na^+) plus maintenance Na^+ (24 mEq [Na^+]) or 49 mEq Na^+: 49 mEq Na^+ in 906 mL, or Na^+ ~55 mEq/L.
- In the second 24 hrs, give maintenance plus the remaining half of the FWD: 906 mL with Na^+ ~25 mEq/L.
- Add dextrose, K^+, Ca^{++} and Mg^{++} and balance the anion content of the fluid as needed.
- Replace ongoing losses via a separate solution, similar in composition to that being lost.
- Monitor progress carefully by serial measurements of electrolytes to ensure a safe decline in Na^+ concentration. If the serum [Na^+] decreases at a rate >0.5 mEq/L/hr, the rate of volume delivery should be decreased and the sodium content of the IVF should be re-evaluated for an increase in Na concentration. If [Na^+] fails to decrease appropriately or increases, the rate of volume delivery or replacement of ongoing losses may be insufficient. Alternatively, the sodium content of the IVF may need to be decreased. Failure of an elevated BUN to decrease should prompt evaluation for a need for increased fluid delivery, or may indicate renal insufficiency.

6.2   Electrolyte Disturbances

Clinical laboratories routinely measure electrolyte concentrations in serum (that portion of the ECF minus coagulation factors) or plasma (ECF that contains coagulation factors). Abnormal concentrations of electrolytes are among the most common problems in PICU patients. Accuracy of laboratory data may be distorted by problems such as sampling techniques, sample mishandling, assay errors, and presence of interfering substances. Clues to these problems include evidence of hemolysis in the specimen, prolonged tourniquet application and a subnormal anion gap. Unanticipated results should be re-checked before laboratory error is assumed.

6.2.1   Hyponatremia (serum [Na⁺]
< 135 mEq/L; Box 6.2.2)

As serum sodium concentration decreases, water moves from ECF to ICF causing cellular swelling. Brain cell swelling leads to CNS mediated problems such as altered mental status, subnormal body temperature, seizures, raised ICP, and respiratory failure; non-cardiogenic pulmonary edema may also occur. Based on animal and human data, gradual development of hyponatremia (over >1–3 days) results in loss of intracellular solute (K^+, Na^+, amino acids, myoinositol, *et al.*) and therefore loss of water, which minimizes brain swelling. If hyponatremia is corrected rapidly (>10 mEq/L in the first 24 hrs or >18 mEq/L in the first 48 hrs), the risk of osmotic demyelination from brain cell dehydration increases.

Diagnostic and Therapeutic Steps. Compare measured osmolality with calculated osmolarity (*Dehydration, 6.1, Box 6.1.2*; also *Box 6.2.1*) to identify true hyponatremia. Identify the volume status as hypo-, hyper-, or euvolemic.

- Hypovolemic: Signs of volume depletion are present. Resuscitate shock with 0.9% NaCl; correct dehydration as described (*Dehydration, 6.1*).
- Hypervolemic: Edema and/or hypertension may be present.
- Euvolemic: No signs of volume depletion or overload.

Box 6.2.1	How to Identify True Hyponatremia		
	Measured Osm*	Calc. Osmolarity**	Causes
Apparent hyponatremia	↑	↑	Hyperglycemia[†];
Unmeasured osmoles causing apparent hyponatremia	↑	↓	Mannitol
Pseudo-hyponatremia	N	↓	Hyperlipidemia[‡]; hyperproteinemia (*e.g. after IVIG* infusion)
True hyponatremia	↓	↓	See **Box 6.2.2**

N, normal; ↑ increased; ↓ decreased; *Measured osmolality;
** Calculated osmolarity (**Box 6.1.2**)
[†] For every 100 mg/dL increase in glucose above normal (100 mg/dL), the measured [Na^+] decreases by 1.6 mEq/L
[‡] Serum Na^+ is ↓ by ~2 mEq/L for every 1 gm/dL ↑ in serum lipids; serum is often lipemic.

- Water restriction generally means delivery of ≤2/3 the maintenance requirement (same as ≤ the basal requirement; *Dehydration, 6.1, Box 6.1.3*). Half the basal allotment (= insensible losses) or less (*e.g.* no fluid) may be appropriate in acute hyponatremia due to water intoxication or acute ADH excess. Additional needs (glucose, potassium and other medications) must be met and should be delivered in a maximally concentrated solution, particularly in SIADH which may last days to weeks.
- Review causes of hyponatremia to determine the appropriate management strategy (**Box 6.2.2**).
- Note conditions associated with increased ADH effect (**Box 6.2.3**).
- Review management of hyponatremia with refractory shock and/or severe neurologic symptoms (**Box 6.2.4**).

Box 6.2.2   Causes of True Hyponatremia (Measured mOsm +/− 10 mOsm of Calculated Osm)

Hypovolemic States TBW ↓ and TB$_{Na}$ ↓↓	Hypervolemic States TBW ↑↑ and TB$_{Na}$ ↑	Euvolemic States TBW ↑ and TB$_{Na}$ ~ Normal
Renal loss *Urine [Na$^+$]* *> 20 mEq/L** • Osmotic diuresis • Cerebral salt wasting • Adrenal insufficiency • Salt-losing nephropathy • Metabolic alkalosis • Diuretics • Pseudohypo-aldosteronism • Proximal RTA **Extra-renal loss** *Urine [Na$^+$] < 20** • Gastrointestinal losses • Third space collections (*e.g.* effusions, intestinal obstruction) • Sweat	**Oliguric Renal Failure** *Urine [Na$^+$]* *> 20 mEq/L** **Edematous states** *Urine [Na$^+$]* *< 20 mEq/L** • Congestive failure • Nephrotic syndrome • Hepatic cirrhosis	**Water retention in excess of Na$^+$** *Urine [Na$^+$]* *>20 mEq/L** • ↑ ADH secretion ▸ Appropriate ▸ Inappropriate (SIADH) ▸ Drug-related ▸ Stress-related (*e.g.* pain) **Water intoxication** **Hypothyroidism** **Reset Osmostat** **Glucocorticoid deficiency** ** Note: Estimates of urine [Na$^+$] are approximate; interventions prior to urine collection may alter results.*

⇓ | ⇓ | ⇓

| Salt and water repletion (*Dehydration*, 6.1 *Hypotonic dehydration*) | Salt and water restriction | Water restriction |

Box 6.2.3 Conditions Associated with Increased Antidiuretic Hormone Secretion in the Absence of Hypovolemia and Hypertonicity ("SIADH")

- CNS disease: *e.g.* infections, TBI, HIE, ↑ ICP, intracranial hemorrhage, tumors or pituitary disease
- Hormone therapy with vasopressin, oxytocin
- Mechanical ventilation
- Lung disease: *e.g.* asthma, pneumonia, CF, pneumothorax
- Pain
- Hereditary
- Idiopathic
- HIV infection
- Drugs: *e.g.* opiates, amiodarone, methotrexate, carbamazepine, vincristine, haloperidol, nicotine, phenothiazines, barbiturates, salicyclates, bromocriptine, tricyclic antidepressants, serotonin reuptake inhibitors

6.2.2 Hypernatremia (serum $Na^+ > 150$ mEq/L; Box 6.2.5)

Sodium is the primary determinant of ECF volume; it indicates hypertonic conditions, and obligates the movement of water from the intracellular to the extracellular space. Hypernatremia most frequently results from loss of water in excess of salt with inability to drink sufficient replacement fluids such as occurs in diarrheal disease with vomiting (which may be exacerbated by increased free water loss from fever) or diabetes insipidus (DI). Hypernatremia is also caused by sodium intake in excess of water (treatment with NaCl 3%; salt poisoning). Hypernatremia is a hypertonic state that ultimately results in a decrease of TBW (dehydration) regardless of its cause, although circulatory volume may be maintained at the expense of ICF. An exception would be the rapid occurrence of salt poisoning associated with renal failure. Serum $[Na^+]$ returns to normal only if sufficient free water is provided for salt excretion.

If hypernatremia develops rapidly, movement of intracellular water to the ECF space results in brain shrinkage; if hypernatremia is severe, bridging blood vessels may be torn as they are displaced from

Box 6.2.4

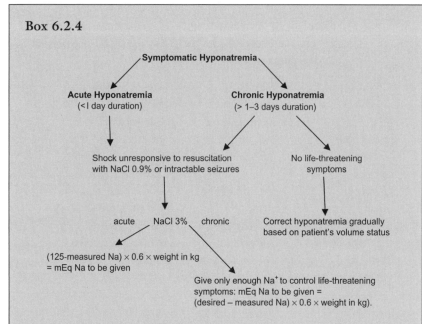

NOTE: *Acute water intoxication* in infants caused by diluted feedings or copious water intake often leads to seizures. These infants may have puffy eyelids and a full fontanel on presentation. Typically, they have diapers soaked with dilute urine. Hyponatremia corrects spontaneously with fluid restriction. In *chronic hyponatremia*, if serum [Na+] increases too rapidly, ICF water shifts to the ECF space, causing acute dehydration of brain cells, increasing the risk of osmotic demyelination syndrome, particularly in pre-pubertal children and adults. Hyponatremia should be corrected by no more than 10 mEq/L in the first 24 hrs and 18 mEq/L in 48 hrs.

a shrinking brain causing hemorrhage. When hypernatremia develops gradually (over hours) brain cells generate intracellular osmoles which decrease the osmotic gradient between ICF and ECF, preserving brain cell size, shape and probably, function. Intracranial bleeding is less likely. In this setting, treatment requires gradual rehydration to prevent a sudden decrease in osmolality with movement of water into osmotically adapted brain cells and brain swelling.

The pathophysiology, symptoms and treatment of hypernatremic dehydration are described in *Dehydration, 6.1*. When hypernatremia

---

Box 6.2.5   Main Causes of Hypernatremia (with Examples)

Primary Loss of Water:

- Lack of water intake (vomiting, breast-fed newborns taking concentrated human milk, lack of access to water)
- Lack of normal thirst response (hypothalamic dysfunction)
- ↑ Insensible losses
- Central DI: congenital; acquired (post-TBI, HIE, CNS infections, vascular lesions, tumors, Guillain-Barre Syndrome, ethanol; opioid antagonists, idiopathic)
- Nephrogenic DI, congenital; acquired (Amphotericin B, lithium; propoxyphene, rifampin, colchicine)

Net Loss of Water in Excess of Salt:

- Gastrointestinal losses (diarrhea, vomiting, enteric drainage) osmotic laxatives
- Renal losses (polyuric renal failure, loop diuretics and osmotic diuretics such as mannitol; glycosuria; primary renal disease)
- Burns
- Sweating

Salt Gain

- Administration or ingestion of hypertonic salts (NaCl 3% infusions, hypertonic $NaHCO_3$; hypertonic feedings, hypertonic dialysate); sodium polystyrene
- Primary hyperaldosteronism ("reset-osmostat") and Cushing Syndrome

---

develops gradually, sodium should be decreased by 10–12 mEq/L/ 24 hours *evenly*, or by 1 mEq/L every 2 hours. When hypernatremia develops acutely, as with hypertonic "pushes" of sodium chloride or bicarbonate, a more rapid correction is appropriate.

If hypernatremia is extreme (>180–200 mEq/L) and renal failure is present, dialysis should be considered. In rare cases of acute salt poisoning associated with volume overload or cardiac compromise, a loop diuretic and/or dialysis may be indicated.

Neurogenic or central diabetes insipidus is caused by lack of antidiuretic hormone (ADH) and is most commonly seen in the PICU post-TBI, or in association with tumors, infiltrative disease, inflammation, hypoxic-ischemic injury or surgery involving the posterior pituitary. Diagnosis is suspected in this setting when urine output (UOP) is inappropriately increased, urine specific gravity is < 1.010, serum [Na$^+$] is > 145 mEq/L and serum osmolality is greater than urine osmolality. The condition may be very transient (lasting a few hours), temporary (lasting days to weeks) or permanent. Treatment with vasopressin (**Box 6.2.6**) should be coupled with close monitoring of UOP and serum sodium.

Box 6.2.6   Management of Central Diabetes Insipidus

Fluid needs and administration of aqueous vasopressin:

- Maintenance fluids = insensible losses + UOP replacement. Insensible losses = one half the basal allotment (**Box 6.1.3**).
- Urine losses are typically close to pure water, which cannot be given i.v.; replacement needs can be met with 2.5% dextrose + NaCl 20 mEq/L + K$^+$ 25–40 mEq/L.
- Deficit: If volume depletion has occurred, estimate the deficit and replace as described in *Dehydration, deficit replacement, 6.1.3*) If shock is present, volume resuscitation with 0.9% NaCl should proceed as in any other cause of hypovolemic shock.
- Ongoing losses: Polyuria in central DI is curtailed with aqueous vasopressin:
  ▶ The usual antidiuretic dose is 0.5–10 milliunits (mU)/kg/hr but doses > 40 mU/kg/hr may be necessary in some PICU patients. Starting doses should be small (0.5 mU/kg/hr) and ↑ by 50–100% every 30 mins until ongoing losses are controlled.
  ▶ Adjust dose to effect a UOP ~2 mL/kg/hr.
  ▶ Monitor serum [Na$^+$] to achieve an appropriate decline to normal.
  ▶ Monitor UOP closely; vasopressin dose requirements may change abruptly and a relatively high dose may need to be decreased and vice-versa.
  ▶ DI may result in very rapid increases in serum [Na$^+$]; since cerebral osmoprotection likely occurs over hours, abrupt changes in serum Na$^+$ may be well tolerated.
- Transition to enteral or intranasal DDAVP once DI is well established and controlled with aqueous vasopressin and it is clinically practical.

Nephrogenic DI results from lack of renal responsiveness to antidiuretic hormone. This disorder is seen in tubulointerstitial disease of the kidney, lithium therapy, hypercalcemia, the resolution phase of acute tubular necrosis and post-obstructive uropathy. More rarely, it is congenital and associated with mutation of the V2 AVP receptor or aquaporin 2. These patients do not respond to exogenous vasopressin. Thiazide diuretics and non-steroidal anti-inflammatory agents (indomethacin) are among the therapeutic strategies.

6.2.3 Hypokalemia (serum K^+ < 3.5 meq/L; Boxes 6.2.7 and 6.2.8)

The normal distribution of potassium is ~98% intracellular and 2% extracellular. This gradient is maintained by the Na-K-ATPase pump

---

Box 6.2.7 Main Causes of Hypokalemia

- ↓ Intake
- Shift of K^+ into cells:
  - ▶ Alkalosis
  - ▶ ↑ Insulin
  - ▶ ↑ β-adrenergic activity (stress)
  - ▶ β-agonist therapy
  - ▶ ↑ RBC production
  - ▶ Hypothermia
  - ▶ Hypokalemic periodic paralysis
- Gastrointestinal losses
  - ▶ Vomiting, diarrhea, intestinal drainage
  - ▶ Laxative abuse
- Drug related
- Hyperthyroidism

- Increased urinary losses
  - ▶ Diuretics
  - ▶ Primary mineralocorticoid excess
  - ▶ In response to metabolic alkalosis and chloride depletion
  - ▶ Metabolic acidosis
  - ▶ Magnesium depletion
  - ▶ Amphotericin B
  - ▶ Polyuria from any cause
  - ▶ Salt-wasting nephropathies
  - ▶ Liddle's syndrome
  - ▶ 11β-hydroxy-steroid dehydrogenase deficiency
  - ▶ Bartter's syndrome; Gitelman's syndrome
- ↑ Losses through sweat
- Plasmapheresis
- Dialysis

Box 6.2.8   Signs and Symptoms of Hypokalemia* (K⁺ mEq/L)

- K⁺ 3.5–3.0: Usually, no symptoms
- K⁺ < 3.0: Generalized weakness; constipation
- K⁺ < 2.5: Muscle necrosis
- K⁺ < 2.0: Paralysis; respiratory muscle weakness; respiratory arrest
- ECG changes
  ▶ U waves in lateral precordial leads (shown)
  ▶ ↑ QRS duration (not illustrated)
  ▶ Flattening followed by inversion of T waves
  ▶ Pulseless electrical activity (PEA)

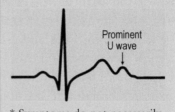

Prominent U wave

* Symptoms do not necessarily correlate with ECG changes

---

in the cell membrane. The ratio of intra- to extracellular concentrations of K⁺ determines the resting membrane potential, impacting primarily on muscle and most critically, on cardiac conduction. Aldosterone is the primary regulator of total body K⁺ stores; it increases in response to hyperkalemia and is suppressed by hypokalemia. Even mild hypokalemia may trigger arrhythmias in patients with cardiac disease. Low potassium potentiates arrhythmogenic effects of digoxin; simultaneous use of diuretics may warrant empiric supplementation with potassium (**Box 6.2.9**).

Treatment of Hypokalemia (Box 6.2.9). The therapeutic approach depends on the cause and severity of hypokalemia: *e.g.* serum [K⁺] 3.0–3.4 mEq/L with normal acid-base status and without abnormal on-going losses in the urine may be easily corrected with enteral supplementation if appropriate, or by low dose IV supplementation with potassium salt (KCl or K-acetate), or addition of K⁺ to maintenance IVF. If the same degree of hypokalemia is present during metabolic acidemia, serum K⁺ will decrease further as K⁺ moves intracellularly in exchange for H⁺ as blood pH is corrected; this situation warrants more aggressive K⁺ supplementation. Alternatively, the same degree

---

Box 6.2.9   Potassium Supplementation in Hypokalemia

IV: Usually: KCl or K-acetate 0.25–0.5 mEq/kg ideal body weight; **maximum** 1 mEq/kg/hr or 40 mEq/hr. This maximal infusion must include K^+ sources already infusing such as TPN. The dose is based on serial measurements of serum K. Potassium infusions containing ≤80 mEq/L in 0.9% NaCl are required for peripheral infusion. Usual concentration for central infusion is 20 mEq/100 mL; K^+ 20 mEq per 50 ml should be given by CVL if fluid restriction is essential. Continuous ECG monitoring is required for doses >0.5 mEq/kg/hr.

Enteral: Preferred route when hypokalemia is mild. Usual dose: KCl or K-acetate 2–5 mEq/kg/day in divided doses, or added to 24 hrs of continuous feedings. Maximum single dose: 2 mEq/kg/dose.

---

of hypokalemia in the presence of renal failure or tumor lysis may be viewed as desirable.

6.2.4 Hyperkalemia (serum $K^+ > 5.5$ mEq/L; Boxes 6.2.10 and 6.2.11)

Hyperkalemia results from an increased burden or decreased excretion of potassium. True hyperkalemia is most commonly associated with renal failure, because either filtration or renal tubular secretion of K^+ is impaired. Specimen hemolysis and prolonged tourniquet application proximal to the site of venipuncture may cause "pseudohyperkalemia" which should be distinguished from true hyperkalemia by optimal sampling techniques and/or ECG changes. If hyperkalemia requires treatment (**Box 6.2.12**), continuous ECG monitoring is essential; also ensure that all sources of potassium are eliminated.

6.2.5 Magnesium (Mg^{++}, Boxes 6.2.13 and 6.2.14)

Normal serum or plasma Mg^{++} ranges from 1.7 to 2.2 mg/dL but does not dependably reflect body stores. However, $Mg^{++} < 1$ mg/dL

Box 6.2.10   Main Causes of True Hyperkalemia

↑ **K⁺ burden/K⁺ release from cells**
- Acidemia (↓ blood pH)
- Insulin deficiency, hyperglycemia and hyperosmolality
- Tissue catabolism; tumor lysis
- Drugs: β-blockers; succinylcholine
- Iatrogenic
- Strenuous exercise; rhabdomyolysis
- True hemolysis
- Hyperkalemic periodic paralysis
- Acute digitalis poisoning

↓ **K⁺ excretion**
- Acute or chronic renal failure
- Congenital adrenal hyperplasia
- Pseudohypoaldosteronism
- Volume contraction
- Renal tubular acidosis, type 1
- Drugs: *e.g.* angiotensin converting enzyme inhibitors (captopril, enalapril); cyclosporine, spironolactone, amiloride, triamterene

---

Box 6.2.11   Signs and Symptoms of Hyperkalemia (K in mEq/L)

Clinical findings:	ECG changes:
K⁺ < 7.0: Usually no symptoms	K⁺ 5.5–6.5: Tall, peaked T-waves ↓ P–R +/− ↓ QT$_c$ interval
K⁺ > 7.0: Muscle weakness which progresses to flaccid paralysis	K⁺ 6.5–7.5: ↑ P–R interval and widened QRS
K⁺ > 9.0: ↑↑ Risk for ventricular fibrillation and asystole	K⁺ > 7.5: flattening of P waves; ↑QT$_c$ interval; S–T changes (↑ or ↓)
	K⁺ > 8.0: absent P waves; ↑↑ QRS to sine wave appearance; bundle branch block or AV nodal block pattern; ventricular fibrillation and asystole may follow.

Box 6.2.12 Treatment of True Hyperkalemia

Intervention	Indication	Onset	Duration	Advantages and Limitations
Calcium gluconate 10% 0.5 mL/kg up to 10 mL; repeat in 5 mins if ECG changes persist.	ECG changes other than peaked T waves; whenever an immediate effect is needed	minutes	30–60 mins	Stabilizes cardiac muscle; Transient effect; supplement with treatments that will shift K^+ into cells and aid in removal of K^+; use caution if given by peripheral vein.
$NaHCO_3$ 7.5% (1 mEq/mL) 2–3 mEq/kg	Moves K^+ intracellularly; patient need not be acidemic	30–60 mins	1–4 hrs	Most effective if patient is acidemic; may promote renal excretion of K^+.
Glucose 1 g/kg IV infused over 15–30 mins followed by regular insulin 0.1 Units per kg subQ or IV	Serum $K^+ \geq 6.5$ if ECG changes are present. If chronic renal failure is present + there are *no* ECG changes, dialysis is the treatment of choice.	15–30 mins	1–4 hrs	Shifts K^+ into cells; may result in K^+ inavailability during hemodialysis.
Albuterol 0.5% (aerosolized) 0.1–0.3 mg/kg	To supplement other treatments by shifting K^+ intracellularly	20–30 mins Peak at 90 mins	1–4 hrs Most effective when given continuously	Same as for glucose and insulin.

(Continued)

Box 6.2.12	Treatment of True Hyperkalemia (Continued)			
Intervention	Indication	Onset	Duration	Advantages and Limitations
Sodium polystyrene sulfonate given with (Kayexalate) 1 g/kg up to 30 gm PO or PR	To remove K^+ through the gastrointestinal tract	1–2 hrs	~4 hrs depending on cause of hyperkalemia	Decreases the total body K^+ burden; cannot be given if bowel integrity is lacking or ileus is present. Most preparations contain sorbitol. See specifications of product used.
Loop diuretics: *e.g.* Furosemide 1–2 mg/kg IV	To remove K^+ through the kidney	5 mins	2 hrs	Volume repletion may be required; ↑ doses may be required in renal insufficiency; not useful in renal failure.
Renal replacement therapy	To remove K^+ if above measures fail; especially effective when K^+ from tissue break-down is on-going.			

is always indicative of deficiency. Hypomagnesemia occurs in ~11% of critically ill children. Low fractional excretion of magnesium may be useful to distinguish true depletion ($FE_{Mg} < 2\%$) with borderline serum levels from magnesium sufficiency, provided renal function is normal.

Treatment of symptomatic hypomagnesemia: $MgSO_4$ 25–50 mg/kg IV (max dose 2 gm) infused over 2 to 4 hrs; do not exceed 125 mg/kg/hr). If not symptomatic, enteral supplementation is preferred if possible.

Hypermagnesemia is uncommon in the absence of renal failure. The normal kidney readily excretes Mg^{++} excess. Symptoms, signs and

Box 6.2.13   Symptoms of Hypomagnesemia

- Trousseau sign: spasm of hand and forearm muscles with BP cuff inflated >SBP for 3 min
- Chvostek sign: twitching of facial muscles by tapping over facial nerve
- Apathy
- Parasthesias
- Depression
- Delirium
- Muscle weakness
- Seizures
- Peaked T waves
- Widening of PR interval
- Ventricular arrhythmias
- Appearance of U waves
- Prolongation of QRS

Box 6.2.14   Causes of Hypomagnesemia

- Gastrointestinal losses (diarrheal disease; ostomy drainage; malabsorption; primary Mg malabsorption)
- Malnutrition (enteral and/or parenteral)
- Renal losses; osmotic diuresis, esp. if chronic as in diabetes; DKA; renal tubular defects; hypercalciuric states (hyperparathyroidism); chronically increased total body volume (hyperaldosteronism and inappropriate ADH secretion); hyperthyroidism; Bartter's syndrome; drugs such as diuretics, aminoglycosides, amphotericin B, cisplatin, cyclosporine
- Hypoparathyroidism
- Acute pancreatitis
- Insulin therapy; hyperinsulinism
- Respiratory alkalosis
- Severe burns
- Chelation of Mg by transfusion with large volumes of citrated blood
- Critical illness

causes of hypermagnesemia are listed (**Box 6.2.15**). Treatment includes elimination of intake of magnesium, ensure euvolemia and correct the cause of hypermagnesemia if possible. Dialysis should be considered in patients with renal failure. If cardiac arrhythmias develop, treat with calcium gluconate 60–100 mg/kg/dose IV (max 3 g/dose).

Box 6.2.15   Hypermagnesemia

Symptoms and Signs	Causes
• Nausea; vomiting	• Renal dysfunction
• Lethargy; coma	• Volume depletion
• Respiratory depression	• Excess administration (*e.g.* TPN)
• Hypotension	• Acidosis; shock; trauma; burns
• Muscle weakness	• Antacid or cathartic overdose
• Prolonged PR/QT/QRS	• Hypothyroidism
with Mg >8 mg/dL	• Hypoaldosteronism
• Paralysis of respiratory and	• Rhabdomyolysis
voluntary muscles with	• Lithium therapy
Mg >12 mg/dL	

6.2.6 Calcium and phosphorus homeostasis

Calcium (Ca) and phosphorus (Phos) availability and regulation are critical to energy production and expenditure (including muscle contraction), and bone formation (leading to growth). Disturbances in Ca or Phos homeostasis may be the primary reason for PICU admission, or may occur secondary to critical illness. While imbalances in each ion are discussed separately to some extent, an understanding of the relationship between calcium and phosphorus is helpful in analyzing the cause of a disturbance in one or the other ion (**Box 6.2.16**).

Causes, symptoms and signs of hypocalcemia are listed in **Boxes 6.2.17 and 6.2.18**. The assessment of calcium disturbances should include a thorough dietary, growth and family history, and review of medications. Simultaneously obtained measurements of ionized calcium (iCa), Phos, Mg^{++}, urea nitrogen, creatinine, liver enzymes and function tests, alkaline phosphatase, intact PTH, 25(OH) vitamin D and 1,25(OH)$_2$ vitamin D. "Spot" urine for urine calcium: creatinine ratio identifies hypercalciuric states. In an infant, a single AP view of one knee is sufficient to R/O active rickets.

Treatment of hypocalcemia should be directed at the cause. Symptomatic hypocalcemia should be treated with calcium gluconate

Box 6.2.16   Key Points Regarding Calcium and Phosphorus Relationships

- Total Ca (tCa) measures the calcium bound to organic and inorganic anions (~15%), calcium bound to albumin (~40%) and the ionized calcium (iCa, ~45%). Normal parathyroid hormone (PTH) secretion requires Mg^{++} and controls the serum iCa concentration tightly. Hypocalcemia causes ↑PTH secretion leading to:

  ▸ Increased renal tubular reabsorption of Ca.
  ▸ Increased calcium mobilization from bone.
  ▸ Decreased renal tubular reabsorption of Phos (causing phosphaturia).
  ▸ Promoting conversion of 25-OH vitamin D to $1,25(OH)_2$ Vitamin D resulting in ↑ intestinal absorption and ↑ renal tubular reabsorption of Ca and Phos, and solubilization of bone. Enteral calcium is poorly absorbed when "the active" vitamin D is deficient.

- For every 1 g/dL decrease in the serum albumin, the tCa is lowered by ~0.8 mg/dL; however, the iCa may be normal. (Note that serum albumin varies slightly with age.)
- The normal serum iCa varies little with age after the newborn period, when it stabilizes at ~4.2–5.2 mg/dL (laboratory dependent). However, normal Phos varies with age and is higher in younger patients. The younger the child, the greater the phosphorus requirement to build bone; of note, less Phos is lost in urine due to a lower GFR in infants.

Age	Normal Serum Phosphorus (mg/dL)
Newborns	4.2–9.0
10 days–24 mos	4.5–6.7
24 mos–12 yrs	4.5–5.5
>12 yrs	2.7–4.5

(Continued)

Box 6.2.16   Key Points Regarding Calcium and Phosphorus Relationships (Continued)

- The [tCa] × [Phos] product in mg/dL: If either Ca *or* Phos concentrations sufficiently alter the Ca × Phos product, soft tissue calcification *vs.* mineralization *vs.* bone resorption may be favored. If the [tCa] × [Phos] product is:
  - 40–60 mg/dL, this indicates the normal range.
  - < 30 mg/dL, rickets or "biochemical rickets" is present. The latter means that if these conditions persist, there will be insufficient Ca and Phos for bone deposition and rickets will result.
  - 30–40 mg/dL, a "gray zone" for development of metabolic bone disease is present.
  - >70 mg/dL (beyond the newborn period) an ↑ risk for soft tissue calcification exisits.

- Phosphate absorption from the GI tract is largely passive, but is enhanced by vitamin D. Phosphate absorption from the GI tract is curtailed by the presence of polyvalent cations such as calcium, aluminum and magnesium in the gut lumen.

- Calcitonin responds to increased iCa, causing a decrease in Ca release from bone and a decrease in renal tubular reabsorption of Ca and Phos; Calcitonin release is also stimulated by glucocorticoids, glucagon, β-adrenergic agents, *et al.*

10% (100–200 mg/kg) or calcium chloride (10–20 mg/kg) IV; dosing may be repeated as needed (usually, every 6 hrs) or given by continuous IV infusion (*e.g.* calcium gluconate 10% 400–600 mg/kg/day); the dose should be adjusted based on close monitoring of serum [iCa]. Intravenous calcium therapy should be provided through a central venous catheter because peripheral tissue infiltration with calcium causes tissue necrosis. Hypomagesemia should be corrected since this disturbance itself can lead to hypocalcemia. Treatment of asymptomatic hypocalcemia with enteral calcium supplements alone will be ineffective if malabsorption, vitamin D deficiency or hypoparathyroidism is operative. Both vitamin D deficiency and hypoparathyroidism require treatment with vitamin D, the latter requiring treatment with calcitriol

Box 6.2.17   Causes of Hypocalcemia

- Inadequate PTH production, secretion and/or reponse to PTH:
  ▸ Transient neonatal hypoparathyroidism, early: infants of diabetic mothers; maternal hypercalcemia (due to hyperparathyroidism); stressed newborns (sepsis; hypoxia, prematurity, *etc*)
  ▸ Transient neonatal hypoparathyroidism; late: usually due to phosphate loading
  ▸ Hypomagnesemia
  ▸ Gram negative sepsis, toxic shock syndrome, AIDS (cytokine-mediated?)
  ▸ Congential hypoparathyroidism: parathyroid agenesis or hypoplasia (*e.g.* diGeorge syndrome)
  ▸ Mitochondrial disorders
  ▸ Acquired hypoparathyroidism *e.g.* parathyroid gland injury (surgical, radiation), hemochromatosis, Wilson's disease, autoimmune
  ▸ Pseudohypoparathyroidism (end-organ unresponsiveness to PTH)
- Vitamin D deficiency, genetic or acquired: *e.g.* nutritional deficiency or malabsorption of vitamin D; inability to 1-α hydroxylate vitamin D in the kidney (vitamin D-dependent rickets, type 1; severe renal disease); end-organ-unresponsiveness to 1,25 $(OH)_2$ vitamin D (vitamin D resistant rickets). These disorders are associated with secondary hyperparathyroidism, *i.e.* the parathyroid gland is normal, and PTH secretion is ↑↑ in response to low iCa.
- Inadequate intake and/or malabsorption of calcium
- Hyperphosphatemia: lead to rapid precipitation of Ca and Phos, first into bone, then into soft tissues (this risk may be increased when [Ca] × [Phos] in mg/dL exceeds 70); may occur with PN errors, repeated or high dose phosphate enemas; tumor lysis.
- Chelation of Ca by citrated blood products; lipid administration; pancreatitis.
- Alkalemia: For each 0.1 unit ↑ in blood pH, the measured iCa ↓ by 0.16 mg/dL due to ↑ protein binding.
- Drug-related liver enzyme induction (via the cytochrome P-450 system) causing ↑ vitamin D catabolism: phenytoin, phenobarbital, carbamazepine, rifampin, isoniazid, *et al.*
- Calcitonin excess
- Critical illness

Box 6.2.18   Signs and Symptoms of Hypocalcemia

- Chvostek sign
- Trousseau sign (carpopedal spasm)
- Parasthesias
- Lethargy; irritability
- Poor feeding
- Apnea
- Seizures (focal or generalized)
- Bronchospasm
- Laryngospasm (recurrent "croup")
- Prolonged QT_c interval

- Signs of long-standing hypocalcemia (or hypophosphatemia) in growing patients include the manifestations of rachitic bone disease:
  ▸ Bowing of the legs with weight-bearing
  ▸ Widening of the wrists
  ▸ Rachitic rosary
  ▸ Craniotabes
  ▸ Growth retardation
  ▸ X-ray: metaphyseal cupping, fraying and cortical spurs at the growing ends of long bones, especially those that are normally flat (*e.g.* ulna, fibula) but can also be seen in the distal radius, femur and tibia
- Osteopenia; pathologic fractures

(1,25(OH)$_2$ vitamin D). Consultation with a pediatric endocrinologist is recommended for these patients.

Hypercalcemia (tCa >11 mg/dL) should be evaluated by measuring iCa and serum albumin to R/O hyperalbuminemia as a cause of factitious hypercalcemia (for each 1 g/dL increase in serum albumin, the tCa is increased by ~0.8 mg/dL). Serum [tCa] >15 mg/dL is associated with severe, life-threatening symptoms. Causes, symptoms and signs of hypercalcemia are listed in **Boxes 6.2.19 and 6.2.20**. Treatment of hypercalcemia is directed at the cause and is dependent on severity. Emergent treatment is outlined in **Box 6.2.21**.

Hypophosphatemia is common among PICU patients. Risk factors common in this population include poor nutrition, acute respiratory disease, diuretic use, chronic osmotic diuresis (*e.g.* poorly controlled diabetes mellitus), insulin, dopamine, antacid therapy, sepsis and volume loading. Phosphorus unavailability has potential to affect energy production when hypophosphatemia is accompanied by depletion of intracellular phosphates resulting in decreased 2, 3 DPG in red blood cells (*Oxyhemoglobin dissociation curve, Appendix, part 2, III*) and a fall in ATP leading to energy failure for all ATP-dependent cell functions. Acute signs and symptoms (**Boxes 6.2.22 and 6.2.23**) may not apparent until deficiency is severe (Phos <1 mg/dL).

Box 6.2.19 Causes of Hypercalcemia

- Excessive intake of Ca ("milk-alkali syndrome") and/or vitamin D; excessive administration of Ca in IVF or TPN
- Primary Hyperparathyroidism (↑PTH *not* in response to hypocalcemia): Includes multiple endocrine neoplasia syndromes, parathyroid adenomas, Ca-sensing receptor mutations, lithium toxicity
- Familial hypocalciuric hypercalcemia
- Sarcoidosis (↑ production of 1,25(OH)$_2$ vitamin D)
- Increased bone resorption: Hyperparathyroidism; immobilization hypercalcemia; hypervitaminosis A; hyperthyroidism; malignancy; cytokine-mediated
- Thiazide diuretics (↑ renal tubular reabsorption of Ca)
- Aluminum toxicity
- Idiopathic infantile hypercalcemia (William's Syndrome)
- Subcutaneous fat necrosis

Box 6.2.20 Signs and Symptoms of Hypercalcemia

- Lethargy
- Headache
- Poor feeding, nausea, vomiting
- Constipation
- Hypercalciuria (leads to polyuria and dehydration)
- Hypertension
- ECG abnormalities including ↓ QT$_c$ interval, bundle-branch block, ventricular arrhythmias, widened T waves
- Bone pain
- Pathologic fractures
- Ectopic calcifications; nephrocalcinosis
- Renal stones
- Renal insufficiency or failure
- Alterations in mental status, including hallucinations, psychosis, coma
- Hyporeflexia
- Seizures

Box 6.2.21   Emergent Treatment of Hypercalcemia

- Ensure adequate circulating volume; correct dehydration.
- For [tCa] >13 mg/dL, renal excretion may be enhanced by saline diuresis. Administer NaCl 0.9% at 2–3 times the maintenance fluid requirement.
- Addition of a loop diuretic (*e.g.* furosemide) to promote excretion of Ca during saline loading may be required. Avoid thiazide diuretics.
- If renal failure is present, or cardiopulmonary disease prohibits volume loading, hemodialysis should be considered.
- Calcitonin and bisphosphonates (*e.g.* pamidronate IV) may be helpful in reducing calcium mobilization from bone.
- Glucocorticoids may be helpful in decreasing Ca absorption from the GI tract in sarcoidosis and hypervitaminosis D.
- Parathyroidectomy may be indicated for: hyperparathyroid crises; "tertiary hyperparathyroidism" (the autonomous hyperparathyroidism resulting from prolonged secondary hyperparathyroidism seen in chronic renal failure) with multi-organ system sequelae, *et al.*

Box 6.2.22   Signs and Symptoms of Severe Hypophosphatemia (Phos ≤ 1 mg/dL)

- Irritability
- Paresthesias
- Altered in mental status; coma
- Seizures
- ↓ Diaphragmatic strength
- ↓ Myocardial contractility
- Proximal skeletal muscle weakness
- ↓ RBC deformability (hemolysis)

- Smooth muscle dysfunction; dysphagia, ileus
- Rhabdomyolysis (seen primarily in alcoholics)
- Hypercalciuria (seen in prolonged hypophosphatemia)
- Rickets; osteomalacia in prolonged hypophosphatemia (not necessarily severe hypophosphatemia)

Box 6.2.23 Causes of Hypophosphatemia (Low [Phos] in Serum for Age)

- ↓ **Intake or fat malabsorption:** Chronic diarrhea; TPN with inadequate provision of Phos; chelation of Phos in the GI tract by calcium, aluminum or magnesium.
- **Renal Phos wasting:** Osmotic diuresis; acetazolamide; metolazone; acute volume expansion; renal tubular defects causing impaired Phos reabsorption; primary or secondary hyperparathyroidism; Familial X-linked hypophosphatemia (mutation in PHEX gene) causes rickets without hypocalcemia; Fibroblast growth factor 23 mutation impairs renal tubular reabsorption of Phos and $1,25(OH)_2$ vitamin D synthesis; post-partial hepatectomy; Fanconi syndrome; tumor-induced osteomalacia; post-transplantation.
- **Redistribution of Phos from extra- to intracellular compartments:** During treatment of DKA with insulin; during refeeding of malnourished patients; acute respiratory alkalosis; post-parathyroidectomy or post-thyroidectomy (Hungry bone syndrome).

Treatment of hypophosphatemia is dependent on its cause and severity. The cause is usually identifiable by history and clinical context. If the cause is unclear, renal wasting of Phos should be ruled out. Calculate the fractional excretion of Phos (FE_{phos}; U, urine; P, plasma; cr, creatinine):

$$(U_{phos}/P_{phos}) \div (U_{cr}/P_{cr})$$

FE_{phos} is 5–20% if serum Phos is normal. The normal renal response to hypophosphatemia is conservation of filtered Phos ($FE_{phos} < 5\%$). If FE_{phos} is $\geq 5\%$ despite hypophosphatemia, renal Phos wasting is present.

Phosphate supplementation (**Box 6.2.24**) is indicated for symptomatic hypophosphatemia (usually Phos < 1–2 mg/dL) and may be considered for subnormal concentrations of Phos (**Box 6.2.16**) particularly when renal function is normal and critical illness may cause further declines in serum Phos. Most enteral feedings are rich in phosphorus. Enteral Phos supplements should be considered as soon as feasible but may cause diarrhea, limiting their use.

Box 6.2.24   Suggested Supplementation with Sodium or Potassium Phosphate (IV) Based on Degree of Hypophosphatemia

Low dose: 0.08 mmol/kg over 6 hrs.
Intermediate dose: 0.16–0.24 mmol/kg over 6 hrs.
High dose: 0.36 mmol/kg over 6 hrs.

Note: Dosing may be ↑ by 25–50% if patient is symptomatic (0.5 mmol/ kg over 4 hrs if serum phosphorus is <0.5 mg/dl) and ↓ by 25–50% if hypercalcemia is present. Dose may also be increased (to the next degree of severity) if ongoing urinary losses are a concern.

When even mild degrees of hyperphosphatemia occur, normal renal function and PTH secretion trigger decreased renal tubular reabsorption of Phos, increasing Phos excretion. Factitious hyperphosphatemia may occur due to specimen hemolysis, assay-related interferences in the presence of hyperlipidemia, hyperbilirubinemia, hyperglobulinemia and high dose liposomal Amphotericin B. Causes of hyperphosphatemia are summarized (**Box 6.2.25**).

Treatment of hyperphosphatemia depends on its cause and degree. Hyperphosphatemia increases the [Ca] × [Phos] product and may lead to soft tissue calcification if the product exceeds 70. Hypocalcemia results as Ca and Phos precipitate (into bone and possibly soft tissues). Induction of a high Ca and Phos ion product complicates the treat-

---

Box 6.2.25   Causes of Hyperphosphatemia

- **Acute ↑ in Phos load:** tumor lysis, rhabdomyolysis, severe hemolysis, transfusion of large volume of stored RBC's; diabetic ketoacidosis or severe hyperglycemia prior to treatment with insulin; lactic acidosis, administration of excessive amount of phosphate (IV; enterally including laxatives and phosphate-containing enemas).
- **Renal failure**
- **↑ Renal tubular reabsorption of Phos:** Hypoparathyroidism, vitamin D toxicity, bisphosphonates, familial tumoral calcinosis.

ment of the resulting hypocalcemia, making the correction of hyper-phosphatemia essential for correction of hypocalcemia. All sources of phosphate intake should be curtailed or discontinued. Food is rich in phosphate; low phosphate feedings and Phos binders may be given to minimize Phos absorption if intake is permitted. Phosphate can be renally excreted if hydration is maintained and GFR is sufficient. Hyperphosphatemia causing hypocalcemia is an indication for dialysis in renal failure acute kidney injury.

6.3 Acid-base Imbalance

Acidosis is a decrease in total carbon dioxide (tCO_2) buffering capacity without a decrease in blood pH; alkalosis is an increase in tCO_2 buffering capacity without an increase in blood pH. "Acidemia" and "alkalemia" describe states of subnormal (<7.35), or supranormal (>7.45) blood pH, respectively. Primary alterations in respiration or metabolism drive the direction of pH change (**Box 6.3.1**). Secondary changes often only partially compensate the pH toward normal range.

Box 6.3.1   Acidosis and Alkalosis

Disorder (normal)	Blood pH (7.35–7.45)	Total CO$_2$* (22–29 mEq/L)	PaCO$_2$ (35–45 mmHg)	Base Excess (+) or Deficit (−) (+ or −3 mEq/L)
Metabolic Acidosis	↓	Primary ↓	Secondary ↓	Negative
Respiratory Acidosis	↓ if acute; low normal if chronic	Secondary ↑	Primary ↑	Positive; may be normal if acute
Metabolic Alkalosis	↑	Primary ↑	Secondary ↑	Positive
Respiratory Alkalosis	↑	Secondary ↓	Primary ↓	Negative

* The clinical laboratory measures total carbon dioxide, most of which is the form of bicarbonate. The terms total CO_2 and bicarbonate sometimes are used interchangeably.

Calculation of pH involves understanding of the Henderson-Hasselbalch equation: $[H^+]$ $[HCO_3^-]/[H_2 CO_3]$ = K (dissociation constant).

$$pH = pK + \log ([HCO_3^-]/[H_2 CO_3])$$
$$pH = 6.1 + \log ([HCO_3^-]/(PaCO_2 \times 0.03))$$

Under normal conditions,

$$pH = 6.1 + \log ([\ 24/40 \times 0.03\ ]) = 6.1 + 1.3 = 7.40$$

Calculation of contributions of respiratory and metabolic factors that impact on acid-base balance can be accomplished. If the ABG reveals pH 7.26 and $PaCO_2$ 50 mmHg:

(1) Estimate the contribution of $PaCO_2$ to pH: for each 10 mm Hg change in $PaCO_2$ the pH should change by 0.08. In the above example, since the $PaCO_2$ is 10 mmHg above 40, the pH is expected to decrease by 0.08 from a normal value of 7.40 or to 7.32. The pH of 7.26 therefore suggests a mixed disturbance, *i.e.* the pH is lower than can be explained by the elevated $PaCO_2$.

(2) Estimate the base excess: Take the estimated pH calculated from contribution of $PaCO_2$ subtract the calculated pH(7.32) from the ACTUAL pH (7.26–7.32 = –0.06); multiply –0.06 by 67 to give the base excess of –4 (or base deficit of 4 mEq/L). In other words, a pH change of 0.01 units should result in a $[HCO_3^-]$ change of 0.67 mEq/L.

(3) The amount of base required to initiate correction of metabolic acidosis (*Appendix, part 2, V*) is approximately one-third the total body base deficit, or: Amount of base to be given (in mEq) = base deficit × weight (kg)/3.

Metabolic acidosis may present with Kussmaul breathing and compensatory hypocapnea (in the absence of lung disease). If acidosis is prolonged, fatigue, weakness and malaise may occur. Metabolic acidosis is categorized by the presence or absence of an "anion gap" (AG; **Box 6.3.2**) calculated as follows:

$$AG = [Na^+] - ([HCO_3^+] + [Cl^-]);$$
the normal AG is 12 +/− 4 mEq/L.

Box 6.3.2   Causes of Metabolic Acidosis Categorized by Anion Gap (AG)

Normal AG ([HCO$_3^+$]
loss or dilution):
- Prolonged infusion of fluid without base (acetate or bicarbonate; *e.g.* 0.9% NaCl)
- Bicarbonate loss in stool or in urine (RTA)
- Pancreatic fistula
- Uretero-sigmoidostomy
- Renal failure (occasionally)
- Intoxication: glue sniffing, NH$_4$Cl, acetazolamide, bile acid sequestrants, isopropyl alcohol

Elevated AG ([HCO$_3^+$]
consumption by acid production or ingestion):
- Renal failure (excess phosphate, sulfate, urates)
- Ketoacidosis
- Lactic acidosis (**Box 6.3.3**)
- Massive rhabdomyolysis
- Intoxication: salicylates, ethanol, methanol, ethylene glycol, formaldehyde, paraldehyde, INH, toluene, metformin

Treatment of acute severe metabolic acidosis (arterial pH < 7.1) may help improve cardiovascular stability by decreasing dilation of arterioles and increasing blunted cardiac contractility. Infusion of 1 mEq/kg of Na$^+$HCO$_3^-$ (preferably over ≥ 30 mins) or infusion of IV fluid with most or all the anion as base (*e.g.* 150 mEq/L of Na$^+$HCo$_3^-$) may be helpful. Rapid infusions ("IV pushes") of hypertonic sodium bicarbonate should be avoided unless responsiveness to life-threatening interventions is impaired by severe acidemia (usually a pH < 7.00). The goal pH after correction should be 7.20–7.30. Monitor for hypokalemia, hypocalcemia and hypophosphatemia resulting from increases in blood pH.

Respiratory acidosis may be present with either increased or decreased work of breathing depending upon the underlying pathology (**Box 6.3.4**).

Treatment of severe respiratory acidosis may require supplemental oxygen (CO$_2$ may displace O$_2$ in the alveolar space and result in

Box 6.3.3   Causes of Lactic Acidosis

Type A lactic acidosis is caused by tissue hypoxia. Examples include:

- Circulatory shock
- Respiratory failure
- Low cardiac output states (*e.g.* CHF; LV dysfunction)
- Sepsis
- Cardiopulmonary arrest
- Strenuous exercise
- Excessive muscle activity (*e.g.* status epilepticus)
- Carbon monoxide poisoning
- Methemglobinemia
- Cyanide poisoning
- Severe metabolic alkalemia

Type B lactic acidosis is usually toxin-induced or associated with regional ischemia or metabolic defects.

- Drug-related (*e.g.* biguanides such as metformin; isoniazid)
- Toxins (*e.g.* ethanol; methanol; ethylene glycol; papavarine)
- Malignancy
- Renal failure
- Inborn Errors of Metabolism (*e.g.*):
  ▶ Type 1 glycogen storage disease
  ▶ Pyruvate carboxylase deficiency
  ▶ Pyruvate dehydrogenase deficiency

Type D lactic acidosis is a direct result of jejuno-ileal bypass or short-gut syndrome. Normally, the small bowel absorbs nutrients capable of producing the *d*-isomer of lactic acid. In short-gut, carbohydrate is delivered to the colon in large amounts. Overgrowth of Gram positive anaerobes such as *Lactobacillus acidophilus* which possess *d*-lactic acid dehydrogenase (*d*-LDH) leads to production of *d*-lactate, which cannot be metabolized by *l*-LDH (mammalian LDH is specific for the *l*-isomer). Levels of *d*-lactic acid may be increased in patients with short-gut, but this may not be problematic unless symptoms (primarily neurologic and usually after high carbohydrate intake) result. It is unclear whether toxicity is directly related to *d*-lactic acid or if *d*-lactic acid is a marker for other toxic product(s) from the colon.

Box 6.3.4 Causes of Respiratory Acidosis

- Respiratory center dysfunction
- Chest wall deformities
- Pneumothorax
- Airway obstruction
- Parenchymal lung disease
- Defects in nerves and muscles of respiration

---

hypoxemia) and/or mechanical ventilatory support. Simultaneous treatment of metabolic acidosis with sodium bicarbonate will increase tCO_2 and therefore, $PaCO_2$; tromethamine decreases $PaCO_2$ while simultaneously increasing plasma bicarbonate.

Respiratory alkalosis (acute) may present with sensations of breathlessness, choking, dizziness, nervousness, parethesias of extremities and around the mouth, altered level of consciousness and tetany (**Box 6.3.6**). Treatment of respiratory alkalosis involves treating the underlying cause.

Box 6.3.5 Causes of Metabolic Alkalosis*

Chloride responsive (Urine Cl⁻ typically low *e.g.* <10 mEq/L)	**Chloride unresponsive (Urine Cl⁻ variable)**
• Chloride loss: *Post*-diuretic use, vomiting (esp. pyloric stenosis), gastric drainage without salt replacement; if diuretic therapy is still in progress, urine Cl⁻ may be increased despite total body Cl⁻ depletion.	• Edema forming states (urine Cl⁻ <10 mEq/L)
	• K⁺ depletion, hypermineralocorticoidism, hypercalcemia/ hyperparathyroidism (urine Cl >10 mEq/L)
• Salt restriction: Post-hypercapneic alkalosis without chloride repletion or after administration of alkali	• Advanced renal failure with extrarenal generation of bicarbonate (urine Cl⁻ unpredictable)
• Congenital chloridorrhea	

* Metabolic acidosis may or may not be lessened after chloride administration.

Box 6.3.6   Causes of Respiratory Alkalosis

- Anxiety or voluntary hyperventilation
- Septicemia and/or hypotension
- Pregnancy or progesterone exposure
- Iatrogenic hyperventilation
- Hepatic failure/encephalopathy
- Lung edema, pulmonary emboli, interstitial lung disease
- Neurologic disorders: trauma, infection, tumors, stroke, pain

- Fever/heat syndromes
- Congenital heart disease
- Severe anemia
- High altitude exposure
- Hemodialysis
- Hypoxia of any cause; carbon monoxide poisoning
- Drugs: salicylate, nicotine, exogenous catecholamines, methylxanthines

---

Metabolic alkalosis may present with altered mental status (even coma), apnea, neuromuscular excitability (tetany, seizures) and presence of hypokalemia, hypochloremia, hypocalcemia or hypophosphatemia. Causes of metabolic alkalosis are categorized as chloride responsive or unresponsive (**Box 6.3.5**). Treatment includes: (1) resolution of underlying cause whenever possible; (2) enhancement of renal excretion of HCO_3^- by correction of hypovolemia, hypokalemia (with KCl), hypercalcemia or use of acetazolamide in edema-forming states; (3) chemical buffering by titration of HCO_3^- with HCl or NH_4Cl (if renal insufficiency or hypovolemia cannot be corrected by volume expansion) and (4) removal of excess HCO_3^- by dialysis.

6.4   Hypoglycemia and Hyperglycemia

Maintenance of normoglycemia results from proper balance of glucose availability and glucose utilization; imbalance on either side of the metabolic scale leads to hypo- or hyperglycemia. Both conditions are eventually toxic, and require recognition with identification of the cause and treatment. Glucose should be measured by both rapid bedside and laboratory assays. The latter requires that the specimen be placed in sodium fluoride preservative ("gray-top" tube) or an iced heparinized sample be brought immediately to the laboratory.

Bedside glucose meter readings may differ from more accurate laboratory measurements within a range of 20%.

Hypoglycemia is variably defined, with general agreement that serum or plasma glucose ≤40 mg/dL at any age should be thoroughly evaluated. Glucose ≥60 mg/dL is expected after the first six hrs of life in a healthy term newborn. Values between 40–60 mg/dL may indicate hypoglycemia warranting evaluation. At a minimum, serum glucose should be maintained above this range in patients who are critically ill. Maintenance of normoglycemia (80–120 mg/dL) depends on:

- Adequate glucose supply: nutrition, glycogen and fat stores, and gluconeogenic substrate (amino acids, glycerol, lactate).
- Metabolic machinery to conduct: absorption, glycogenesis and glycogenolysis, glycolysis, gluconeogenesis and oxidation.
- Hormonal control to regulate glucose homeostasis: insulin, glucagon, catecholamines, cortisol, growth hormone.
- Other factors such as autonomic input, glucagon-like peptide 1, and cytokines may play important roles.

Infants and children utilize glucose 2–3 times faster than adults (~4–6 mg/kg/min vs. 2–2.5 mg/kg/min, respectively); the brain utilizes glucose ~20 times faster than other tissues. Therefore, vulnerability to neurologic injury from hypoglycemia is heightened in

---

Box 6.4.1   Signs and Symptoms of Hypoglycemia

Autonomic response to hypoglycemia:
- Tachycardia
- Tachypnea
- Tremulousness, agitation
- Sweating
- Pallor
- Cyanosis
- Nausea and vomiting

Neurologic effects of hypoglycemia:
- Lethargy; altered mental status; visual disturbances; attention deficits; headache; incoordination
- Poor feeding; dysarthria
- Hypothermia
- Apnea
- Seizures; parasthesias; stroke
- Hypotonia; posturing
- Coma

Box 6.4.2   Causes of Hypoglycemia

- R/O "artifactual hypoglycemia" by repeating the bedside glucose test and sending a specimen to the laboratory if time permits. Samples that remain on the test strip >10–15 min may result in a falsely low glucose value. Treatment of hypoglycemia should not await confirmatory data.
- Stress with ↑ glucose utilization: Sepsis, shock, severe trauma, surgery
- Liver disease: Hepatitis, α-1-antitrypsin deficiency, Reye's syndrome
- Congenital heart disease: Possibly due to hepatic congestion or poorly perfused liver
- Toxic ingestions: Determine access to oral hyperglycemic agents and insulin, alcohol (including mouthwash), β-blockers, aspirin, quinine, iron, hydrocarbon exposure, *et al.*
- Endocrinopathies:
  ▶ Growth hormone deficiency
  ▶ Cortisol deficiency (CAH, Addison's disease, ACTH deficiency or unresponsiveness)
- Hyperinsulinism: Exogenous insulin administration or endogenous production: insulinoma; persistent hyperinsulinemic hypoglycemia of infancy
- Ketotic hypoglycemia: Usually occurs during fasting in patients 18 mos – 5 yrs with spontaneous resolution prior to 10 yrs of age
- Inborn errors of metabolism:
  ▶ Disorders of carbohydrate metabolism: Defects in glycogenolysis, gluconeogenesis, galactosemia, hereditary fructose intolerance
  ▶ Disorders of protein metabolism: Organic acidemias such as maple syrup urine disease, propionic acidemia, glutaric aciduria, *et al.*
  ▶ Disorders of fatty acid metabolism: may have ↑ FFA; alterations in mental status do not improve with correction of hypoglycemia; abnormal acylcarnitine profile.

---

the pediatric population; management is directed to protecting the brain and identifying the cause. Symptoms, signs, causes, clinical and laboratory evaluation and treatment of hypoglycemia are outlined in **Boxes 6.4.1 through 6.4.4**.

Box 6.4.3   Diagnostic Evaluation for Hypoglycemia

- History: Past, current and family; particularly relevant are age of onset, nutritional history, growth history, acute vs. chronic nature of symptoms, circumstances of symptoms, family history of childhood deaths, hypoglycemia and possible metabolic errors.
- Physical findings: Nutritional status, hyperpigmentation (hypoadrenalism), dysmorphism, midline defects suggesting pituitary abnormalities, hepatomegaly, macroglossia suggesting glycogen storage disease, ambiguous genitalia, suggesting congenital adrenal hyperplasia.
- Obtain bedside and laboratory glucose values; glucose should be processed in a heparinized syringe or tube and kept on ice, or transported in a sodium fluoride-treated tube ("gray-top").
- R/O intoxication, especially in previously healthy patients >6 mos.
- Obtain serum electrolytes, liver enzymes and function tests including arterial ammonia (on ice; must be processed quickly), bilirubin, PT, PTT and fibrinogen.
- Perform the following tests when the cause of hypoglycemia is uncertain and while the patient is hypoglycemic. Do not give dextrose or food until laboratory studies are obtained UNLESS the patient is unstable/seizures are present. Vascular access that permits readily obtainable samples allows timely specimen collection without potentially dangerous prolongation of hypoglycemia. Appropriate specimen containers should be available at the bedside. Consultation with a pediatric endocrinologist will help focus the evaluation:
  - ▸ Bedside and laboratory glucose as described above
  - ▸ Serum insulin; also obtain C-peptide (secreted with endogenous insulin) if exogenous insulin is taken (or is suspected). Insulin glargine, insulin aspart and insulin lispro may not be detectable depending on the assay
  - ▸ Free fatty acids (FFA)
  - ▸ β-hydroxybutyrate
  - ▸ Growth Hormone
  - ▸ Lactic acid (arterial; place on ice; must be processed quickly)
  - ▸ Cortisol
  - ▸ ACTH
  - ▸ Plasma amino acids
  - ▸ Carnitine, free and total
  - ▸ Acylcarnitine profile
- Urine obtained close to the time of hypoglycemia for ketones and reducing substances other than glucose; urine for organics acids.
- Additional studies that may be helpful include serum T4, TSH, FSH, LH, testosterone; these may be obtained during normoglycemia.

Box 6.4.4   Management of Hypoglycemia

- If IV insulin is infusing, discontinue the infusion.
- Dextrose: If asymptomatic or mildly symptomatic and able to take by mouth, simple sugars such as juice, honey, glucose tablet or gel, cake-icing, *etc.* may be given. If symptoms are marked or the mental status is altered or the patient is unable to take by mouth, administration of dextrose IV is indicated:

  Dextrose 0.25–1 g/kg has been recommended. Doses >0.25 gm/kg should be reserved for profound or symptomatic hypoglycemia. For infants, $D_{10}W$ 2.5 mL/kg (0.25 g/kg) given slowly via peripheral IV typically provides sufficient glucose without causing hyperglycemia and rebound insulin secretion. Beyond infancy, solutions containing up to 25% dextrose (and up to 50% dextrose for adolescents and adults) may be given via peripheral IV for emergency correction of hypoglycemia (so-called "bolus" dosing).
- Glucagon (0.3 mg/kg; maximum 1 mg IM or subQ): Useful if hyperinsulinemia is the cause of hypoglycemia and if oral intake is not possible and IV access is not available. The effect is transient and depends on adequate glucagon stores. Glucagon does not replace appropriate administration of glucose. Glucagon may cause vomiting.
- Maintain glucose in the range of 70–120 mg/dL.
- Recheck glucose 10 min (after IV) or 15 min (after enteral) treatment of hypoglycemia to ensure adequate response; follow IV dextrose rescue with a continuous infusion of dextrose-containing IVF. Concentrations in excess of 5% dextrose may be required. Some patients may require central venous access for sustained infusion of concentrations in excess of 12.5% dextrose.
- Frequent monitoring (every 30–60 mins) is warranted until stability is achieved.
- If dextrose >10 mg/kg/min is required to maintain normoglycemia, hyperinsulinemia is likely.

Hypoglycemia is most frequently encountered in the PICU in the context of sepsis, septic shock, insulin therapy or inadvertent interruption of dextrose supply in a patient with poor glycogen stores or relative hyperinsulinemia due to high rates of IV glucose delivery (*e.g.* TPN). These situations require emergency correction of low glucose values to avoid CNS consequences. Glucose monitoring is important in all critically ill pediatric patients, particularly in the first 24 hrs of PICU stay. Once stability is achieved, monitoring may be less intensive. In addition, glucose should be checked whenever there is a change in vital signs, mental status, or any suggestive symptomatology (**Box 6.4.1**). New onset hypo- or hyperglycemia in an established PICU patient may be the first sign of nosocomial infection, particularly in fungal infections.

Hyperglycemia in the general pediatric population (including term infants) is defined as a fasting glucose >125 mg/dL. Hyperglycemia is a common finding among sick pediatric patients. Patients deprived of intake because of illness may have ketonemia as well, particularly at the time of hospital admission. Most PICU patients with hyperglycemia, with or without ketones *and* an accompanying acute, severe illness have stress-related hyperglycemia. While hyperglycemia may be present on admission, most of these elevations self-resolve in the first hours as therapy proceeds. Patients with diabetic ketoacidosis (*DKA, 6.6*) latent diabetes, or inborn metabolic errors (*Inborn Errors of Metabolism, 6.5*) should be identifiable by history, physical examination and laboratory evaluation. The differential diagnosis of hyperglycemia in the PICU is listed (**Box 6.4.5**). The underlying cause of hyperglycemia should be addressed and treated as indicated. Acute hyperglycemia can be distinguished from more chronic hyperglycemia (as in diabetes) by measuring Hb A_{1C} (reflects glucose values over the previous 1–3 mos). Fructosamine is potentially useful in reflecting glucose elevations during the prior ~2 weeks.

Hyperglycemia in critically ill adults has been associated with increased morbidity and mortality. Among adult critically ill surgical patients, those treated with insulin to achieve strict glucose control (80–110 mg/dL) demonstrated a 43% decrease in mortality compared with more permissive control (<215 mg/dL). In other studies of mixed populations (adult surgical, medical and trauma patients) strict control was either of no benefit or associated with increased mortality and/or an increase in incidence of hypoglycemia

---

Box 6.4.5   Causes of Hyperglycemia in the PICU

- Stress-related: Suspected to result from ↑ counter-regulatory hormones +/− insulin resistance. Common stressors include infection, enteritis, respiratory distress, hypoxia, sepsis, shock, trauma, burns, surgery, cardiopulmonary arrest, CPR *et al.*
- Medications such as corticosteroids, vasoactive drugs, calcium channel blockers, antipsychotics, certain chemotherapeutic agents *et al.*
- Pancreatitis
- Diabetes (Hgb A_{1C} ≥ 6.5%) with or without DKA
- Insulin-resistance associated with metabolic syndrome, endocrinopathies such as Cushing's syndrome
- ↑ Glucose delivery (PN, medications dissolved in dextrose solution, *etc.*)
- Inborn metabolic errors: these usually present with hypoglycemia; occasionally, hyperglycemia may be present in isovaleric acidemia, methylmalonic acidemia, proprionic acidemia; defects in ketolysis and in L-isoleucine catabolism.

---

when compared to more permissive strategies. However, adult patients demonstrated improved survival when glucose was maintained <180 mg/dL. This trend is similar among critically ill pediatric patients; however, the optimal degree of glucose control during pediatric critical illness has not yet been defined. Normalization of serum glucose appears to be of greater importance in the presence of brain injury as opposed to illness that does not involve the CNS. Therefore, there may be a role for more intensive glucose control among brain injured patients. An approach used in our practice is outlined in **Box 6.4.6**.

Box 6.4.6 **Management Guidelines for Hyperglycemia of Critical Illness Not Associated with Primary Diabetes:**

- R/O "artifactual hyperglycemia" (*e.g.* blood tested from an extremity/IV catheter with a dextrose-containing infusion).
- R/O readily reversible causes such as excessive infusion of glucose. Check for "occult" glucose administration such as use of dextrose solution as a diluent for medications. If glucose supply cannot be curtailed, administration of insulin should be considered.
- Treat glucose ≥150–180 mg/dL* that persists (>6–8 hrs), is increasing, or is not expected to resolve spontaneously because of underlying illness or risk factors (*e.g.* pancreatitis, obesity).
  - ▶ Start continuous infusion of insulin IV 0.025 Units/kg/hr.
  - ▶ Check rapid bedside glucose hourly and more frequently if glucose is declining by >50 mg/dL/hr until stability is achieved.
  - ▶ Add dextrose to IVF for infants or young children unless the serum glucose is very high (*e.g.* >300 mg/dL).
  - ▶ Add dextrose to the IVF (and increase insulin delivery as needed) if urine ketones are present.
  - ▶ Increase insulin progressively by 0.01–0.05 Units/kg/hr until glucose is in the desired range (*usually* ~120–180 mg/dL). See below for patients with brain injury.*
  - ▶ Decrease or discontinue insulin for glucose <120 mg/dL unless there is a demonstrated need for continued insulin therapy.
- If the insulin requirement is stable over several days and changing needs are not anticipated, consideration may be given to once daily administration of long-acting basal insulin (*e.g.* insulin glargine or insulin detemir). These insulins work particularly well if glucose supply is constant, as during PN or continuous enteral feedings. A regimen of supplemental or correction doses of insulin using shorter-acting insulin may be required.
- Consultation with a diabetologist or endocrinologist is helpful, particularly if subcutaneous insulin administration is warranted.

* For brain injured patients, consider more aggressive control, *e.g.* maintain glucose in the 100–150 mg/dL range.

6.5   Inborn Errors of Metabolism (IEM)

Despite advances in early diagnosis of IEM through screening of the newly born, pediatric patients *of any age* may still present with an acute neurologic and/or metabolic crisis due to IEM's that may escape early detection. These genetic disorders are caused by the complete or partial deficiency of an enzyme or its cofactor resulting in either accumulation of a metabolite or deficiency of the normal product(s) of a given biochemical reaction. Such biochemical aberrations require recognition and intervention to prevent potential metabolic deterioration, irreversible neurologic damage and death (**Box 6.5.1**). A high index of suspicion is required since the presentation of an IEM is most often nonspecific and the presenting signs and symptoms can be mistaken for the more common causes of acute illness such as sepsis, congenital heart disease, CNS infection, idiopathic epilepsy, enteritis, toxin exposure, or primary diseases of the liver. Non-acute features such as developmental delay and myopathy may provide clues to the presence of an IEM. Categorization of the defect is often possible based

---

Box 6.5.1   Typical Ages at Presentation of Various Inborn Errors of Metabolism

Age of Onset	Disorder
12–72 hrs	Non-ketotic hyperglycinemia; Urea cycle disorders; Branched chain organic acidemias
1st week	Maple syrup urine disease
1st–2nd week	Galactosemia
After the 1st week	Tyrosinemia
After the 3rd week	Alpha-1-anti-trypsin deficiency
1–2 yrs	Mucopolysaccharidosis type II (Hunter's Syndrome)
Anytime (1yr through the 7th decade)	Mitochondrial disorders;urea cycle defects; partial defects of any metabolic disease

on the presence or absence of hypoglycemia, hyperammonemia, metabolic acidosis and elevated serum lactate (**Box 6.5.2**). The participation of an expert in genetics and metabolism is essential when an IEM is suspected.

Since fetal metabolism is shared by maternal hepatic and renal function, most newborns with IEM are normal at birth; hence, screening for IEM's is performed after several days of age or after feedings are established. Among the notable exceptions are non-ketotic hyperglycinemia, the sulfatase deficiencies, glycogen-branching enzyme deficiency, and certain lysosomal and

---

Box 6.5.2 Typical Clinical Characteristics of Selected IEM's by Category of Disorder

Metabolic Defect Category (Examples)	Signs and Symptoms	Characteristic Initial Laboratory Findings
Aminoacidopathies (also called **Aminoacidemias/ aminoacidurias**) (Maple syrup urine disease; tyrosinemia; phenylketonuria)	Newborns: ↓ feeding, lethargy, encephalopathy, coma, death. Children: developmental delay or regression +/− Hepatosplenomegaly	+/− Metabolic acidosis* +/− Lactic acidosis +/− Hypoglycemia +/− Ketosis +/− Hyperammonemia Abnormal LFT's Non-glucose reducing substances in urine
Organic acidemias (also called **Organic acidurias**) (Methylmalonic acidemia; propionic acidemia)	Same as above	Metabolic acidosis* +/− Lactic acidosis +/− Hypoglycemia +/− Ketosis Hyperammonemia +/− Abnormal LFT's +/− ↓Carnitine
Urea Cycle Defects (Ornithine transcarbamylase deficiency; Citrullinemia)	Usually presents in newborns after protein feeding: lethargy, poor feeding, vomiting, failure to thrive	Ketosis Hyperammonemia Respiratory alkalosis (due to ↑ NH_3) +/− Abnormal LFT's

(Continued)

Box 6.5.2   Typical Clinical Characteristics of Selected IEM's by Category of Disorder (Continued)

Metabolic Defect Category (Examples)	Signs and Symptoms	Characteristic Initial Laboratory Findings
Disorders of Carbohydrate Metabolism (Galactosemia; glycogen storage diseases; pyruvate carboxylase deficiency)	Lethargy; encephalopathy +/− Hepatomegaly +/− Splenomegaly +/− Myopathy +/− Cardiomyopathy	+/− Metabolic acidosis* ↑ Lactate (usually) Hypoglycemia Ketosis +/− ↑ Triglycerides +/− ↑CK and/or ↑ aldolase +/− ↑LDH +/− Abnormal LFT's +/− Non-glucose reducing substances in urine +/− Urine myoglobin
Fatty Acid Oxidation Defects (Medium chain acyl-Co-A-dehydrogenase ("MCAD") deficiency)	Encephalopathy during period of ↓ CHO intake +/− Hepatomegaly +/− Dilated cardiomyopathy +/− Myopathy	+/− Metabolic acidosis* +/− Lactic acidosis Hypoglycemia (usually) Ketones: appropriately ↑ or ↓↓ +/− Hyperammonemia Abnormal LFT's
Mitochondrial Disorders (Cytochrome C oxidase deficiency: Mitochondrial encephalopathy, lactic acidosis and stroke-like episodes "MELAS")	Poor feeding, vomiting, CNS dysfunction, blindness, deafness, myopathy, cardiomyopathy; renal Fanconi syndrome; multisystem involvement	+/− Metabolic acidosis* Lactic acidosis (usually) +/− Hypoglycemia +/− Ketosis +/− Abnormal LFT's
Peroxisomal Disorders (Adreno-Leukodystrophy; Zellweger syndrome; Refsum disease)	May include: microcephaly, dysmorphic facies, seizures, hypotonia, developmental delay/ regression, hepatosplenomegaly	↑ Very long chain fatty acids in plasma

(Continued)

Box 6.5.2   Typical Clinical Characteristics of Selected IEM's by Category of Disorder (Continued)

Metabolic Defect Category (Examples)	Signs and Symptoms	Characteristic Initial Laboratory Findings
Lysosomal Storage Disorders [Mucopolysaccharidoses (MPS); cystinosis; sphingolipidoses; oligosaccharidoses; mucolipidoses]	May include: loss of milestones, coarse facial features, short stature, peripheral neuropathy, ataxia, hypertrophic cardiomyopathy, hepatosplenomegaly, loss of range of motion.	Absence of specific enzyme in serum, white blood cells, or skin fibroblasts: *e.g.* in Hurler's syndrome (MPS 1): there is a deficiency of α L-iduronidase.
Disorders of Purine and Pyrimidine Metabolism (Lesch Nyhan Disease; adenosine deaminase (ADA) deficiency)	May include: neurologic dysfunction, developmental delay, self-mutilation, renal stones, hemolytic anemia, immune defects	Disease-specific enzyme deficiencies. Uric acid: ↓ in purine metabolism defects and ↑ in Lesch-Nyhan and glycogen storage diseases.
Disorders of Metal Metabolism (Wilson's disease; hemochromotosis)	Disease-specific	*E.g.* Wilson's Disease: ↓ serum ceruloplasmin and ↑ urine copper. ↑ copper deposits on liver biopsy is the "gold standard."
Porphyrias: Seven types depending on the effected enzyme in heme synthesis	Abdominal pain; neuropsychiatric disease	Type specific; *e.g.* acute porphyria (rapid diagnosis) ↑ urinary porphobilinogen; confirmatory testing needed.

* The metabolic acidosis of IEM's typically demonstrates an ↑ in anion gap.

peroxisomal disorders. Perinatal clues for IEM's are decreased fetal movement, prolonged labor, maternal "HELLP" syndrome (hemolysis, elevated liver enzymes and low platelets), acute fatty liver of pregnancy (the fetal liver may or may not be affected), maternal hyperemesis and fetal hydrops. Beyond the immediate newborn period, signs and symptoms that should prompt consideration of an IEM are listed (**Box 6.5.3**). Symptoms of IEM are often precipitated by ingestion of a challenging nutrient (*e.g.* disorders of carbohydrate metabolism, urea cycle defects, organic acidemias and amino acidemias), or an acute stress such as infection or surgery (*e.g.* amino acidemias, organic acidemias, fatty acid oxidation defects, urea cycle disorders, *etc.*). Certain drugs may precipitate symptoms of diseases such as glucose-6-phosphate dehydrogenase deficiency and the porphyrias. Accurate diagnosis requires expertise in assessment, specimen acquisition during periods of symptomatology, reliable processing of laboratory specimens and skilled interpretation of results. Selection of an appropriate metabolic laboratory supervised by a medical director with expertise in the relevant metabolic assays and their interpretation

---

Box 6.5.3   Common Features, Signs and Symptoms Suggesting an IEM

- Recurrent vomiting, diarrhea and/or dehydration
- Poor feeding
- Failure to thrive
- Recurrent hypoglycemia
- Recurrent metabolic acidosis
- Metabolic acidosis precipitated by mild intercurrent illness
- Recurrent or difficult to control seizures (**Box 6.5.4**)
- Cataracts; corneal opacities; lens dislocation; retinal abnormalities; strabismus

- Hemolysis
- Cardiomyopathy
- Acute life-threatening events (ALTE)
- Sudden infant death (SIDS)
- Developmental delay/regression
- Muscle cramping, weakness
- Recurrent abdominal pain
- Consanguinity
- Abnormal odor (**Box 6.5.5**)
- History of fetal and or childhood deaths in the family
- History of thrombotic events (personal or familial)

Box 6.5.4   IEM's Presenting with Seizures/Status Epilepticus

- Pyridoxine deficiency
- Urea cycle disorders
- Aminoacidemias
- Mitochondrial disorders
- Nonketotic hyperglycinemia
- Gangliosidoses

- Biotinidase deficiency
- Molybdenum cofactor deficiency
- Copper metabolism disorders (Wilson's disease)
- Creatine metabolism disorders
- Purine metabolism disorders
- Pyrimidine metabolism disorders

Box 6.5.5   Characteristic Odors Associated with Certain IEM's

Fruity or ammonia-like: Propionic and methylmalonic acidemia; (also, DKA)
Musty; "dead mouse" or mouse urine: Phenylketonuria
Sweaty sock, sneaker or cheese: Isovaleric acidemia
Maple syrup or curry: Maple syrup urine disease
Cat urine: 3-Methylcrotonic acidemia; 3-Hydroxy, 3-methyl glutaric aciduria
Fishy: Trimethylaminuria; Carnitine excess
Cabbage or rotten egg: Tyrosinemia

---

is critical to arriving at a diagnosis. Therapy is based on symptomatology and sometimes on the suspected diagnosis until a final diagnosis is determined.

During evaluation for an IEM, it is important to consider alternative diagnoses such as infection or sepsis, heart disease, primary neurologic disease, *et al.* that require specific investigation, intervention and sometimes empiric treatment until a final diagnosis is made. Concomitant infection may trigger manifestations of an IEM, therefore, antibiotics should be considered in all cases. The suggested laboratory evaluation for suspected IEM is described in **Box 6.5.6.** Severe problems such as hypoglycemia

(*Hypo- and Hyperglycemia, 6.4*), seizures (*Status Epilepticus, 5.2*) and hyperammonemia require immediate treatment. Recurrent or difficult to control seizures frequently result in PICU admission; the possibility of an IEM should be considered in each patient for which the cause of seizures has not been identified (**Box 6.5.4**). Serum ammonia (NH_3) $\geq 120\,\mu mol/L$ in the newborn or $\geq 80\,\mu mol/L$ in

---

Box 6.5.6   Suggested Laboratory Evaluation for an IEM

- ABG*
- Glucose
- Electrolytes, urea nitrogen, creatinine
- Uric acid
- Liver enzymes (AST, ALT, Alkaline phosphatase)
- Liver function tests (bilirubin, PT, albumin)
- Arterial ammonia*
- CBC
- Urinalysis: note color, odor, specific gravity (consider renal tubular defects), pH, presence or absence of ketones and non-glucose reducing substances
- For symptoms of myopathy:
  ‣ Creatine kinase
  ‣ Aldolase
  ‣ Lactate dehydrogenase
  ‣ Urine myoglobin
- During symptoms:**
  ‣ Plasma amino acids (quantitative)
  ‣ Urine organic acids (qualitative)
  ‣ Free and total carnitine
  ‣ Acyl carnitine profile
  ‣ Arterial lactate and pyruvate[†]

(Continued)

Box 6.5.6   Suggested Laboratory Evaluation for an IEM (Continued)

- Additional studies:
  ▶ Ophthalmology evaluation for corneal opacities, Kayser-Fleischer ring, cherry red spots, retinitis pigmentosa, lens dislocations
  ▶ Echocardiogram (R/O cardiomyopathy)
  ▶ Brain MRI (R/O basal ganglia abnormalities associated with mitochondrial disorders)
  ▶ CSF for glucose, protein, lactate, pyruvate, glycine (CSF: plasma glycine >0.8 is consistent with nonketotic hyperglycinemia), serine, alanine, neurotransmitters, pterins
  ▶ Urine sulfocysteine (sulfite oxidase and molybdenum cofactor deficiencies)
  ▶ Urine glycosaminoglycans, oligosaccharides (lysosomal storage diseases)
  ▶ Urine purine and polyol analyses (disorders of purine and polyol metabolism)
  ▶ Urine and plasma creatine and guanidinoacetate (defects in creatine metabolism)

---

* Freely flowing arterial blood should be obtained via arterial puncture. The specimen should be placed on ice and assayed immediately.

** Specimens may be obtained and stored based on the specific handling prescribed by the laboratory.

† Pyruvate requires special handling (perchlorate or similar medium). The normal lactate:pyruvate ratio is 10–20:1; This ratio is ↑ in mitochondrial disorders and pyruvate carboxylase deficiency; normal or ↓ in glycogen storage diseases and pyruvate dehydrogenase deficiency.

infants and children can cause brain swelling and is neurotoxic. Acute hyperammonemia requires aggressive therapy (**Box 6.5.7**). Management "pearls" are summarized (**Box 6.5.8**). See *Appendix, part 2, IX* for clinical decision trees in evaluation of IEMs.

Box 6.5.7   Approach to Management of Acute Hyperammonemia in Urea Cycle Defects

• Monitor airway stability, oxygenation and ventilation. Assist ventilation when necessary to prevent ↑ work of breathing.
• Restore circulating volume and monitor urine output; avoid over-hydration and hypo-osmolality because these may exacerbate brain swelling.
• Discontinue oral intake and all intake of protein.
• Prevent catabolism by provision of adequate dextrose in isotonic fluid (*e.g.* $D_{10}W$ 0.9% NaCl)
• If possible, avoid drugs that ↑ protein catabolism (*e.g.* steroids), inhibit urea synthesis (*e.g.* valproate) or are hepatotoxic.
• Give NH_3 scavengers sodium phenylacetate and sodium benzoate (available in combination) IV until the enteral preparation can be tolerated. These require ~24–48 hrs to take effect.
• Remove ammonia until $NH_3 < 200\,\mu mol/L$:
  ‣ Continuous renal replacement therapy (CRRT) *with hemodialysis* is the treatment of choice for rapid NH_3 removal. Hemodialysis is not effective at concentrations of $NH_3 < 200\,\mu mol/L$.
  ‣ CRRT with hemofiltration if hemodialysis is not available. This is not as effective as hemodialysis for very high levels of NH_3, but is useful while awaiting efficacy of scavenging therapy (see above) once NH_3 is $< 200\,\mu mol/L$ and to help clear ongoing NH_3 being produced.
  ‣ Peritoneal dialysis is suboptimal because removal of NH_3 may take days.
• Arginine deficiency results in ↑ protein breakdown and ↑ NH_3 production in urea cycle defects. Administration of arginine hydrochloride curtails protein breakdown and promotes formation of water-soluble compounds (ornithine, citrulline, argininosuccinic acid) resulting in ↑ excretion of NH_3.
• During dialysis, ammonia should be measured hourly. During sodium phenylacetate-sodium benzoate therapy, electrolytes should be monitored closely, and hypokalemia should be corrected.
• Management plans and nutrition recommendations and should be designed in conjunction with a metabolic expert.
• Additional therapy is disease-specific.

Box 6.5.8   Pearls in the Management of IEM

- Fundamental respiratory and circulatory care remains the first priority in caring for patients with IEM. Hypoglycemia should be corrected immediately and anticonvulsant therapy should be initiated to stabilize the patient.
- Obtain necessary laboratory studies during the acute phase of illness. Obtain serum for necessary studies before treating hypoglycemia provided this does not delay administration of glucose (*Hypo- and Hyperglycemia, 6.4*).
- If significant hyperammonemia is present, multidisciplinary involvement may be required to determine the most efficient strategies to lower the ammonia.
- The neurologic outcome of patients with acute ↑ammonia correlates with duration of hyperammonemia and encephalopathy.
- Consider IEM in the differential diagnosis of patients with unexplained hypoglycemia, acidosis, recurrent seizures, abnormal liver function, encephalopathy, cardiomyopathy and SIDS.
- In cases of SIDS, consult a metabolic specialist regarding appropriate post-mortem studies. Aminoacids, lactate, pyruvate and carnitine are not accurate when obtained after death.
- Administration of sodium bicarbonate should be avoided in treatment of metabolic acidosis when it co-exists with hyperammonemia.
- Bicarbonate does not reverse the acidosis of organic acidemias. If given, it should be given slowly, preferably as a component of IVF (*e.g.* $NaHCO_3$ 150 meq/L at a maintenance rate).
- Provide dextrose (~8–10 mg/kg/min) to discourage breakdown of protein and fat. Insulin infusion may be necessary to maintain glucose in the 100–120 mg/dL range.
- Co-factor supplementation may be important in the following settings:
  - ▶ Pyridoxine: refractory seizures
  - ▶ Folinic acid: refractory seizures not responsive to pyridoxine
  - ▶ Cobalamine: methylmalonic acidemia may be vitamin B_{12} responsive.
  - ▶ Biotin: multiple carboxylase deficiency
  - ▶ Carnitine: cardiomyopathy, organic acidemias, fatty acid oxidation disorders, carnitine deficiency.
- Early consultation with a metabolic expert in genetics and metabolism is essential when an IEM is suspected.

6.6 Diabetic Ketoacidosis (DKA)

DKA is a life-threatening metabolic disturbance caused by insulin deficiency and counter-regulatory hormone excess resulting in ketoacidosis, a paradoxical state of hypertonic dehydration and possibly, symptomatic brain swelling ("cerebral edema"). Although rare, brain herniation during treatment is the most frequent cause of morbidity and mortality. DKA is most common among type 1, but may be seen in type 2 diabetics.

Absolute or relative insulin deficiency causes impaired transport of glucose into cells resulting in hyperglycemia, glycosuria, cellular starvation and metabolic stress.

- The associated surge of counterregulatory hormones (*e.g.* glucagon, epinephrine, cortisol and growth hormone) leads to lipolysis, proteolysis, glycogenolysis and gluconeogenesis.
- The resulting high glucagon: insulin ratio in the portal circulation promotes ketogenesis and contributes to hyperglycemia.
- Osmotic diuresis leads to dehydration.
- Non-compliance with home diabetes care and/or problems with insulin delivery are the most common causes of DKA among known diabetics. Infections and emotional stress are also important triggers.
- Disturbances in blood brain barrier permeability, cytotoxic processes and changes in osmolality are among suspected causes of raised ICP associated with DKA.

Assessment and Management (Key Findings, Box 6.6.1)
Airway/Breathing. Severe DKA is associated with highly efficient respiratory compensation; $PaCO_2$ may be as low <10 mmHg. Tracheal intubation is rarely required; when indicated, it should be performed to guard against:

- Increased ICP: Use neuroprotective techniques. (*Bag-Mask Ventilation and Tracheal Intubation, 15.2*).
- CNS acidosis: Physiologic hyperventilation should be maintained if mechanical ventilation is required. Untoward increases in $PaCO_2$ may exacerbate CNS acidosis and brain swelling.

Box 6.6.1   Key Findings

Commonly present:

- Polyuria, polydipsia, appetite changes, weight loss, abdominal pain, vomiting, weakness
- Hyperglycemia, glycosuria and ketonuria
- Varying degrees of dehydration; Kussmaul breathing with parched oral mucosa
- Ketoacidosis; lactic acid is typically normal or only mildly elevated.
- Total body potassium depletion
- Altered mental status

Sometimes present:

- Perineal candida, oral thrush; fruity odor on the breath
- Shock; decompensated shock is uncommon.
- Hyponatremia; Hypernatremia
- Hypophosphatemia
- Increased BUN and creatinine (creatinine may be artifactually increased due to ketonemia)
- Dyslipidemia (esp. in the obese patient)
- Increased amylase and/or lipase without acute pancreatitis

Circulation (Fig. 6.6.1):

- Severe ketonemia (*e.g.* arterial pH <7.15) causes vasoconstriction and may complicate assessment of circulation in DKA; cool mottled skin may be due to acidemia rather than hypovolemia (**Box 6.6.2**).
- If shock is present after 20–30 ml/kg resuscitation fluid is given, a complicating illness (*e.g.* pancreatitis, sepsis) may be present.
- **For obese patients, use ideal body weight for fluid and electrolyte calculations.**

Insulin Administration (Box 6.6.3). The acidosis of DKA is a ketoacidosis; insulin is required for its reversal. Begin insulin after shock is corrected, by the end of the first treatment hour. Blood gases are useful to measure progress in correction of the acid-base disturbance. For DKA patients using an **insulin pump**, assume the pump is not working; treat with continuous regular insulin IV and discontinue the insulin pump.

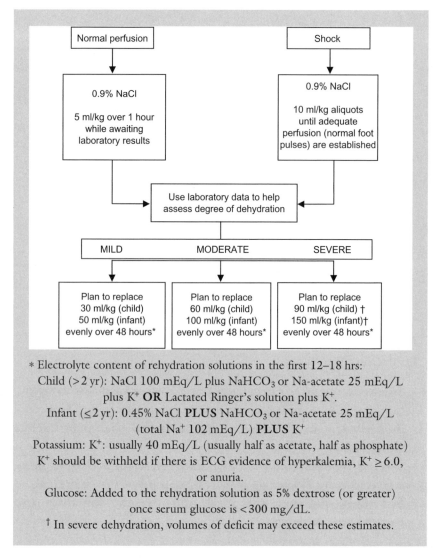

* Electrolyte content of rehydration solutions in the first 12–18 hrs:
Child (>2 yr): NaCl 100 mEq/L plus NaHCO$_3$ or Na-acetate 25 mEq/L
plus K$^+$ **OR** Lactated Ringer's solution plus K$^+$.
Infant (≤2 yr): 0.45% NaCl **PLUS** NaHCO$_3$ or Na-acetate 25 mEq/L
(total Na$^+$ 102 mEq/L) **PLUS** K$^+$
Potassium: K$^+$: usually 40 mEq/L (usually half as acetate, half as phosphate)
K$^+$ should be withheld if there is ECG evidence of hyperkalemia, K$^+$ ≥ 6.0,
or anuria.
Glucose: Added to the rehydration solution as 5% dextrose (or greater)
once serum glucose is < 300 mg/dL.
† In severe dehydration, volumes of deficit may exceed these estimates.

Fig. 6.6.1. Rehydration in the Normally Nourished Infant or Child with DKA. Modified from Harris GD, Fiordalisi I, Shah BR. Diabetic ketoacidosis, in Shah BR, Lucchesi M (eds.), *Atlas of Pediatric Emergency Medicine*, McGraw Hill, NY, p. 559, 2006.

Box 6.6.2 Guidelines for Estimating Volume of Deficit (DEGREE DEHYDRATION) in DKA

Guideline Measures	Degree of Dehydration		
Volume of deficit*	Mild	Moderate	Severe**
> 2 yr	30 ml/kg	60 ml/kg	90 ml/kg
≤ 2 yr	50 ml/kg	100 ml/kg	150 ml/kg
Clinical measures			
Peripheral perfusion†			
Palpation of peripheral pulses (pulse volume)	N	N to ↓	↓ to absent
Heart rate	N to ↑	↑	↑↑
Blood pressure	N	N to ↑	↓ to↑
Biochemical measures in serum			
Urea nitrogen (mg/dL)	N to ↑	↑	↑↑
	e.g. <20	*e.g.* 20–25	*e.g.* 30
Predicted Na⁺ (meq/L)	Usually N	Usually N	N to ↑
Glucose (mg/dL)	Mildly ↑	Moderately ↑	Severely ↑
	e.g. 400	*e.g.* 600	*e.g.* 800

N, normal; ↑, increased; ↓, decreased

* **Use actual weight for normally nourished patients; for obese patients, use ideal body weight.**

** In some instances, severely dehydrated patients may exceed these volumes of deficit.

† If peripheral (foot) pulses are easily palpable on presentation but skin is cool to cold and capillary refill time is delayed, give NaCl 0.9% (or LR) 10 ml/kg. If the patient has easily palpable peripheral (foot) pulses with cool to cold skin and delayed capillary refill time after 10–20 ml/kg resuscitation fluid, these findings are most likely due to severe ketonemia and should be treated with insulin and serial reassessments, not *necessarily* more fluid!

Modified from Harris GD, Fiordalisi I, Harris WL *et al.*, Minimizing the risk of brain herniation during treatment of diabetic ketoacidemia: a retrospective and prospective study, *J. Pediatr*, **117**:28, 1990.

Box 6.6.3 Guidelines for Insulin Administration

- Mix regular insulin 1 unit/ml 0.9% NaCl; waste ~50 ml of solution to saturate potential binding sites in tubing.
- Usual starting dose: 0.1 unit/kg/hr based on **actual** body weight, even for obese patients. An initial loading dose is not indicated.
- The t½ of i.v. insulin is 5–10 mins; any interruption in continuous insulin infusion ≥ 15 mins results in further ketoacid production and potentially, worsening metabolic acidemia. Intermittent i.v. "pushes" of insulin are ineffective in treating DKA because of its short half-life.
- Measure bedside glucose hourly during i.v. insulin infusion. If glucose is <200–250 mg/dL in the presence of ketonemia, increase dextrose delivery to allow continuation of an adequate insulin dose.
- The dose of insulin should be based on response; expect an improvement in base deficit by at least 1 mEq/L/hr. Improvement in measured tCO_2 usually lags behind improvement in the base deficit and blood pH. If the expected rate of improvement is not demonstrated, check for problems with:

  (1) Insulin delivery: *e.g.* medication error, tubing disconnection, i.v. pump malfunction, venous access (i.v. infiltration)
  (2) Insulin resistance: some patients may require insulin >0.1 unit/kg/hr, particularly those with type 2 diabetes, severe infection or inflammatory processes, those receiving medications such as steroids, vasoactive drugs, or if the blood pH is <7.0.

Rehydration:

(1) Once shock, if present, is reversed, estimate the degree of dehydration based on physical findings and laboratory data (**Box 6.6.2**).

(2) Use solutions as described in **Fig. 6.6.1**.

(3) Subtract emergency volumes given from the estimated volume of deficit; plan infusion of the remainder evenly over 48 hrs.

(4) Give deficit plus maintenance allotments. While $PaCO_2$ is <30 mmHg, give 25–30% more than the usual maintenance requirement because of increased insensible losses associated with hyperventilation.

> **Box 6.6.4 Biochemical Monitoring and Data Interpretation During Treatment of DKA**
>
> - **Hourly blood glucose during continuous i.v. insulin:** the serum glucose concentration is determined by both dextrose and insulin delivery. Volume resuscitation may also lower the serum glucose.
> - **Hourly blood gases:** the dose of insulin controls the correction of the base deficit and tCO_2
> - **Serum electrolytes every 2 hrs:** The volume of fluid/hr controls the trend of the concentration of sodium and urea nitrogen. Potassium supplementation in excess of 40–80 mEq/L delivered in the rehydration solution may be required (see **Box 6.2.9**)
> - **Serum Mg and phosphorus every 4–8 hrs:** Depletion of these electrolytes is common; supplement as needed. See *Magnesium, 6.2.5 and Box 6.2.24.*
> - Serum ketones and lactate as indicated.

(5) Monitor electrolytes and the trend of the serum sodium concentration at least every 2 hrs during treatment (**Box 6.6.4**). Calculate the predicted concentration of sodium (Na^+_p) for each simultaneously measured sodium-glucose pair (with Na in mEq/L and glucose in mg/dL):

$$Na^+_p = \text{measured } Na^+ + 1.6\,[(\text{glucose} - 100)/100]$$

The decline in osmolality caused by normalization of glucose during treatment is offset if $[Na^+]_p$ remains relatively constant. If $[Na^+]_p$ decreases during therapy ("negative sodium trend"), the patient should be re-evaluated for a decrease in the hourly rate of fluid infusion. Provided the rehydration solution contains ~125 mEq/L Na^+, the trend of the concentration of serum sodium is controlled by the rate of fluid delivery, not by further increase in the sodium concentration of the IV fluid (rehydration solution). If an initially normal Na^+_p concentration increases during treatment (*e.g.* >145 mEq/L) the patient should be re-evaluated for an increase in the hourly rate of fluid infusion. The trend of the concentration of urea nitrogen should also be considered in these decisions.

(6) If the initial predicted sodium is ≥ 150 meq/L, correct hyperglycemia first; then correct hypernatremic dehydration by decreasing the content of sodium in the rehydration solution. If the Na^+_p rises during the correction of hyperglycemia, consideration should be given to decreasing the concentration of sodium in the rehydration fluid (*e.g.* from Na^+ 125 meq/L to 75 meq/L).

Glucose. Add dextrose to the rehydration solution once glucose is < 250 mg/dL. Some patients require as much as D12.5% or more in the rehydration solution to provide sufficient substrate for the required dose of insulin.

Potassium. The initial concentration of serum K^+ may be elevated and does not reflect total body stores. Treatment with fluids, insulin and the correction of acidosis cause the serum K^+ to move into cells. Total body K^+ depletion is common and K^+ 40 meq/L (or greater) is typically required to prevent hypokalemia (**Fig. 6.6.1**).

Magnesium and Phosphorus. Hypomagnesemia and/or hypophosphatemia in the setting of DKA may indicate severe total body depletion of these ions and require treatment. Mg^{++} depletion exacerbates K^+ losses and should be considered if hypokalemia is not responsive to potassium supplementation.

Neurologic monitoring. Monitor for symptoms or signs of raised ICP, and treat with mannitol (or NaCl 3%; see below) if raised ICP is suspected. Symptomatic brain swelling typically occurs after treatment has begun; rarely, it occurs prior to treatment. Patients at risk for brain herniation are not readily identifiable; all pediatric patients with DKA require close neurologic monitoring. Symptomatic brain swelling and brain herniation are associated with young age, new-onset diabetes, very low $PaCO_2$ (< 18 mmHg), high urea nitrogen concentration, and failure of the serum sodium concentration to rise as glucose declines during treatment (negative sodium trend). Provided the rehydration solution contains approximately 125 meq/L Na^+, a negative sodium trend is associated with an increased incidence of symptomatic brain

---

Box 6.6.5 Signs and Symptoms of Raised ICP

- Systemic hypertension
- New onset or worsening headache
- Any deterioration in mental status during treatment
- Slurred speech

- Any new focal neurologic finding
- Pupillary changes: anisocoria; sluggish response to light
- Actual or relative bradycardia
- Any deterioration in breathing pattern
- Age-inappropriate unawareness of incontinence

---

swelling and is directly related to volume delivery. If symptomatic brain swelling is suspected (**Box 6.6.5**):

- Treat with mannitol 20–25% 0.5–1 gm/kg i.v. depending on the severity of symptoms.
- Alternatively, 3% NaCl (3–10 mL/kg) should be considered if raised ICP is suspected in the presence of hemodynamic instability (*e.g.* shock is present).
- The patient should be evaluated for a decrease in fluid administration.
- Brain imaging should not delay therapy for raised ICP; after stabilization, imaging is important to support clinical suspicions or identify other complications such as stroke, thrombosis, acute hydrocephalus, hemorrhage.

The Resolution of DKA and Transition from Intravenous Fluids and Insulin to Subcutaneous Insulin and Oral Intake (Box 6.6.6). DKA is resolved when normal acid base balance is restored and/or serum ketones are undetectable. Residual hyperchloremic acidosis in patients who have recovered from DKA may be treated with sodium bicarbonate (*e.g.* 1 mEq/kg up to 50 mEq i.v. over 1 hr) if the disturbance is significant. Discontinuation of i.v. insulin should occur after DKA is resolved. In uncomplicated episodes, this is usually near the time the patient is free of complaints, interested in taking a meal, and when i.v. fluids can be discontinued safely.

Box 6.6.6   Guidelines for Transition from IV to Subcutaneous Insulin

- Anticipate the need for a basal insulin and give an appropriate dose at a strategic time *e.g.* about 6–12 hrs before DKA is expected to be resolved.
- If the pre-meal glucose is relatively low (<100 mg/dL), i.v. insulin may be discontinued within 30 mins of ingesting the meal. If the pre-meal glucose is elevated (>150 mg/dL), i.v. insulin may be continued for 1–2 hrs after the fast-acting insulin is given, while the patient eats.
- "Cover" carbohydrate intake with an appropriate dose of fast-acting insulin based on grams of carbohydrate ingested (or, if reliable, grams to be ingested).
- For older children and adolescents, fast-acting insulin should be given before meals; for infants and young children or "picky eaters", a fast-acting insulin should be given after meals (to ensure food has been eaten).
- After i.v. insulin is discontinued, check glucose prior to meals, mid-afternoon snack, at bedtime and at two o'clock A.M. to best assess insulin requirements. Treat occurrences of hyperglycemia with a correction dose of insulin.
- If a correction dose of insulin is needed at bedtime or during the night, blood glucose should be checked at a time when the insulin given would be expected to peak: *e.g.* 1–2 hrs after a dose of insulin aspart.

All patients need circulating insulin at all times. This is achievable in most diabetics by resuming an appropriate insulin pump regimen or by subcutaneous administration of a basal-acting insulin (*e.g.* insulin glargine, insulin detemir) at least 6 hrs prior to the anticipated resolution of DKA. In both type 1 and type 2 diabetics, DKA is associated with a transient but significant increase in insulin resistance for ~24 hrs, often requiring subcutaneous doses larger than those required subsequently. In addition to basal insulin, patients should have a specifically designed regimen using fast-acting insulin to correct occurrences of hyperglycemia ("correction dose") and to help metabolize ingested carbohydrate ("carbohydrate exchange dose"). See **Box 6.6.7** for "Pearls" in management of DKA.

Box 6.6.7   "Pearls" in Management of DKA

- Prevention of DKA is the primary goal.
- Correction of shock, if present, and treatment with insulin are essential for correction of DKA
- The degree dehydration does not correlate with the degree of acidosis and should be assessed in each individual patient to avoid over- or under-hydration.
- The most common cause of morbidity and mortality among pediatric patients with DKA is brain swelling with raised ICP.
- Close monitoring of VS and mental status, a physiologic approach to rehydration and early intervention if raised ICP is suspected are the cornerstones of therapy.
- Recurrent DKA may have its root cause in depression and/or child abuse
- Consultation with a diabetologist or endocrinologist, a diabetes educator, nutritionist, social worker and/or discharge planner, and child psychologist when indicated, are important for successful problem resolution.

6.7   Adrenal Insufficiency

The adrenal cortex regulates the secretion of aldosterone, cortisol and adrenal androgens. Cortisol secretion is under the control of the hypothalamic-pituitary-adrenal axis (**Fig. 6.7.1**). Signs and symptoms of

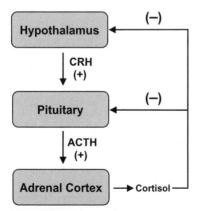

Fig. 6.7.1.   Hypothalamic-Pituitary-Adrenal Axis (HPA).
CRH, corticotropin releasing hormone; ACTH, adrenocorticotropic hormone

---

Box 6.7.1   Signs and Symptoms of Adrenal Insufficiency

Chronic Adrenal Insufficiency

- Weakness
- Malaise
- Lethargy
- Failure to thrive/weight loss
- Anorexia
- Nausea/vomiting
- Abdominal pain
- Hyperpigmentation (primary)
- Salt craving (primary)

Acute Adrenal Insufficiency

- Dehydration
- Tachycardia
- Hypotension
- Seizures
- Somnolence/coma
- Respiratory distress
- Shock/cardiovascular collapse
- Death

---

adrenal insufficiency occur when the adrenal gland is unable to secrete adequate cortisol in response to the physiologic need (**Box 6.7.1**). Etiologies can be either congenital or acquired and can be due to either primary adrenal failure or secondary to a deficiency of either pituitary adrenocorticotropic hormone (ACTH) or hypothalamic corticotropin-releasing hormone (CRH; **Box 6.7.2**). In primary adrenal failure, concomitant aldosterone deficiency can also lead to a salt wasting crisis. This is not seen with secondary adrenal insufficiency because aldosterone secretion is primarily under the control of the renin-angiotensin system and is not dependent on ACTH stimulation. A patient with chronic adrenal insufficiency may present with an acute adrenal crisis when an intercurrent illness, surgery or other physiologic stressor is superimposed on a setting of limited adrenal reserve. Although controversial, a relative adrenal insufficiency for the physiologic condition may occur in a previously normal patient during critical illness and should be suspected in a child that is persistently hypotensive despite treatment with fluids and vasoactive drugs.

Treatment for suspected adrenal insufficiency in an unstable, critically ill patient should not be delayed. However, obtaining random serum cortisol, ACTH, glucose and electrolytes **prior** to a therapeutic trial of exogenous steroids may help confirm the diagnosis (**Box 6.7.3**; **Fig. 6.7.1**). While random cortisol values are often difficult to

---

Box 6.7.2   Etiologies of Adrenal Insufficiency

Primary Adrenal Insufficiency (high ACTH +/– salt wasting)
- Congenital adrenal hyperplasia (CAH)
- Congenital adrenal hypoplasia
- Autoimmune Addison Disease (isolated or in association with autoimmune polyglandular syndrome 1 or 2)
- Adrenoleukodystrophy or Wolman Disease
- Infiltrative/Infectious diseases of the adrenal cortex: tuberculosis, histoplasmosis, coccidioidomycosis, CMV, sarcoidosis, neoplasm, hemochromatosis
- Hemorrhage: Waterhouse-Friderichsen syndrome (in sepsis)
- Medications: ketoconazole, etomidate, mitotane
- ACTH resistance syndromes: Triple A syndrome (achalasia, alacrima, addisonianism)
- Isolated hypoaldosteronism or pseudohypoaldosteronism (normal ACTH with defective responsiveness to aldosterone)

Secondary Adrenal Insufficiency (low ACTH)
- Congenital hypopituitarism: genetic defects and structural abnormalities
- CNS tumor
- Inflammatory/infiltrative diseases of the hypothalamus/pituitary: histiocytosis, hypophysitis, sarcoidosis, hemochromatosis
- CNS surgery that impacts the hypothalamic-pituitary axis
- Cranial radiation
- Head trauma
- Chronic glucocorticoid use

---

interpret in isolation, a very low cortisol (<5 mcg/dL) with a simultaneously high ACTH (>100 pg/ml) is highly suggestive of primary adrenal insufficiency. Alternatively, a very high cortisol (>30 mcg/dL) in the setting of critical illness suggests normal adrenal function. If the patient is clinically stable, additional studies including an ACTH stimulation test (**Box 6.7.4**) should be obtained prior to treatment to help establish a diagnosis and etiology.

Box 6.7.3   Initial Laboratory Evaluation of Suspected Adrenal Insufficiency:

- Cortisol: low for the clinical situation
- ACTH: high if primary adrenal insufficiency; low if secondary adrenal insufficiency
- Serum glucose: low
- Serum sodium: low or normal
- Serum potassium: high (if primary) or normal
- Serum calcium: high or normal

Box 6.7.4   Additional Laboratory Evaluation for Adrenal Insufficiency

These studies should be obtained prior to treatment whenever possible:
Confirmation of cortisol and/or aldosterone deficiency:

- ACTH stimulation tests:
  ▶ Measure serum cortisol (and aldosterone) immediately prior to giving cosyntropin.
  ▶ Give cosyntropin 250 mcg IV push or IM. If secondary adrenal insufficiency is suspected (*e.g.* hypopituitarism), consider stimulation testing with cosyntopin 1 mcg IV or a CRH stimulation test.
  ▶ Measure serum cortisol (and aldosterone) at 30 and 60 mins after giving cosyntropin
  ▶ Cortisol $> 18 \mu g/dL$ or an increase of $> 9 \mu g/dL$ indicates normal adrenal function
- Plasma renin activity
- Aldosterone

Evaluation for CAH for patients < 1 year of age or with history of ambiguous genitalia/virilization:

- 17-OH progesterone
- 17-OH pregnenolone
- Dehydroepiandrosterone (DHEA)
- Dehydroepiandrosterone-sulfate (DHEA-s)
- Androstenedione
- Testosterone
- 11-deoxycortisol
- Deoxycorticosterone

Box 6.7.5   Treatment of Acute Adrenal Insufficiency

- Hydrocortisone: $100 \, mg/M^2$ IV or IM once, followed by $50–100 \, mg/M^2/day$ divided every 4–6 hrs IV OR every 8 hrs *PO* for 24 hrs or until physiologic stress has resolved. Alternatively, hydrocortisone may be given as $50 \, mg/M^2$ IV followed by $25–100 \, mg/M^2/24$ hrs by continuous infusion. Consider using equivalent doses of dexamethasone because it will not interfere with cortisol (or aldosterone) assay.
- Fluid resuscitation: D_5 0.9% NaCl $500 \, ml/M^2$ or 20 ml/kg over 30–60 mins to correct shock followed by deficit volume replacement.
- Hyponatremia: Consider 3% NaCl if seizures are present (*Hyponatremia, 6.2.1*).
- Hypoglycemia: $D_{10}W$ 2 ml/kg if hypoglycemia fails to correct with initial fluid resuscitation (*Hypo- and Hyperglycemia, 6.4*).
- Hyperkalemia: If fluid resuscitation and hydrocortisone do not correct hyperkalemia or there are EKG changes caused by hyperkalemia, definitive treatment to lower serum K^+ should be considered (*Hyperkalemia, 6.2.4, Boxes 6.2.11 and 6.2.12*).

Box 6.7.6   Maintenance Hormone Replacement Therapy in Adrenal Insufficiency

- Hydrocortisone: $6–12 \, mg/M^2/day$ divided every 8 hrs orally
- Fludrocortisone: 0.05–0.2 mg/day orally (if aldoseterone deficiency is also present)
- Sodium chloride: 2–4 g per day (for an infant with aldosterone deficiency)

Patients with possible adrenal insufficiency and clinical instability should receive stress doses of steroids until the physiologic stress has resolved (**Box 6.7.5**). At that point, patients with suspected or confirmed chronic adrenal insufficiency should be placed on maintenance doses of glucocorticoids and mineralocorticoids if indicated (**Box 6.7.6**). If the underlying adrenal reserve is not known, steroids can be weaned and once they are discontinued, the HPA axis should be evaluated. Until the adrenal reserve status is determined, stress doses of steroids should be restarted on patients who become clinically unstable again.

6.8 Thyroid Emergencies

Thyroid hormone is responsible for a variety of metabolic and physiologic functions including thermoregulation, growth and development. A balance between the stimulatory effects of thyroid releasing hormone (hypothalamic; TRH) and thyroid stimulating hormone (pituitary; TSH) and the negative feedback of T3 and T4 on the pituitary maintains thyroid hormone levels within the normal physiologic range. A disruption in this balance can lead to clinically significant hyper- or hypothyroidism. Hypothyroidism rarely presents emergently in the pediatric population. Hyperthyroidism and thyroid storm may present at any age with a metabolic crisis requiring intensive care.

Hyperthyroidism describes the effects of excess thyroid hormone (elevated T4 and/or T3) on target tissues. The most common cause of hyperthyroidism is autoimmune Graves' disease in which antibodies to the TSH receptor in the thyroid gland lead to excessive and uncontrolled secretion of thyroid hormone (**Boxes 6.8.1 and 6.8.2**).

While hyperthyroidism usually has an insidious onset and can be treated in the outpatient setting, life-threatening thyroid storm can

---

Box 6.8.1   Signs and Symptoms of Hyperthyroidism

- Weight loss
- Frequent stools
- Palpitations
- Tachycardia
- Jitteriness
- Tremor

- Heat intolerance
- Smooth, moist skin
- Difficulty concentrating or increased activity
- Emotional lability
- Goiter
- Exophthalmos (Graves' disease)

6.8.2   Etiologies of Hyperthyroidism

- **Conditions associated with suppression of TSH:**
  - ▶ Graves' Disease
  - ▶ Subacute or suppurative thyroiditis
  - ▶ Hyperfunctioning thyroid nodule
  - ▶ TSH Receptor Activating Mutation (McCune-Albright Syndrome)
  - ▶ Exogenous thyroid hormone administration (Thyroiditis factitia)
  - ▶ Destructive: Post radio-ablation or thyroidectomy

- **Conditions associated with elevated or normal TSH:**
  - ▶ Pituitary T3 Resistance
  - ▶ TSH Secreting Pituitary Tumor

develop requiring intensive care treatment. Thyroid storm is an acute clinical condition of decompensated thyrotoxicosis which is usually the result of an intercurrent illness, diabetic ketoacidosis, surgery, radioablation or withdrawal of anti-thyroid medications in the setting of long-standing and possibly unrecognized hyperthyroidism. The clinical presentation and treatment are outlined (**Boxes 6.8.3 and 6.8.4**).

Box 6.8.3   Clinical Presentation of Thyroid Storm

- Cardiac: ↑HR, ↑BP, widened pulse pressure, high output heart failure, arrhythmias
- Thermoregulatory: high fever, sweating
- Gastrointestinal: nausea, vomiting, dehydration, diarrhea, abdominal pain, jaundice
- CNS: disorientation, agitation, restlessness, psychosis, seizures or coma
- Metabolic/Hematologic: hyperglycemia, hypercalcemia, ↑ LDH, AST, ALT and alkaline phosphatase; leukocytosis

---

Box 6.8.4   Treatment of Thyrotoxicosis and Thyroid Storm

- Treat precipitating condition.
- Treat systemic disturbances and provide supportive therapy:
  - ▶ Fever: Antipyretics (acetaminophen); external cooling (ice packs, hypothermia blankets); avoid shivering
  - ▶ Dehydration: Restore fluid balance and correct electrolyte abnormalities
  - ▶ Heart failure: Treat CHF with diuretics; digoxin (cardiology consultation recommended)
- Reduce thyroid hormone synthesis and secretion. Strategies include:
  - ▶ Thionamides: Propylthiouracil (PTU; 6–10 mg/kg/day up to 200–300 mg divided every 6 hrs) or methimazole (0.6–0.7 mg/kg/day divided every 8 hrs): both drugs are given PO, NG or PR; While PTU may be favored because it reduces extrathyroidal conversion of T4 to T3, its use in children has been questioned due to associated liver toxicity.
  - ▶ Potassium iodide and iodine therapy [*e.g.* Lugol's solution 5 drops PO; saturated solution of potassium iodide (SSKI) is among the alternatives]. Thionamide therapy should be given 30–60 mins prior to giving iodide therapy to prevent stimulation of thyroid hormone synthesis. Consider lithium therapy and/or thyroidectomy if clinical condition does not improve.
- Block peripheral actions of thyroid hormone
  - ▶ Beta-blockade (*e.g.* esmolol by continuous IV infusion; or propranolol: 2–3 mg/kg/day PO divided every 6 hrs).
  - ▶ Dexamethasone: 1–2 mg PO every 6 hrs for patients >2 yrs
  - ▶ Consider dialysis or plasmapheresis.

The diagnosis of thyrotoxicosis is suspected based on clinical findings and confirmed by an elevated T4 and/or T3. Serum electrolytes, glucose, liver enzymes and function tests, chest X-ray, and ECG should also be obtained to evaluate for systemic abnormalities. An echocardiogram should be considered. The distinction between severe thyrotoxicosis and thyroid storm is often subjective; all thyrotoxic patients should be treated without delay.

6.9 Hypopituitarism

The anterior pituitary gland normally secretes six major hormones: adrenocorticotropic hormone (ACTH), growth hormone (GH), thyroid stimulating hormone (TSH), luteinizing hormone (LH), follicle stimulating hormone (FSH) and prolactin (PRL). The first five hormones enter the peripheral circulation and stimulate target organs to secrete additional hormones and growth factors such as cortisol, insulin-like growth factor-1 (IGF-1), thyroid hormone and estrogen and testosterone. This system is tightly regulated by the hypothalamus through the secretion of inhibitory and releasing factors into the hypophyseal portal circulation and by the negative feedback effect of peripheral hormones secreted by the target organs on both the hypothalamus and the pituitary gland.

The posterior pituitary secretes antidiuretic hormone (ADH) primarily in response to increasing plasma osmolality and/or hypovolemia. It acts on the collecting ducts of the kidney to reabsorb water through aquaporin-2 channels.

Box 6.9.1   Etiologies of Hypopituitarism

Congenital
- Genetic defects in pituitary/hypothalamic development or hormone production (isolated and combined hormone deficiencies)
- Structural abnormalities: holoprosencephaly, septo-optic dysplasia, hydrocephalus

Acquired
- Tumors: pituitary/hypothalamic (craniopharyngioma, germinoma, optic glioma, meningioma, large pituitary adenomas, cystic lesions, metastatic disease)
- Infection: tuberculosis, fungi, syphilis, toxoplasmosis, meningitis, encephalitis
- Infiltrative: sarcoidosis, histiocytosis, lymphocytic hypophysitis
- Vascular abnormalities and infarction
- Head trauma
- Post-surgery: stalk resection/radiation

Box 6.9.2   Signs and Symptoms of Hypopituitarism by Hormone Deficiency

↓ ACTH*	↓ GH**	↓ TSH†	↓ LH/FSH‡	↓ ADH^
Weakness	Growth	Growth	Delayed	Polyuria
Malaise	failure	failure	puberty	Polydipsia
Lethargy	Delayed	Cold	Menstrual	Failure to
Failure to	bone	intolerance	irregularities	thrive
thrive	age	Fatigue	Micro-phallus	Weight
Weight loss	Hypoglycemia	Constipation	(infant)	loss
Anorexia	(infant)	Dry skin/		Vomiting
Nausea/	Micro-phallus	thin hair		Hypernatremia
vomiting	(infant)	Delayed puberty		
Abdominal		Menstrual		
pain		irregularities		
Adrenal Crisis:		Bradycardia		
Hyponatremia		Anemia		
Hypoglycemia		Prolonged		
Hypotension		jaundice		
Circulatory		(infant)		
shock				

* Secondary adrenal insufficiency (*Adrenal Insufficiency, 6.7*)
** Growth hormone deficiency
† Secondary hypothyroidism
‡ Hypogonadotropic hypogonadism
^Central diabetes insipidus (*Hypernatremia, 6.2.2*)

Hypopituitarism can result from pituitary dysfunction, disruption of the hypothalamic-pituitary connection or hypothalamic dysfunction (**Box 6.9.1**). The secretion of single or multiple hormones may be altered. The signs and symptoms of hypopituitarism are due to loss of target organ function (**Box 6.9.2**). In the PICU it is important to note that these signs and symptoms can contribute to the presentation of an acquired intracranial lesion (tumor, infection or infiltrative process) or can be the result of treatment (surgery, radiation); pituitary function should be investigated in each case.

Hypopituitarism is diagnosed by demonstrating low levels of both pituitary hormones and the products of peripheral target organs

Box 6.9.3   Diagnosis of Hypopituitarism

Secondary Adrenal Insufficiency

- Low 8 a.m. cortisol (< 5–9 mcg/dL in non-stressed patient > ~6 mos) with low or low-normal ACTH. Cortisol level depends on the assay used, time of day and clinical situation. If 8 a.m. cortisol is low, it should be confirmed with a provocative test:
  ▶ Low dose ACTH (1 mcg) stimulation test (**Box 6.7.4**): cortisol <18 mcg/dL
  ▶ Corticotropin Releasing Hormone (CRH) stimulation test*: cortisol < 18 mcg/dL

Growth Hormone Deficiency

- Low insulin-like growth factor 1 (IGF-1)
- Low insulin-like growth factor binding protein-3 (IGFBP-3)
- Low peak GH (<10 ng/mL) during two provocative tests (*i.e.* arginine and clonidine)

Hypothyroidism

- Low total T_4 with low T_3 resin uptake
- Low free T_4
- TSH can be low, inappropriately normal or mildly elevated (TRH deficiency)

Hypogonadism in the setting of delayed puberty or menstrual irregularities

- Low LH and/or FSH
- Low estradiol/testosterone

Central Diabetes Insipidus

- Hypernatremia
- Elevated serum osmolality
- Inappropriately dilute urine (low specific gravity or low osmolality)
- Low ADH
- Loss of T1-weighted bright spot on MRI of the pituitary
- May need to perform water deprivation test to confirm diagnosis

Note: Prolactin may be elevated due to disruption of the pituitary stalk and loss of dopamine inhibition from the hypothalamus

* CRH stimulation test: measure baseline ACTH and cortisol; give CRH 1 mcg/kg IV and re-measure ACTH and cortisol at 15 mins, 30 mins and 60 mins.

Box 6.9.4   Treatment of Hypopituitarism

Adrenal Insufficiency (*Adrenal Insufficiency, Boxes 6.7.5, 6.7.6*)

- Hydrocortisone: physiologic or stress doses as appropriate for the clinical situation

Growth Hormone Deficiency

- Infants with hypoglycemia: subcutaneous GH
- Children and adolescents: consider treatment with growth hormone if clinical condition allows (>1 yr after successful treatment of a malignancy; consult with endocrinologist)

Hypothyroidism

- Levothyroxine: 6–15 mcg/kg per day enterally if <12 months and 2–6 mcg/kg per day enterally if >12 mos. Relatively higher doses per kg are used in younger patients; divide dose in half for IV administration.
- Adrenal insufficiency should be treated first to avoid precipitation of adrenal crisis.

Hypogonadism in the setting of delayed puberty.

- Initiate sex steroid replacement when age appropriate (consult with endocrinologist)

Central Diabetes Insipidus (*Electrolyte Disturbances, 6.2; Box 6.2.6*)

- Fluid management (*Hypernatremia, 6.2.2*)
- Vasopressin (IV, SubQ) or DDAVP (enteral, intranasal, SubQ) as appropriate for the clinical situation

---

(**Box 6.9.3**). For assessment of ACTH and GH, provocative testing may be needed to document deficiencies in these hormones due to their episodic secretion. A water deprivation test with a vasopressin trial may be needed to confirm the presence of central diabetes insipidus.

Treatment of the pituitary hormone deficiencies should take the following into consideration (**Box 6.9.4**):

- In the setting of acute illness, it is important that adrenal insufficiency and diabetes insipidus (DI) be treated immediately to avoid the development of life-threatening dehydration and shock. Adrenal insufficiency may mask the symptoms of DI, and polyuria may become evident once cortisol replacement is initiated.

- When managing diabetes insipidus, it is important to note that patients post head trauma/neurosurgery can have a triphasic response with transient DI occurring within 24–48 hrs of the injury followed by an SIADH-like phase several days later and ultimately permanent DI. Patients should be monitored closely in the post-operative period to avoid both dehydration and water intoxication.

- Thyroid hormone replacement can be initiated if indicated once the possibility of adrenal insufficiency has been addressed.

- Treatment of GH deficiency and hypogonadism should be addressed once the acute clinical situation has resolved. The clinical condition, the age of the patient and family/patient preferences should be considered. One exception is that growth hormone treatment should be initiated early in any infant with congenital hypopituitarism and growth hormone deficiency to prevent hypoglycemia.

Chapter 7

Renal Disease

7.1 Acute Kidney Injury (AKI; Acute Renal Insufficiency or Failure)

The normal kidney functions to (1) maintain normovolemia, (2) maintain normal water, electrolyte and acid-base balance, and (3) to remove metabolic waste and other toxins. AKI refers to an acute impairment or loss of ability to perform these functions independent of the volume of urine produced. Absence or nearly complete absence of renal function is renal failure. All of these conditions are characterized by a decrease in glomerular filtration rate (GFR), which is eventually clinically evident by an increase in the serum creatinine (Scr). Elevation of Scr lags behind any reduction in GFR. The result of AKI may be oliguria [urine output (UOP) < 500 ml/1.73 m²/24 hr or < 1 ml/kg/hr in infants and young children], anuria, or non-oliguria (any volume, from appropriate to excessive UOP). The onset of AKI may be indicated by a progressive increase in Scr even though the absolute value may be within the normal range (**Box 7.1.1**).

A standardized classification for AKI among adults was adopted ("RIFLE" classification; acronym for Risk; Injury; Failure; Loss of kidney function; End-stage renal disease; The Acute Dialysis Quality Initiative, 2002) and modified (The Acute Kidney Injury Network, 2005) to establish uniformity of definition, permit data interpretation, and allow study across large populations. Among critically ill pediatric patients, secondary renal injury appears to be more common than primary renal disease, although its true incidence is not known. AKI is common among critically ill pediatric patients and is associated

Box 7.1.1   Normal Serum Creatinine (Scr) Concentrations
Based on Age (mg/dL)*

Age	Serum Creatinine (mg/dL)
Birth	Equal to the creatinine of the mother; usually < 1.0 mg/dL
1 wk: Term infants	0.3–0.5
2–3 wks: Pre-term infants	0.3–0.5
Infants	0.2–0.4
Children	0.3–0.7
Adolescents	0.5–1.0
Adult Males	0.7–1.3
Adult Females	0.6–1.1

*Scr is proportional to the lean body muscle mass. Its measurement may be altered (an ↑ in Scr without a ↓ in GFR) in the presence of ketonemia (acetoacetate), rhabdomyolysis, icteric serum (as occurs in hyperbilirubinemia), hemolysis, lipemia, cephalosporins (esp. cefoxitin), ascorbic acid, trimethoprim, hydantoin, methyldopa, uric acid, pyruvate, glucose, cimetidine, *et al.* An ↑ in Scr attributed to the benign effect of any such factors should be a diagnosis of exclusion.

with an increase in mortality; early recognition and institution of potentially preventative strategies is essential. Modified pediatric RIFLE criteria have been proposed (**Box 7.1.2**).

The causes of AKI in pediatric patients are diverse (**Box 7.1.3**). The development of AKI during critical illness is often multifactorial and results from a coalescence of hypoperfusion, medication and sepsis-related injury. The goals of the critical care team are:

- To identify risk factors (**Box 7.1.4**) for AKI and reverse them if possible (*e.g.* correct hypovolemia) or strategize to prevent its occurrence (*e.g.* monitor levels of nephrotoxic drugs; prepare for tumor lysis (*Oncologic Emergencies, 9.7*), etc.
- To recognize adverse changes in renal function, initiate evaluation (**Box 7.1.5**) and consult a pediatric nephrologist when appropriate.

Box 7.1.2 Modified RIFLE Criteria for Children*

	Estimated Creatinine Clearance (Clcr)	Urine Output (UOP)
At Risk	↓ by 25%	<0.5 ml/kg/hr for 8 hrs
Injury	↓ by 50%	<0.5 ml/kg/hr for 16 hrs
Failure	↓ by 75% *or* <35 ml/min/1.73m^2	<0.3 ml/kg/hr for 24 hrs *or* anuria for 12 hrs
Loss	Persistent failure for >4 weeks	
End Stage	Persistent failure for >3 months	

* Adapted from Akcan-Arikan A *et al*. Modified RIFLE criteria in critically ill children with acute kidney injury, *Kidney International* 71:1028–1035, 2007.

Note: Volume status may influence the Scr and hence the Clcr and other factors besides AKI may influence UOP. A reduction in UOP, however, should prompt evaluation for a cause.

- To provide supportive care (**Box 7.1.6**) and be prepared to provide **renal replacement therapy (RRT)** when indicated (**Box 7.1.7**).

The goal of RRT in AKI is removal of endogenous (and/or exogenous) toxins, restore normovolemia, and restore normal electrolyte and acid-base balance. The method chosen depends on patient factors such as degree of urgency, patient age and size, hemodynamic stability, potential efficacy of the peritoneum, vascular access, the cause of AKI and availability of the specialized personnel required for each modality.

Peritoneal dialysis (PD) requires placement of a catheter in a well perfused, intact peritoneal space. PD may be performed continuously (and therefore is a form of continuous renal replacement therapy or CRRT), is relatively safe, usually well tolerated in hemodynamically unstable patients, and heparinization is not required. However, correction of metabolic disturbances is gradual, and recent abdominal surgery,

Box 7.1.3   Common Causes of Acute Kidney Injury (AKI) in the Critically Ill

- **Pre-renal:**

  ▶ **Intravascular volume depletion** from any cause, including edematous states in which circulating blood volume may be depleted. The route/nature of volume depletion (*e.g.* poor intake, GI losses, hemorrhage, burns, osmotic diuresis, renal salt wasting, diabetes insipidus, *etc.*) should be identified.

  ▶ **Inadequate renal perfusion** due to low cardiac output states caused by pericardial effusion; cardiogenic shock; regional ↓ in perfusion such as abdominal compartment syndrome.

  ▶ **Pre-renal vascular compromise:** Renal artery stenosis; renal artery thrombosis

- **Intrinsic Renal Disease:**

  ▶ **Primary infectious:** Pyelonephritis; sepsis.

  ▶ **Acute tubular necrosis (ATN)** secondary to hypoxic-ischemic injury (including pre-renal AKI); nephrotoxic agents, rhabdomyolysis (myoglobinuria), hemoglobinuria (intravascular hemolysis); NSAIDS and radioconrast media are also suspected to cause renal vasoconstriction, enhancing their potential to cause AKI during hypovolemia.

  ▶ **Tumor lysis syndrome/uric acid nephropathy**

  ▶ **Interstitial nephritis:** Usually secondary to drugs (*e.g.* penicillins, NSAIDS, *et al.*), *but* may be primary (idiopathic).

  ▶ **Glomerular disease:** Acute glomerulonephritis (*e.g.* post-streptococcal); SLE; Henoch-Schönlein purpura *et al.*

  ▶ **Vascular:** Hemolytic uremic syndrome; malignant hypertension; vasculitis.

- **Post-renal:** Renal vein thrombosis
- **Obstructive uropathy:** Obstruction must affect both kidneys (*e.g.* posterior urethral valves) *OR* create unilateral obstruction of a solitary functioning kidney.

Box 7.1.4 Factors Associated with Increased Risk for Acute Kidney Injury*

• Hypovolemia	• Trauma	• Hepatorenal
• Low CO states	• Rhabdomyolysis	syndrome
• Sepsis	($\uparrow$CK)	• Nephrotoxic
• Underlying renal	• Abdominal	medications such as:
disease or history	compartment	NSAIDS
of AKI	syndrome	aminoglycosides
• Tumor lysis	• Radiocontrast dye	chemotherapy
• Cardiopulmonary	esp. hyperosmolar	amphotericin B
bypass	agents	

* Risk factors for the critically ill pediatric population are incompletely identified; these risk factors are extrapolated from both adult and pediatric series.

Box 7.1.5 Initial Evaluation of Suspected Acute Kidney Injury

- History: Complete, with special attention to events surrounding the suspected injury, drug exposures, volume loss, quantity and quality of urine output (UOP); past medical and family history.
- Physical examination: Complete, with special attention to blood pressure, volume status, presence of edema, hepatomegaly, abdominal or flank mass, evidence of coagulopathy.
- CBC with peripheral smear; platelet count.
- Serum urea nitrogen (SUN; more commonly called BUN) and creatinine. The ratio of urea nitrogen to Scr may be useful in older children and adolescents; > 20:1 is consistent with pre-renal AKI; < 20:1 is consistent with AKI.
- Urinalysis; Evaluate for cells, casts and evidence of tubular dysfunction. Eosinophils suggest drug-induced tubulointerstitial nephritis.
- Serum electrolytes, tCO_2, phosphorus, calcium, magnesium.
- Uric acid and creatine phosphokinase (CK).
- Fractional excretion of sodium (FE_{Na}): (Urine [Na] $\div$ Plasma [Na]) $\div$ (Urine [creatinine] $\div$ Scr) $\times$ 100 with Na in mEq/L and creatinine in mg/dL. In infants and children, values < 1% are most consistent with pre-renal AKI; values > 2% are most consistent with ATN; FE_{Na} between 1–2% may occur in either type of AKI. The newborn's ability to concentrate sodium is decreased, so FE_{Na} in pre-renal AKI is typically < 2.5% and in ATN > 2.5–3.5%.

(Continued)

Box 7.1.5   Initial Evaluation of Suspected Acute Kidney Injury (Continued)

- Urine osmolality: > 500 mOsm/kgH$_2$O is indicative of pre-renal AKI; < 500 mOsm/kgH$_2$O may be found in pre-renal disease as well as ATN.
- Estimate the clearance of creatinine (Clcr; *Appendix, part 2, V*).
- Renal ultrasonography if cause of AKI is unknown. R/O structural abnormalities, obstructive lesions, vascular disorders (*e.g.* thrombosis).
- CXR for pulmonary edema and heart size, if indicated.
- Determine levels of any potentially nephrotoxic drugs (*e.g.* aminoglycosides) and adjust their administration as needed.
- Review all medications being given and determine if dosing adjustments are needed based on Clcr.

Box 7.1.6   Acute Interventions and Supportive Care for Patients with AKI

- Ensure normovolemia and maintain renal perfusion. Dehydration and hemodynamic instability may lead to or exacerbate AKI; empiric administration of isotonic fluid (*e.g.* NaCl 0.9% 20 ml/kg) is warranted to attempt restoration of UOP *provided* there are no contraindications to fluid administration (*e.g.* CHF or signs of hypervolemia). This fluid challenge may be repeated. CVP monitoring may be indicated if intravascular volume status is difficult to determine; echocardiogram is helpful in assessment of cardiac function and volume status. Vasoactive medications may be indicated.
- If the history and findings are consistent with volume overload (*e.g.* hypertension, edema, pleural effusions) and the patient is oliguric, a trial of furosemide (2–5 mg/kg) IV may be given. If there is no response, diuretics should be discontinued.
- Address hypertension: Hypervolemia is the most common cause of ↑BP in AKI; however, some patients require antihypertensive therapy.
- Address serum potassium: Remove all sources of potassium where possible (IVF, TPN; minimize dietary potassium) and monitor serum K$^+$ closely.

(Continued)

Box 7.1.6   Acute Interventions and Supportive Care for Patients with AKI (Continued)

- Hyperphosphatemia and hypocalcemia: As GFR declines, serum phosphorus rises. Hyperphosphatemia may lead to hypocalcemia acutely. In more long-standing disease, hypocalcemia may result from deficient 1,25 $(OH)_2$ vitamin D and/or PTH unresponsiveness. Phosphorus and calcium should be monitored closely.
- Monitor acid-base balance: Mild acidosis ($tCO_2 \geq 15\,mEq/L$) does not require correction in the context of AKI. However, if hyperkalemia is a problem, administration of sodium bicarbonate (1 mEq/kg over 30–60 mins) may be indicated; raising the blood pH may precipitate hypocalcemia.
- See *Electrolyte Disturbances, 6.2* for management of hyperkalemia, hyperphosphatemia and hypocalcemia.
- After normovolemia is achieved, fluid administration should provide:

  ▶ Replacement of insensible losses (half the basal allotment *or* ~500 ml/m^2/day) plus UOP replacement. Abnormal ongoing losses should be replaced ml for ml with a fluid of similar composition. The volume of required medications should be considered a "contribution" toward insensible loss replacement, UOP replacement or other required input.

  ▶ Provide nutrition: Give at least maintenance calories as soon as possible. If oliguria does not permit provision of adequate caloric intake, renal replacement therapy may be warranted if recovery is likely to be prolonged. Protein, potassium and phosphate intake should be guided by the consulting nephrologist and nutritionist.

  ▶ Control glycemia (*Hypo- and Hyperglycemia, 6.4*)

- Avoid nephrotoxic drugs.
- Dopamine in low doses ("renal dosing") does not prevent AKI and should not be used for that purpose.
- Mannitol neither treats nor prevents AKI and may lead to complications.

Box 7.1.7   Indications for Renal Replacement Therapy

- Uremia: altered mental status, pericarditis
- Hypertension, pulmonary edema or CHF associated with volume overload not responsive to diuretic therapy.
- Hyperkalemia not reversible with medical therapy.
- Hyper- or hyponatremia not reversible with medical therapy.
- Refractory metabolic acidosis.
- Fluid needs, including nutrition, that present a volume in excess of that manageable by the kidney, despite supportive care.

---

presence of an enterostomy, abdominal mass or marked organomegaly may prohibit its use. Absolute contraindications include diaphragmatic hernia, gastroschisis, and draining (post-surgical) abdominal wounds. Potential complications are listed in **Box 7.1.8**.

Hemodialysis (HD) requires vascular access and usually, systemic heparinization, although regional heparinization, citrate anticoagulation or heparin-free dialysis can be used when heparinization is contraindicated. HD is highly effective in the rapid removal of toxins and is the method of choice for removal of certain toxins (*e.g.* lithium, ethylene glycol, methanol). It is also rapidly effective in removing endogenous toxins (ammonia, urea nitrogen) and fluid. HD is typically performed intermittently, and while rapid removal of certain substances may be desirable, rapid ultrafiltration may result in hemodynamic instability; other potential complications include osmotic disequilibrium syndrome which can result in cerebral edema and raised ICP.

Hemofiltration is a form of rapidly effective continuous renal replacement therapy (**CRRT**) commonly chosen for unstable PICU patients. It effects a less abrupt fluid and electrolyte shift as compared to HD, and generally allows for greater hemodynamic stability. In addition to the listed goals and indications (**Box 7.1.7**), CRRT is beneficial in tumor lysis syndrome (for removal of uric acid, phosphorus, potassium), post-cardiopulmonary bypass, inborn errors of

Box 7.1.8   Potential Complications of Peritoneal Dialysis (PD)

- Peritonitis: Usually fever, abdominal pain with peritoneal signs and cloudy peritoneal fluid are present. **Peritonitis is a potentially life-threatening infection and suspicion of its presence requires appropriate cultures (peritoneal fluid and blood) and treatment for infection until proven otherwise.**
  - ▶ Infectious: Neutrophils typically predominate in the peritoneal fluid, but lymphocytes commonly predominate in the presence of fungal, or very rarely, mycobacterial, infections.
  - ▶ Aseptic peritonitis: An inflammatory response for which there is no identified pathogen. This reactive peritonitis may be infectious, secondary to dialysate, peritoneally-instilled medications, the catheter itself, *et al.* A variety of cells may be seen in the peritoneal fluid. When occuring shortly post-catheter placement, a predominance of eosinophils typically represents a self-limited foregin body reaction to the catheter commonly referred to as eosinophilic peritonitis, although this cell type may be seen from other causes as well.

- Catheter-related complications:
  - ▶ Malfunction:
    - ■ "Omental wrap" (more common in infants), usually occurring 1–15 days after catheter placement; omentectomy is usually required.
    - ■ Intraluminal thrombus
    - ■ Adhesions
    - ■ Catheter malposition (usually evident within days of placement). The catheter tip should lie in the lower quadrant opposite that of the exit site.
    - ■ Kinking of the catheter
- Dialysate leak at insertion or exit site
- Traction on catheter leading to cuff extrusion
- Shoulder pain or tenesmus may occur secondary to catheter position (despite a well placed catheter) or as referred pain (or sensation) due to the presence of dialysate. These typically occur early after catheter placement (days), are transient and self-resolve with symptomatic care.
- Bleeding

> **Box 7.1.9   Potential Complications of Hemodialysis and Hemofiltration**
>
> - Clotting of the circuit, filter, or catheter is possible even with anticoagulation.
> - Bleeding diatheses from anticoagulation or clotting is possible but uncommon.
> - Embolism from air or clots returning from the circuit is possible but rare.
> - Access complications include clotting, venous stasis, thrombosis of the vessel, and insertion site infections.
> - Hypotension with initiation of CRRT may occur but is uncommon with proper priming of the circuit and gradual increase of pump flow to target flow; may be less of a problem with newer technology.
> - Hypothermia from extracorporeal cooling of the patient's blood is less common with newer CRRT pumps which allow temperature regulation. However, this regulation may also mask fever.
> - Equipment malfunction is possible and may require replacement of the circuit. Blood and/or volume loss may occur.
> - Bradykinin release from the filter membranes in the setting of acidosis or blood priming may cause symptoms including nausea, hypotension and anaphylaxis.
> - Sudden electrolyte changes are uncommon but may occur in the setting of dialysate preparation errors. Use of commercially available premix dialysate preparations may be preferable to decrease this risk.

metabolism (ammonia, lactic acid, organic and amino acids, *etc.*) and in acute volume overload; it may be beneficial in disease states such as sepsis and SIRS (inflammatory mediators). The most commonly used mode of CRRT is continuous venovenous hemofiltration (CVVH) or variations thereof. Complications are listed in **Box 7.1.9**.

7.2 Hypertension

Hypertension in pediatrics is defined based upon the normative distribution of blood pressure in healthy children. The prevalence of hypertension in the pediatric population is estimated at 1–2%. The

National High Blood Pressure Education Program Working Group on High Blood Pressure in Children and Adolescents (NHBPEP), armed with recent data from the National Health and Nutrition Examination Survey (NHANES), recently published the Fourth Report on the Diagnosis, Evaluation, and Treatment of High Blood Pressure in Children and Adolescents. This report provides an update and recommendations to the clinician, incorporating the rapid advances in the detection, evaluation, and management of hypertension in the pediatric population (Pediatrics, **114**:555–576, 2004).

Criteria for diagnosis of hypertension and pre-hypertension are outlined in (**Box 7.2.1**). Blood pressure (BP) is classified by systolic

---

Box 7.2.1   Classification of Hypertension in Pediatric Patients

Status	Percentile* of SBP and/or DBP
Normal	< 90th
Pre-hypertension	90th to < 95th *OR* > 120/80 mmHg but < *95th*
Hypertension	
▸ Stage 1 (mild)	95th to 99th + 5 mmHg
▸ Stage 2 (severe)	> 99th + 5 mmHg
Hypertensive urgency	Severe hypertension without evidence of end-organ damage or dysfunction. May be associated with nonspecific symptoms (*e.g.* headache, blurred vision, nausea, vomiting) without evidence of target organ injury; usually develops over days to weeks.
Hypertensive emergency	Severe hypertension with evidence of end-organ injury. Associated with rapid, progressive damage to end organs such as the heart, kidney, brain and large arteries. The absolute level of hypertension is not as important as the evidence of complications in other organ systems.

---

* Percentiles are based on age, gender and height. See *Appendix, part 2, I* or http://www/nhlbi.nih.gov/guidelines/hypertension/child/_tbl.htm

Box 7.2.2   Guidelines for Diagnosis of Hypertension in Infants (< 1 year)*

AGE	Significant Hypertension**		Severe Hypertension†	
	SBP (mmHg)	DBP (mmHg)	SBP (mmHg)	DBP (mmHg)
Newborn–7 days	≥ 96		≥ 106	
8–30 days	≥ 104		≥ 110	
Infants	≥ 110	≥ 63	≥ 118	≥ 82

* From Report of the Second Task Force on Blood Pressure Control in Children–1987, *Pediatrics* 79(1):1–25, 1987.
** Average systolic and/or diastolic BP between 90th and 95th percentiles.
† Average systolic and/or diastolic BP ≥ 95th percentile.

BP (SBP) and diastolic BP (DBP) percentiles for age, sex and height (*Appendix, part 2, I or at*: http://www/nhlbi.nih.gov/guidelines/hypertension/child_tbl.htm). In infants < 1 year, hypertension is defined by SBP alone (**Box 7.2.2**). Routine blood pressure measurement has not been recommended in otherwise healthy infants due to technical difficulties in obtaining accurate measurements and the overall low incidence of hypertension among healthy newborns; normative data for this population are therefore scarce.

Essential (idiopathic) hypertension is recognized with increasing frequency in children, and now accounts for the majority of pediatric hypertension, and is associated with the rising prevalence and severity of obesity in the pediatric population. The *metabolic syndrome*, also associated with obesity, is a constellation of cardiovascular risk factors that includes insulin resistance, abnormal glucose tolerance, dyslipidemia, and hypertension. Metabolic syndrome is associated with a higher risk for cardiovascular and metabolic diseases such as diabetes mellitus type 2 and atherosclerosis. The syndrome is present in 30% of overweight children.

Children who suffer from sleep apnea associated with hypoxia have elevated BP during wakefulness that is independent of their degree of obesity; hence a brief sleep history should be obtained in a child who has hypertension.

Secondary hypertension is more common among hypertensive children than among hypertensive adults. These children are usually younger, and are more likely to have both systolic and diastolic hypertension. In contrast to those with essential hypertension, children with secondary hypertension have relatively higher BP and high morbidity and mortality. Renal abnormalities account for approximately 60–70% of cases, with reflux nephropathy and obstructive uropathy as the most common causes. Another 10% of cases are caused by renovascular disease. The mechanism causing secondary hypertension varies depending upon the primary disease process, such as vascular obstruction in coarctation, volume overload in renal diseases and catecholamine excess in pheochromocytoma. **Box 7.2.3** shows the most common causes of hypertension by age group.

Box 7.2.3   Most Common Causes of Hypertension in Children by Age Group

Newborns	Renal artery thrombosis; renal artery stenosis; congenital renal malformations; coarctation of the aorta; bronchopulmonary dysplasia
Infancy–6 yrs	Renal parenchymal diseases; renal scarring due to reflux nephropathy; coarctation of the aorta; obstructive renal disease
6–10 yrs	Essential hypertension; renal artery stenosis; renal parenchymal disease
Adolescents	Essential hypertension; renal parenchymal disease; ingestions and drug use

Blood pressure is the result of the interaction of two main factors: cardiac output and peripheral vascular resistance. An increase in one factor while the other factor remains unchanged will result in an increase in blood pressure. The renin-angiotensin-aldosterone system plays an important role in the development of high BP by affecting peripheral vascular resistance. Renin is an enzyme produced in the kidney that converts angiotensinogen to angiotensin I. Its production is influenced by several factors, including arteriolar perfusion of the kidneys and the sympathetic nervous system. Angiotensin I is converted rapidly to angiotensin II by the angio-converting enzyme (ACE). Angiotensin II is a potent vasoconstrictor that stimulates the production of aldosterone, which further increases BP by causing salt and water retention. Both of these substances increase BP by increasing vascular resistance. Other factors that influence BP include the activity of the autonomic nervous system, renal regulation of sodium, and compliance of both resistance and capacitance vessels.

The pathophysiologic mechanisms causing acute hypertensive urgencies and emergencies are complex and not well understood. Hypertensive urgencies occur as a result of acute changes in vascular resistance secondary to secretion of catecholamines, angiotensin II, vasopressin, endothelin, thromboxane or decreased production of nitric oxide and PGI_2 (prostacyclin). Typically, end-organ vessels remain uninjured. In hypertensive emergencies, endothelial control of vascular tone is overwhelmed, leading to end-organ hyperperfusion, arteriolar fibrinoid necrosis and increased endothelial perfusion resulting in end-organ injury. The rate of rise in BP determines the clinical presentation. Organs at greatest risk for injury are brain, heart and kidneys. An increase in afterload causes LV dysfunction, an increase in myocardial oxygen demand, and decreased coronary blood flow. Hypertension causes decreased blood flow to the kidneys as manifested by a deterioration of renal function.

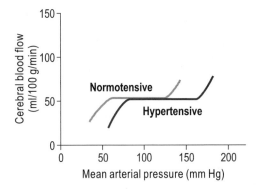

Fig. 7.2.1. The Relationship Between Mean Arterial Pressure and Cerebral Blood Flow When Hypertension is Chronic. Cerebral blood flow is maintained constant at a higher mean arterial pressure.

Hypertensive encephalopathy is a constellation of signs and symptoms of severe hypertension due to hyperperfusion of the brain. Normally, brain perfusion is controlled by autoregulatory processes over a wide range of mean arterial pressure (MAP), usually between 60 and 125 mmHg. In chronically hypertensive patients, this steady state perfusion is shifted to the right so that cerebral blood flow is regulated at a higher than normal range of MAP, usually from 80 to 160 mmHg (**Fig. 7.2.1**). However, a rapid increase in MAP can overwhelm cerebral autoregulatory capacities. This loss of autoregulation and disruption of the blood brain barrier permits excessive blood flow to the brain (**Fig. 7.2.2**) that may lead to cerebral edema, raised ICP, intracranial hemorrhage and eventually death. Retinal changes usually mirror other changes in the brain as encephalopathy progresses. Eye findings include areas of arteriolar vasospasm and dilatation, hemorrhage, exudates, and papilledema. Symptoms of hypertensive encephalopathy include severe headache, visual disturbance, vomiting, seizures, lethargy, confusion, or coma.

Evaluation. Accurate BP measurement is essential for diagnosis (*General Approach to the Critically Ill Child, 1.2*). BP should be

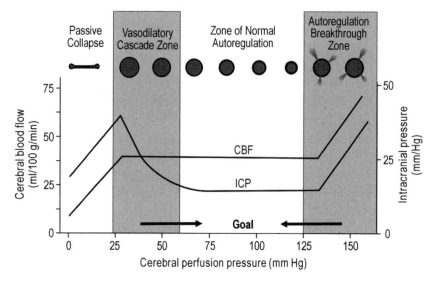

Fig. 7.2.2.   The Relationship Between Mean Arterial Pressure and Cerebral Perfusion Pressure When Hypertension is Acute. Note that vascular leak and ↑ICP occur as the zone of normal autoregulation is exceeded. Adapted from Rose JC, Mayer SA, Optimizing blood pressure in neurological emergencies, *Neurocritical Care* 1:287–299, 2004.

measured in all four extremities to identify possible aortic coarctation (lower extremity SBP > 10 mmHg lower than upper extremity SBP suggests coarctation of the aorta). Discrepancies in BP between cuff and arterial catheter readings should be reconciled. Oscillometric readings are particularly inaccurate at the extremes of measurement (very low or very high BP). If an indwelling arterial catheter is functioning well, provides a normal arterial waveform and is properly "zeroed" with its transducer correctly positioned, it has been our practice to rely on these readings rather than oscillometric determinations.

History should be geared toward identifying risk factors for secondary hypertension and co-morbidities in essential hypertension (**Box 7.2.4**). Physical examination should focus on identification of a cause for secondary hypertension or end-organ damage (**Box 7.2.1**).

Box 7.2.4   Some Causes and Risk Factors for Hypertension

- Neonates

  Prematurity
  Steroids used to treat chronic lung disease
  Low birth weight (independent of prematurity)
  Umbilical artery catheterization
  Sympathomimetic medication for apnea of prematurity
  Prenatal cocaine exposure

- Renal disease

  AKI; renal scarring or thromboemboli; acute tubular necrosis; fibromuscular dysplasia; polyarteritis nodosa; vasculitides

- Congenital heart disease

  Coarctation of the aorta (even without residual obstruction); mid-aortic syndrome

- Medications

  Sympathomimetics
  Dietary supplements (*e.g.* to enhance atheletic performance or promote weight loss)
  Recreational drugs: cocaine, amphetamines, phencyclidine; drug over-dose

- Endocrinopathies

  Hyperthyroidism/thyroid crisis
  Cushing Syndrome
  Hyperreninism; renin-secreting tumors
  Pheochromocytoma
  Conn disease

- Pregnancy

  Pre-eclampsia

- Being a PICU Patient

  Pain; anxiety
  Medications (*e.g.* steroids; cyclosporine; tacrolimus; sympathomimetics)
  Poisoning; illicit drug exposure
  Obstructed urinary catheter
  Raised ICP
  Autonomic dysfunction associated with injury, manipulation of the spine or neurologic disease
  Occult seizure activity (*e.g.* seizure in a muscle-relaxed patient, akinetic seizures or non-convulsive status epilepticus).
  Volume overload
  New onset renal dysfunction; acute kidney injury

Patients with a hypertensive emergency may present with altered mental status, seizures, LV failure (pulmonary edema, MI), aortic dissection, oliguria, and focal neurologic findings that may indicate raised ICP, intracranial hemorrhage, lacunar infarcts, stroke or evidence of hypertensive encephalopathy ("PRES" or posterior reversible encephalopathy syndrome). The examination should include a thorough assessment to identify heart murmurs, gallops, abdominal bruits, weak femoral pulses, poor peripheral perfusion, subtle nerve deficits, visual field deficits, abnormalities on fundoscopic examination and evidence of hemolytic anemia.

Infants with severe hypertension may present with apparent shock, CHF or simply irritability or failure to thrive. Renal or cardiac pathology may be present. Bell's palsy is an uncommon presenting symptom of pediatric hypertension. Autonomic dysfunction is common in Guillian-Barre syndrome, occurring in up to 67% of patients; hypertension may be identified before or after neurologic findings are present. Conversely, hypertension may be unrelated to the apparent presenting disease process, making retrieval of any BP data for all health care encounters helpful in evaluation (**Box 7.2.5**).

Box 7.2.5.   Initial Diagnostic Evaluation of Hypertension in the PICU

- Measure BP in all four extremities.
- Urinanalysis (identify proteinuria, hematuria, casts, *etc.*)
- Electrolytes, urea nitrogen and creatinine
- CBC with examination of the peripheral smear (R/O microangiopathic process as seen in hemolytic uremic syndrome)
- CXR
- 12-lead ECG
- Urine beta-HCG as indicated
- Brain imaging (CT or MRI) as indicated for neurologic symptoms
- Search for illicit drug use as indicated
- Consider ultrasonography of the urinary tract and/or heart.
- Consider pediatric cardiology and/or nephrology consultation as appropriate.

Management and Therapy. A hypertensive emergency in a child is life threatening and requires treatment in the PICU. Patients with hypertensive urgency may receive treatment and be observed for a response (emergency department or pediatric ward). Children with a hypertensive emergency should have an indwelling arterial catheter placed for continuous blood pressure monitoring. The radial artery is the preferred location, but occasionally other sites (*e.g.* dorsalis pedis, axillary, and femoral arteries) must be utilized. A central venous catheter may also be warranted in order to deliver continuous IV antihypertensive medications as well as to accurately monitor CVP.

The clinician treating a hypertensive crisis (an emergency or urgency) should consider the underlying disease process when choosing initial therapy. Associated congenital or acquired heart diseases (arrhythmia or heart block), underlying renal disease (renal artery stenosis), or co-morbid CNS disease (cerebral hemorrhage or infarct) are just a few of the concerns that the practitioner should attempt to address prior to initiation of therapy.

The goal for antihypertensive therapy is to safely lower the blood pressure at a rate that arrests or alleviates end-organ damage without causing ischemia of vital organs. This usually translates to a reduction of MAP by 20–25% over 2–3 hrs for treatment of a hypertensive emergency. If the patient is clinically stable, the BP may be further decreased toward normal over the next 24–48 hrs. Intravenous nitroprusside, labetalol, or nicardipine are the typical first line, titratable agents for treatment of a hypertensive crisis (**Box 7.2.6**). A majority of children with hypertensive crisis have acute or chronic renal disease and therefore diuretics may be helpful adjunctive therapy.

Box 7.2.6   Selected Antihypertensive Agents* in the PICU

Class	Drug	Usual Dose (Duration)	Comments
Alpha and Beta blockers	Labetalol	Acute: 0.2–1 mg/kg per dose IV; max 20 mg per dose or 0.4–3 mg/kg per hour (2–4 hr for a single IV dose)	Contraindications include CHF, bradycardia, heart block; relative contraindications include obstructive airway disease.
Beta-blocker	Esmolol	500 mcg/kg min for one min, then 50–1000 mcg/kg per min; the loading dose is sometimes omitted. (10–30 min)	Selective β-1 blocker; very brief duration making it a good choice if response is undesirable. Relatively c/i in severe asthma, heart block and diabetes.
Vasodilation of arterioles and venules	Sodium nitro-prusside (SNP)	Initial: 0.25 mcg/kg/min IV; max. 8–10 mcg/kg/per min; doses >4 mcg per kg/min are rarely required. (1–10 min)	No direct ionotropic or chronotropic effects. If high doses (>3–4 mcg/per kg/min), infusion >72 hrs *or* renal impairment is is a factor, addition of thiosulfate (1 gram per 100 mg SNP) or hydroxocobalamin can prevent cyanide accumulation. However, *thiocyanate* toxicity can develop despite normal kidneys.

(Continued)

Box 7.2.6 Selected Antihypertensive Agents* in the PICU (Continued)

Class	Drug	Usual Dose (Duration)	Comments
Arterial dilator	Hydralazine	0.1–0.2 mg/kg per dose IV or IM, initially; max single dose 20 mg; up to 1.7–3.5 mg/kg per day in divided doses (2–6 hr)	Avoid in pre-existing heart disease (esp. LVH), ↑ICP, pulmonary HTN or HTN associated with CNS disease. Reflex tachycardia common; generally used as an "add-on" agent.
	Diazoxide	1–3 mg/kg IV; max dose 150 mg; may repeat q 5–15 min until adequate BP control achieved (3–12 hr)	Avoid in renal or liver disease, diabetes, ↑ uric acid, CHF or gout
	Minoxidil	0.1–0.2 mg/kg PO once daily initially; max initial dose 5 mg/day (12–24 hr)	Same as hydralazine; 3% develop pericardial effusion; c/i in pheochromocytoma; reserved for resistant HTN.
Calcium channel blocker	Nicardipine	0.5–5 mcg/kg per min IV (Effect ↓s by 50% within ~30 min of discontinuation of infusion.)	Afterload reduction by ↓ing peripheral vascular resistance without ↓ing CO; rapid onset and brief duration make it ideal for immediate treatment; ↓s HTN-associated cardiac and cerebral ischemia. (See nifedipine).

(Continued)

Box 7.2.6   Selected Antihypertensive Agents* in the PICU (Continued)

Class	Drug	Usual Dose (Duration)	Comments
Calcium-channel blocker	Nifedipine	0.25–0.5 mg/kg per dose PO; max 10 mg/dose (4–8 hr)	This class generally exhibit greater BP lowering effects as compared to ACE inhibitors in females and black patients. Use extended release formulations for chronic therapy.
Dopamine receptor (DA$_1$) agonist	Fenoldopam	0.2–0.8 mcg/kg per min; limited to short-term (4 hr) use (5–60 min)	Acts at post-synaptic DA receptors in renal, coronary, cerebral and splanchnic vasculature causing vasodilation and ↓MAP. Peak effects in 5–15 mins, with steady state in 30–60 min. Effects dissipate rapidly upon discontinuation of infusion. Causes ↑ renal blood flow and Na$^+$ excretion
Central alpha agonist	Clonidine	5–10 mcg/kg per day PO in divided doses q 8–12 hr (8–12 hr)	Stimulates α2-adreno-receptors in the brainstem, ↓ing sympathetic outflow.
ACE Inhibitors**	Enalaprilat	5–10 mcg per kg/dose IV (8–24 hrs)	Preferred initial agent in diabetics, micoalbuminuria, proteinuria. ↑ Risk of neutropenia in renal disease. ↑ Scr and K$^+$ common and transient. (Continued)

Box 7.2.6   Selected Antihypertensive Agents* in the PICU (Continued)

Class	Drug	Usual Dose (Duration)	Comments
	Captopril	0.05 (neonates) to 0.5 mg/kg/dose PO q 8–24 hr; max 6 mg/kg/day; max adult dose 450 mg daily (6–24 hr depending on age)	Same as enalaprilat. Rash in ~5% of patients is usually mild and disappears within a few days of ↓ing dose or discontinuation.
Diuretics	Furosemide	1–2 mg/kg/dose IV (4–6 hrs.)	Electrolyte monitoring required. Leads to K⁺ depletion and metabolic alkalosis. Useful in CHF and renal impairment; causes calciuria.
	Hydrochloro-thiazide	1–2 mg/kg/dose PO (12–24 hrs.)	Electrolyte monitoring required. Ineffective in moderate – severe renal impairment. Avoid if Clcr < 10 ml/min/1.73 m²; ↑ renal tubular reabsorption of calcium.

* Careful monitoring is essential; profound, acute hypotension may occur with recommended doses.

** Use with caution and modify dosage in renal impairment, esp. renal artery stenosis.

7.3 Hemolytic-Uremic Syndrome (HUS)

HUS is characterized by non-immune microangiopathic hemolytic anemia, (hematocrit < 30% with schistocytes or helmet cells on blood smear), thrombocytopenia (platelet count $< 150 \times 10^3/\text{mm}^3$), and renal dysfunction (Scr > upper limit of normal for age; *Box 7.1.1*). The disorder occurs most frequently in children < 5 yrs. The presentation is generally heralded by diarrhea, which is often bloody. Most pediatric cases (90%) are secondary to infection with *Escherichia coli* which produce Shiga-like toxin ("STEC"; serotypes 0157:H7, 0111:H8, 0103:H8, 0123, 026). This "typical" HUS is often referred to as diarrhea (+) HUS and accounts for 90% of cases. The remainder are classified as "atypical" or "diarrhea (–) HUS", since they are not caused by Shiga-like toxin producing bacteria (**Box 7.3.1**). Atypical HUS has a poorer prognosis, with morality rates as high as 25% and progression to end-stage renal disease in up to 50% of patients. Research has linked atypical HUS to uncontrolled activation of the complement system (Noris M, Remuzzig G. Atypical hemolytic uremic syndrome, *N Engl J Med* **361(17):**1676–1687, 2009).

Box 7.3.1   Causes of Atypical HUS ["Diarrhea (–)"]

• Infection-induced
  ▸ *S. pneumoniae*
  ▸ Group A *Streptococcus*
  ▸ HIV
• Genetic Forms
  ▸ Complement pathway mutations
  ▸ Complement Factor H deficiency
  ▸ von Willebrand factor cleaving protease (ADAMTS 13) deficiency
  ▸ Intracellular defects of vitamin B_{12} metabolism
  ▸ Membrane cofactor protein deficiency
  ▸ Idiopathic autosomal dominant disease
	• Drug-induced
	  ▸ Cyclosporine, tacrolimus
	  ▸ Sirolimus
	  ▸ Mitomycin C, cisplatin, bleomycin
	  ▸ Ticlodipine
	  ▸ Quinine
	• Autoimmune Diseases
	  ▸ Systemic lupus erythematosus
	  ▸ Antiphospholipid syndrome
	• Other associations
	  ▸ Pregnancy
	  ▸ Organ transplant
	  ▸ Cancer

Box 7.3.2   Relative Risk for Death in HUS Based on Clinical
             Illness at Time of Admission*

Critical Illness at Admission	Relative Risk of Mortality
Oliguria	1.79
Anuria	2.58
Seizures	8.5
Coma	9.36
Dehydration	1.91
Lethargy	1.39
WBC > 20 × 10³/mm³	2.58

* Oakes RS, Siegler RL, McReynolds, Pysher T, Pavia AT, Predictors of fatality in postdiarrheal hemolytic uremic syndrome, *Pediatrics* 117(5):1659, 2006.

Signs and symptoms. HUS is characterized by the sudden onset of pallor, decreased activity, and an ill-appearing child. Intravascular volume status may be low, normal, or expanded. A microangiopathic hemolytic anemia is uniformly present, with numerous fragmented RBC's on peripheral smear, typically negative Coombs test, and very elevated serum lactate dehydrogenase (LDH). There may be mild elevation of indirect bilirubin and decreased haptoglobin concentrations. The platelet count averages ~ 40,000 per mm³ on presentation. Leukocytosis, reported in 20–25%, has been associated with a worse outcome (**Box 7.3.2**). Renal involvement ranges from isolated hematuria and proteinuria to oliguric or anuric renal failure. Multiple changes are present in the glomerular walls and fibrin thrombi may be found in the glomerular capillaries. Over 50% of patients require some form of renal replacement therapy for an average of 10 days before the recovery of renal function. The severity of anemia and thrombocytopenia do not correlate with the severity of renal involvement. Although the kidney is most commonly affected, numerous other organs may be involved (**Box 7.3.3**).

Reports from large outbreaks suggest that HUS will develop in approximately 5–10% of those infected with STEC. STEC infection undergoes an incubation period of 2–5 days, most commonly followed

---

Box 7.3.3   HUS: Other Organ System Involvement and Complications

- CNS
  - ▶ 20–25% of patients; lethargy, irritability, seizures, hemiparesis, cortical blindness, coma, stroke
  - ▶ ↑ Incidence of death if CNS is involved
- GI
  - ▶ More likely in diarrhea (+) HUS; vomiting, crampy abdominal pain
  - ▶ Intussusception, bowel necrosis, bowel perforation with septicemia
  - ▶ Severe colitis is predictive of prolonged renal failure
- Pancreas
  - ▶ 20% of patients
  - ▶ ↑Amylase and lipase
  - ▶ Pancreatic pseudocyst
  - ▶ Transient and/or permanent diabetes mellitus in 4–15% of patients
- Cardiac
  - ▶ Hypertension
  - ▶ Severe myocardial dysfunction with ↑ troponin I
- Respiratory
  - ▶ Pleural effusion
  - ▶ Pulmonary hemorrhage is rare

---

by crampy abdominal pain and watery diarrhea without fever, progressing to bloody diarrhea in > 50% of cases. HUS develops in those affected approximately 1 week after the onset of diarrhea. However, recent studies suggest that endothelial injury has already occurred in patients who go on to develop HUS within the first 2 to 4 days of the onset of diarrhea. In addition to direct endothelial injury from shiga-like toxin, release of cytokines from damaged cells appears to be of importance. Interleukins 6, 8 and TNF-α have been implicated. By the time of presentation with HUS, STEC are often no longer present in the stool.

The frequency of *S. pneumoniae*-induced HUS is increasing. In one recent study, 0.6% of children with invasive pneumococcal infections developed HUS. The pneumococcus produces a circulating neuraminidase, which cleaves N-acetyl neuraminic acid from the glycoproteins on the cell membrane of RBCs, platelets, and glomerular capillary walls. Different strains likely produce different amounts. This exposes the Thomsen-Freidenreich antigen (T-antigen), which can react with IgM normally circulating against the T-antigen. Intravascular hemolysis ensues. In a recent study, 6 of 10 patients with pneumococcal-induced HUS were positive for RBC T-antigen activation. Numerous groups have reported higher mortality rates from pneumococcal-induced HUS, ranging from 29–50% of patients.

Treatment. Despite numerous approaches to specific therapies for HUS, there is currently no definitive therapy other than supportive care for patients with diarrhea (+) HUS. Fresh frozen plasma (FFP) and/or plasmapheresis have been reported to benefit certain patients with diarrhea (−) HUS. Critical care and early dialysis have resulted in a dramatic fall in mortality. Careful attention to fluid and electrolyte disturbances is of utmost importance. After adequate volume replacement has been achieved, fluid restriction to insensible losses plus UOP replacement may be required if oliguria or anuria ensue. A trial of loop diuretics may be warranted. Parenteral nutrition may be needed because of intolerance to enteral feedings.

PRBC transfusions may be necessary for symptomatic anemia. Platelet transfusion may promote the pathologic process and should be reserved for procedures associated with significant bleeding risk or for profound thrombocytopenia (*e.g.* < 10–$20 \, k/mm^3$). Corticosteroids, prostacyclin, anticoagulants, and thrombolytics have not been shown to be helpful. Plasmapheresis is usually unnecessary in the diarrheal form of HUS. Plasmapheresis is warranted for HUS following bone marrow transplant, or the adult counterpart of HUS, namely, thrombotic thrombocytopenic purpura.

The need for dialysis has been reported in 50–60% of patients. Use of PD has been most often reported, although contraindicated in the setting of severe colitis. Both hemodialysis and continuous hemofiltration have also been used. A combination of dialysis modalities is often required.

Patients who develop CNS involvement require careful attention to detection and control of seizures. Cerebral edema is a common feature of severe CNS involvement. Use of mannitol in patients with renal failure may result in hyperosmolality (*Raised Intracranial Pressure, 5.5*). Hypertonic saline would be an acceptable alternative therapy.

Inotropic agents may be required in patients with cardiomyopathy. Hypertension may respond to a decrease in intravascular volume in the presence of volume overload. Antihypertensive medicines may also be required (*Hypertension, 7.2*).

The use of antibiotics in patients with STEC infection is discouraged. Potential therapies under investigation include synthetic toxin binders, probiotic bacteria, and monoclonal antibodies against Shiga toxin.

7.4 Rhabdomyolysis

Rhabdomyolysis is the necrosis of skeletal muscle characterized by an influx of calcium into the sacrolemma due to failure of ATP-dependent pumps, channels and exchangers in the muscle cell. Direct muscle injury or energy (ATP) depletion from any cause may result in leakage of myoglobin and other intracellular components (*e.g.* potassium, phosphate, urate, creatine kinase (CK), lactate, aldolase and other proteins) into plasma. Myoglobin is a heme-protein; it contains iron (Fe^{2+}) which can be oxidized to ferric (Fe^{3+}) oxide. Under normal conditions, intracellular antioxidants prevent accumulation of oxygen free radicals, which can cause cell injury. Normally, myoglobin in plasma is filtered by the glomerulus and metabolized in the renal tubule epithelial cell. When rhabdomyolysis is severe, myoglobin leaves the renal tubule cell and spills into the tubular lumen causing leakage of free radicals into the environment with resultant oxidative injury and a classic reddish-brown discoloration of the urine.

The cause of AKI resulting from myoglobin appears to be multifactorial. *Volume depletion* (due to fluid accumulation in injured muscle as well as other associated fluid losses) and the ensuing physiologic responses of the sympathetic nervous system, the renin-angiotensin system and ADH secretion lead to renal vasoconstriction. Release of oxygen free radicals favors local vasoconstriction and causes *direct tubular injury* associated with *local inflammation* in the kidney. In addition, *tubular obstruction* (primarily in distal tubules) is caused by sloughed renal tubule cells and precipitation of Tamm-Horsfall protein-myoglobin complexes, the formation of which is favored by acidic urine. Therefore, renal ischemic and inflammatory injuries as well as tubular obstruction contribute to AKI in severe rhabdomyolysis.

AKI is reported in as many as 50% of adults with rhabdomyolysis, but its incidence in children is not known. A majority of adult cases are associated with drug (cocaine) and alcohol abuse, trauma (especially crush injuries) and toxic effects of medications. The causes in children are more diverse (**Box 7.4.1**). Key points and findings are summarized

---

Box 7.4.1 Causes of Rhabdomyolysis

- Direct muscle trauma; crush injuries
- Muscle ischemia; compartment syndrome
- Infections causing myositis:
  ‣ Influenza A and B
  ‣ EBV
  ‣ Parainfluenza
  ‣ CMV
  ‣ Coxsackie virus
  ‣ Herpes viruses
  ‣ HIV
  ‣ *Legionella*
  ‣ Group A Streptococcal disease
  ‣ Salmonella
  ‣ *Francisella tularensis*
  ‣ *Plasmodium falciparum*
- Septic shock
- Severe exertion, esp. in hot environments (Patients with sickle cell trait may be at especially increased risk)

- Seizures, esp. if prolonged
- Certain IEM's: *e.g.* Disorders of glycogenolysis, glycolysis, lipid metabolism, purine metabolism and any disturbance in ATP production and/or utilization (mitochondrial defects)
- Electrolyte disturbances including: hypophosphatemia, hypocalcemia, DKA, hypokalemia, nonketotic hyperosmolality
- Respiratory failure, esp. status asthmaticus with use of corticosteroids and NMB.
- Heat stress, including malignant hyperthermia and neuroleptic malignant syndrome (*Drug-Induced Toxic Hyperthermic Syndromes, 13.2*)
- Cold stress
- Snake or insect envenomation
- Drug (cocaine) or alcohol abuse
- Lipid-lowering drugs (statins; fibrates)

(**Box 7.4.2**). The cause of rhabdomyolysis should be identified in each case. Sources of muscle injury that require urgent intervention (*e.g.* compartment syndromes) should be addressed urgently with the appropriate consultant. Treatment is outlined in **Box 7.4.3**. Experimental therapies have included treatment with antioxidants and free-radical scavengers; these novel approaches are promising but require more rigorous investigation to determine efficacy (Suggested reading: Bosch X, Poch E, Grau JM, Rhabdomyolysis and acute kidney injury, *N Engl J Med*, **361**(**14**): 62–72, 2009).

Box 7.4.2   Rhabdomyolysis: Clinical Manifestations and Key Points

- Risk factors are usually but not always present (**Box 7.4.1**).
- The hallmark of myoglobinuria is a reddish-brown urine with a positive reaction for blood on "urine dipstick" testing but an absence of RBC's on urine microscopic examination.* This occurs because myoglobin cross-reacts with hemoglobin on the dipstick. This finding is present ~ 80% of the time; therefore a negative test for heme on urine dipstick does not R/O myoglobinuria.
- Myoglobin (not CK) is the offending toxin in the kidney. An increase in plasma myoglobin is inferred if CK is elevated. (The $t_{1/2}$ of myoglobin in plasma is very brief (1–3 hrs) and its metabolism is variable; the $t_{1/2}$ of CK is ~ 36 hrs). Urine myoglobin is typically assayed in reference laboratories and may be helpful when concomitant hematuria is present.
- CK < 15,000 to 20,000 U/L is usually not associated with sufficient myoglobinuria to cause AKI; however, concentrations as low as 5,000 U/L may be associated with AKI, particularly when other risk factors (*e.g.* sepsis, dehydration and acidosis) are present.
- AKI due to myoglobinuria is usually associated with oliguria or less frequently, anuria (Scr may be mildly increased without AKI in rhabdomyolysis *i.e.* a low BUN/creatinine ratio).
- A low FE_{Na} (< 1%) is more common in rhabdomyolysis-associated AKI, esp. in the earlier phases of injury. Once ATN is established, the FE_{Na} typically increases.

(Continued)

Box 7.4.2   Rhabdomyolysis: Clinical Manifestations and Key Points (Continued)

- Electrolyte disturbances may be manifest prior to Acute Kidney Injury and should be monitored:
  ‣ Hyperkalemia
  ‣ Hyperphosphatemia [which may lead to hypocalcemia via precipitation of calcium phosphate deposits in soft tissue and through inhibition of formation of 1,25 $(OH)_2$ vitamin D]
  ‣ Hyperuricemia
  ‣ Hypocalcemia may occur secondary to hyperphosphatemia (as above) or due to Ca^{++} entry into injured muscle cells
  ‣ Hypercalcemia may be seen in the recovery phase as the above processes leading to hypocalcemia reverse.

* Other causes of a positive dipstick test for blood in urine include hemoglobinuria (no RBC's on microscopic examination) and blood (+ RBC's on microscopic examination). Other causes of red to brown urine with negative dipstick test for blood and no RBC's in urine include porphyria, bile pigments, certain foods (*e.g.* blackberries, beets, fava beans, food colorings) and certain drugs (*e.g.* rifampin, ibuprofen, deferoxamine *et al.*)

Box 7.4.3   Approach to Treatment of Rhabdomyolysis

- Assess airway, breathing and circulation; intervene as indicated. Monitor the ECG.
- Measure serum creatine kinase (CK), electrolytes including sodium, potassium, chloride, tCO_2, ionized Ca^{++}, Mg, phosphorus; also: uric acid, BUN, creatinine and albumin. Obtain blood gases if indicated.
- Obtain CBC, PT, INR, and PTT.
- Urinalysis, with bedside dipstick.
- Aggressive hydration: Early restoration of intravascular volume and promotion of generous UOP (usually > 2 ml/kg/hr) is the cornerstone of therapy.
- The content of IVF for rehydration is dependent on the clinical setting (nature of the volume of deficit); the content of IVF used for promotion of adequate UOP is controversial.
  ‣ Both NaCl 0.45% and 0.9% have been recommended.

(Continued)

Box 7.4.3   Approach to Treatment of Rhabdomyolysis (Continued)

▸ Alkalinization of the urine is controversial. In animal models, alkalinization:

- Minimizes precipitation of the Tamm-Horsfall protein myoglobin complex (promoted by acidic urine primarily in the distal renal tubule).
- Inhibits lipid peroxidation and oxidation–reduction recycling of myoglobin.
- Limits metmyoglobin (the oxidized form of myoglobin)-induced renal vasoconstriction in the isolated rat kidney.

▸ The main disadvantage of alkalinization is the potential aggravation of hypocalcemia.

▸ Note that administration of large volumes of IVF containing chloride as the only anion (*e.g.* NaCl 0.9%) typically leads to hyperchloremic acidosis via dilution of serum bicarbonate. Whether or not alkalinization is a goal, acidosis should be avoided. If alkalinization of the urine is *not* a goal, consideration should be given to providing about 1/3 the anion as base (*e.g.* NaCl 100 mEq/L plus NaHCO$_3$ 50 mEq/L).

▸ If the urine pH is < 6.5 or 7.0, some experts recommend alkalinization to urine pH > 6.5, depending on severity of rhabdomyolysis. If alkalinization is instituted, monitor urine pH closely, since urine pH in the 8–9 range may ↑ complications and is of no proven benefit.

▸ If alkalinization is a goal, consider providing all or most of the sodium salt as bicarbonate.

▸ Do not include lactate or potassium in the IVF's; if hypokalemia occurs it should be managed based on individual patient circumstances.

▸ Dextrose should be provided as needed to maintain normoglycemia; if fluid is infused at a high rate (*e.g.* twice the normal maintenance rate); dextrose at half the usual concentration (*e.g.* Dextrose 2.5% PLUS appropriate electrolytes) may be required to avoid hyperglycemia.

(Continued)

Box 7.4.3   Approach to Treatment of Rhabdomyolysis (Continued)

- Monitor UOP hourly.
- Use of diuretics is controversial; however, if considered, they should only be given after volume repletion is assured. Mannitol may have advantages over other diuretics in this setting.
- Monitor electrolytes (at least every 4 hrs), with special attention to K^+ and ionized Ca^{++}
- Monitor CK serially; failure of CK to decline suggests ongoing muscle injury.
- Correct electrolyte abnormalities: (*Electrolyte Disturbances, 6.2; Box 6.2.10*): If [K+] > 6.0 mEq/L give glucose and insulin, a beta-agonist (albuterol) and $NaHCO_3$ (if acidemia is present); administration of $NaHCO_3$ may worsen hypocalcemia. Remove K^+ from the body via sodium polystyrene sulfonate or renal replacement therapy (*Acute Kidney Injury, 7.4*).
- Hypocalcemia exacerbates the dysrhythmic effects of hyperkalemia; correct hypocalcemia only if the patient is symptomatic (tetany, seizures, arrhythmias attributable to hypocalcemia).
- Consult a pediatric nephrologist early in the course of disease.

Chapter 8

Gastrointestinal Disorders and Nutrition

8.1 Nutritional Requirements in the Hospitalized and Critically Ill Child

Children admitted to the PICU are at risk for poor and potentially worsening nutritional status, a factor that further increases co-morbidities and complications, prolongs the hospital stay, increases costs and increases mortality. One in five children admitted to the PICU experience acute or chronic malnutrition. Poor nutrition is associated with loss of integrity of the normal gastrointestinal barrier and impairment of other defenses such as cell-mediated immunity, phagocytic function, and the complement system. In addition, the increased energy demands secondary to the metabolic stress response to critical illness add to the nutritional shortfall, especially when nutrition requirements are inadequately estimated or nutritional support is inadequate.

Critical illness is characterized by a unique set of alterations in hormonal and inflammatory mediators, including elevation in serum levels of insulin, glucagon, cortisol, catecholamines, and proinflammatory cytokines. Elevation of serum counterregulatory hormone concentrations induce insulin and growth hormone resistance, resulting in the catabolism of endogenous protein, carbohydrate, and fat to provide energy and micronutrient needs. A large amount of free amino acids are dumped into the circulation and serve as substrate for inflammatory response mediators that participate in tissue repair. The remaining amino acids are cycled though the liver where they contribute to gluconeogenesis.

The metabolic response to trauma, including surgery, inflammation, or other stress varies greatly, and it is generally proportional to the severity and duration of stress. However, the energy and nutrient requirements resulting from this stress are difficult to estimate. Of note, nutritional support *per se* will not reverse or prevent the metabolic stress response.

Careful nutritional evaluation upon admission to the PICU is essential for optimizing clinical care. This assessment includes standard anthropometrics (length, weight, weight/length or height), and routine laboratory studies including lymphocyte count (immune status), and hemoglobin (iron status); serum albumin (half life 2–3 weeks) reflects visceral protein status, prealbumin (half life 1–2 days) reflects the acute visceral protein status. History and physical examination may dictate the need for specific laboratory assessment of micronutrients.

Provision of optimal dietary protein does not eliminate the negative protein balance associated with the catabolic response to injury, but it can slow the rate of net protein loss. Carbohydrate turnover is simultaneously increased during the metabolic response, with a significant increase in glucose oxidation and gluconeogenesis. However, the administration of exogenous glucose does not blunt the elevated rates of gluconeogenesis, and net protein catabolism continues unabated. A combination of dietary glucose and protein may improve protein balance during critical illness, primarily by enhancing protein synthesis. During stress there are also increased rates of fatty acid oxidation and consumption of lipid stores, which does not slow down with provision of glucose; this increases the risk for essential fatty acid deficiency, particularly in premature and young infants.

Children with severe burn injury exhibit the highest rates of hypermetabolism, particularly in the early stages of injury; it is important not to underestimate energy requirements, which can result in rapid consumption of lean body mass. Caution should also be exerted not to overestimate requirements with stress factors that range typically from 1.2 to 2 times the basal metabolic rate (BMR). Decreased metabolic expenditure from decreased physical activity, decreased insensible fluid losses, growth cessation during stress, mechanical ventilation, sedation, and other alterations from the normal increase the risk of overestimation of requirements and may lead to overfeeding.

In turn, overfeeding may increase CO_2 production causing an increase in the work of breathing or prolong mechanical ventilation in certain patients. Overfeeding may induce hepatic steatosis, cholestasis and increase the risk for infection from hyperglycemia.

Energy Requirements. For any patient, total energy expenditure (TEE) determines energy needs:

TEE = BMR + SDA + Energy for activity + Energy for growth + Energy for thermoregulation

BMR (*i.e.* energy expenditure at rest in a neutral thermal environment after food has been processed) is the largest component of TEE; SDA (Specific Dynamic Action) is the energy produced and lost as heat from digestion and metabolism of food. Thermoregulation losses are increased energy expenditures that occur when ambient temperatures are below the zone of thermoneutrality. There are various ways to estimate energy requirements in infants and children. In healthy populations, dietary reference intakes are appropriate. For hospitalized adults, it is best to estimate BMR (calculated using standard equations depending on weight, height, age, gender) by the "Harris Benedict Equations". For pediatric patients, the equations from Schofield provide a better approximation for BMR (*Appendix, part 2, VI*). Alternatively, reported BMRs based on ideal weight (*Appendix, part 2, VI*) or estimations of basal caloric expenditure (*Dehydration, 6.1, Box 6.1.3*) can be multiplied by a stress factor (*Appendix, part 2, VI*).

Note that in general, hospitalized infants have a lower energy requirement than healthy infants. Of the 5 components of TEE, four are significantly reduced in the hospital (activity, specific dynamic action, growth and thermoregulation), especially if a patient is receiving parenteral nutrition. For this reason, in more critically ill patients, most of these equations tend to overestimate energy needs. Reasonable estimated initial target energy values can be based simply on the daily recommended value for a child of similar age and weight.

While useful and practical, these estimations all have varying levels of inaccuracy. The most reliable estimate of energy requirements come from indirect calorimetry (IC). IC, using a metabolic cart, can be performed at the bedside, and measures the volume of oxygen consumed (VO_2) and the volume of carbon dioxide produced (VCO_2). The respiratory quotient (RQ), defined by the ratio of VCO_2 to VO_2, is partially determined by substrate administered to the patient. The RQ of metabolizing carbohydrate is usually approximately 1.0 whereas the metabolism of protein usually results in an RQ of 0.9. IC can help identify overfeeding from underfeeding. Underfeeding, which promotes use of endogenous fat stores, should cause decreases in the RQ (RQ 0.7), whereas overfeeding (which results in lipogenesis) and anaerobic metabolism should cause increases in the RQ (RQ > 1.0). Accurate IC data are dependent upon an airtight system from which the RQ is determined and usually requires a low delivered FiO_2; expertise for interpretation, experience in applying the equipment and resource availability are additional factors.

Protein Requirements. During disease, protein requirements typically will be higher than in health due to increased GI and skin losses, increased urinary nitrogen losses from the catabolic state, and increased needs for protein synthesis. In severe injury, endogenous protein from lean tissues is used for synthesis of proteins, enzymes, and as energy for tissue repair. During stress, this response does not halt with provision of glucose, but can be ameliorated with provision of protein, allowing for continued synthesis of proteins needed in the stress response. Protein requirements for most hospitalized patients varies between 100–150% of protein RDA for age. Nitrogen balance is the most reliable way of measuring adequacy of protein administration; however it is not always practical. Serum albumin, prealbumin and retinol binding protein are reasonably useful markers of visceral protein status.

Whenever possible, protein should be delivered enterally. Amino acids provided parenterally will be utilized for lean body mass accretion and functional protein synthesis when adequate energy is also delivered. When non-protein parenteral substrates provide less energy than BMR, parenteral amino acids will be used as energy substrate. For this reason, the ratio of non-protein energy to nitrogen intake is used as a measure of adequate energy-protein balance. A ratio of 150–250:1 is generally considered acceptable. It is calculated as follows:

calories from carbohydrate
+ calories from fat: (gm of protein/6.25)

Carbohydrate Requirements. Provision of carbohydrate is critical in retarding protein catabolism, and is most effective when provided with amino acids. However, as with energy requirements, carbohydrate requirements are often overestimated, with risk of hyperglycemia, and increased CO_2 production. Careful glucose monitoring is mandatory (*Hypo- and Hyperglycemia, 6.4*).

Lipid Requirements. Lipids are also quickly metabolized during stress, providing free fatty acids as a form of energy. Essential fatty acid deficiency is more likely in infants who do not receive linolenic and linoleic acid. Lipids should provide up to 30–40% of total energy, starting at 1 gram/kg/d, and gradually advancing this amount while monitoring serum triglyceride levels.

Feeding Route. When oral feeding is impaired, enteral tube feeding is preferred to the parenteral route for the following reasons: (1) maintenance of gut barrier integrity; (2) reduction of infection risk; (3) reduced fluid and metabolic abnormalities; (4) less cost. Enteral tube feeding should be instituted in any infant or child not able to feed orally, but who has a functional GI tract. Enteral tube feedings should also be used in situations when there is inability to fully meet nutritional needs orally (*e.g.* patients with burns, trauma, infection, congenital heart disease) and in malabsorptive states (*e.g.* chronic diarrhea, short bowel syndrome, IBD, pancreatitis, cystic fibrosis, *et al.*). Enteral tube feedings can also help bypass anatomic abnormalities or oral impediments and are often needed in CNS disorders interfering with the ability to eat.

8.1.1 *Enteral feeding*

Enteral feeding can be instituted by one of several methods (**Box 8.1.1**) Formula considerations are listed (**Box 8.1.2**).

Box 8.1.1   Methods of Enteral Feeding

- Intragastric: Use small bore (5–6Fr) polyurethane or silicone tube passed nasally or orally; nasal tubes may remain for 2–3 months. Severe GER or gastric motility disorders may necessitate continuous rather than bolus feedings.
- Transpyloric (directly into small bowel): May be useful for gastric dysmotility and if increased risk of aspiration exisits; only continuous infusions (not boluses) are tolerated.
- When intragastic feeding is needed for over 3 months, gastrostomy is often indicated, and may be placed endoscopically (Percutaneous Endoscopic Gastrostomy, PEG).
- Prolonged need for transpyloric feeding may warrant a jejunostomy or a gastric jejunal tube that can be placed through a gastrostomy site.

Box 8.1.2   Factors in Enteral Formula Selection for PICU Patients

- Age: macro and micronutrient composition varies for infants vs. older children; infants < 12 mos should receive human milk or an appropriate infant formula.
- Energy concentration: use of calorically dense formula may be useful in provision of high caloric intake for patients who are volume-sensitive and require low volume delivery.
- Protein type/concentration: higher protein concentration is useful during times of acute stress. Hydrolyzed formula (especially whey based or whey-predominant) may aid gastric emptying. Extensively hydrolyzed formula may be absorbable in malabsorbtive states or cow milk protein allergy.
- Osmolality: Hyperosmolar feedings (> 300 mOsm/L) are important to consider, and avoid, particularly in upper GI dysmotility, delayed gastric emptying, or in severe diarrhea.
- Carbohydrate: Use a lactose free preparation in diarrheal disease and malabsorption.
- Fat: Mid chain triglycerides may be helpful in steatorrhea; these are sometimes used in patients with chylothorax to decrease the burden of long-chain fatty acids trafficking the lymphatics.

Select special nutritional considerations in diarrheal disease (*8.3*) hepatic disease (*8.10*), acute kidney injury/renal failure (*7.1*), and pancreatitis (*8.9*) are addressed within respective sections and include:

- **Hepatic disease (severe dysfunction, liver failure)**

  ▸ Energy requirements may be increased *e.g.* 100–150% of daily recommended intake (DRI)

  ▸ Protein intake should be reduced to 0.5–1 gm/kg day in hepatic encephalopathy, and returned to 2–3 gm/kg/day when stable.

  ▸ Parenteral nutrition *per se* may cause cholestasis

  ▸ Standard amino acid solutions are generally acceptable. Use of branched chain amino acids as nitrogen source may be beneficial, although there is no consensus. Enteral and parenteral alternatives with high branched chain amino acids are available.

  ▸ Mid chain triglycerides in oral/enteral feeding facilitate absorption in cholestasis.

  ▸ Fat soluble vitamins may require supplementation in chronic liver disease.

- **Acute kidney injury/renal failure**

  ▸ In persistent/chronic renal disease, protein and energy requirements estimated are based on DRIs. There is no evidence that protein intake below recommended daily allowance delays progression of AKI.

  ▸ Emphasis should be on adequate protein and energy intakes, avoiding excesses that may exacerbate uremia or hyperphosphatemia.

  ▸ In severe acute kidney injury protein intake may need to be reduced until resolution or until renal replacement therapy is instituted.

  ▸ Acidosis may require bicarbonate or citrate supplementation

  ▸ Decreased phosphate excretion and consequent decreased serum calcium leading to secondary hyperparathyroidism, require phosphate restriction and calcium supplementation as Ca-carbonate, Ca-acetate.

▶ Supplementation with active vitamin D [1,25(OH)$_2$ cholecalciferol] may be required.

▶ Decreased excretion of K^+ and Mg^{++} may require restriction of intake.

▶ Parenteral nutrition in end stage renal disease should be initiated without addition of potassium, magnesium or phosphate.

▶ Fluid retention or hypertension may require fluid and sodium restriction

▶ In dialysis, water soluble vitamin supplementation may be required.

- **Acute pancreatitis**

  ▶ There are few evidence based recommendations regarding feeding in acute pancreatitis in pediatrics. There is general agreement that nutritional support should be initiated very early in the course, and many advocate early "pancreatic rest". However adult studies suggest that there is little or no benefit to parenteral nutrition (*i.e.* pancreatic rest), over enteral feedings in the clinical outcomes of acute pancreatitis, when initiated within 48–72 hrs of admission.

  ▶ Complication rates (*e.g.* infection and hyperglycemia) are significantly higher in parenteral nutrition compared to early enteral nutrition.

  ▶ There is little evidence that post pyloric or more distal feedings are superior to NG feedings in decreasing recurrence of symptoms or clinical outcomes.

  ▶ There is no evidence that "low fat" feeding or "low fat" enteral diets are of any benefit compared to standard enteral feedings. Elemental or semi-elemental tube feedings may be better suited for jejunal feedings than polymeric feedings for digestive reasons rather than for concerns regarding outcomes in pancreatitis.

The above suggests that cautious initiation of feedings in the first 72 hrs, NG or NJ, may be adequate and potentially beneficial. If feedings are delayed or full feedings are not achieved or expected in this scenario, parenteral nutrition maybe initiated, ideally for only a short time. Standard polymeric diet, or semi-elemental diet if fed jejunally, is recommended.

8.1.2 *Parenteral nutrition*

When nutritional support cannot be safely administered or adequately tolerated via the enteral route, parenteral nutrition (PN) is indicated. Although adults can often tolerate inadequate nutrition without damaging effects for up to 7 days, critically ill infants and children often do not have adequate physiologic reserves, requiring more immediate attention to the provision of protein and calories to prevent malnutrition, which may adversely affect clinical outcomes. Specific indications for PN in the PICU are listed in **Box 8.1.3**.

Venous Access. PN may be provided via peripheral or central venous access. Peripheral access is sufficient for short-term or supplemental (but not total) PN support. Patients with peripheral venous access must be able to tolerate large fluid volumes to receive adequate

---

Box 8.1.3   Indications for Parenteral Nutrition

- Malabsorption
- Congenital gastrointestinal anomalies requiring surgery
- Enteral fistulas
- Intestinal obstruction (prolonged)
- Paralytic ileus (prolonged)
- Short gut syndrome
- Radiation enteritis
- Chylothorax unresponsive to a high concentration medium chain triglyceride diet
- Severe Stevens-Johnson syndrome (Toxic epidermal necrolysis, TEN)
- Severe burns
- Severe acute pancreatitis
- Severe trauma
- Severe sepsis

calories. All PN solutions, even at low dextrose concentrations, are relatively hypertonic solutions. If it is anticipated that a patient may need total PN support or supplemental PN support for > 7 days, central venous access is recommended. Central venous access allows delivery of hypertonic solutions for long-term nutritional support (>7 days). It is especially helpful for those patients who are fluid-restricted, have limited peripheral access, or are being considered for home PN therapy.

Estimating Energy Requirements. (*Nutritional Requirements in the Hospitalized and Critically Ill Child, 8.1*)

Fluids. When ordering PN fluid, other sources of fluid such as continuous infusions of sedatives and analgesics, arterial and CVP fluids, and medications (*e.g.* antibiotics) should be considered. The total volume of fluid per day determined to be acceptable for a given patient minus the obligatory volume for essential medications determines the volume of fluid available for PN (*Fluids, Electrolytes and Metabolism, Chapter 6*).

Protein. Provision of dietary protein is the most important nutritional intervention in critically ill children. During critical illness, especially during recovery from trauma or surgery, there is increased protein catabolism related to the metabolic stress response. Muscle protein is utilized to generate glucose and inflammatory response proteins. Unlike during starvation, provision of dietary carbohydrate (CHO) is ineffective in reducing endogenous glucose production via gluconeogenesis in the metabolically stressed state. Ongoing negative nitrogen balance contributes to skeletal muscle wasting, weight loss, and immune dysfunction. The optimal amount of protein required to enhance protein accretion is higher in critically ill than in healthy children. Exogenous protein must be provided in amounts sufficient to optimize protein synthesis, facilitate wound healing and the inflammatory response, and prevent the loss of endogenous protein mass over time. Excessive protein administration, however, has been shown to have detrimental effects, particularly in patients with renal and hepatic dysfunction. The practice of gradually increasing protein amounts over several days is no longer recommended. Estimated protein requirements for critically ill infants and children are tabulated (**Box 8.1.4**).

Box 8.1.4	Estimated Protein Requirements in Critically Ill Patients
Age	Protein (gm/kg/day)
0–2 yrs	2–3
2–13 yrs	1.5–2
13–18 yrs	1.5

Carbohydrate (CHO). Once protein needs have been addressed, energy can be delivered and utilized via CHO and lipid sources. Dextrose is the source of CHO in PN solutions, providing the primary source of energy utilized by the brain, erythrocyte, and renal medulla. Glucose is also useful in the repair of injured tissue. In healthy infants and children, initiation of CHO calories may begin at 10 gm/kg/day (4–7 mg/kg/min) and increased by 5 gm/kg/day (3–4 mg/kg/min) to reach the desired caloric goal. Stated differently, in patients receiving maintenance IVF of standard dextrose 5%, PN may be started with dextrose 10% and advanced by 5% each day (with central IV access) until nutritional goals are met. Because many PICU patients are fluid-restricted or are receiving IVF from other sources, the glucose infusion rate (GIR in mg/kg/min) is a helpful way to calculate glucose delivery since using percentages of dextrose may be misleading.

$$\text{GIR in mg/kg/min} = \frac{\text{Fluid rate (ml/hr)} \times \% \text{ Dextrose} \times 0.167}{\text{Weight (kg)}}$$

PICU patients are at risk for hyperglycemia due to glucose intolerance from the metabolic stress response and may not tolerate full rates of CHO infusion without administration of exogenous insulin. Overfeeding CHO beyond the maximal glucose oxidation rate can increase the production of CO_2 and impair sufficiency of pulmonary function in critically ill patients. Excessive glucose administration also promotes fat deposition, particularly in the liver. Maximal glucose oxidation rates vary based on age and clinical status, therefore strict monitoring of tolerance to infused dextrose is mandatory. If hyperglycemia occurs even in the absence of apparent excessive CHO infusion, reducing the rate of glucose delivery or addition of low dose insulin (*e.g.* 0.025 units/kg/hr) IV, adjusting the dose as needed, is recommended.

$$\text{CHO kcal} = \{[\text{Total volume (ml)} \times \% \text{ Dextrose (gm/100 ml)}] \div 100 \text{ ml}\} \times 3.4 \text{ kcal/gm}$$

Fat. Intravenous fat emulsions (IVFE), composed of soy- or soy/safflower-based emulsions, are administered to prevent essential fatty acid deficiency (EFAD) and to provide a concentrated source of calories. IVFE are initially given in low doses and advanced based on serum triglyceride measurements. Most patients can tolerate initial doses of 1 gm/kg/day, increasing by 1 gm/kg/day until the caloric goal is reached. The maximum recommended dose of IVFE is 4 gm/kg/day but calories from fat should not exceed 40% of total kcals (or 500 ml IVFE per day). IVFE are best tolerated when infused over 20–24 hrs (and not less than 12 hrs).

Critically ill patients are at increased risk for hypertriglyceridemia, a marker of IVFE intolerance. The risk of hypertriglyceridemia is increased in patients with sepsis or trauma, hyperglycemia, renal failure, pancreatitis, and in those receiving corticosteroids. In addition, some medications, such as the anesthetic propofol and the new IV calcium channel blocker clevidipine, are formulated in lipid emulsions and can contribute to the total daily lipid dose. Failure to account for these additional sources of lipid can contribute to the development of IVFE intolerance. Although the serum triglyceride level that indicates adequate IVFE clearance differs according to laboratory assay and time of sample in relation to IVFE dose, it has been our practice to hold or decrease the dose of IVFE if the triglyceride concentration exceeds 200 mg/dL. IVFE may be administered via dedicated IV tubing or mixed with the CHO and protein solution as a total nutrient admixture; IVFE are isotonic and may be delivered peripherally at any rate of infusion. It is our practice to administer IVFE separately for IV compatibility reasons so that the entire PN infusion does not

Box 8.1.5   Daily Electrolyte and Mineral Requirements

Electrolyte	Preterm Neonate	Infants/Children	Adolescents
Sodium	2–5 mEq/kg	2–5 mEq/kg	1–2 mEq/kg
Potassium	2–4 mEq/kg	2–4 mEq/kg	1–2 mEq/kg
Calcium	2–4 mEq/kg	0.5–4 mEq/kg	10–20 mEq
Phophorus	1–2 mMol/kg	0.5–2 mMol/kg	10–40 mMol
Magnesium	0.3–0.5 mEq/kg	0.3–0.5 mEq/kg	10–20 mEq
Acetate	As needed to maintain acid-base balance		
Chloride	As needed to maintain acid-base balance		

have to be interrupted if a medication is incompatible with the IVFE. Calculation of fat calories from IVFE:

Fat kcal (20% IVFE) = Total volume (mL) × 2 kcal/ml

Electrolytes and Minerals. Daily electrolyte and mineral requirements are shown in **Box 8.1.5.** Although the dose ranges of calcium and phosphorus are wide, in general, rapidly growing neonates and infants require higher doses than older children and adolescents. In monitoring adequate calcium and phosphorus delivery in infants, serum calcium levels may appear normal due to the activity of parathyroid hormone, which stimulates mobilization of calcium from bone; therefore, serum concentrations may not reflect actual calcium needs.

In addition to daily maintenance requirements, electrolyte deficiencies resulting from excessive body fluid losses (*e.g.* nasogastric, ostomy and CSF drainage, diarrheal stool, *etc.*) should be replaced separately with a comparable electrolyte solution (*Appendix, part 2, V*). When losses are chronic and predictable, these losses may be incorporated into the PN plan. When determining adequate electrolyte and mineral requirements for patients, risk factors for depletion should be taken into account. Medications (*e.g.* diuretics, amphotericin B, prior chemotherapy regimens), end-organ function (*e.g.* renal insufficiency), and baseline nutritional status should influence dosing of electrolytes and minerals. In patients who are severely malnourished, the "refeeding syndrome" may occur if delivery of nutrients is too rapid. As phosphorus, potassium, and magnesium are mobilized into cells to produce energy, serum concentrations of these ions may plummet, resulting in cardiac arrhythmias and sudden death. For patients at risk for refeeding syndrome, it is recommended to start nutrient repletion slowly and advance carefully over several days while maintaining adequate serum levels of phosphorus, potassium and magnesium.

Vitamins and Trace Elements play a key role in the metabolic processes. Many parenteral vitamins have greater bioavailability than oral forms; therefore, a lower dose than the Recommended Daily Allowance is needed to meet metabolic needs. Standard amounts in commercially available multivitamin products are listed (**Box 8.1.6**). Patients >40 kg or >11 yrs should receive the adult product.

Daily trace element requirements are listed (**Box 8.1.7**). Trace element supplementation may require modification for post-surgical patients and patients with renal, intestinal, or liver dysfunction. Additional zinc may be needed in children with prolonged diarrhea or

---

Box 8.1.6   Recommended Daily Allowance of Vitamins

Vitamin	Pediatric Dose (5ml)	Adult Dose (10 ml)
Vitamin A	2,300 IU	3,3000 IU
Vitamin C (ascorbic acid)	80 mg	100 mg
Vitamin D	400 IU	200 IU
Vitamin E	7 IU	10 IU
Vitamin K	200 mcg	150 mcg
Folic Acid	140 mcg	400 mcg
Thiamin (B_1)	1.2 mg	3 mg
Riboflavin (B_2)	1.4 mg	3.6 mg
Niacin (B_3)	17 mg	40 mg
Pyridoxine (B_6)	1 mg	4 mg
Cyanocobalamin (B_{12})	1 mcg	5 mcg
Pantothenic acid	5 mg	15 mcg
Biotin	20 mcg	60 mcg

Box 8.1.7	Daily Requirements of Trace Elements*			
Trace element	Preterm Neonates < 3 kg	Term Neonates 3–10 kg	Children 10–40 kg	Adolescents > 40 kg
Units		(mcg/kg/day)		Total per day
Zinc	400	50–250	150–125	2–5 mg
Copper	20	20	5–20	200–500 g
Manganese	1	1	1	40–100 mcg
Chromium	0.05–0.2	0.2	0.14–0.2	5–15 mcg
Selenium	1.5–2	2	1–2	40–60 mcg

*Assumes normal age-related organ function and normal losses. Recommended doses cannot be achieved with the use of a single pediatric multiple trace element product. Recommended doses can only be delivered by using an individualized trace element product.

large ileostomy fluid losses in the NPO state. Copper and manganese can accumulate in patients with cholestatic liver disease. These trace elements may need to be administered less frequently or witheld in patients with cholestasis. Similarly, chromium and selenium are renally excreted and may require dose-adjustment in patients with renal failure.

Suggested **monitoring parameters** for patients receiving PN are listed (**Box 8.1.8**). Because of the constantly changing clinical status of PICU patients, frequent use of diuretics, and potential end organ dysfunction, electrolytes are often monitored more frequently than other patients who are receiving PN. For more stable, long-term PN patients, frequent monitoring of electrolytes may not be indicated. Although albumin and prealbumin levels are often measured to assess and guide nutrition support therapy, these markers may not be accurate in the stress phases of critical illness, particularly in burns or sepsis, as the liver increases production of acute phase proteins. These

---

Box 8.1.8   Suggested Monitoring for PICU Patients Receiving Parenteral Nutrition

Measure	Frequency
Weight	Daily (as clinical status allows)
Length and head circumference (infants)	Weekly
Electrolytes	At least daily, with potassium more frequently as indicated
Calcium, Phosphorus, Magnesium	At least daily until stable, then at least weekly thereafter
Liver function tests	Baseline, then at least weekly
Albumin	Consider baseline, then at least weekly
Prealbumin	Consider baseline, then 1–2 times weekly
Triglycerides	Daily with changes in lipid dosing, then at least weekly
CBC with differential	As clinically indicated
Iron studies	As clinically indicated

Box 8.1.9   Metabolic Complications of Parenteral Nutrition

- Hyper- or hypoglycemia
- Acid-base imbalance
- Azotemia
- Hyper- or hypokalemia

- Hypo- or hypocalcemia
- Hypo- or hyperphosphatemia
- Hypo- or hypermagnesemia
- Hypertriglyceridemia

---

levels may become more useful in guiding nutrition therapy, however, when the stress response diminishes.

Complications of PN therapy include metabolic (**Box 8.1.9**), infectious, cholestatic, and mechanical (*Vascular Access 15.3, Box 15.3.6*). Infusion of PN fluid via a CVC has been associated with sepsis. Fever, new-onset glucose or lipid intolerance, and/or glycosuria may be indications for obtaining appropriate cultures and initiation of appropriate antimicrobial therapy. In order to minimize the infectious and other risks of PN, attempts to establish enteral access and advance enteral feeding should be ongoing.

8.2 Acquired Constipation/Obstipation in the PICU

Constipation is the difficult passage of hard/firm stool or difficult or painful passage of hard stools following a period of stool retention for various reasons; obstipation refers to long intervals between stool passages, although the term "constipation" has been applied to both situations. Infants normally pass 1–9 stools/day; beyond infancy, this decreases to 3 per day to 3 per week. Some situations associated with decreased GI motility and decreased stool output common in the PICU are listed (**Box 8.2.1**).

Complications of constipation include feeding intolerance, abdominal distension, delayed gastric emptying, fecal stasis which may induce overgrowth of Gram-negative bacteria, and potential translocation of gut organisms. Correlation reported between constipation, organ dysfunction, prolonged length of stay and failure to wean from mechanical ventilation has been reported.

Management. Recognition of risk factors that may lead to insufficient stool output and institution of a preventive strategy for this problem is the most efficient approach for patients with an intact GI tract. Circulatory and electrolyte stabilization should always precede any management of constipation. It is important to differentiate

---

Box 8.2.1   Conditions Associated with Constipation or Obstipation in the PICU

• Drugs	• Shock and other causes of splanchninc hypoperfusion
▶ Narcotics	
▶ Benzodiazepines	• Electrolyte imbalances (hypokalemia, hypomagnesemia)
▶ Anticholinergics	
▶ Anticonvulsants	• Underfeeding
• Immobilization	• Low fiber diet

obstipation (*e.g.* from lack of enteral feedings for significant periods of time), which may resolve following institution of enteral feedings, from fecal retention, recognizable by abdominal exam, rectal exam, and/or plain abdominal films. The latter requires maneuvers to disimpact and help maintain defecation regularity. The possibility of intestinal obstruction or medical ileus should be considered and ruled out before proceeding with efforts to evacuate the bowel.

A maintenance program should be instituted if no stool is passed within 3 days of initiation of enteral feedings. Disimpaction should proceed if there is evidence of significant fecal retention with hard stools (**Box 8.2.2**).

Box 8.2.2   Maintenance of Regularity and Treatment of Constipation/Obstipation*

- **Maintain regularity   Dose/comments**

  ▸ Fiber content in diet; adequate fluid intake

  Additional fluids beyond feedings are not necessary. Orally, increased insoluble fiber in diet or supplements (*e.g.* psyllium, wheat dextrin). Tube feedings containing fiber (soy polysaccharide, guar gum, wheat dextrin or fructo-oligosaccharides "FOS")

  ▸ Docusate (Stool softener)

  < 3 yr: 10–40 mg/day, 3–6 yr: 20–60 mg/day; 6–12 yr: 40–150 mg/day; > 12 yr and adult: 50–400 mg/day enterally; divided once daily to QID

  ▸ Senna (Colonic stimulant)

  1 mo–1 yr: 55–109 mg PO QHS to max dose: 218 mg/24 hr; 1–5 yr: 109–218 mg PO QHS to max. dose: 436 mg/24 hr, 5–15 yr: 218–436 mg PO QHS to max dose: 872 mg/24 hr Useful in conjunction with docusate for patients at "high risk" (*e.g.* receiving narcotics and immobilized).

(Continued)

Box 8.2.2   Maintenance of Regularity and Treatment of Constipation/Obstipation* (Continued)

▶ Polyethylene glycol 3350 (PEG) (Electrolyte lavage solution)	1 gm/kg/day enterally, divided BID (range: 0.25–1.5 gm/kg/day). Do not exceed 17 gm/day for maintenance therapy. For > 20 kg use adult dose. Adult: 17 gm in 240 ml of water/day. No adverse effects recognized. Increasingly the agent of choice for disimpaction as well as maintenance.

• **Disimpaction:**

▶ Polyethylene glycol 3350	1–1.5 gm/kg/day (max dose: 100 gm/day) orally or by enteral tube × 3 days OR PEG solution with electrolytes (20–25 ml per kg/h for 4 hrs (max 4L)
▶ Sodium- phosphate enemas (Osmotic effect)	3 ml/kg (up to 130 ml). Monitor carefully for hyperphosphatemia, hypocalcemia, hypernatremia.
▶ Milk and molasses enemas	1:1 ratio; 600 ml; For older children, up to 1000 ml. Reserve for patients >2 yrs

* **Mineral oil** in critically ill patients is of limited use; it has greater risks if there is any possibility of aspiration, although it is useful in overcoming stool withholding in management of chronic constipation. **Lactulose** increases gas significantly, and has little advantage over PEG. **Enteral naloxone** may be effective in ↑ing stool output in narcotic-induced constipation but carries the risk of introducing withdrawal symptoms. Studies in pediatrics are limited, and superiority over other approaches is not established.

8.3   Diarrhea

Diarrhea is a symptom, not a disease. Fluidity of stool, indicating an increase in the water content is the essential characteristic of diarrhea. Stool frequency and stool amount (weight) are surrogate markers of diarrhea. Normally, the small intestine and colon absorb > 95% of both oral intake and endogenous GI secretions, thus, a reduction as little as 1% in water absorption can result in diarrhea. Diarrhea is typically classified according to its mechanism:

- Predominantly secretory (**Box 8.3.1**).
- Predominantly osmotic (**Box 8.3.2**).
- Inflammatory diarrhea (**Box 8.3.3**).

Box 8.3.1   Secretory Diarrhea

Definition and Description: Watery diarrhea that results from disordered electrolyte transport. This includes ↓ electrolyte absorption (a net inhibition of sodium absorption, which is more common) as well as from net secretion of anions (chloride or bicarbonate). In the critically ill child the most common cause of secretory diarrhea is toxin mediated from an infection; most secretory diarrheas are acute.

Common Causes:

- Bacterial toxins: *V. cholera*, enterotoxigenic *E. coli*, *Cryptosporidium parvum*, *Shigella*, *Salmonella*, *Campylobacter*
- GI peptides/hormones: Hypergastrinemia, hyperthyroidism, vasoactive intestinal peptide-producing tumor (VIPoma), ganglioneuroblastoma, Zollinger-Ellison syndrome
- Ileal bile acid malabsorption
- Congenital syndromes: congenital chloridorrhea

Box 8.3.2   Osmotic Diarrhea

Definition and Description: Diarrhea that results from an osmotically active substance that retains fluid within the lumen to maintain osmotic equilibration with fluids, thereby reducing water absorption. It is due either to ingestion of non-nutritive osmotically active substances (*e.g.* magnesium, lactulose), or a reduction in nutrient absorptive capacity (particularly of carbohydrates), leaving unabsorbed nutrient in the lumen and which exerts an osmotic effect. Electrolyte absorption is not impaired in osmotic diarrhea, and electrolyte concentrations in stool water are usually low.

(Continued)

Box 8.3.2 Osmotic Diarrhea (Continued)

Outside osmotically active medications, the delivery of oral or enteral feedings that surpass the absorptive capacity of the gut, particularly of enteral carbohydrate at any given time, is the most common cause of diarrhea in this population. Causes of ↓ absorptive capacity can be acute (*e.g.* rotavirus infection, intestinal ischemia), or chronic (bowel resection, inflammatory GI conditions). Providing substrate like lactose to an older infant or adult with normal decreases in lactase activity will also cause osmotic diarrhea.

Often both secretory and osmotic mechanisms co-exist. However, osmotic diarrhea, or an osmotic component to diarrhea, when present, will drastically decrease or disappear with cessation of ingestion of the offending substance or nutrient, while secretory diarrhea will not.

Carbohydrate malabsorption not only exerts an osmotic effect in the lumen but fermentation of unabsorbed carbohydrate in the distal gut by distal intestinal flora leads to release of CO_2 and H_2 gases, increased intraluminal water, and short-chain fatty acids. This increases stool fluidity and volume, as well as signs of intolerance (gas, bloating, acid stool [$pH < 5.5$], and in some cases metabolic acidosis).

Common Causes:

- Medication and drugs: Osmotic laxatives (*e.g.* magnesium, phosphate, sulfate salts)
- Lactose malabsorbtion (normal lactase decline with increasing age)
- Pancreatic exocrine insufficiency (*e.g.* cystic fibrosis, Shwachman Diamond syndrome, pancreatitis)
- Mucosal injury

  ‣ Infectious: Virus (rotavirus, norovirus), parasites (*Giardia lamblia*), small intestine overgrowth
  ‣ Radiation enteritis
  ‣ Mesenteric ischemia
  ‣ Celiac disease

- Inadequate luminal bile acid concentration
- Loss of mucosal surface: Short bowel syndrome, dumping syndrome

---

Box 8.3.3   Inflammatory Diarrhea

Definition and Description: Occurs secondary to acute or chronic intestinal injury, and stools typically contain white blood cells, mucus, and/or blood. Inflammation can induce both secretory and malabsorptive diarrhea, often depending on the course and duration of illness.

In general, fluid loss is milder than in non-inflammatory causes of diarrhea, but occasionally these conditions may induce a secretory component with minimal markers of inflammation in the stool (*e.g.* infectious enterocolitis). Malabsorption and attendant osmotic diarrhea can be more prominent particularly when the inflammatory process is chronic (*e.g.* celiac disease, IBD). Intestinal ischemia may develop in some patients during hypotension or shock. Bloody diarrhea may result from ischemic bowel (colon/small intestine).

Common Causes:

- Infectious diseases

  ‣ Invasive bacterial infections: *Shigella, Salmonella, Yersinia, E coli, C. difficile, Campylobacter, Mycobacterium avium intracellulare*
  ‣ Invasive parasitic infections: *Entamoeba, Strongyloides*
  ‣ Pseudomembranous colitis: *Clostridium difficile* infection
  ‣ Ulcerating viral infecftions: Cytomegalovirus, herpes simplex virus

- Food allergy   • Inflammatory bowel diseases
- Celiac disease   • Radiation enteritis & colitis
- Ischemic colitis

- Associated with intestinal dysmotility. Abnormal or disordered motility may lead to diarrhea that has secretory and osmotic components. Dysmotility may occur from acute infection and altered peristalsis, or from poor perfusion (post mesenteric ischemia), ileus, or persistent or intermittent obstruction (*e.g.* toxic megacolon from Hirschsprung's disease. "Accelerated transit" may decrease opportunities for nutrient absorption and increase the risk of osmotic diarrhea. Conversely, stasis can lead to bacterial overgrowth which can cause altered electrolyte transport.

Endocrine diarrheas (*e.g.* peptide-secreting tumors or hyperthyroidism), may lead to diarrhea not only by affecting intestinal electrolyte transport, but also by accelerating intestinal motility.

Other considerations. Antibiotics may alter the colonic bacterial flora and change in patterns of fermentation of carbohydrate or permit overgrowth of toxin-producing *C. difficile*. Chemotherapeutic agents are associated with a high frequency of diarrhea, which may result from disruption of the delicate balance between enterocyte proliferation and apoptosis, leading to what has been termed an *apoptotic enteropathy*.

Maldigestion of carbohydrate significantly correlates with severity of associated diarrhea; fat maldigestion does not. Loss of fluid related to undigested fat is relatively small, and of less clinical consequence to fluid balance. Diarrhea associated to carbohydrate requires decreasing amount or rate or type of carbohydrate enteral delivery. Steatorrhea, on the other hand requires maintaining or increasing fat in the diet or feedings, to maintain adequate energy delivery. This may change stool character, but not fluid balance.

Low serum albumin, and gut edema can exacerbate malabsorption.

Bile acid malabsorption from decreased gut absorptive capacity (of many etiologies) allows excessive amounts of conjugated bile acid to enter the colon, and this can inhibit electrolyte absorption and stimulate secretion by the colonic mucosa. For this reason cholestyramine and other binding agents have been used. However in pediatrics this is of limited benefit and is potentially detrimental in prolonged diarrhea. Enterohepatic circulation is low, due to malabsorption, the bile acid pool is diminished, decreasing digestive capability further. So bile sequestration further depletes the bile acid pool and worsens digestive and absorptive capacity of the gut.

The approach to diagnosis and management is outlined (**Boxes 8.3.4 and 8.3.5**).

Enteral nutrition in diarrheal disease. Key points include:

- Oral feedings are always preferable when possible.
- In critically ill patients with or without diarrhea, enteral feedings should always be preferred to parenteral feedings.

Box 8.3.4   Diagnosis of the Cause(s) of Diarrhea

- History should help elicit potential underlying and triggering factors.
- Observation of stool output in relation to feeding or enteral delivery helps discriminate osmotic from secretory diarrhea. In some difficult cases a brief NPO period will be helpful in determining if diarrhea is induced by feeding; this will help guide appropriate choice of enteral nutrition. If the conditions warrant, PN should be provided during this diagnostic period.
- Stool examinations:

  ‣ Samples should be examined for WBCs and blood, and sent for culture, including parasite examination when suspected.
  ‣ Patients who have been treated with antibiotics in the preceding three months or those in whom diarrhea develops in the institutional setting should be tested for *C. difficile* toxin
  ‣ Enzyme-linked immunosorbent assays (ELISAs) for rotavirus, giardiasis and cryptosporidiosis and serologic testing for amebiasis can be helpful.
  ‣ Stool pH < 5.5 and > 0.5% reducing substances provides useful information about the possibility of carbohydrate malabsorption if dietary disaccharides (such as lactose or sucrose) or glucose are present. Reducing substances may be less sensitive in detecting carbohydrate malabsorption in enteral feedings with maltodextrins or long carbohydrate polymers (due to fewer reducing terminals available for reduction).
  ‣ In persistent diarrhea of unclear etiology, and no evidence for infection, proctoscopy or flexible sigmoidoscopy with biopsies may be helpful.

- Abdominal radiographs can be helpful in unstable or toxic patients to assess for colitis and to look for evidence of ileus or megacolon.
- Documentation of steatorrhea by use of a Sudan stain on a random specimen, or preferably a timed (48–72 hrs) collection may help guide both diagnosis and management.

(Continued)

Box 8.3.4   Diagnosis of the Cause(s) of Diarrhea (Continued)

- Upper endocopy may be diagnostic for multiple mucosal conditions that may lead to diarrhea.
- The occurrence of bacterial overgrowth requires a high index of suspicion. Dysmotility, persistent ileus, significant feeding intolerance, immunodeficiency, should all trigger consideration of this diagnosis. Diagnosis is not always simple (fasting breath hydrogen test, endoscopic duodenal aspirate for culture). Empiric antibiotics in persistent cases may be warranted occasionally.

Box 8.3.5   Management of Diarrhea

- Always first assess and correct any fluid and electrolyte imbalance (*Dehydration, 6.1; Electrolyte Disturbances, 6.2; Acid-Base Imbalance, 6.3*).
- In critically ill patients the majority of cases will be explained by
  ▶ Medication
  ▶ Infection
  ▶ Dysmotility from electrolyte imbalance, and/or poor perfusion and hemodynamic instability
  ▶ Malabsorptive (osmotic) intolerance to oral or enteral feedings following acute or chronic mucosal, pancreatic, or hepatobiliary injury or dysfunction
- Not to forget, paradoxical overflow loose stool around fecal impaction can appear to be "diarrhea", particularly in neurologically impaired children, and requires disimpaction. (*Acquired Constipation in the PICU, 8.2*).
- Discontinue potentially causative medication (laxatives, antacids).
- Treat infectious and parasitic causes (antibiotics, antiparasitics).
- Aggressive therapy of *C. difficile* with metronidazole (enterally or parenterally) or vancomycin (enterally) is critical in the toxic patient, with severe pain, abdominal tenderness.
- Manage underlying hemodynamic problems (ischemia), surgical causes (obstruction), Hirschsprung's disease; correct hypoalbuminemia, *etc.*

(Continued)

Box 8.3.5   Management of Diarrhea (Continued)

- Opiates such as loperamide or diphenoxylate with atropine are not indicated and are of little effectiveness in most acute cases, and not indicated for chronic diarrhea in pediatrics.
- Intraluminal agents, such as bismuth subsalicylate (Pepto-Bismol®) and adsorbents (*e.g.* kaolin), also may help reduce the fluidity of bowel movements in *mild* osmotic or secretory diarrhea.
- Octreotide, a somatostatin analog, has been shown to improve diarrhea in patients with endocrinopathies, dumping syndrome, chemotherapy-induced diarrhea
- Cholestyramine is rarely of benefit in suspected bile acid related diarrhea (see above).
- Most often, the emphasis of management is in maximizing tolerance of oral or enteral feedings.

- Parenteral nutrition should always be considered if tolerance and diarrhea are impediments to deliver full requirements enterally; one route of feeding is not exclusive of the other.
- Preferred choices in enteral feeding formulations in diarrheal disease:
  - ▶ Isotonic, or minimally hypertonic feedings
  - ▶ Semi-elemental formulas (hydrolyzed whey or whey-predominant protein source) may facilitate digestion and absorption.
  - ▶ Lactose-free to minimize chance of lactose intolerance
  - ▶ Medium chain (6–12 carbon atoms) triglycerides to facilitate fat absorption.
  - ▶ Fiber containing formulations can improve stool consistency.
  - ▶ Use of prebiotics (fructo-oligosaccharides) may help balance intestinal microflora towards preferable species (lactobacilli and bifidobacteria)
  - ▶ Tolerance and decreased stool output can be significantly improved with continuous enteral ("drip") feedings compared to bolus feedings.
  - ▶ Interest in and evidence to support the use of probiotics, (*e.g.* certain strains of bifidobacteria or lactobacilli) as part of the

management of diarrhea and enteral tolerance has increased but awaits better documentation in the critically ill population.

8.4 Gastroesophageal Reflux Disease (GERD)

Gastroesophageal reflux (GER) refers to passage of gastric contents into the esophagus; this is physiologic, occurs post-prandially at all ages but is particularly common among infants. The vast majority of infants with GER are content, healthy, and grow adequately. **GERD** refers to GER that causes objective symptoms or pathology (**Box 8.4.1**) some of which can result in admission to the PICU.

Box 8.4.1 GERD: Signs, Symptoms, and Diseases or Presentations

Signs and Symptoms:

- Persistent, recurrent regurgitation
- Heartburn, chest pain, abdominal pain
- Hoarseness; recurrent stridor
- Vomiting
- Dysphagia
- Hematemesis

- Chronic cough
- Recurrent pneumonia
- Respiratory distress
- Infant sleep apnea
- Irritability
- Food refusal; poor growth

Diseases or Presentations:

- Related to regurgitation: failure to thrive
- Related to the respiratory system:
  ▶ Laryngeal obstruction, apnea (laryngospasm); ALTE
  ▶ Laryngitis; supraglottitis
  ▶ Wheezing
  ▶ Aspiration pneumonia
  ▶ Central apnea and bradycardia (relationship less clear)
  ▶ Possibly otitis media, sinusitis

- Related to esophageal diseases:
  ▶ Dysphagia
  ▶ Chest or abdominal pain
  ▶ Reflux esophagitis
  ▶ Peptic stricture
  ▶ Barrett's esophagus
- Other:
  ▶ Sandifer syndrome
  ▶ Rumination
  ▶ Failure to thrive

Box 8.4.2   Normal Protective Mechanism that Prevent GERD and Conditions that Increase the Risk for GERD

Esophageal Protection

- Normal lower esophageal sphincter function
- Esophageal capacitance and clearance
- Mucosal mucus and bicarbonate secretion
- Swallowing of saliva to clear residual acid

Airway Protection

- Upper esophageal sphincter
- Esophageal-glottal closure reflex
- Reflex apnea
- Pharyngeal clearance
- Effective cough
- Ciliary airway clearance

Conditions that increase the risk for GERD

- Neurologic and neuromotor impairment (GERD occurs in ~ 50% of those with IQ < 50)
- Esophageal/upper GI anatomic disorders (*e.g.* esophageal atresia, diaphragmatic hernia), especially post surgical intervention.

- Pulmonary disease (*e.g.* cystic fibrosis, post-lung transplant)
- Prematurity
- Presence of hiatal hernia
- Obesity; ↑intra-abdominal pressure
- GER and GERD can present together with, or as consequence of, milk protein allergy

---

Certain populations are at increased risk for GERD (**Box 8.4.2**). **Regurgitation** ("spitting up") refers to reflux of material into the oro- and/or nasopharynx, sometimes with ejection of the regurgitated matter, usually effortlessly. Less than 20% of episodes of reflux result in regurgitation; if severe, failure to thrive may result. Regurgitation is infrequent after 12 mos of age in the absence of underlying disease. **Vomiting** is the forceful ejection of gastroduodenal contents via the mouth and is associated with distress and retching.

  Diagnosis of GERD ideally uses tests that determine the likelihood that GER is causing the specific symptom and would predict that treatment of GERD would alleviate that symptom. History and

---

Box 8.4.3   Options Used in the Evaluation of GERD

- **UGI contrast and Radiography Studies:** Not strictly useful for diagnosing GERD; can detect anatomic abnormalities that may cause/explain respiratory complications, dysphagia or vomiting; can provide documentation of aspiration during swallowing, tracheal-esophageal fistula, esophageal webs and rings and gastroduodenal abnormalities (antral webs, hiatal hernia, malrotation).
- **Esophageal pH monitoring:** Determines the degree of exposure of the distal esophagus to a low pH (< 4); clinical utility in acute care is generally limited. A reflux score is calculated (% of time in 24 hrs that pH < 4) which may suggest, but is not predictive of esophagitis. A symptom score (% GER episodes associated with symptoms) may be useful in correlating GER to respiratory events, but predictive value has been poorly established.
- **Upper endoscopy with biopsies** can evaluate for the presence of espophagitis or UGI conditions predisposing to GER.
- **Bronchoscopy with lavage** and evaluation of lipid-laden macrophages may suggest aspiration during swallowing or following GER and explain GERD associated respiratory complications.
- **Trial of gastric acid anti-secretory therapy:** Short-term use of acid suppressant therapy has been validated in adults with GERD symptoms; but results are less clear in children.

---

physical findings may uncover signs and symptoms potentially associated with GERD, but are not diagnostic. Ancillary studies are described in **Box 8.4.3**.

Apparent Life Threatening Events (ALTEs; see *Apparent life threatening events, 2.1.1*) and GERD. These episodes usually occur in the first 2 months of life and are rare after 8 months of age. ALTEs coinciding with reflux episodes have been documented, including in awake infants. Reflex laryngospasm is the most common type of reflux-associated apnea. However, a causal relationship between acid or non-acid GER and prolonged apnea or bradycardia is often difficult to establish. Diagnosis of reflux-related apnea can be made with concomitant pH probe, polysomnography, and thoracic impedance, but requires episodes frequent enough to be identified within a short (~24 hr) period of monitoring. Though highly variable, evidence for the response to GERD therapies (thickened feedings, acid suppression, or prokinetic agents) is poor.

Recurrent pneumonia or interstitial lung disease may be associated with GERD, although it is often associated with aspiration during swallowing rather than due to GER alone. In high risk populations, particularly infants and children with neurologic disease, empiric therapy with acid suppression or nasogastric (or naso-jejunal) feeding to exclude direct aspiration during swallowing, may be useful

---

Box 8.4.4   Management of GERD

- Non-Pharmacologic:

  ▸ Position changes; prone positioning is acceptable in the closely monitored infant, particularly in the post-prandial period. This should be considered only in infants with upper airway disorders in which the risk of death from GERD may outweigh the risk if SIDS. Prone positioning may be beneficial in patients > 1yr since the risk of SIDS is negligible.

  ▸ Efficacy of "reflux slings" is controversial.

  ▸ Formula thickening (↓s episodes of regurgitation, but not esophageal acid exposure)

  ▸ Trial of a hypoallergenic formula (A time limited trial of at least 2 weeks with an extensively hydrolyzed formula or an amino acid based formula may show ↓ in symptoms.)

  ▸ Increasing caloric density of formula if poor weight gain present

  ▸ NG/ND/NJ feedings may help with feeding delivery in poor growth. Continuous gastric feedings may help decrease regurgitation in some cases, and may reduce respiratory symptoms when associated with aspiration, especially in neurologically impaired patients. Transpyloric feedings should never be delivered in bolus form and should always be given continuously.

(Continued)

Box 8.4.4   Management of GERD (Continued)

- **Pharmacologic**
  - ▶ Antacids: Effective in older children on as needed basis. Limited usefulness for prolonged use given high doses necessary chronically to achieve similar effect when compared to acid suppression medications available.
  - ▶ Surface agents: *e.g.* sucralfate; useful in treatment of childhood esophagitis; limited evidence of efficacy or safety for prolonged use.
  - ▶ Motility agents: *e.g.* metoclopramide, domperidone, bethanechol, erythromycin, baclofen, and cisapride have limited evidence of efficacy in management of GERD.
  - ▶ Acid suppressive agents:
    - ▪ Histamine-2 receptor antagonists (H2RA; *e.g.* cimetidine, ranitidine, famotidine, nizatadine); all are effective in acid suppression and treatment of esophagitis and related symptoms. Efficacy onset is faster than with proton pump inhibitors, but tolerance can develop with chronic use.
    - ▪ Proton pump inhibitors (*e.g.* omeprazole, lanzoprazole, pantoprazole, esomeprazole). High efficacy for acid-related signs and symptoms of GERD, particularly esophagitis, including H2RA- resistant disease. All have good safety profiles for infants, including premature infants, and children, with omeprazole being the most extensively studied. Sudden discontinuation may cause acid rebound; tapering is recommended if use has been prolonged.

- **Surgical**

Current pharmacologic therapy is uniformly effective in the management of esophageal complications of GER. Surgical approaches are most often considered for those with respiratory complications of GERD, and should be individualized. Medical therapies should always be optimized before considering surgery.

- ▶ Fundoplication (multiple techniques, including laparoscopic)
- ▶ Gastrostomy/jejunostomy for feeding (when chronic aspiration is documented)
- ▶ Esophago-gastric dissociation procedures.

(1) to establish a correlation of GER with symptoms (2) as therapy or (3) to demonstrate whether or not surgical correction of GERD may be useful in individual cases.

Asthma. It is often quite difficult to establish a relationship between GER and asthma. GER may trigger respiratory symptoms via aspiration and airway inflammation, or esophago-vagal reflexes, and asthma *per se* can exacerbate reflux due to increased intra-abdominal and increased negative intrathoracic pressures. Generally, GERD management is still only erratically and modestly useful in these situations, and should be individualized.

Management of GERD should be tailored to age and the presenting disorders accompanying GER. These are listed in **Box 8.4.4**.

8.5 Gastrointestinal (GI) Bleeding

Upper Gastrointestinal (UGI) bleeding originates above the ligament of Treitz. Hematemesis (vomiting of bright red blood) generally indicates rapid more active bleeding. "Coffee ground" emesis usually suggests a slower bleeding event, with time for a digestive coagulative effect of gastric contents and acid on blood. Melena, passage of black tarry stools, can occur following even relatively small amounts (50–100 ml) of blood in the UGI tract, and can persist for two to three days following an UGI bleeding episode. While UGI bleeding is relatively rare in pediatrics, hematemesis has been documented in 6–25% of critically ill pediatric patients; life threatening UGI bleeding occurs in <1% of this group.

Lower GI (LGI) bleeding originates below the ligament of Treitz. Hematochezia is the passage of bright red blood per rectum, alone, or mixed in the stool. It commonly indicates distal GI bleeding, often colonic; if blood is seen without stool it is likely rectal or perianal. Severe proximal/upper GI bleeding may present occasionally as hematochezia, particularly in young infants, due to rapid transit and the cathartic effect of blood in the GI tract. Melena is the passage of foul-smelling black tarry stools. It usually indicates bleeding proximal to the ileocecal valve and is black because the blood has been digested. Uncommonly mild colonic bleeding with delayed stool passage can present as melena. Lastly, non-visible (occult) LGI bleeding may manifest as anemia with physical signs of pallor and tachycardia.

The general approach to assessment of GI bleeding is outlined (**Box 8.5.1**). As for all critical illnesses, assessment and management

---

Box 8.5.1   General Approach to the Assessment of UGI Bleeding in Pediatric Patients

- Confirm that the observed GI content is blood. Common substances that can be confused with blood include red food coloring in beverages, gelatins and desserts, strawberries, beets, tomato skins. Common substances causing appearance of melanotic stools include spinach, blueberries, licorice, bismuth, iron. Confirmation of the presence of blood is easiest at bedside, using a technique to identify hemoglobin:

  ▶ Gastrocult® (Smith Kline Diagnostics) for gastric contents, and Hemoccult® (Smith Kline Diagnostics), are based on the blue quinine compound resulting from oxidation of guaiac by H_2O_2, which is catalyzed by the peroxidase activity of the heme portion of hemoglobin. False positive guaiac testing is rare, but can result from red meat and foods with significant peroxidase activity (melon, grape, radish, cauliflower, and broccoli).

  ▶ HemoQuant® (Biosafe Medical Technologies) identifies sequences of antigens on the globin chains of hemoglobin, and may be slightly more effective as it does not depend on heme compound peroxidase activity, which may be ↓ by GI or bacterial flora digestion.

  ▶ Iron does not cause false positive results with these tests.

- Confirm that the blood is originating from either the UGI or LGI tract. Non-GI causes of UGI of LGI are blood found in the oral cavity include blood originating from the lungs, epistaxis, oropharyngeal bleeding from inflammation, trauma, arteriovenous malformations, *etc.* LGI bleeding may be confused with severe diaper rash, hematuria, or menarche.

(Continued)

Box 8.5.1   General Approach to the Assessment of UGI Bleeding in Pediatric Patients (Continued)

- Identify and correct coagulopathy (*Hematology-Oncology Emergencies, 9.1*).
- Severe bleeding is manifest as tachycardia, followed by hypotension, requiring correction of volume loss and anemia (*Shock, 3.5*) and **surgical consultation** for potential need of exploratory surgery.
- Correct blood, fluid and electrolyte loss; replace red blood cells, platelets and plasma as indicated. When bleeding is rapid, blood loss may not acutely be reflected by the hemoglobin/hematocrit; platelets are usually maintained $> 50 \, K/mm^3$ and INR < 1.5.
- Monitor and replace calcium if massive transfusion is required.

---

often occur in parallel, since life-threatening problems require intervention before diagnostic certainty may be possible. Attention to airway, breathing and circulation is a priority.

Common causes of severe rapid bleeding include esophageal or gastric varices, deep ulcers or mucosal tears penetrating into arterial vasculature. Causes of UGI bleeding (from the more commonly to the less frequently identified) vary significantly by age. These are listed (**Box 8.5.2**).

In neonates, ingested maternal blood swallowed during birth or from cracked or inflamed nipples can be differentiated from the newborn's own blood with the Apt test. Drug-induced bleeding in neonates is rare, but has been associated with indomethacin given to close a patent ductus arteriosus.

In infants, stress gastritis, peptic-acid gastritis-esophagitis are common etiologies of UGI bleeding but rarely are significant enough to cause hemodynamic instability. Hemangiomas are the most common vascular anomalies causing bleeding, are often associated with skin lesions; most will regress over time.

In older children and adolescents, Mallory-Weiss tear from vomiting caused by multiple etiologies is the most common cause for

Box 8.5.2   Causes of Upper GI Bleeding by Age Group

Newborn Neonate	• Swallowed maternal blood • Vitamin K deficiency • Stress gastritis/stress ulcer	• Acid-peptic disease • Vascular anomalies • Coagulopathy • Milk protein sensitivity
Infant	• Stress gastritis or ulcer • Acid-peptic disease • Mallory-Weiss tear • Vascular anomalies • GI duplications • Gastro-esophageal varices	• Milk protein sensitivity • Hypertrophic pyloric stenosis • Duodenal or gastric webs • Bowel obstruction (*Acute Abdomen, 8.6*)
Older Child Adolescent	• Mallory-Weiss tear • Acid-peptic disease • *H. pylori* gastritis • Gastro-esophageal varices • Stricture/tear from caustic ingestion	• Henoch-Schonlein purpura • Crohn's disease • Bowel obstruction • Hemophilia

minor esophago-gastric bleeding. Esophageal varices are the most common cause of severe UGI bleeding, and most often are secondary to portal hypertension from hepato-biliary disease (**Fig. 8.5.1**). Variceal bleeding will spontaneously stop in about half of patients, and re-bleeding is common. **Bleeding secondary to medications** (aspirin, NSAIDS) should always be considered, especially in the PICU environment. Foreign body ingestion can be a rare cause of bleeding. Recommended laboratory studies are listed (**Box 8.5.3**); further evaluation and management strategies for UGI bleeding are described in **Boxes 8.5.4 and 8.5.5**.

Lower GI Bleeding. Causes by age group are listed (**Box 8.5.6**) and evaluation and management strategies are described (**Box 8.5.7**).

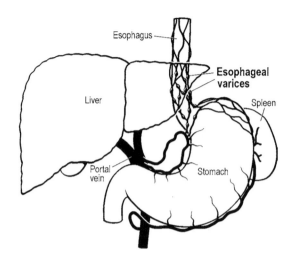

Fig. 8.5.1. Esophageal Varices. Increased portal venous blood volume and obstruction to outflow via the portal vein can result in portal venous hypertension. When portal venous pressure exceeds a critical level, collateral veins develop to divert blood into the *vena cavae*. As these small, thin-walled vessels distend they take on the appearance of varices. Varices typically develop in the rectum, stomach and lower esophagus. Bleeding may occur from any site. Esophageal varices have relatively scant supportive tissue and can bleed massively.

Box 8.5.3   Laboratory Studies Useful in Evaluation of GI Bleeding*

- CBC and differential
- Reticulocyte count
- PT and PTT
- Liver enzymes, albumin
- SUN, creatinine

- Aspiration of gastric contents helps confirm gastric and/or esophageal source. Negative results do not rule out a duodenal source. The presence of esophageal varices is not an absolute contraindication to gastric aspiration.

---

* **Blood for typing and cross-matching should be obtained along with studies for evaluation of bleeding.**

Box 8.5.4   Evaluation of Upper GI Bleeding

Evaluation

- **Endoscopy:** Esophagogastroduodenoscopy (EGD) is the most valuable adjuvant tool in assessing UGI bleeding. It is particularly effective in identifying the bleeding source (~90% of cases), particularly of mucosal origin (the majority of pediatric etiologies). Endoscopy is generally indicated in acute GI bleeding requiring transfusion, and in unexplained recurrent UGI bleeding. EGD should generally be performed only when the patient is hemodynamically stable. Emergency endoscopy is indicated in situations where it will influence an immediate therapeutic decision, particularly the need for surgical intervention.
- **Radiographic studies:** These have a limited role in early management of UGI bleeding. Plain films may identify foreign bodies, obstruction, and perforation. Barium studies can obscure mucosal lesions (sometimes for days) and therefore should be avoided if EGD is planned. Angiography may be considered for identifying the source in severe bleeding (typically at least 0.5 ml/min blood loss) and may be used therapeutically to embolize a localizable vascular source.

Box 8.5.5   Management Strategies in Upper GI Bleeding

- Instability despite transfusion requires surgical consultation and potential intervention.
- Acid suppression (H-2 receptor antagonists, PPIs) should be initiated as soon as possible for suspected peptic-related or peptic-exacerbated mucosal disease.
- Ice saline lavage is not effective in the management of UGI bleeding.
- Vasoconstriction with octreotide can be useful in severe bleeding associated with ↑ portal pressure by ↓ing splanchnic blood flow, without compromising renal perfusion.

(Continued)

Box 8.5.5   Management Strategies in Upper GI Bleeding (Continued)

• Endoscopic management: Multiple methods of endoscopic hemostasis are available.

▶ Injection of sclerosing agents (*e.g.* ethanol, ethanolamine, sodium morrhuate) for esophageal varices is a well established and effective procedure in pediatrics.

▶ Other hemostatic endoscopic procedures are used but await additional validation of efficacy in pediatric populations. These include:

  ▪ Local injection of epinephrine for non-variceal bleeding
  ▪ Thermal hemostasis: monopolar and bipolar probes, and argon plasma coagulation, which pass electrical current to mucosal cells leading to coagulation.
  ▪ Mechanical hemostasis: endoscopic metallic clips; banding of esophageal varices.

Box 8.5.6   Causes of LGI Bleeding by Age Group

Newborn	• Vitamin K deficiency • Necrotizing enterocolitis • Malrotation/midgut volvulus	• Milk protein sensitivity • Vascular anomalies • Hirschsprung's enterocolitis
Infant	• Anal fissure • Infectious colitis • Allergic proctocilitis • Intussusception • Lymphonodular hyperplasia	• Malrotation with volvulus • Hirschsprung's enterocolitis • Vascular anomalies • GI duplications • Meckel's diverticulum • Bowel obstruction

(Continued)

Box 8.5.6   Causes of LGI Bleeding by Age Group (Continued)

Older child-
Adolescent

- Anal fissure
- Infectious colitis
- Intestinal polyps
- Henoch-Schonlein purpura
- Inflammatory bowel disease (Crohn's disease, ulcerative colitis)
- Neoplasia
- Hemobilia

- Hemolytic uremic syndrome
- Hemorrhoids
- Angiodysplasia
- Dieulafoy lesion (bleeding arteriole in stomach wall without underlying ulcer defect)
- Solitary rectal ulcer syndrome
- Telangiectasia

Box 8.5.7   Evaluation and Management Strategies in LGI Bleeding

Evaluation

- **Gastric aspiration:** by NG or OG helps to rule out an UGI bleeding source
- **Anoscopy:** Mandatory for any patient with hematochezia (fresh blood)
- **Endoscopy:**
  ▶ Proctosigmoidoscopy is indicated when hematochezia is present and bleeding of rectosigmoid origin is suspected. Helpful in diagnosing polyps, proctitis and colitis of various etiologies. Mucosal biopsies may be critical in confirming diagnosis.
  ▶ Colonoscopy is indicated in patients with melena, in whom nasogastric aspiration has ruled out UI bleeding, and with negative proctosigmoidoscopy.
  ▶ Colonoscopy is **not** generally indicated in acute onset bloody diarrhea, until stool and infectious work up have been done, nor in cases of suspected intestinal obstruction, bowel ischemia, toxic megacolon (Hirschsprung's disease), or intussusception

(Continued)

Box 8.5.7   Evaluation and Management Strategies in LGI Bleeding (Continued)

▶ Enteroscopy: Several techniques with long enteroscopes, as well as wireless capsule endoscopy are now available. Their use may be helpful in diagnosis of obscure sources of chronic and/or recurrent small bowel bleeding. However, their evaluation and efficacy in pediatrics await further study.

• **Biopsy:** can be an effective adjunct during endoscopy for assisting in diagnostic considerations *e.g.* colon biopsy during colonoscopy.
• **Radiographic studies:** Limited role in early management

▶ Plain films may identify foreign bodies, obstruction, perforation, pneumatosis intestinalis (newborns with necrotizing enterolcolitis).

▶ Barium studies of LGI tract are seldom used in initial etiologic diagnosis of LGI bleeding and may actually delay subsequent endoscopic evaluation because of barium in the visual field. Following acute bleeding and stabilization it may be useful in subsequent etiologic evaluation (*e.g.* malrotation, inflammatory bowel disease, Hirschsprung's disease).

▶ Radionuclide scanning and angiography have similar applications and limitations as for UGI bleeding.

Management
• Attend to airway, breathing and circulation (*Shock, 3.5*).
• Instability despite transfusion requires surgical consultation and potential intervention.
• Endoscopy provides therapeutic options of hemostasis in specific cases of bleeding and polypectomy when polyps are found.

8.6 Acute Abdomen

An "acute abdomen" refers to any rapidly progressing abdominal pathology which requires emergency evaluation, diagnosis and often, surgical intervention. An acute abdominal process is usually associated with pain, distension, inflammation, and a catastrophic or potentially catastrophic event such as perforation, obstruction, infarction, hemorrhage and/or rupture of abdominal organs. In the general pediatric population, most instances of abdominal pain reflect non-surgical, self-limited processes; this section highlights the clinical manifestations of an acute abdomen, and outlines its evaluation and management. Key historical information and clinical signs and symptoms are listed in **Box 8.6.1**. In most cases the likely diagnosis is identifiable by history and (often serial) physical examinations, with ancillary testing specific for clinical presentation. Surgical consultation should be sought early in the course when an acute abdomen is suspected.

Box 8.6.1   Key Historical Data in the Patient with Suspected Acute Abdomen

- **Past medical history** with special attention to risk factors such as known systemic illness (*e.g.* sickle cell disease with cholelithiasis; DKA with pancreatitis, immunosuppression with typhlitis, SLE with vasculitis, *et al.*) or prior abdominal surgery (*e.g.* adhesions with intestinal obstruction; potentially dislodged gastrostomy or enterostomy tubes, *etc.*); chronic constipation (Hirschsprung's disease)
- **Markers in the history of present illness:**
  ‣ Age (**Box 8.6.4**)
  ‣ History of trauma
  ‣ Anorexia is common but not universally present.
  ‣ Vomiting: Clear: vomitus originates proximal to the Papilla of Vater: Bilious: consistent with bowel obstruction below the Papilla of Vater; may occur with ileus or other medical disease. Bloody or coffee-ground: suggests lesion within the enteric tract (*e.g.* trauma, ulcer) swallowed blood from the upper airway or mouth; coagulopathy, *et al.*
  ‣ Fecaloid emesis: obstruction
  ‣ Diarrhea: More common in enteritis than with surgical disease; present in up to 15% of patients with appendicitis; bloody, mucoid stools are seen in intussusception; mucoid diarrheal stools may be seen in appendicitis, esp. with abscess formation. Bloody diarrhea is also typical in infectious enterocolitis, HUS and inflammatory bowel disease (*Diarrhea, 8.3*).

(Continued)

Box 8.6.1   Key Historical Data in the Patient with Suspected Acute Abdomen (Continued)

▶ Abdominal pain: Inferred in infants and toddlers; usually verbalized in children; non-specific. Urinary tract infection or obstruction and disease of the reproductive system can present with abdominal pain. Types of pain:

  - Poorly localized or diffuse: **visceral** (caused by stretching of the peritoneum or organ capsules).
  - Sharp; well localized: **somatic** (caused by inflammation of parietal peritoneum or diaphragm).
  - Perceived at a distance from the involved organ: **referred**. The origins may be "distant" from the abdomen (*e.g.* lower lobe pneumonia, pericarditis or myocarditis) or within the abdomen but "referred to another abdominal site" (*e.g.* appendicitis).
  - Peritoneal inflammation typically results in reluctance to move about; vasculitic pain can result in writhing.
  - Determine duration (greater than 6 hrs is more consistent with a surgical problem); whether intermittent or continuous; whether associated with precipitants (*e.g.* bowel movements; feeding, *etc.*); whether radiation of pain is present *e.g.* right scapula: gallbladder; left scapula and shoulder: spleen; back: pancreas; flank to groin: kidney and ureter.

▶ Determine urinary habits (including color, odor, frequency of voiding or diaper changes and urgency of voiding in the older child, enuresis, dysuria).

▶ Gynecologic history in pubertal girls: Ectopic pregnancy; salpingitis; tubo-ovarian abscess. Lower abdominal pain in a female of child-bearing age is ectopic pregnancy until proven otherwise whether or not menses are present.

The most common non-surgical cause of abdominal pain in children is gastroenteritis whereas the most common surgical cause is appendicitis. An acute surgical abdomen will often present with pain before vomiting while in medical conditions, vomiting will often precede onset of pain. Findings most consistent with an acute abdomen include severe or rapidly worsening pain, abdominal findings in the setting of trauma, bilious or feculent emesis, marked abdominal distension, involuntary guarding, rebound tenderness and evidence of sequestration of blood or acute accumulation of fluid in the abdomen.

Key findings, laboratory and imaging evaluation, common diagnoses and management guidelines are listed in **Boxes 8.6.2 through 8.6.5**.

Box 8.6.2   Key Physical Findings in the Patient with Suspected Acute Abdomen

The physical examination should be complete and a focused examination should be repeated frequently (*General Approach to the Critically Ill Child, 1.2*)

- Vital signs: Consistent with stress (tachycardia); compensated or decompensated shock may be present; fever, normothermia or hypothermia may be present; tachypnea is common and may signal pulmonary involvement, metabolic acidosis, presence of reactive pleural effusion, anemia from intra-abdominal hemorrhage, *etc*. BP may be ↑ from pain.
- Mental status: Normal or altered. Patients with intussusception may have fluctuating mental status (normal between episodes of obstruction and altered during episodes of obstruction).
- Icterus (suggests biliary obstruction, hemolysis, hepatic dysfunction, *etc.*).
- Abdominal findings: Optimal yield during periods of quiescence, distraction; analgesia prior to surgical evaluation has been controversial. Administration of morphine (0.05–0.1 mg/kg) did not obscure the physical findings sufficiently to change the surgical impression in two series: Kim MK *et al.*, A randomized clinical trial of analgesia in children with acute abdominal pain, *Academic Emerg Med*, 9(4):281–287, 2002 and Green R, Early analgesia for children with acute abdominal pain, *Pediatrics* 116(4):978–983, 2005.

  ▪ Position and general appearance: Refusal to move is consistent with inflammation/peritonitis; restlessness is consistent with hollow viscus obstruction.

(Continued)

Box 8.6.2   Key Physical Findings in the Patient with Suspected Acute Abdomen (Continued)

- Discoloration: Erythema (inflammation); bruising (trauma; coagulopathy); venous congestion (mass; portal hypertension; thrombosis)
- Distension: suggests obstruction; a taught abdomen may indicate a surgical emergency; R/O abdominal compartment syndrome
- Absent bowel sounds: suggest ileus or peritonitis; ↑ bowel sounds may be present in obstruction.
- If stability and developmental age permit, the patient may be able to localize the source of pain.
- Percussive tenderness is typical for peritonitis; dullness is consistent with a mass.
- Tenderness: Localization requires skill; serious pathology rarely results in a soft easy-to-palpate abdomen. Peritoneal signs may or may not be present. Right lower quadrant localization may not occur in infants or young children (<8 yrs).
- Rectal examination: An integral part of the abdominal examination and in some cases may avoid need for imaging. Particularly informative if right lower quadrant pain is present. Swelling and tenderness suggests an abscess, esp. in infants with symptoms for several days. Pelvic appendicitis in a teen may have more impressive findings on rectal examination than on anterior abdominal examination.
- Scrotal tenderness and swelling suggests an incarcerated hernia or testicular torsion.
- Pubertal females who are sexually active should have a pelvic examination to R/O gynecologic causes of acute abdominal symptoms: pelvic inflammatory disease, ectopic pregnancy, masses, cysts, *etc.*

Box 8.6.3   Laboratory and Imaging Data Potentially Useful in Evaluation of the Acute Abdomen

• CBC	• Lipase
• Urinalysis	• Coagulation studies
• Electrolytes, glucose, BUN and creatinine	• Blood for type and cross match if indicated
• Lactic acid	• CXR
• Pregnancy test in post-menarchal girls	• Plain abdominal radiograph: Identifies "free air" (gas outside the intestinal lumen) and obstructive patterns;
• Liver enzymes and function tests	may indicate ileus or identify mass effect. A fecalith suggests appendicitis.

Consultation with a surgeon experienced in the care of pediatric patients is advisable prior to selecting an imaging study.

- Upper GI contrast series allows visualization of the duodeno-jejunal junction to assess for malrotation and mid-gut volvulus.
- Ultrasound (USG) of the abdomen: This may be very useful in the hands of experienced sonographer and radiologist. There is limited experience in children with the "FAST" examination (Focused abdominal sonography for trauma) used in the ED to rapidly R/O massive intra-abdominal hemorrhage in the unstable adult trauma patient with shock. Abdominal USG may identify:
  1) Gynecologic pathology such as ovarian cysts, ovarian torsion, ectopic pregnancy, *et al.*
  2) Appendicitis with peri-appendiceal involvement in children.
  3) Intussusception ("target sign"); an attempt at contrast or air-enema reduction of an intussusception should be pursued only with the participation of a surgeon.
  4) Volvulus (abnormal position of the superior mesenteric vein; "whirl pool sign" caused by twisted vessels at the base of the pedicle). A dilated duodenum caused by obstruction from Ladd's bands (malrotation) may be evident.
  5) Abscess
  6) Renal or perinephric lesions
  7) Gallstones
  8) Testicular torsion

(Continued)

Box 8.6.3   Laboratory and Imaging Data Potentially Useful in Evaluation of the Acute Abdomen (Continued)

- CT scan is useful in:

  1) Acute abdominal trauma (identifies solid organ and intestinal injury, active bleeding)
  2) Distortion or disease of the intestinal wall (*e.g.* typhlitis)
  3) Appendicitis (>90% sensitivity and 85–90% specificity)
  4) Abscess or other mass
  5) Inflammatory changes
  6) Abnormal morphology

Suggested Approach to Imaging for Right Lower Quadrant Pain

Girls	Boys
• ≥12 yrs: USG	• <25 kgs: USG
• <25 kg: USG	• >25 kgs: CT
• >25 kg AND <12 yrs: CT	

Box 8.6.4   Common Considerations Among Causes of Acute Abdomen by Age

- Neonate: Necrotizing enterocolitis; malrotation with mid-gut volvulus (esp. <1 mos)
- 2 mos–2 yrs: Intussusception (esp. 5–9 mos); incarcerated inguinal hernia (esp. <1 yr); tumor; complications of Hirschsprung disease; appendicitis is rare in this age-group.
- 2–5 yrs: Intussusception; appendicitis; abscess; tumor; ovarian torsion; primary bacterial peritonitis
- > 5 yrs: Appendicitis (peaks at 10–12 yrs); abscess; perforated ulcer; ovarian torsion; testicular torsion; complications of inflammatory bowel disease

(Continued)

Box 8.6.4   Common Considerations Among Causes of Acute Abdomen by Age (Continued)

- Any age: Trauma; adhesions; gastric or enteric feeding tube complications; abdominal compartment syndrome; cholelithiasis/cholecystitis; complications from foreign body ingestion. The latter are rare once the foreign body passes into the stomach. An exception would be button battery ingestion, in which injury can be caused by leakage of battery contents (*e.g.* potassium, sodium hydroxide, heavy metals) electrical injury and pressure necrosis. Although infrequent, ulceration, fistula formation, perforation, mediastinitis, hemorrhage and other life-threatening complications may occur. These are dependent upon the type of battery and its location/duration in the GI tract.

Box 8.6.5   Guidelines for the Medical Support of the Patient with an Acute Abdomen

- Assess airway, breathing and circulation. Support oxygenation, ventilation and resuscitate shock as indicated.
- Monitor vital signs with continuous ECG, respiratory rate, pulse oximetry, blood pressure and temperature. Intervene as indicated. Consider invasive blood pressure monitoring in hemodynamically unstable patients.
- Decompress the stomach (NG or OG tube to continuous low wall suction).
- Correct hypoglycemia and electrolyte disturbances; if hyperglycemia persists consider treatment with insulin (*Hypo- and Hyperglycemia, 6.4*)
- Correct acid-base disturbances (*Acid-Base Disturbances, 6.3*). If serum lactic acid is increased, this often indicates the need for volume resuscitation; alternatively, its elevation may be secondary to sepsis, necrotic tissue or other considerations in lactic acidosis (*Acid-Base Disturbances, 6.3, **Box 6.3.3***).

(Continued)

> **Box 8.6.5   Guidelines for the Medical Support of the Patient with an Acute Abdomen (Continued)**
>
> • Place a urinary catheter to monitor UOP.
> • Obtain blood cultures and consider empiric antibiotic administration based on age and most likely pathology (*Appendix, part 2, XII*).
> • Consider the need for blood products based on CBC and coagulation studies.
> • Address vascular access needs.
> • Discuss the scope of supportive measures required with the surgeon.

8.7   Abdominal Compartment Syndrome (ACS)

The abdominal compartment syndrome is the end-stage result of progressive intra-abdominal hypertension (**Boxes 8.7.1 and 8.7.2**). It manifests a loss of compliance of the abdominal wall and a pressure transfer to organ systems beginning with intra-abdominal organs, namely the intestines and extending to the brain. ACS was initially shown to effect pulmonary inspiratory pressure, but subsequently decreased preload, cardiac contractility, renal perfusion and increased vascular resistance were demonstrated.

Normal intra-abdominal pressure (IAP) is <10 mmHg. IAP is considered increased if >20 mmHg. However, in infants, normal IAP may be as low as 1–3 mmHg, and deleterious effects may be seen with IAP >12 mmHg. IAP >30 mmHg at any age is unsustainable without intervention. Abdominal perfusion pressure (APP = MAP − IAP) is a predictor of mortality. Abdominal perfusion pressure >50 mmHg

> **Box 8.7.1   Stages of Intra-abdominal Hypertension Based on Intra-abdominal Pressure**
>
> • Grade I   12–15 mmHg
> • Grade II   16–20 mm Hg
> • Grade III   21–25 mm Hg
> • Grade IV   > 25 mmHg

Box 8.7.2   Characterisitics of Abdominal Compartment Syndrome

- Pulmonary dysfunction: ↑ PIP, ↓ FRC, ↑ PVR, ↓ alveolar oxygen tension, ↓ PaO_2, ↑ $PaCO_2$.
- Cardiac dysfunction: ↓ venous return, ↓ SV, ↓CO, ↑ afterload, compression of the inferior vena cava and aorta; lactic acidosis due to shock.
- Renal dysfunction: ↓ UOP, azotemia, anuria secondary to ↓ renal perfusion, ↓ GFR, and ↑ Na and H_2O retention.
- Visceral dysfunction: ↓ intestinal, hepatic and portal blood flow; ↓ gastric pH.
- CNS dysfunction: ↑ CVP leading to ↑ ICP and ↓ CPP.
- Extremity dysfunction: ↓ femoral pulses, livid discoloration of the lower extremities, scrotal and perineal edema.

Box 8.7.3   Causes of Abdominal Compartment Syndrome

- Intra-abdominal   Intestinal perforation (NEC), trauma, Hirschsprung's enterocolitis, liver transplant.
- Retroperitoneal   Tumors (Wilm's; neuroblastoma), spinal fusion for scoliosis, pancreatitis, pelvic trauma.
- Abdominal wall   Primary closure of omphalocele, gastroschisis or diaphragmatic hernia; thermal injury.
- Secondary ACS   May result from hemorrhagic or septic shock; massive resuscitation with intra-abdominal accumulation of fluid.
- Chronic ACS   Pregnancy, ascites, and morbid obesity.
- Iatrogenic ACS   May result from prolonged pneumoperitoneum related to laparoscopic surgery.

---

increased chances of survival among adults with ACS. Causes of acute ACS are listed (**Box 8.7.3**). Clinical assessment over time is essential to interpret IAP values for individual patients. Initial studies that may be helpful in evaluation and management are listed in **Box 8.7.4**.

Box 8.7.4   Initial Studies in the Evaluation of Suspected Abdominal Compartment Syndrome*

- ABG
- CBC
- PT, PTT, INR, Fibrinogen
- Electrolytes, urea nitrogen, creatinine
- Lipase
- Lactic acid
- Urinalysis

- Abdominal plain film *may* identify a cause such as free air
- Abdominal ultrasound may identify a cause such as mass, ascites, *etc.*
- Abdominal CT may identify a cause such as edema of bowel; mass; blood, *etc.*
- The following may identify additional associated organ injury due to ACS:
  ‣ Troponin I
  ‣ CK, total and MB fraction

---

*Note that neither laboratory data nor imaging can confirm a diagnosis of ACS. The data may support or refute its presence or absence, or in the case of imaging, identify a cause.

The reader is referred to the website of the World Society of the Abdominal Compartment Syndrome (www.wsacs.org) for additional data and information.

Various methods of measuring IAP have been advocated. Intraperitoneal pressure is the most accurate, but involves placing a catheter into the abdomen. Urinary bladder pressure is a suitable alternative which is highly correlated (r = 0.98) with IAP. The technique is simple and involves filling the bladder with a small volume of sterile saline through an indwelling bladder catheter (**Fig. 8.7.1**). Gastric pressure can be measured by a similar technique. The bladder or stomach must be free of inherent disease affecting their wall; patients should be mechanically ventilated and sedated with appropriate analgesia. Inferior vena cava pressure is also a useful monitor. A falling gastric pH has been associated with progressive worsening of organ perfusion and function in IAH. This technique indirectly measures pH by allowing equilibration of the gastric luminal CO_2 concentration with that of an inserted balloon. As

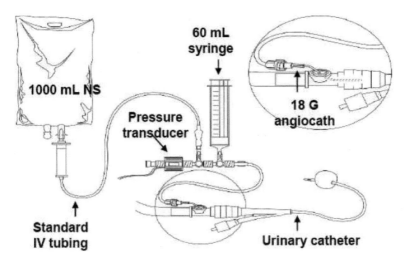

Fig. 8.7.1. **Measurement of Bladder Pressure**: an indirect but accurate measure of intra-abdominal pressure. Sterile technique is mandatory. An indwelling urinary catheter is clamped immediately distal to the specimen collection (instillation) port. Instill 1 ml/kg (maximum of 25 ml)* of 0.9% NaCl. The tubing should be completely filled with saline; if not, briefly unclamp the catheter to allow escape of any residual air. The head of the bed should be at 0 degrees, or a flat as possible. Attach a pressure transducer to an 18 gauge needle and insert the needle into the collection port. The pressure transducer should be zeroed at the level of the pubic symphysis. Pressure is measured at end-expiration. PEEP should be subtracted from the observed pressure. Contractions of abdominal muscles, or a neurogenic or small, contracted bladder prevent accurate measurement of IAP.

* This volume is recommended by the WSACS. However, recent data suggest that much smaller volumes (3 ml in children 2.6–50 kg) can be instilled into the bladder to accurately measure IAP, and that larger volumes may introduce error by causing false elevation of IAP. (Ejike JC, Bahjri K, Mathur M, What is the normal intra-abdominal pressure in critically ill children and how should we measure it? *Crit Care Med*, **36**(7):2157–2162, 2008.)

mucosal perfusion decreases, CO_2 production increases. Other non-invasive means of assessing ACS include comparative abdominal CT scans showing organ and/or vascular compression. Abdominal ultrasonography may demonstrate drainable fluid collections.

Without intervention, well founded clinical experience documents 100% mortality in the setting of severe IAH. Despite aggressive intervention, there is still a mortality of 30–40%, indicating widespread metabolic dysfunction and multiple organ failure. There are three possible treatment approaches that have been utilized with success: hemodynamic, drainage and decompression.

Hemodynamic and ventilation management strategies include (1) increased preload to improve end diastolic filling. Ionotropic agents may increase cardiac output once the volume status has been normalized; (2) afterload reduction agents may also improve cardiac performance and organ perfusion.

Secondly, **drainage** of accumulated blood, pus or necrotic material may lessen the IAP and should be considered based on the clinical situation. Paralysis and sedation may improve compliance of the abdominal musculature if edema is not prohibitive. Changes in body position may aid in the dependent drainage of interstitial fluid.

Lastly, if the IAP >25 mmHg, **opening of the abdomen to decompress the viscera** into an artificial silo will reduce IAP. There are many methods to perform this procedure, depending on the underlying condition. Spring loaded silos are manufactured for gastroschisis, while silastic sheeting or even IV bags (Bogota Bag®) can be used for trauma patients. A wound vacuum assisted closure ("wound VAC") is used for this purpose. Strict sterility is imperative and generally a suction device is employed. Eventual abdominal closure is undertaken when the clinical condition permits. This can be performed at once or stepwise using a Velcro® system, while monitoring the IAP. Diuretic treatment and even venovenous hemofiltration may decrease tissue edema enough to alter the course of the patient. Decreasing dead space ventilation through changes in the ventilator mechanics will improve gas exchange. These are the temporary measures employed until definitive decompression can be accomplished.

8.8 Pancreatitis

Pancreatitis is a disease characterized by inflammation of the pancreas. Pathophysiology is depicted in **Fig. 8.8.1**.

Acute pancreatitis (**Box 8.8.1**) refers to self limiting inflammation of the pancreas, associated with nausea, vomiting, anorexia,

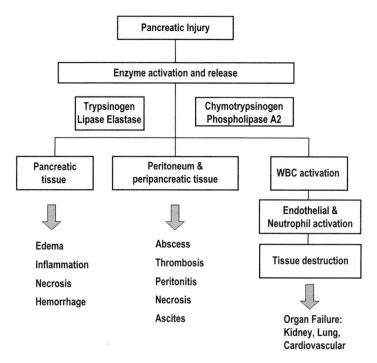

Fig. 8.8.1. Pathophysiology of Pancreatitis.
Modified from Werlin SL, Pancreatitis, in Wyllie R, Hyams JS (eds.), *Pediatric Gastrointestinal Disease*, WB Saunders, Philadelphia, 2006.

abdominal pain and marked elevations in amylase and lipase. Mild pancreatitis leads to minimal organ dysfunction, and eventual complete recovery. Severe pancreatitis indicates organ failure and local complications (*i.e.* necrosis, abscess, and/or pseudocyst).

Chronic pancreatitis refers to a progressive inflammatory process with debilitating pain, morphologic changes, and possible fibrosis and loss of exocrine and endocrine function; protein ductal plugs may calcify in the gland leading to chronic calcific pancreatitis.

Necrotizing, hemorrhagic pancreatitis describes an inflamed gland vulnerable to infection with bacteria leading to sepsis, multiple organ failure (and often death).

Herediatry pancreatitis is an autosomal dominant condition that is characterized by recurrent attacks of pancreatitis.

Box 8.8.1   Conditions and Drugs Most Commonly Associated with Pancreatitis*

Conditions (Approximate Incidence)		Drugs (The Ten Most Common)
Idiopathic	(20–25%)	• Valproate (most common)
Systemic	(20%)	• L-asparaginase
e.g. HUS; KD; IBD		• Prednisone
Trauma	(20%)	• Azathioprine and mercaptopurine
Structural	(10%)	• Metronidazole
e.g. Pancreas divisum		• Acetaminophen
Medications	(10%)	• Furosemide
Infectious	(8%)	• Cocaine
e.g. Mumps, Hepatitis A, EBV, Coxsackie B		• Macrodantin
Familial	(2%)	• Phenytoin
Post ERCP	(1–5%)	
Cystic fibrosis	(<1%)	
Hypercalcemia	(<1%)	
Hypertriglyceridemia	(<1%)	
DKA	(<1%)	

*Adapted from Whitcomb DC, Lowe ME, Pancreatitis in Kleinman, *et al.* (eds.), *Walker's Pediatric Gastrointestinal Disease*, BC Decker Inc, Hamilton, Ontario, 2008.

Symptoms, physical findings and key laboratory data are outlined in **Box 8.8.2**; diagnostic imaging and procedures are described in **Box 8.8.3**. Principles of management are listed in **Box 8.8.4**. Approximately 15% of patients may develop severe pancreatitis. The major cause of mortality in acute pancreatitis is septic complications, believed to arise from bacteria that have translocated from the small or large intestine via the mesenteric lymph nodes and lymphatics resulting in septic shock, cardiovascular collapse, and multisystem organ failure (*Septic Shock and Multiple Organ Dysfunction Syndrome, 3.6*).

Box 8.8.2 Clinical and Laboratory Findings in Pancreatitis

Symptoms:
- Abdominal pain: sharp and sudden, constant, epigastric or right upper quadrant, periumbilical area, back or lower chest
- Nausea
- Vomiting aggravated by eating
- Anorexia

Signs:
- Abdominal tenderness
- Abdominal distension
- Low-grade fever, tachycardia and hypotension
- Diminished or absent abdominal bowel sounds
- Grey Turner sign (blue discoloration of the flanks)
- Cullen sign (blue discoloration around the umbilicus) in hemorrhagic pancreatitis
- Ascites, palpable pseudocyst or pulmonary findings (left sided pleural effusion) may be present in advanced disease

Laboratory Data:
- CBC: ↑ WBC with bandemia and hemoconcentration
- Chemistries: Hyperglycemia, hypocalcemia, ↑ alkaline phosphatase (AP), ↑ alanine aminotransferase (ALT), ↑ aspartate aminotransferase (AST), ↑ total bilirubin
- Advanced disease: Hypoalbuminemia, hypocalcemia, azotemia, hyperglycemia and ↑ lactate dehydrogenase (LDH)
- Serum pancreatic enzymes:
  - Amylase (low sensitivity and specificity); typically ↑ within 2–12-hrs after pancreatic insult; peaks at 12–72 hrs, and remains elevated for 4–5 days. Specificity is higher when level is at least three-fold normal. Hyperamylasemia may occur in many diseases in the absence of pancreatitis (*e.g.* DKA, abdominal surgery, renal failure, burn patients).
  - Lipase (higher specificity and sensitivity); remains ↑ in plasma longer than amylase, beginning to increase 4–8 hrs after insult, peaking at 24 hrs and decreasing over 8–14 days. Specificity increased also with at least three-fold increase. After 24 hrs of illness onset, lipase level has a higher sensitivity than amylase level.
  - Use of both amylase and lipase levels increases the sensitivity for diagnosis of pancreatitis to 94%; degree of enzyme elevation does not reflect the severity of pancreatic disease.

Box 8.8.3   Imaging and Interventions Useful in Diagnosis of Pancreatitis

- Plain abdominal radiograph: May show sentinel small bowel loop (distended small bowel loop adjacent to pancreas), colon cut-off sign (air in the splenic or hepatic flexure with absent distal colonic gas), ileus, obscured psoas margins, or a radiolucent "halo" around the left kidney are suggestive of disease; ascites; all are non-specific.
- Abdominal ultrasonography: May reveal changes in pancreatic size, contour and echotexture, presence of dilated ducts, associated cholelithiasis, pseudocysts, abcesses, ascites.
- Abdominal CT: Provides limited additional information in early phases of illness; may reveal pancreatic and peripancreatic inflammatory signs. Up to 20% of CT scans are normal in acute pancreatitis.
- Magnetic resonance cholangiopancreatography (MRCP): Performed when ductal abnormalities are suspected.
- Endoscopic retrograde cholangiopancreatography: (ERCP): Reserved for unexplained persistence or recurrent episodes of pancreatitis with suspicion of ductal obstruction or structural defect.

Box 8.8.4   Management of Pancreatitis: Key Points

- Management is generally supportive.
- Assess airway, breathing and circulation; intervene as indicated for cardio-respiratory insufficiency.
- Analgesia (*e.g.* narcotic analgesics)
- Monitor volume status and consider needs for "third space" losses; severely ill patients may require invasive hemodynamic monitoring (CVP); marked instability may indicate infectious complications.
- Monitor electrolytes serially.
- Low measured total calcium due to low serum albumin may be present; no treatment is required so long as the ionized calcium is normal. If hypomagnesemia coexists, consider first correction of magnesium; and if signs of neuromuscular irritability persist, then consider careful correction of calcium levels with calcium gluconate.

(Continued)

> **Box 8.8.4   Management of Pancreatitis: Key Points (Continued)**
>
> - Hyperglycemia may present in the first few days, and typically subsides along with the inflammation. Careful insulin therapy may be required (*Hypo- and Hyperglycemia, 6.4*).
> - Correction of hypoalbuminemia is sometimes warranted but there is no consensus on the degree of hypoalbuminemia that should be tolerated.
> - NG suction may relieve vomiting, but does not accelerate recovery.
> - "Pancreatic rest" is considered by some to be helpful. However early enteral feedings (~72 hrs. after onset), may be appropriate provided there is no evidence of organ failure and no deterioration ensues. Enteral feedings are generally well tolerated and may improve outcomes, without recurrence of pain. Post pyloric enteral feedings may offer some advantage over gastric feeding if nausea or vomiting are persistent when enteral feedings are attempted. Re-feeding should definitively commence once symptoms and amylase are declining. (*Nutrition, 8.1*)
> - Parenteral nutrition should be initiated to prevent protein catabolism if expected to be without enteral feedings for more than 72 hrs (*e. g.* patients with evidence of organ failure).
> - Acute mild pancreatitis generally requires no antibiotic therapy, although there is no uniform consensus. Antibiotics are indicated when there are clinical signs of sepsis, necrotic pancreatitis or multiorgan system failure. Antibiotic choices include a carbapenem (*e.g.* meropenem), or ciprofloxacin + metronidazole.

8.9 Fulminant Hepatic Failure

Fulminant Hepatic failure (FHF) is the *severe* impairment of hepatic functions in the absence of pre-existing liver disease. Current classification includes:

- Hyperacute liver failure: Coagulopathy (prolongation of prothrombin time, PT) due to acute liver dysfunction of ≤ 10 days total duration; jaundice is often clinically absent initially and encephalopathy varies.

- Acute liver failure: Coagulopathy due to acute liver dysfunction of more than 10 days, but less than 30 days total duration; encephalopathy is absent or unrecognizable, especially in younger children.
- Subacute liver failure: Coagulopathy due to acute liver dysfunction of more than 31 days, but less than 6 months total. Jaundice is almost always present and encephalopathy often marks pre-terminal deterioration.

Chronic hepatic failure (CHF) is the development of advanced signs of liver disease in the presence of pre-existing liver disease. Virtually any cause of chronc liver injury may result in fibrosis, eventually cirrhosis and CHF. These include cholestatic diseases (*e.g.* biliary atresia, Alagille syndrome, sclerosing cholangitis, PN-associated cholestasis), hepatocellular disease (*e.g.* neonatal hepatitis, hepatitis B, C), and genetic metabolic diseases (*e.g.* galactosemia, tyrosinemia, lipid storage disease).

   Pathophysiology (Box 8.9.1). Hepatic failure usually begins with exposure of a susceptible person to an agent capable of producing severe hepatic injury, although the exact etiology remains unidentified in many cases. Ten percent of patients with CHF and up to 50% with FHF develop renal compromise. The mechanisms are multiple, and still not totally understood. Likewise, the mechanism that leads to hepatic encephalopathy has not been fully defined. A possible explanation is the effect of the neurotoxic or neuroactive substances as a consequence of hepatocellular failure; these substances include false neurotransmitters, ammonia, increased gamma-aminobutyric acid receptor activity and increased circulating levels of endogeneous benzodiazepine-like substances. Viral agents may cause damage to the hepatocyte either by direct cytotoxic effect or as a result of a hyperimmune response; the interaction between agent and host determines the incidence of FHF. Hepatotoxic metabolites (which accumulate as a result of errors in metabolism or of taking hepatotoxic drugs) are among the often identifiable causes of liver failure. Causes of liver

Box 8.9.1   Pathophysiology and Circulatory Changes in Fulminant Hepatic Failure*

Portal hypertension and hyperdynamic circulation, secondary to possible etiologies including infectious, metabolic, autoimmune or and acetaminophen poisoning

High cardiac output and low systemic vascular resistance (SVR) Vasodilation leading to sodium retention, ECF expansion, intravascular volume depletion

Decreased renal perfusion pressure
Pulmonary arteriovenous shunting (specially in CHF) resulting in hypoxemia

⇓

Marked renal vasoconstriction, rise in renal vascular resistance, fall in glomerular filtration rate, and acute tubular necrosis (ATN), sodium and fluid retention

---

* Note that in liver failure, synthetic, excretory and metabolic functions are impaired. Bacterial translocation, endotoxemia, activation of macrophages, cytokine release, initiation of inflammatory cascade, circulatory compromise, tissue hypoxia and end organ injury result.

failure and key historical and clinical data are listed in **Boxes 8.9.2 and 8.9.3**.

Broad Diagnostic Evaluation. A multidisciplinary team approach and early referral to liver transplant center is critical for optimal patient management.

Key points regarding this evaluation include:

• Aminotransferase levels do not correlate well with the severity of the disease; they are elevated in patients with metabolic disorders and decreased with progressive necrosis of the liver.

• Bilirubin: Elevated serum direct and indirect bilirubin are typical.

Box 8.9.2   Most Common Causes of Fulminant Hepatic Failure Based on Age*

- Neonate/Infant
  - ▶ Infection: Septicemia; hepatitis B; adenovirus; parvovirus B19; echovirus; coxsackievirus
  - ▶ Metabolic: Neonatal hemochromotosis; tyrosinemia type1; mitochondrial disorders; fatty acid oxidation defects
  - ▶ Poisoning: Acetaminophen

- Older children
  - ▶ Infection: Viral hepatitis A-G, EBV
  - ▶ Acetaminophen intoxication
  - ▶ Metabolic: Wilson's disease
  - ▶ Autoimune hepatitis

---

*These patients differ from those with CHF, who most often present to the PICU with a known diagnosis (*e.g.* biliary atresia).

- Electrolyte abnormalities: hyponatremia, hyperkalemia, respiratory alkalosis or metabolic acidosis, decreased glucose concentrations, especially in infants.
- Coagulopathy: PT is prolonged, and does not improve with vitamin K.
- Viral studies: hepatitis A; hepatitis B; hepatitis C; Epstein-Barr virus; cytomegalovirus; herpesvirus; adenovirus.
- Other serological tests: acetaminophen level; serum copper, ceruloplasmin (>3 yrs); autoantibodies (anti SLA, ANA, ASM) and immunoglobulins; serum amino acids.
- Urine studies: drug metabolites as indicated; amino acids, succinyl acetone; organic acids; reducing sugars (*e.g.* galactose, fructose, glucose, *etc.*).
- Radiology: CXR, doppler abdominal sonography, echocardiogram, head CT.
- Liver biopsy: In the presence of coagulopathy, transvenous biopsy is a safe route for obtaining liver tissue to assist in reaching a likely diagnosis or in preparation for liver transplantation.

Box 8.9.3   Key Historical and Clinical Findings in Fulminant Hepatic Failure

- FHF may occur in previously healthy children with no recognized risk factors for liver disease. Can present with hepatitis-like clinical picture and worsening of symptoms over a period of several days to a few weeks. A prodrome of flulike illness may precede jaundice; fever, anorexia, vomiting, abdominal pain, fatigue and fetor hepaticus may be present.
- Identify risk factors for hepatitis based on common causes (**Box 8.9.2**), risk factors for HIV exposure, history of anesthesia or drug ingestion, depression, suicidal behavior, neuropsychiatric symptoms.
- Note past medical history of acute or chronic liver disease
- Family History: Liver disease, neurologic disease, emphysema, hepatitis, deaths in infancy
- **Physical Findings and Laboratory Correlates**: GI bleeding may occur because of severe coagulopathy; liver size may be normal, large, or small (shrunken with deterioration of the overall condition of the patient).

▸ **Jaundice** is the presenting symptom in most patients; have elevated aminotransferases and progressively rising bilirubin levels. Low transaminase values with elevated bilirubin and prolonged prothrombin time indicate significant deterioration.

▸ **Altered consciousness**: Mental status changes occur in most children within 2–3 weeks of the onset of jaundice; euphoria, belligerence, foul language, altered sleep, confusion, slurred speech, disorientation, hyperventilation, lethargy, hyperreflexia, unarousablity and posturing may be seen. See **Box 8.9.4**. Evaluate for evidence of cerebral edema; specifically, arterial hypertension, any alteration of mental status, seizures, ↑ muscle tone, sluggish pupillary response to light.

▸ **Increased bruisability:** Coagulopathy (PT >20 sec) not correctable with parenteral vitamin K.

▸ **Other findings:** Malnutrition, low cholesterol, portal hypertension, rickets, spider angioma, clubbing.

Box 8.9.4   Clinical Stages of Hepatic Encephalopathy*

Stage	Clinical Findings	Asterixis	EEG Changes
I (Prodrome)	Slowness of mentation, disturbed sleep-wake cycle.	Slight	Minimal
II (Impending coma)	Drowsiness, confusion, inappropriate behavior, disorientation, mood swings	Easily elicited	Generalized slowing
III (Stupor)	Very sleepy but arousable; unresponsive to verbal commands, markedly confused, delirious, hyperreflexia, positive Babinski sign.	Present	Grossly abnormal slowing
IV (Coma)	Unconscious, decerebrate posturing, response to pain present or absent.	Absent	Appearance of delta waves, ↓ amplitudes

*Modified from Suchy FJ, Sokol RJ, Balistreri WF (eds.), *Liver Disease in Children*, 3rd ed., Cambridge University Press, NY, 2007.

Medical Care. The management and anticipated complications of acute liver failure are numerous and complex; a pediatric ICU and pediatric hepatology service with facilities for liver transplantation should be available to assume or participate in care. The main complications include: GI bleeding, fluid imbalance and nutritional compromise, coagulopathy and encephalopathy. Management strategies that address these anticipated problems are outlined in **Box 8.9.5**.

Box 8.9.5 Key Management Strategies in Liver Failure	
Upper GI bleeding	▶ Hemodynamic stabilization. ▶ Proton pump inhibitor by continuous infusion. ▶ Banding of esophageal varices. ▶ Sclerotherapy for esophageal varices.
Fluid balance and nutrition	▶ In general, provide a low Na, low protein diet (see below). ▶ Enteral nutrition is preferred. ▶ Enteral formulations with mid-chain triglycerides. Include supplementation of fat soluble vitamins (A, D, E, K). ▶ When hepatic encephalopathy is present, mild protein restriction (0.8–1 gm/kg/d) may be beneficial. ▶ TPN may be required in advanced disease: Give highest concentration of glucose tolerated with insulin as needed; amnio acid (0.5–1.0 gm/day); lipids (20% solution) (0.5–3 gm/kg/day). ▶ While definitive benefit is still unclear, some advocate solutions with high levels of branched chain amino acids (BCAA), of 35% (compared to 15–25% in standard solutions). Objective is to decrease concentration of aromatic AA and increase that of BCAA, which may decrease formation of false neurotransmitters associated with encephalopathy. ▶ Maintain UOP: fluid restriction (50–75% of maintenance) using either dextrose or high calorie enteral feeds; restrict hydration up to 2 ml/kg/hr. ▶ Correct electrolyte disturbances (IV administration of calcium, phosphorus, magnesium). ▶ Correct hypoglycemia (infusion of 10–20% glucose). ▶ Monitor central venous pressure. ▶ Parenteral proton pump inhibitors or H2-receptor blocker administered prophylactically to prevent potential GI bleeding; maintain gastric pH > 4.0.

(Continued)

Box 8.9.5	Key Management Strategies in Liver Failure (Continued)
Coagulopathy	▸ Parenteral vitamin K (0.2 mg/kg/day, max 10 mg IV) × 3 days, then every other day. ▸ Maintain PT at 20–25 sec (if no active bleeding) or < 20 sec (if active bleeding). ▸ Platelet transfusion to maintain platelet count > 50,000/mm³. ▸ PRBC transfusion to maintain Hct > 30%. ▸ Plasmapheresis to correct coagulopathy. ▸ FFP infusions for active bleeding. ▸ More aggressive measures to correct coagulopathy may be required if an invasive procedure is planned.
Encephalopathy	▸ Management of cerebral edema is critical for survival; avoid manipulations that ↑ ICP (*Raised Intracranial Pressure, 5.5*). ▸ Fluid restriction and head elevation. ▸ Elective mechanical ventilation is recommended by some in ≥ Grade II hepatic encephalopathy (**Box 8.9.4**), keeping $PaCO_2$ ~ 30 mmHg; Excessive hyperventilation should be avoided as it may compromise cerebral perfusion. ▸ Lactulose 0.5 ml/kg/dose (max 30 ml/dose) PO/NG every 6 hrs. ▸ Oral antibiotics (*e.g.* vancomycin, metronidazole or neomycin) may be useful to decrease the population of enteric bacteria that produce ammonia. These are given for encephalopathy ≥ Stage II.
	(Continued)

Box 8.9.5	Key Management Strategies in Liver Failure (Continued)
	▶ Initiation of ICP monitoring is individualized, and if performed is generally instituted for patients with ≥ Grade II encephalopathy. ▶ Mannitol (0.5 gm/kg as 20% solution over 15 min) should be given for patients with signs or symptoms of raised ICP or measured intracranial hypertension (ICP > 20 mmHg). ▶ Avoid sedation and analgesia; use intermittent and low doses of benzodiazepine (midazolam) and opiates (fentanyl); continuous infusions are contraindicated.
Specific treatment	▶ Hepatitis: herpesvirus (acyclovir); autoimmune (prednisone and azathioprine). ▶ Acetaminophen overdose (N-acetylcysteine) ▶ Metabolic: *e.g.* galactosemia, fructosemia, hereditary tyrosinemia (dietary elimination).
Surgical care	▶ Orthotopic liver transplantation remains the only effective mode of treatment. ▶ Consider: disease etiology, prognostic factors, presence/absence of multisystem disease or reversible brain damage. ▶ Immediate transplantation: PT > 50, ↑ing bilirubin and ↓ing transaminases.

Chapter 9

Hematology-Oncology Emergencies

9.1 Bleeding Disorders

Excessive bleeding is common in critically ill patients and its management can be challenging. Appropriate hemostasis requires a complex interaction between platelets, vascular surface factors and plasma clotting factors as illustrated in **Fig. 9.1.1**. Defects in any of these processes can lead to excessive bleeding and frequent causes of excessive bleeding are listed (**Box 9.1.1**).

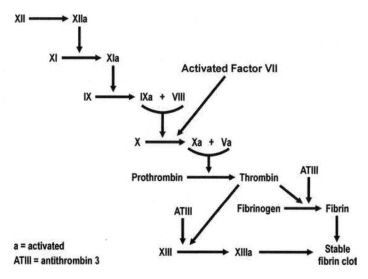

Fig. 9.1.1.   The Coagulation Cascade.

Box 9.1.1   Frequent Causes of Excessive Bleeding

- Consumptive coagulopathy: DIC (typically associated with sepsis, trauma, malignancy)
- Systemic fibrinolysis: Thrombolytic therapy, liver disease, surgery, amyloidosis, malignancy, plasminogen activator inhibitor-1 (PAI 1) or α-2 antiplasmin inhibitor defects)
- Vitamin K deficiency
- Liver disease
- Dilutional coagulopathy; massive blood transfusion
- Heparin excess
- Coagulation factor deficiency : Hemophilia, von Willebrand disease, hypofibrinogenemia, dysfibrinogenemia
- Coagulation factor inhibitors: Antiphospholipid antibody syndrome
- Thrombocytopenia

  ▶ Decreased platelet production: Amegakaryocytic thrombocytopenia; thrombocytopenia with absent radius (TAR); aplastic anemia; malignancy; chemotherapy; other drug-induced; radiation of bone marrow

  ▶ Increased platelet destruction: Splenomegaly, congenital heart disease, Kasabach-Merritt Syndrome, thrombotic thrombocytopenic purpura, immune thrombocytopenic purpura, neonatal alloimmune thrombocytopenic purpura

- Platelet dysfunction: Bernard-Soulier syndrome; drug-induced
- Connective tissue abnormalities: Ehlers-Danlos syndrome
- Vascular malformation
- Others: Malignancy, renal disease, metabolic disorders, graft vs. host disease

---

Evaluation of a child with a potential bleeding disorder requires a detailed personal and family medical and surgical history (**Box 9.1.2**). Clinical presentation varies depending on the etiology of the bleeding disorder (**Figs. 9.1.1 and 9.1.2**). Physical examination should determine whether bleeding is appropriate for the circumstance. Clothing and bedding should be evaluated for blood soaking. Patients should be assessed for presence of bruising, oozing from catheter sites,

Box 9.1.2   Important History in Evaluation of a Child with a Suspected Bleeding Disorder

Nature of Bleeding	Past History	Medication	Family History
• Prolonged, recurrent delayed or profuse? • Single or multiple sites? • Related to surgery or trauma? • Excessive for severity of injury?	• Bleeding with surgery or trauma? • Bruising, epistaxis? • Problems with wound healing?	• Use of NSAID's (including aspirin), anti-coagulants; use of herbal supplements?	• Known bleeding problems? • Gender and age of onset? • Site, duration and frequency? • Pedigree?

hepatomegaly, splenomegaly, and lymphadenopathy. Flank bruising may suggest retropharyngeal hemorrhage.

Laboratory Evaluation. Basic laboratory tests should include: CBC with peripheral blood smear, PT/INR, APTT and fibrinogen. Laboratory abnormalities commonly present in specific bleeding disorders are listed (**Boxes 9.1.3 and 9.1.4**). If DIC is suspected, d-dimer should be obtained. If systemic fibrinolysis is suspected, the euglobulin lysis time (ELT) should be performed (*Appendix, part 1, ELT*).

In the interpretation of laboratory results, it should be noted that normal PT and APTT do not necessarily denote normal factor levels. Mild factor deficiencies may not be reflected in these assays. Some coagulation factors do not attain adult levels until age 6–12 months. If hemophilia or inhibitors to specific coagulation factors is suspected, mixing studies (*Appendix, part 1, mixing study*) and assays for specific factor levels may be necessary.

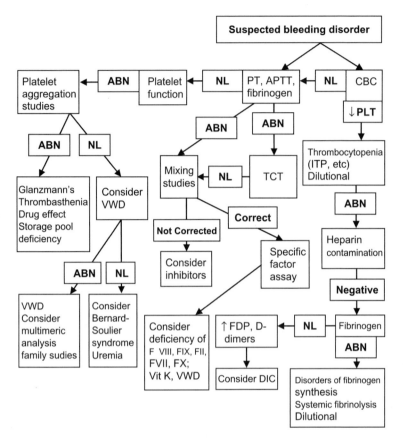

Fig. 9.1.2.   Decision-making-tree in the Evaluation of a Bleeding Disorder. PT, Prothrombin Time; aPTT, activated partial thromboplastin time; TCT, thrombin clotting time, F, Factor; CBC, Complete Blood Count; PLT, Platelet count (normal white blood count and hemoglobin are assumed); VWD, Von Willebrand disease; FDP, fibrin degradation products; DIC, disseminated intravascular coagulation; NL, Normal; ABN, Abnormal; ITP, Idiopathic Thrombocytopenic Purpura. **Note**: Bold captions denote findings. Arrows point to recommended actions or possible diagnoses.

Management of Bleeding Disorders. In active bleeding the first priorities are: maintain airway, breathing, circulation and control bleeding. Where possible, compression should be applied, with caution taken to limit damage to vital structures. If a patient has a known

Box 9.1.3 Common Clinical Features of Common Bleeding Diatheses in Children

Thrombocytopenia	Von Willebrand Disease	Hemophilia	Others
• Petechiae • Ecchymosis • Epistaxis • Intra-operative bleeding • Bleeding is rare if platelet count >50,000/µL.	• Mostly autosomal dominant • Epistaxis • Menorrhagia • Post-surgical bleeding • Joint and muscle bleeding if severe • Factor VIII may be ↓ • Platelet count may be ↓ • PT usually normal • APTT is usually ↑ but may be normal • Von Willebrand antigen is an acute phase reactant and may be falsely ↑ during illness, and/or with use of oral contraceptives.	• Deficiency of Factor VIII or IX • X-Linked; boys primarily affected. • Joint bleeding • Soft tissue bleeding • Intracranial hemorrhage • Post surgical/circumcision bleeding • PT usually normal • APTT usually ↑	• Factor XIII deficiency may present with delayed post-surgical bleeding. • Factor VII deficiency may present with severe bleeding. • Vitamin K deficiency can lead to severe bleeding as in hemorrhagic disease of the newborn. Beware of a neonate born at home presenting with bleeding. • DIC may present with oozing from catheter sites.

Box 9.1.4	Basic Laboratory Findings in Common Bleeding Disorders*					
Disorder	Platelet count	PT	APTT	TCT	Fibrinogen	D-dimer
Vitamin K deficiency	N	↑	↑	N	N	N
Liver disease	↓ to N	↑	↑	↑	↓	↑
DIC	↓	↑	↑	↑	↓	↑
Systemic fibrinolysis	N	↑	↑	↑	↓	↑
Dilutional coagulopathy	↓	↑	↑	N	↓	N
Excessive heparin	N	N or ↑	↑	↑	N	N
Connective tissue disorder	N	N	N	N	N	N
Thrombocytopenia	↓	N	N	N	N	N
Platelet dysfunction	N	N	N	N	N	N
Hemophilia	N	N	↑	N	N	N
FVII deficiency	N	↑	N	N	N	N
Von Willebrand Disease	Usually N	N	N to ↑	N	N	N

*N, Normal; ↑, increased or prolonged; ↓, decreased.

specific hemostatic defect, specific treatments should be administered as soon as possible. To accelerate diagnosis, basic laboratory tests may be sent prior to detailed evaluation of the patient. Dilutional and massive transfusion induced coagulopathy should be treated with platelet transfusion and infusions of FFP or cryoprecipitate. These infusions should be laboratory guided. If the patient is hemodynamically unstable, consider transfusion with PRBC, platelets and fresh frozen plasma.

Activated FVII has been demonstrated to control bleeding and decrease the need for transfusion in trauma patients and other conditions of acute bleeding but given the associated risk of thromboembolism, its use is discouraged especially in conditions with increased risk of thromboembolism.

Patients with thrombocytopenia and bleeding should be transfused with platelets. Platelet transfusions are not effective in ITP and should be avoided except in life threatening bleeding in which case, continuous platelet infusions should be considered. Intramuscular injections should generally be avoided in patients with hemorrhagic disorders.

Disseminated Intravascular Coagulation (DIC; Fig. 9.1.3). An attempt should be made to identify and treat the underlying cause and to provide supportive care. This frequently reverses DIC and further treatment is not necessary. If hemorrhage is ongoing, laboratory guided replacement therapy with fresh frozen plasma, cryoprecipitate and platelet concentration should be considered. Heparin should be considered if DIC is severe or complicated by thrombosis. Unfractionated heparin 5–10 units/kg/hr (based on adjusted body weight; *Appendix part 1*) by continuous infusion should be given and benefits should carefully be weighed against the potential risk of bleeding. Neonates and infants with severe DIC may benefit from exchange transfusion.

Systemic Fibrinolysis. If systemic fibrinolysis is suspected during thrombolytic therapy, the thrombolytic agent should be discontinued. Since most thrombolytic agents have short half lives, this is frequently sufficient to arrest fibrinolysis. Fresh frozen plasma provides coagulation factors. If fibrinolysis persists, anti-fibrinolytic agents such as epsilon aminocaproic acid can be administered. In some circumstances fibrinolysis is protective. In the face of thrombolytic therapy and other conditions of systemic fibrinolysis, the risk and extent of bleeding must be weighed against the risk of re-thrombosis.

Vitamin K Deficiency and Liver Disease. Hemorrhagic disease of the newborn can be prevented by the administration of vitamin K

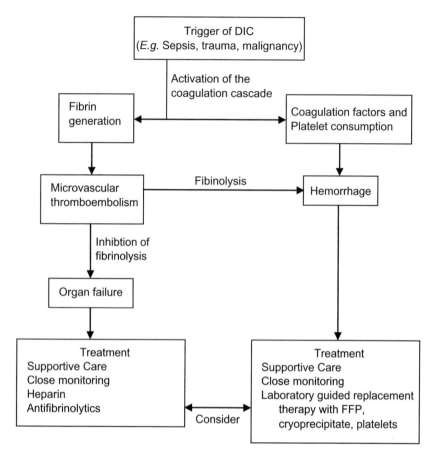

Fig. 9.1.3. Pathophysiology and Treatment for DIC.

1 mg IM or 2 mg orally. Bleeding patients with vitamin K deficiency should be treated with vitamin K subcutaneously or *slowly* IV: 1–5 mg for infants and 5–10 mg for older children and adults. The dose should be repeated in days to weeks as indicated. Response with visible cessation of bleeding occurs within 8 hrs.

In liver disease, vitamin K replacement should be considered early when PT and APTT prolongation occur. In acute bleeding, FFP should be considered. Patients with liver disease and bleeding should be transfused platelet concentrates if the platelet count falls below 50,000/µL.

Hemophilia and Von Willebrand Disease. Recombinant FVIII and FIX are the treatments of choice for hemophilia A and B respectively. The dosing range for recombinant FVIII is 20–50 units/kg every 8–12 hrs depending on severity of bleeding. For recombinant FIX the dosing range is 40–200 units/kg every 18–24 hrs depending on severity of bleeding. Abnormal bleeding in Von Willebrand disease may be treated with antihemophilic factor/Von Willebrand factor complex (Humate–P®) 20–50 units/kg depending on severity of bleeding every 8–12 hours. Dosing should be based on the Von Willebrand component of Humate–P®. DDAVP IV or nasal spray (Stimate®) is the preferred method of treatment for Type I Von Willebrand Disease. DDAVP is not effective in type 3 Von Willebrand disease and is contraindicated in type 2B Von Willebrand disease. DDAVP may cause hyponatremia and seizures especially if given IV and should not be given more often than every 24 hrs or in children younger than 2 yrs. Given the possibility of hyponatremia with DDAVP, IV fluids should be given judiciously.

Amicar® (epsilon-aminocaproic acid; anti-fibrinolytic agent) can be used for bleeding with a loading dose PO or IV 100–200 mg/kg (max 10 gm) followed by 50–100 mg/kg (max 5 gm) every 6 hrs not to exceed 30 gm/day. For oral bleeding, it can be used as swish (for 2 min) and spit. Patients should remain NPO at least one hour after "swish and spit." Amicar® is contraindicated in patients with hematuria.

For patients with hemophilia A, B or Von Willebrand disease with inhibitors who are experiencing life threatening bleeding, activated FVII 100 mcg/kg (range 90–240 mcg/kg) every 6 hrs (range 2–12 hrs) should be used. If bleeding persists, consider activated prothrombin complex concentrates (APCC) 75 units per kg and monitor closely for DIC and thrombosis. APCC should not be given to patients with a history of anaphylaxis to FIX. Patients with established hemophilia should carry a medical alert bracelet bearing their diagnosis and any allergies.

9.2 Anemia

Physiologically, anemia is defined as inadequate hemoglobin to meet oxygen requirements. Practically, anemia is defined as a hemoglobin concentration or hematocrit less than two standard deviations below the mean for age, gender and race. Causes of anemia are listed (**Box 9.2.1**).

Box 9.2.1   Causes of Anemia

- Blood loss: Trauma, surgery, internal organ rupture, gastrointestinal blood loss, bleeding diathesis.
- ↑ RBC destruction: Immune mediated hemolysis, red blood cell enzyme defects, red blood cell membrane defects, hemoglobinopathies, medication, infection.
- ↓ RBC production: Aplastic anemia, Diamond Blackfan anemia (DBA), transient erythroblastopenia of childhood (TEC), chronic illness, infection, malignancies, storage disease disorders, chemotherapy, nutritional deficiencies.

Box 9.2.2   Hemoglobin, Hematocrit and Mean Corpuscular Volume by Age and Gender

	Hemoglobin (g/dL)		Hematocrit (%)		MCV (fL)	
Age	Mean	−2SD	Mean	−2SD	Mean	−2SD
Birth	16.5	13.5	51	42	108	98
2 mos	11.5	9	35	28	96	77
6–24 mos	12.5	11	37	33	77	70
2–6 yrs	12.5	11.5	38	34	79	73
6–12 yrs	13.5	11.5	40	36	86	77
12–18 Female	14	12	42	37	90	78
12–18 Male	15	12	46	38	88	78

MCV, Mean Corpuscular Volume; −2SD, 2 standard deviations below the mean.

Hemoglobin concentration varies significantly with age, and this must be taken into consideration when analyzing laboratory findings (**Box 9.2.2**). Certain medical conditions may physiologically necessitate higher or lower hemoglobin concentrations.

Signs and symptoms of anemia result from decreased oxygen supply to the tissues. The presentation depends on age and the rapidity of onset of anemia. Signs and symptoms include: decreased energy and endurance, headache, pallor, dizziness, tachycardia, systolic murmur, hypotension, CHF, *etc.*

Evaluation. A comprehensive history, physical examination and laboratory testing often yield clues to the etiology of anemia (**Box 9.2.3** and **Fig. 9.2.1**).

Management. Acute blood loss, especially if symptomatic, should be treated with PRBC transfusions. If there is severe ongoing blood loss it may also be necessary to replace platelets and plasma. Bleeding should be controlled by compression, surgery or treatment of bleeding diathesis as needed.

Box 9.2.3   Etiologies of Anemia: History and Physical Examination

History:
- Excessive milk consumption or unusual cravings may suggest iron deficiency anemia.
- A recent infection may suggest infection induced hypoproliferative or hemolytic anemia.
- Chronic illnesses may suggest anemia of chronic illness. Anemia of chronic illness is usually insidious. If secondary to renal failure, there may be hypoerythropoietinemia.
- A family history of anemia, cholecystectomy, splenectomy may suggest red cell enzyme, red cell membrane or hemoglobin defect.
- Recent use of medication such as sulfa drugs or anticonvulsants may suggest medication induced marrow suppression or hemolysis.

Physical examination:
- Well appearance suggests iron deficiency, thalassemia or chronic hemolysis.
- Jaundice, dark urine, splenomegaly may suggest a hemolytic anemia.
- Brusing, lymphadenopathy, hepatosplenomegaly may suggest malignancy.
- Frontal bossing suggests extra medullary hematopoiesis.
- Skeletal abnormalities may suggest Fanconi's anemia or Diamond Blackfan anemia.

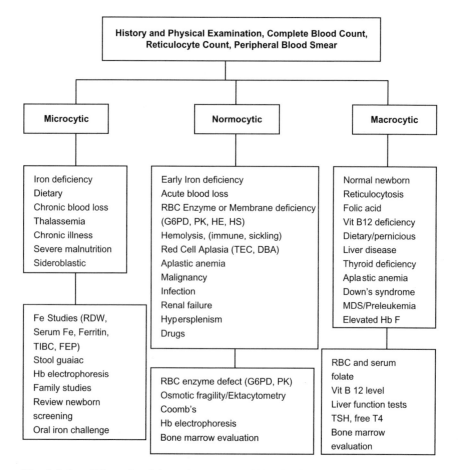

Fig. 9.2.1.   Dignosis of Anemia. RBC, Red blood cell; PK, Pyruvate kinase; HS, Hereditary spherocytosis; HE, Hereditary elliptocytosis; G6PD, Glucouse 6 phosphate dehydrogenase; DBA, Diamond Blackfan anemia; TEC, Transient erythroblastopenia of childhood, MDS, myelodysplastic syndromes; RDW, red cell distribution width; TIBC, total iron binding capacity; FEP, free erythrocyte protoporphyrin.

Progressive and symptomatic hemolytic anemia may require blood transfusions. It may be difficult to find matched blood for patients with autoimmune hemolytic anemia. In such a situation, the least incompatible blood units should be used. Other anemias that may warrant transfusions include aplastic anemia, transient erythroblastopenia of childhood, Diamond Blackfan anemia, chemotherapy induced anemia, marrow infiltration syndromes or severe nutritional anemias (*Transfusion Therapy, 9.3*). Severe autoimmune hemolytic anemia should be treated with steroids: initial dose of prednisone 30 mg/kg *po* or methylprednisolone 30 mg/kg IV followed by 2 mg/kg/day in 1–4 divided doses.

Iron deficiency should be treated with supplemental iron (6 mg/kg/day of elemental iron) best taken with a vitamin C containing juice, preferably "on an empty stomach" since food or milk can inhibit absorption. A rise in hemoglobin and reticulocyte count should be noted within one week of treatment if the diagnosis is correct and patient is compliant.

Anemia of chronic illness frequently resolves with treatment of the baseline condition. However, the baseline conditions can be long standing in which case intermittent transfusions may be warranted. Erythropoietin 250 IU/kg sub-cutaneously three times per week may decrease or eliminate the need for transfusion in anemia of chronic illness and other hypoplastic anemias. However, erythropoietin should be used with caution because it has been shown to increase mortality in certain patient groups (*e.g.* cancer patients). A hematologist should be consulted as needed to aid with management.

9.3 Transfusion Therapy

Despite great improvements, blood products still carry risks of both infectious and non-infectious complications and should be used judiciously and benefits should be carefully weighed against risks. In non-emergent transfusions, an informed consent should be obtained. Whole blood is seldom indicated, but may be used in severe acute blood loss amongst other rare indications. The decision to transfuse should be based on the clinical situation including symptoms, signs (↑HR or acidosis), probable etiology of anemia and the likelihood of progression or recovery rather than on specific hemoglobin/hematocrit values alone.

Packed Red Blood Cells (PRBC). PRBC should be ABO and Rh compatible. For children with sickle cell disease, the blood should also be minor antigen (at least C, E and K) compatible and be sickle

Hb negative. Potential bone marrow transplant candidates, neonates (< 30 days of age, with special consideration given to pre-term infants) and immune compromised patients should preferably receive leukocyte depleted and irradiated products to decrease the risk of CMV transmission and transfusion associated graft *versus* host disease. Leukocyte reduction also decreases the risk of transfusion-related febrile reactions. Washed RBC's are rarely necessary but may be indicated in patients with severe IgA deficiency and certain immune conditions.

The typical unit of PRBC contains 280–340 ml with a hematocrit of 55–65%. The required transfusion PRBC volume can be calculated as follows: PRBC transfusion volume in ml = Ideal body weight in kg × (desired hematocrit – current hematocrit) × 3.5. Where possible, the volume should be rounded up or down to full or half units to avoid waste and unnecessary exposure to multiple donors. The rate of transfusion should not exceed 5 ml/kg/hr (to avoid CHF) except in cases of rapid hemorrhage and rapid hemolysis. Children with chronic anemia and very low hemoglobin concentrations (< 5g/dL) should be transfused more slowly.   Indications for PRBC transfusions are listed (**Box 9.3.1**). Hypocalcemia may develop after massive transfusions due to the anticoagulants in blood products and calcium supplementation may be necessary. Post transfusion hemoglobin level may be checked two hours post transfusion to allow for adequate equilibration. Post transfusion hemoglobin levels should not exceed 12 g/dL in children with sickle cell disease.

Platelet transfusions may be indicated in children with thrombocytopenia secondary to decreased platelet production, non-immune mediated platelet destruction or bleeding in children with platelet dysfunction. Platelet transfusion is generally not indicated in immune mediated thrombocytopenia except in the case of life-threatening bleeding. Platelets are given as random concentrate 5–10 ml/kg to raise the platelet count by ~20,000–50,000/μL. Common indications for platelet transfusions are listed (**Box 9.3.2**).

Patients who are anticipated to have multiple platelets transfusions should preferably be given apheresis platelets to limit exposure

Box 9.3.1 Indications for PRBC Transfusions*

- Acute blood loss with hypovolemia not responsive to fluid replacement alone.
- Acute blood loss >10% of total blood volume (*e.g.* trauma; peri-operative period).
- Chronic symptomatic anemia with hemoglobin <8g/dL without expected rapid response to medical treatment without transfusion.
- Phlebotomy losses >5% of total blood volume and/or symptoms of anemia in neonates.
- Hemoglobin <13 g/dL in infants with severe cyanotic heart disease, severe pulmonary disease or in the first 24 hrs of life.
- Complications of abnormal hemoglobin *e.g.* Sickle cell disease with acute chest syndrome or suspected cerebral infarction. Exchange transfusion may be necessary if hemoglobin >9g/dL to avoid increasing viscosity (*Sickle Cell Disease, 9.4*).
- Chronic transfusions to suppress erythropoiesis such as in some cases of sickle cell disease or thalassemia.
- Hemoglobin <9g/dL prior to surgery in children with sickle cell disease.
- Hemoglobin <7g/dL prior to surgery.
- Hemoglobin <7g/dL and low reticulocyte count post-chemotherapy.
- Hemoglobin <7g/dL in critically ill patients.

*Exchange transfusions** may be indicated in certain complications of sickle cell disease, hyperbilirubinemia, hyperleukocytosis or certain immunologic conditions.

to donor antigens. These are collected from single donors and average 270 ml in volume. A post-transfusion platelet count should be done about one hour post-transfusion. If the platelet count rise is <10,000/μL, platelet refractoriness should be suspected and ABO compatible, leukocyte-depleted platelets, and other immunologic treatments should be considered. Causes of platelet refractoriness include splenomegaly, infections, fever, DIC, immune processes and certain drugs.

Box 9.3.2   Common Indications for Platelet Transfusions*

Platelet Count (per μL) or Condition	Clinical Context
< 10,000	Stable, non-bleeding patient
< 20,000	Septic or febrile patient or pre-IM injection
< 30,000	With a brain tumor or undergoing radiation therapy for any reason
< 50,000	Pre-term, sick infants or in association with bleeding or prior to an invasive procedure or minor surgery
< 100,000	Before major surgery
Any platelet count with qualitative platelet defect	Associated with bleeding or prior to an invasive procedure or surgery

* Platelets should be irradiated for reasons similar to those indications for PRBC irradiation.

Plasma may be used either as fresh frozen plasma (FFP) or cryo-precipitate. FFP is frequently used as a source of plasma protein and coagulation factors; 1 mL of FFP contains 1 IU of each coagulation factor. Cryoprecipitate contains high concentrations of fibrinogen, factors VIII, XIII and Von Willebrand's factor. Cryoprecipitate may be indicated in massive transfusions secondary to blood loss, supportive care in DIC or as a replacement of coagulation and anti-coagulation factors where specific factor preparations are not available. FFP 10–15 ml/kg per dose should be ABO matched; cryoprecipitate 0.15 units/kg (~1 bag/10 kg ideal body weight) and should raise plasma fibrinogen level by 75 mg/dL.

Granulocyte concentrate transfusion is rarely indicated but may be warranted in patients with severe neutropenia (ANC < 100/μL) and persistent Gram negative or fungal sepsis despite appropriate treatment. The donor should be ABO and Rh compatible and the product should be irradiated to eliminate lymphocytes.

Transfusion should proceed as soon as possible after granulocyte collection. Transfusions should infuse at 150 mL/m^2/hr and continue daily until clinical symptoms improve. The blood neutrophil count does not generally rise significantly because transfused neutrophils migrate to the site of infection. Granulocyte transfusions should be accomplished under the direction of the hematologist and the blood bank. Patients should always be pre-treated with an antihistamine (*e.g.* diphenhydramine) and steroids (methylprednisolone 1 mg/kg).

Transfusion reactions occur in up to 5% of transfusions and are most commonly non-serious, febrile, non-hemolytic and urticarial reactions. Delayed hemolytic reactions are rare but may occur as late as 4 weeks post-transfusion. Serious reactions are most commonly due to clerical errors. Whenever a transfusion reaction occurs, a bed-side evaluation to review labeling of products, confirmation of patient ID and compatibility of the blood unit should be conducted. Blood samples from the unit and from the patient should be sent to the blood bank for typing and microbiology for culture.

Urticarial or febrile reactions should be treated by halting the transfusion and administration of an antihistamine such as diphenhydramine (1 mg/kg, max. 50 mg) and acetaminophen (10–15 mg/kg). If symptoms resolve, transfusion may be continued. Patients should be pre-treated with antihistamines and corticosteroids (such as methylprednisolone (1–2 mg/kg IV) prior to subsequent transfusions. Anaphylactoid reactions should be managed by discontinuing the transfusion and treatment with antihistamines, corticosteroids and epinephrine 1:1000 solution (0.01 ml/kg or 0.01 mg/kg to max 0.5 mg subQ every 20 mins as needed). Patients should be evaluated for possible IgA deficiency or other immunologic disorders. These patients may require washed blood products.

Acute hemolytic reactions are characterized by fever, jaundice, dyspnea, rigors, chills, hypertension or hypotension, abdominal pain, back pain, renal failure, etc. Treatment includes immediate cessation of transfusion, fluid resuscitation and vasoactive support as needed, with administration of antihistamines and corticosteroids.

Transfusion related acute lung injury (TRALI) is characterized by pulmonary edema resulting in shortness of breath, tachypnea, hypoxemia, hypotension, and sometimes fever occurring during or within 6 hrs of transfusion of blood products. It is the most frequent cause of transfusion related mortality in the US. It is most commonly seen after cardiac surgery, massive transfusion, sepsis, or hematologic malignancies. If suspected, a CXR should be obtained and other causes of respiratory distress and air space disease should be considered. Treatment is mostly supportive.

Other transfusion reactions include circulatory overload, delayed hemolysis, alloimmunization, transfusion graft versus host disease, bacterial contamination and blood-related infectious diseases. Circulatory overload should be treated with diuresis. Children likely to have repeat transfusions should be screened for the development of alloantibodies 4–6 weeks post transfusion. Children receiving chronic transfusions are at risk of iron overload and may need chelation therapy.

9.4 Sickle Cell Disease (SCD)

The most common sickle cell genotypes are HbSS, HbSC, HbSß° and HbSß⁺. SCD can lead to acute and chronic complications. Severity of symptoms varies, but patients with HbSS and HbSß° generally have more severe symptoms, while patients with HbSß⁺ have milder symptoms. Complications affect almost all organ systems and include infections, acute hemolysis, acute and chronic pain, acute chest syndrome (ACS), splenic sequestration, cerebral infarction, nephropathy, avascular necrosis and retinopathy.

Febrile children with SCD should be treated emergently. Blood culture should be obtained and parenteral antibiotics should be given promptly. Chosen antibiotics should be adequate for treatment of *Streptococcus pneumoniae* amongst others. If there are respiratory symptoms, coverage for Chlamydophila and Mycoplasma should be included.

Vaso-occlusive Pain. Patients with acute pain should be carefully evaluated to rule out other etiologies of pain such as

---

Box 9.4.1.   Management of Vaso-occlusive Crisis

- Fluids: Assess for dehydration and replace any accrued deficits. Maintenance hydration in SCD patients often requires 1–1.5 × the usual maintenance allotment (IV + PO); however, if respiratory symptoms are present, do not exceed the usual maintenance fluid rate to avoid pulmonary edema. Weigh daily and monitor intake/output to help detect fluid overload.
- Analgesia: Options include:
  ▶ Narcotics: scheduled (*e.g.* morphine 0.1–0.15 mg/kg IV every 3–4 hrs)*
  ▶ NSAID's: scheduled PO (*e.g.* ibuprofen 10 mg/kg PO every 6 hrs) OR scheduled IV (*e.g.* ketorolac 1 mg/kg up to 60 mg loading dose followed by 0.5 mg/kg up to 30 mg IV every 6 hrs) may be given. Avoid giving ketorolac for more than 5 consecutive days.
  ▶ Patient controlled analgesia (PCA): *e.g.* morphine 0.1 mg/kg IV loading dose followed by a basal rate of 0.02 to 0.05 mg/kg/hr and an on-demand dose of 0.01 to 0.04 mg/kg/dose every 6 to 10 mins with a total (basal rate + PRN doses) lockout dose of 0.15 mg/kg/hr. After pain has been adequately controlled, narcotics should be weaned slowly to avoid rebound of pain.
- Respiratory care: Initiate incentive spirometry (10 maximal inflations every hour while awake and an appropriate frequency during sleeptime (*e.g.* every 2–4 hrs). Ambulate as soon as possible.
- Supportive care: Consider antihistamines for pruritus, stool softeners for constipation, heat packs and massage for discomfort, physical therapy to address range of motion and facilitate ambulation; child psychology and child life for emotional, developmental and behavioral care.

---

*Hydromorphone or fentanyl may be used instead of morphine. Meperidine should be avoided because it may cause seizures or dysphoria.

appendicitis, osteomyelitis, trauma, *etc.* Pain is a frequent complication of SCD, thus most patients have an out-patient pain management plan. Inpatient vaso-oclusive pain management is detailed in **Box 9.4.1**.

Acute Anemia/Acute Hemolysis. All children with SCD have chronic hemolysis and their metabolism is generally adapted to a decreased hemoglobin concentration at baseline. Severe acute hemolysis (characterized by increased jaundice, bilirubin and reticulocyte counts above baseline) warrants intervention. Patients may exhibit headache, fatigue or other symptoms of severe anemia. Treatment includes careful fluid resuscitation and PRBC transfusion with sickle negative ABO and preferably phenotype specific (minor antigen) compatible blood. The post-transfusion hemoglobin concentration goal should not exceed 12 g/dL.

Aplastic Anemia (AA). Transient RBC aplasia is a common finding in children with SCD. Hemoglobin decreases from baseline level and is associated with a low reticulocyte count. Reticulocytopenia often differentiates AA from splenic sequestration though occasionally splenic sequestration and AA may occur concomitantly; splenomegaly usually is present. Several viruses and bacteria can cause AA; Parvovirus B19 is the most common cause of AA in children with SCD, but it can also precipitate splenic sequestration. Anemia results from ongoing hemolysis with inadequate reticulocytosis.

Perform a thorough physical examination, monitor vital signs, obtain a CBC with reticulocyte count and type and screen for possible transfusion. Blood culture should be done and antibiotics given if fever is present. AA in children with SCD is usually self limited and requires only close monitoring. Patients with severe anemia (hemoglobin < 5 g/dL) or those who are symptomatic should be transfused. If anemia persists for a long period, consider treating with erythropoietin.

Patients with Parvovirus B19 develop lifelong immunity. Individuals of child bearing age who are not immune should take precautions with children infected with parvovirus B19 since the virus can cause birth defects.

Acute Splenic Sequestration. Children with sickle cell disease can develop an acute intrasplenic trapping of RBC's leading to a significant decrease in hemoglobin from baseline; reticulocytosis (not present in pure AA) follows. Thrombocytopenia and/or leukopenia may co-exist. Peak incidence occurs between 2–5 years and is frequently induced by an infection.

Monitor vital signs; obtain a CBC with reticulocyte count, and type and screen for possible transfusion. Blood cultures should be obtained and antibiotics initiated if fever is present. Splenic sequestration is an emergency because hypovolemic circulatory collapse can occur rapidly. Acute management should include volume expansion with 0.9% NaCl or Ringer's lactate® while awaiting compatible blood to initiate transfusion. Target hemoglobin should not exceed 10 mg/dl as there is a risk of trapped intrasplenic RBC's being released into the circulation and leading to hyperviscosity. The required PRBC volume to be transfused can be calculated as follows: PRBC volume (ml) = ideal weight (kg) × (desired − current hematocrit) × 3.5. Splenectomy should be considered in children with more than two episodes of splenic sequestration. Consideration for lifelong penicillin prophylaxis should be given for all children status-post surgical splenectomy.

Acute Chest Syndrome (ACS) is an acute lower respiratory tract illness associated with a new or progressive pulmonary infiltrate on CXR and fever or chest pain, tachypnea, wheezing, hypoxia or increased sputum production. ACS is one of the leading causes of hospitalization and mortality in children with SCD and is a frequent treatment-related or post-operative complication. It also occurs in children with SCD admitted to the hospital for complaints unrelated to the respiratory system. About half of all individuals with SCD will experience at least one episode of ACS in their lifetime. The etiology of ACS remains unclear. A trigger is identified in only 38% of cases; infections account for a majority of these. Children at risk for ACS should be reassessed frequently because its onset can be rapid or it can worsen suddenly.

Evaluation should include a CBC with differential and reticulocyte count, blood cultures and CXR. Blood gases, electrolytes, glucose, urea nitrogen, creatinine and liver enzymes should be considered. Serial CXR's may be necessary because findings can change rapidly. Treatment is multimodal (**Box 9.4.2**).

Neurologic Complications of Sickle Cell Anemia. Acute clinically apparent neurological events occur in about 10% of children with SCD. Common presenting signs and symptoms include: hemiparesis, aphasia or dysphasia, monoparesis, seizures, cranial nerve palsies, headache, stupor or coma. Any child with SCD and a neurologic

---

Box 9.4.2   Key Points in Treatment of ACS

- Administer broad spectrum antibiotics (including a cephalosporin and a macrolide) to treat typical and atypical microorganisms. Vancomycin should be considered for ill-appearing children.
- Indications for simple or exchange transfusions: Multi lobar disease, progressive infiltrates, hypoxia beyond baseline, history of prior ACS or otherwise ill-appearing child. The target hemoglobin level is 10 g/dL, not to exceed 12 g/dL. HbS concentration after transfusion should be less than 30% of total Hb. Transfused blood should be sickle negative, leukoreduced and if possible major (A, B, O, Rh) and minor (C, E, K) antigen matched.
- Hydration goal is euvolemia; avoid fluid overload. If there are signs of fluid overload, furosemide should be considered.
- Supplemental O_2 should maintain Pox reading >91% or at baseline.
- Increased oxygen requirements should prompt reassessment since patients with ACS can worsen precipitously.
- Bronchodilators are indicated for wheezing or bronchospasm; up to 80% of patients with ACS develop bronchospasm.
- Aggressive ventilator support including inhaled nitric oxide may be needed.
- Pain may be treated with opioids and non-opioids; monitor patients for development of excessive sedation.
- Provide incentive spirometry and early ambulation to all patients.
- Frequently reassess to monitor for possible deterioration.
- Children with severe ACS should be considered for chronic transfusion therapy or hydroxurea and monitored for pulmonary hypertension via echocardiogram.

---

event should be evaluated and treated promptly. There should be a high index of suspicion for strokes in children with SCD; otherwise, subtle signs of stroke may be missed. Evaluation should include a CBC, reticulocyte count, hemoglobin electrophoresis, type and cross-match for RBC transfusion. Imaging should include MRI and MRA of the brain. If MRI cannot be performed in the acute setting, a CT scan should be obtained initially; blood transfusions should not be delayed while awaiting imaging.

Management of Stroke. If stroke is suspected in a child with SCD a simple transfusion or exchange transfusion should be initiated as soon as possible. Post-transfusion hemoglobin should not exceed $12 \, g/dL$. If stroke is confirmed on imaging, chronic transfusions should be instituted to suppress hematopoiesis and keep the proportion of hemoglobin S less than 30%. Chronic transfusions are the only therapy that has been proven to decrease the risk of stroke recurrence in children with SCD. Chronic transfusion therapy is frequently complicated by iron overload; if not appropriately managed, hemosiderosis can lead to multi-organ disease.

Hydroxyurea is currently being investigated as a possible alternative to chronic blood transfusions. See also *Transfusion Therapy, 9.3* and *Stroke, 9.6.*

9.5 Methemoglobinemia

The iron of hemoglobin is generally in the ferrous (Fe^{2+}) state, which is essential for oxygen transport and delivery. Slow release of oxygen results in the ferric (Fe^{3+}) state of iron. The combination of hemoglobin iron in the ferric state and water results in the formation of methemoglobin (Met-Hb). The enzyme cytochrome 5b oxidase reduces Met-Hb and maintains a predominant ferrous hemoglobin state. When this balance is disrupted, methemoglobinemia may result. Methemoglobinemia is most commonly acquired; however, rare congenital causes exist (**Box 9.5.1**). The presence of Met-Hb at sufficiently high levels may result in life-threatening failure of oxygen delivery. Methemoglobinemia should be suspected in a child without known cardiopulmonary disease and a cyanotic or slate-gray color.

Acquired methemoglobinemia results from excessive oxidative stress. It may be secondary to oxidizing medications, environmental agents, or with exacerbations of chronic medical conditions (**Box 9.5.2**). **Slate gray** discoloration of the mucous membranes

Box 9.5.1   Causes of Hereditary Methemoglobinemia

- NADH Cytochrome b5 Reductase Deficiencies (most common cause):
  ▶ Type I: Enzyme deficiency in RBCs only.
  ▶ Type II: Enzyme deficiency in all tissues resulting in neurologic manifestations in early infancy (see text).
  ▶ Type III: Enzyme deficiency in leukocytes, platelets and RBC's.
  ▶ Type IV: Enzyme deficiency of only RBC cytochrome b5.
- Hemoglobin M: Congenital methemoglobinemia due to abnormal hemoglobin which is more stable in the ferric (oxidized) state.
- NAPDH-Flavin Reductase Deficiency.

Box 9.5.2   Selected Etiologies of Acquired Methemoglobinemia

Medications:	Predisposing Medical Conditions:	Environmental agents:
• Benzocaine • Phenazopyridine (Pyridium) • Chloroquine • Prilocaine • Dapsone • Primaquine • Flutamide • Riluzole • Lidocaine including Eutectic Mixture of Local Anesthetic (EMLA®) • Rasburicase • Metoclopramide • Silver nitrate • Nitrates • Sulfonamides • Nitroprusside	• Pediatric gastrointestinal infection • Sepsis • SCD-related pain crisis • Glucose-6-phosphate dehydrogenase (G6PD) deficiency	• Recreational drug overdose with amyl nitrate ("poppers") • Fume inhalation (automobile exhaust, burning of wood and plastics) • Industrial chemicals: nitrobenzene, nitroethane (found in nail polish, gasoline octane booster) • Well-water • Aniline dyes • Pesticides/Herbicides • Resins, rubber adhesives

and skin is the most common sign of methemoglobinemia. Blood from patients with methemoglobinemia is frequently **chocolate brown** in color. Infants may present with lethargy and poor feeding. Older patients may report dyspnea, headache, dizziness, exertional fatigue, lethargy, and mental confusion. The ability to tolerate methemoglobinemia depends upon its severity and the rapidity of its development (which can be compared to the ability of a patient to tolerate anemia).

In hereditary methemoglobinemia, cyanosis is the most notable clinical sign. The degree of cyanosis may vary with the season and patient's diet, and high levels of Met-Hb are generally well tolerated. Type II NADH cytochrome 5b reductase deficiency can present in infancy with encephalopathy, spasticity, mental retardation, growth retardation, and cyanosis.

Acquired methemoglobinemia is most frequently encountered in the setting of a young infant with a diarrheal disease. Several factors make newborns and infants particularly susceptible to acquired methemoglobinemia:

- The enzyme cytochrome b5 oxidase is present in all tissues in diminished amounts in the infant, reaching adult levels at approximately 4 months of age.
- Fetal hemoglobin is also more vulnerable to oxidation than hemoglobin A.
- An infant's gastrointestinal tract contains an increase in nitrite-producing Gram negative organisms secondary to its alkaline nature.

Methemoglobin is measured by co-oximetry. Levels >15–20% result in clinical cyanosis, while levels >70% are lethal. Met-Hb levels are reported as a percentage of the normal hemoglobin contained in the blood sample; thus a toxic level of Met-Hb may be lower in an anemic child. Oxygen saturation by pulse oximetry is often low in a patient with methemoglobinemia despite normal PaO_2; saturations will not improve with supplemental oxygen administration. (*General Approach to the Critically Ill Child, 1.2; Box 1.2.4.*) Hemoglobin M may be detected at birth through routine newborn screening for hereditary methemoglobinemia.

Management of Methemoglobinemia. Elimination of exacerbating agent(s) is (are) the most important aspect of management. Individuals with hereditary methemoglobinemia tolerate higher levels, and have a normal life expectancy as long as Met-Hb levels are < 25–40%. For harmful concentrations of methemoglobin (Met-Hb > 30%), management consists of **methylene blue 1–2 mg/kg IV** (max 50 mg/dose) followed by maintenance dosing (100–300 mg PO daily) for chronic cases. Methylene blue in therapeutic doses is a mild but effective oxidizing agent (electron acceptor). In the presence of NADPH and methemoglobin reductase, methylene blue is reduced to leukomethylene blue, which acts as a reducing agent (electron donor) to convert met-Hb (Hb Fe^{+++}) to hemoglobin (Hb Fe^{++}). Methylene blue is a strong oxidant in high doses; doses >7 mg/kg can result paradoxically in methemoglobinemia. Methylene blue is contraindicated in patients with G6PD deficiency because these patients lack sufficient NADPH, which is necessary for the reduction of methylene blue. For mild cases of methemoglobinemia, **ascorbic acid** (200–500 mg PO daily in divided doses) reduces Met-Hb to below 10%. Ascorbic has been associated with renal calculi formation and hyperoxaluria. Along with medication, avoiding intake of nitrite-enriched foods such as beets, spinach and carrots may be warranted. Prognosis for patients with acquired methemoglobinemia depends on the severity of disease and the rapidity with which treatment is initiated.

9.6 Stroke

Stroke is rare in children but when it occurs its effects can be severe with a high incidence of long term sequelae (up to 70% in some studies) and a mortality rate of 10–25%. Stroke is traditionally defined as rapidly developing focal or global brain disturbance lasting more than 24 hrs without an obvious non-vascular cause. This definition does not capture all cases of stroke in children. Some children with transient ischemic attack (TIA)-like syndrome have imaging evidence of cerebral infarction. It is important to consider other causes of brain dysfunction, but even in the presence of other causes of brain dysfunction such as in infections, stroke cannot be ruled out. It is important to recognized symptoms of stroke promptly so that timely intervention can be instituted in an effort to mitigate cerebral damage.

About 55% of pediatric strokes are ischemic in nature; the remainder are hemorrhagic. In a large number of cases the etiology is unknown. The etiology varies with age at presentation and about 50% of cases have a previously diagnosed risk factor for stroke. Common causes are listed (**Box 9.6.1**).

Box 9.6.1   Common Causes of Stroke in Children

Ischemic Stroke	Hemorrhagic Stroke
• Heart disease	• Arteriovenous malformation
• Cerebrovascular malformation	• Aneurysm
• Vasculopathy	• Venous angioma
• Cervicocephalic arterial dissection	• Other cerebrovascular malformation
• Vasculitis	• Trauma
• Idiopathic occlusion of carotid artery	• Thrombocytopenia
• Infections	• Hemophilia
• Primary hypercoagable state	• Vitamin K deficiency
• Secondary hypercoagable state	• Central venous sinus thrombosis
• Sickle cell disease	• Other bleeding diatheses
• Essential thrombocytopenia	• Infections
• Paroxysmal nocturnal hemoglobinuria	• Malignancies
• Hyperlipidemia	
• Elevated lipoprotein (a)	
• Homocystinuria; other metabolic disorders	
• Chemotherapy	
• Thrombotic Thrombocytopenic Purpura	
• Trauma	

The clinical presentation is varied to include severe headaches, altered mental status, hemiparesis, facial asymmetry, asymmetric startle, aphasia, hyperreflexia, spasticity, flaccidity and hemiparesis. Post- ischemia induced cerebral edema and intracranial hemorrhage frequently lead to signs of raised ICP (hypertension, bradycardia, tachypnea, papilledema, seizure, *etc.*)

Evaluation. A rapid but detailed past medical and family history should be performed to determine existing risk factors such as SCD, hemophilia, cardiac disease, medication, fever, *etc.* Physical examination should evaluate stability of airway, breathing, and circulation. A murmur may suggest heart disease, nuchal rigidity may suggest hemorrhage or meningitis, bruising may suggest trauma. Initial laboratory evaluation should include CBC, chemistries, PT, APTT and d-dimer. Blood gases should be obtained to evaluate for hypoxia and/or ventilatory disturbances. Other specific coagulations studies can be deferred initially as these are often not necessary in guiding initial management except in the rare case where a specific factor replacement may be essential for treatment such as the neonate with bleeding or child with purpura and suspected Protein C or antithrombin III deficiency.

Imaging studies should be obtained as soon as feasible but these should not delay management or significantly endanger patient stability. Head CT is helpful in the evaluation of hemorrhage or tumor with mass effect but it is generally not sensitive for recent ischemic events or subtle masses. Ultrasonography and Doppler ultrasonography can be helpful in evaluating blood flow. Magnetic resonance imaging (MRI) often includes MRA and MRV. Nuclear medicine imaging may help evaluate cerebral perfusion and tissue viability. Catheter angiography remains the gold standard for evaluation of cerebral vascular abnormalities but it is invasive and frequently not feasible in the acute setting. Other studies including echocardiography, lumbar puncture, appropriate cultures, metabolic studies, *etc* depend on the above laboratory findings, history, physical examination and imaging studies.

Management. The focus of treatment should be stabilization of vital functions, preservation of neurological function and limitation of

Box 9.6.2   Supportive Care for Patients with Cerebral Hemorrhagic or Ischemic Events

- Correct hypoxia and provide ventilatory support as indicated.
- Control fever, which exacerbates cerebral damage in children with stroke. The efficacy of induced hypothermia is unproven.
- Control of hypertension should be individualized based on the injury and its anatomy.
- Correct anemia.
- In SCD, PRBC transfusion to Hb 10–12 gm/dL as soon as possible. If Hb is > 9g/dL, a partial or full exchange transfusion should be performed as directed by the hematologist (*Sickle Cell Disease, 9.4*).
- Correct dehydration.
- Surgical evacuation of hemorrhage with cerebral ventricular shunt placement should be considered as indicated.
- Surgical treatment of vascular malformations and cardiac anomalies should be considered.
- Children with specific coagulation defects should be treated with appropriate factor replacement.
- Anticoagulation with heparin or low molecular weight heparin should be considered for patients with cerebral venous sinus thrombosis or other ischemic strokes if hemorrhage has not occurred. It is often difficult in the acute setting to exclude hemorrhage. Dosing guidelines for low molecular weight heparin (**Box 9.6.3**) and unfractionated heparin (**Box 9.6.4**) and are listed.
- Thrombolysis is reserved for a very select group of patients such as those with cerebral venous sinus thrombosis. Thrombolysis should be undertaken with extreme caution and under the direction of the hematologist.
- Children with substantial risk of recurrent cardiac embolism, cerebral venous thrombosis and selected hypercoagable states should be considered for long term anticoagulation with low molecular weight heparin, warfarin or aspirin.

long term sequelae. A neurologist should be consulted to participate in management. If hemorrhage or an embolic event is suspected, neurosurgery and hematology consultation should be sought. Supportive measures are listed in (**Box 9.6.2**).

All children with stroke should be considered for physical therapy and rehabilitation. Selected patients should be screened for thrombophilia risk factors and very rarely thrombophilia screening may be considered in family members.

Box 9.6.3 Low Molecular Weight (LMW) Heparin* for Ischemic Stroke			
Obtain results of CBC, PT, PTT; ensure no contraindication exists based on laboratory results (*e.g.* pre-existing coagulopathy)			
Drug	Age	Weight	Dose (Sub Q)
Enoxaparin	<2 months	NA	1.5 mg/kg/dose q12h
	>2 months	NA	1 mg/kg/dose q12h
Reviparin	NA	<5kg	150 Units/kg/dose q12h
	NA	>5kg	100 Units/kg/dose q12h

* Other LMW heparins include dalteparin and tinzaparin. NA, not applicable. Note that doses are for treatment (not prophylaxis).

Box 9.6.4   Unfractionated Heparin Administration and Dose Adjustments for Children with Ischemic Stroke Based on APTT

- Obtain results of CBC, PT and APTT (same as PTT).
- If no contraindication exists based on laboratory results (*e.g.* pre-existing coagulopathy), give unfractionated heparin* 75 units/kg over 10 min. Neonates may require a loading dose of 100 units/kg.
- Begin a continuous infusion of heparin at 28 units/kg/hr. Adults may require 10–30 units/kg/hr.
- **Check APTT 4 hrs after initiation of continuous heparin and 4 hrs after any rate change.**
- The goal APTT of 60–85 sec should reflect an anti-factor Xa level of 0.3–0.7 units/mL (these may vary depending on local laboratory techniques).
- If goal APTT (60–85 sec) is obtained, recheck the APTT in 24 hrs.
- CBC and APTT should be obtained daily. Caution should be taken to avoid heparin contamination of the sample. If heparin contamination occurs, heparinase can be added to the specimen to reverse its effects.
- Adjust heparin dose (infusion rate) as needed based on APTT as indicated below.

APTT (sec)	Loading Dose of Heparin	Hold Heparin Infusion (min)	Rate Change Adjustment
<50	50 units/kg	No	↑ 10%
50–59	None	No	↑ by 10%
60–85	None	No	None
86–95	None	No	↓ by 10%
96–120	None	30 min	↓ by 10%
>120	None	60 min	↓ by 15%

* Base dose of unfractionated heparin on the adjusted body weight (*Appendix, part 1*).

9.7 Oncologic Emergencies

Life-threatening situations can occur in the pediatric oncology patient as a result of the disease itself or as a consequence of treatment. Oncologic emergencies may occur at the time of presentation or at any time during therapy. Pediatric oncologic emergencies may result from structural or functional compromise of the cardiopulmonary or neurologic systems, metabolic abnormalities, or a compromised immune system.

Superior Mediastinal Syndrome (SMS). Masses in the mediastinum have the potential to create life-threatening compromise of the airway or cardiovascular system. SMS refers to compression of the trachea or mainstem bronchi by a mediastinal mass. SMS is closely related to superior vena cava syndrome (SVCS), which refers to compression or obstruction of the vena cava. These two entities often coexist. Masses causing SMS and/or SVCS are frequently malignant; however, certain benign processes should also be considered in the differential diagnosis. Regardless of the cause, children with evidence of SMS or SVCS must be managed with care to avoid complete loss of the airway or cardiovascular collapse. In particular, the use of sedation or general anesthesia should be avoided pending a thorough evaluation of anesthesia risk.

In children, the trachea and mainstem bronchi are very compliant and vulnerable to collapse from external compression. The superior vena cava is a thin-walled vessel with low intraluminal pressure. Compression by a mediastinal mass or obstruction by tumor or thrombosis leads to venous stasis and diminished blood return to the heart. SMS/SVCS generally results from compression from a mass in the anterior compartment of the mediastinum, with lymphoma being the most common cause. The differential of a mediastinal mass depends on the age of the child, the rapidity with which symptoms developed, and the mediastinal compartment that contains the mass (**Box 9.7.1**).

Presentation (Box 9.7.2) and Management. Children with SMS and/or SVCS may be asymptomatic at the time of presentation, or they may come to medical attention just prior to cardiopulmonary collapse. In some cases, the airway may be so tenuous that total airway loss may be precipitated by simply placing the child in a supine or flexed position. Once there is suspicion of a mediastinal process, care must be taken to protect the airway. Diagnosis and initiation of therapy should occur in the most expeditious and least invasive manner possible.

Box 9.7.1 **Differential Diagnosis of a Mediastinal Mass by Location within Mediastinum**

Anterior	Middle	Posterior
• Lymphoma	• Lymphoma	• Neuroblastoma
• Leukemia	• TB	• Ganglioneuroblastoma
• Malignant germ cell tumor	• Histiocytosis	• Sarcoma
• Benign teratoma	• Sarcoidosis	• Duplication cyst
• Thymic lesion (thymic hyperplasia, thymoma, thymic cyst)	• Anomalies of the great vessels	
• Substernal thyroid		

Box 9.7.2 **Signs and Symptoms of Superior Mediastinal (SMS) and Superior Vena Cava (SVCS) Syndromes**

SMS:

- • Cough
- • Dyspnea
- • Orthopnea
- • Wheezing
- • Stridor
- • Dysphagia
- • Anxiety
- • Diaphoresis

SVCS:

- • Facial swelling
- • Upper body edema
- • Cyanosis of the face or upper body
- • Plethora
- • Conjunctival edema or suffusion
- • Headache

In severe cases, empiric therapy (either corticosteroids or occasionally radiation therapy) may need to be employed prior to making a tissue diagnosis. However, in most cases, a tissue diagnosis can be made prior to therapy. The child should be approached in a stepwise manner, considering all potential sources of diagnostic tissue (**Box 9.7.3**). Procedures may be performed using local anesthesia with the child in the sitting position.

Box 9.7.3   Potential Sources of Diagnostic Tissue

- Peripheral blood
- Superficial lymph node (Fine needle aspiration, core needle biopsy, biopsy with local anesthesia)
- Pleural fluid
- Bone marrow
- Mediastinal mass biopsy (image-guided needle biopsy or open biopsy by Chamberlain procedure)

Assesment of Anesthesia/Sedation Risk. Several clinical factors have been associated with an increased risk for life-threatening anesthesia-related complications in the context of SMS (**Box 9.7.4**). There are case reports of anesthesia-related deaths in asymptomatic children with SMS; therefore, in a child with a known mediastinal mass, a CT scan and pulmonary function testing when possible should be performed prior to subjecting the child to anesthetics. Tracheal cross sectional area (TCA) can be assessed by CT scan. Pulmonary function testing may be done fairly easily at the child's bedside, and readings should be done in both the sitting and supine position.

Box 9.7.4   Signs of a Critical Airway in a Child with a Mediastinal Mass

- Orthopnea*
- Upper body edema
- Dyspnea
- Clinical findings of impending respiratory failure
- Tracheal cross sectional area (TCA) can be assessed by CT scan
- Severe compression of one or both mainstem bronchi
- Peak Expiratory Flow Rate of < 50% predicted (performed in sitting and supine position)

---

*Orthopnea most closely correlates with degree of anesthesia risk.

Studies have shown that children with a TCA and peak expiratory flow rate (PEFR) of >50% of normal for age can be given general anesthesia or sedation safely if needed.

Spinal Cord Compression (SCC) may lead to irreversible neurologic damage including permanent paralysis. Early recognition and treatment of cord compression are essential to decrease long-term morbidity. SCC occurs in approximately 3–5% of all pediatric oncology patients from any malignancy and can present either at the time of diagnosis or as the disease progresses. In the pediatric patient, cord compression most frequently results from a paravertebral tumor extending through the intervertebral foramina (*e.g.* soft tissue sarcomas, tumors of neurogenic origin). Tumors growing through the intervertebral foramina initially cause mechanical nerve root compression. If growth continues, transverse myelitis (inflammation of gray and white matter of the spinal cord) may ultimately occur. Also, the venous plexus may be compressed at the intravertebral level, resulting in ischemic injury to the cord. Intradural spinal metastasis from an intracranial process (*e.g.* medulloblastoma) may also lead to cord compromise. These lesions tend to occur in the lumbosacral region. Primary spinal cord tumors, such as an intramedullary astrocytoma, may also be the cause of pain and neurologic symptoms in children. More rarely, infiltration of the *cauda equina* or *conus medullaris* may occur with a leukemic process.

Presentation and Management. Localized or radicular back pain occurs in 80% of children with SCC. Back pain in any child with a malignancy is highly suspicious for SCC and deserves further investigation. Depending on the rate of tumor growth, the pain and deficits may be long-standing and slowly progressive or more acute in nature. History should elicit the time course and include questioning about changes in gait and bowel or bladder habits. Tenderness to palpation tends to localize to the site of the lesion. A thorough neurologic examination should be performed with attention to motor strength, reflexes, gait abnormalities, sensation, and sphincter tone.

If SCC is suspected, dexamethasone should be initiated without delay. Corticosteroid therapy may decrease cord edema and preserve neurologic function while plans for more definitive therapy are underway. Optimal dosing of dexamethasone is not known; a loading dose of 1–2 mg/kg IV followed by 0.25–0.5 mg/kg IV every 6 hrs has been suggested; in our practice, we use a maximum of 4 mg/dose. If lymphoma is the cause of the SCC, dexamethasone is likely to be cytolytic and may lead to TLS.

Imaging studies should be obtained as soon as possible. Plain radiographs are insufficiently sensitive. The optimal study in a patient with potential SCC is an MRI. If MRI cannot be arranged, CT myelography should be performed. Definitive therapeutic options will include surgical resection, radiation therapy, and/or chemotherapy. The optimal choice of treatment is best determined by a multi-disciplinary team including a pediatric oncologist, radiation oncologist, and neurosurgeon. Treatment choice will be influenced by whether a tissue diagnosis has been made, radio- and chemosensitivity of the tumor, extent of disease, and the degree of neurologic compromise present. Studies have suggested that the degree of neurologic deficit at the time of presentation and the duration of symptoms prior to initiating therapy both correlate with the ultimate functional outcome, regardless of the treatment method employed. When planning definitive therapy, both acute relief of SCC as well as long-term sequelae of the treatment modality used need to be considered. Radiation therapy and surgical resection, while offering more immediate benefit in terms of local tumor control, may lead to long-term sequelae in terms of growth problems and scoliosis. For this reason, chemotherapy is generally the treatment of choice in a child with lymphoma, leukemia, or disseminated neuroblastoma who has minimal symptoms of SCC. If SCC occurs in the setting of progressive refractory disease, palliative therapy (*e.g.* radiation or surgical intervention) for SCC should not be withheld, as it may have a substantial impact on the quality of life.

Hyperleukocytosis (HL) is defined as a white blood cell (WBC) count of greater than 100 K/μL. It may result in neurologic abnormalities including stroke, pulmonary compromise, renal insufficiency, and metabolic derangements. HL is present at the time of diagnosis in approximately 10% of cases of ALL, 5–20% of AML, and in virtually all patients with CML.

Children with HL are at increased risk of death during the early phase of induction therapy. The risk of fatal complications is highest in patients with AML and this risk increases with the total WBC count. In patients with HL, early death occurs in approximately 20% of patients with AML and 5% of patients with ALL. Complications of HL are listed (**Box 9.7.5**). HL results in increased blood viscosity and

---

Box 9.7.5   Potential Life-Threatening Complications from Hyperleukocytosis

- **CNS:** Hemorrhage; thrombosis: deaths from intracranial events are most common in AML.

- **CV:** Pericardial hemorrhage

- **Pulmonary:** Hypoxia; pulmonary hemorrhage; respiratory failure

- **Metabolic:** Renal failure; hyperkalemia; hypocalcemia; hyperphosphatemia; hyperuricemia; life-threatening metabolic derangements are most frequent in ALL.

- **GI/Abdominal:** GI bleeding; splenic rupture; splenic rupture is most commonly a danger in CML.

---

leukostasis. End organ damage results from interaction between aggregates of leukemic blasts and injured epithelium. This interaction leads to tissue hypoxia with resultant release of inflammatory cytokines. Myeloblasts are more apt to cause damage due to their larger size and increased adhesiveness. Aggressive supportive care and prompt initiation of cytoreductive chemotherapy reduces the risk of early death in these patients.

Presentation and Management. Signs and symptoms of HL are listed in **Box 9.7.6**. Supportive care is directed at correction and prevention of metabolic abnormalities and coagulopathies. Cranial radiation is of no proven benefit and is not routinely employed. Leukapheresis and exchange transfusion may be considered as temporizing measures however after pheresis the blast count will rise again. Initiation of effective cytoreductive therapy remains critical. Initial imaging and laboratory studies obtained in

Box 9.7.6 Signs and Symptoms of Hyperleukocytosis			
Neurologic:		**Respiratory:**	**Other:**
• Seizure	• Coma	• Dyspnea	• Priapism
• Headache	• Stroke	• Hypoxia	• Dactylitis
• Blurred vision	• Papilledema	• Acidosis	• Clitoral
• Altered mental status	• Retinal artery or vein distension	• Cyanosis	enlargement

HL are listed in **Box 9.7.7** and initial supportive therapies are listed in **Box 9.7.8**.

Neutropenia and Fever. Pediatric oncology patients receiving chemotherapy frequently present with fever in the setting of neutropenia. Clinically significant neutropenia is defined as an absolute neutrophil count (ANC) <500–$1000/\mu L$ that is expected to decline due to recent chemotherapy administration. Those with an ANC

Box 9.7.7   Initial Imaging and Laboratory Studies in the Setting of Hyperleukocytosis

• Peripheral blood for flow cytometry
• Coagulation studies (PT, PTT, Fibrinogen)
• Urea nitrogen, creatinine, potassium, phosphorus, calcium
• Uric acid
• Glucose-6-phosphate dehydrogenase (G6PD) deficiency screen (needed prior to administration of Rasburicase)
• CXR to R/O mediastinal mass

$<200/\mu L$ are particularly vulnerable. Fever in this population should be regarded as a sign of a potentially life-threatening infection, and empiric antibiotic treatment should be initiated without delay. It should also be noted that the absence of fever in a neutropenic patient with generalized malaise or with localizing signs or symptoms (*e.g.* abdominal pain) does not rule out infection. This is particularly true

---

Box 9.7.8   Initial Supportive Therapy in the Setting of Hyperleukocytosis

- Hydration: D_5 0.2% NaCl + $NaHCO_3$ 40 mEq/L at 3000 ml/m^2 per day. No supplemental potassium should be given in anticipation of TLS or renal insufficiency.
- Allopurinol 300 mg/m^2 divided TID.
- Consider administration of Rasburicase if patient is hyperuricemic and not G6PD deficient.
- Transfuse platelets if platelet count is < 25,000/μL.
- Correct other significant coagulopathies.
- Avoid transfusion of PRBCs if hemodynamically stable.

---

if the child is receiving steroids as a part of their treatment. Necessary laboratory studies are listed in **Box 9.7.9**.

Evaluation and Management. A thorough history and physical examination should be performed, with particular attention to potential sites of infection (oral lesions, perirectal tenderness, central venous access sites). Neutropenic patients do not have the ability to mount an inflammatory response to infection. As a result, the localizing signs and symptoms may be subtle (*e.g.* pneumonia may present with mild

---

Box 9.7.9   Febrile Neutropenia: Initial Laboratory Studies

- CBC
- Electrolytes, urea nitrogen, creatinine, calcium, magnesium, phosphorus.
- Blood cultures from a peripheral site, all ports of CVC access, A–line.
- Urinalysis, urine culture.
- CXR in the presence of respiratory signs or symptoms.
- Respiratory tract culture if possible.
- Culture any drainage at a CVC insertion site.
- Stool studies if diarrhea is present (consider bacterial, protozoal, C. difficile toxin and viral studies).
- Lumbar puncture if altered mental status or other symptoms or signs of meningitis are present.

respiratory symptoms, and may not have characteristic findings on examination or CXR). Any reported areas of discomfort should be pursued as potential sites of infection.

Neutropenic patients are at risk for both common and opportunistic infections, therefore the differential diagnosis is broad. Bacterial infection presents the most immediate risk to life. Appropriate cultures should be obtained before antibiotics whenever possible and broad spectrum antimicrobials should be instituted within 30 mins of presentation to a medical facility. The choice of initial antibiotic therapy is guided by institutional and community antibiotic resistance patterns, the presence of localizing signs and symptoms, and the type of chemotherapy that the patient has recently received. In some settings, antibacterial monotherapy will provide sufficient empiric coverage (**Box 9.7.10**); however, if the patient develops clinical sepsis or localizing signs are present,

---

Box 9.7.10   Frequently Chosen Antibiotics for Febrile Neutropenia*

- Broad spectrum: ceftazidime; cefepime; piperacillin-tazobactam; meropenem.
- Additional Gram-negative coverage: amikacin; gentamicin; tobramycin.
- Additional Gram-positive coverage: vancomycin.
- Additional anaerobic coverage: clindamycin; metronidazole.
- Atypical bacterial coverage: azithromycin; clarithromycin.

---

* See *Appendix, part 2, XII.*

additional coverage should be instituted (**Box 9.7.11**). Significant abdominal pain is a particularly ominous sign in the neutropenic patient, as it may indicate the onset of typhlitis (inflammation of cecum) that may be associated with infection.

Prolonged Febrile Neutropenia. The management of febrile neutropenic patients should be reassessed frequently; repeat imaging including CT scans of sinuses, chest, abdomen and pelvis may also be required. Antibiotic regimens should be altered as new clinical evidence becomes available. If fever persists beyond 72 hrs, obtain

> **Box 9.7.11 Indications for Specific Antimicrobial Therapy in Addition to Broad Spectrum Antibiotic**
>
> - **Clinical sepsis:** Broad spectrum antibiotic* + vancomycin + aminoglycoside
> - **High dose cytarabine chemotherapy** *or* mucositis *or* cellulitis *or* concern for CVC infection: Broad spectrum antibiotic + vancomycin
> - **Pulmonary Infiltrates:** Broad spectrum antibiotic + vancomycin + atypical antibacterial agent; if infiltrates are diffuse and hypoxia is present, consider treatment for *pneumocystis jiroveci* pneumonia (formerly, PCP)
> - **Abdominal Symptoms:** Broad spectrum antibiotic + vancomycin + aminoglycoside + metronidazole *or* clindamycin
> - **Perirectal lesions:** Broad spectrum antibiotic + vancomycin + metronidazole *or* clindamycin

* See Box 9.7.10.
** Predisposes to *viridians* streptococcal bacteremia.

appropriate cultures and consider empiric antifungal therapy (*Appendix, part 2, XII*). In the case of sinusitis or pneumonia attempts to obtain diagnostic fluid should be considered in a persistently ill child. In addition to bacterial and fungal infections, oncology patients with prolonged severe neutropenia are also at risk for viral infections (HSV, varicella, CMV) and infection with opportunistic organisms (PCP, toxoplasmosis). When the clinical picture is suggestive of a viral infection, empiric anti-viral therapy should be started. Antifungal and antiviral drugs are listed in **Box 9.7.12**.

Tumor Lysis Syndrome (TLS) is defined as the triad of hyperkalemia, hyperuricemia, and hyperphosphatemia. In conditions of rapid cell turnover, the release of intracellular chemicals (**Box 9.7.3**) may cause these metabolic derangements which cause further metabolic derangement (*e.g.* hypocalcemia), renal dysfunction, and cardiac dysrhythmia.

Presentation and Management. TLS may occur with any malignancy with rapid cell turnover and high tumor burden. It most commonly occurs in the setting of leukemia or high grade

Box 9.7.12   Key Points: Anti-Fungal and Anti-Viral Antibiotic Options

Antifungal agents:

- **Amphoteracin B Liposome:** Often employed as first line agent for presumed fungal infections in the febrile neutropenic patient. Effective against *Candida*, *Aspergillus* and *Cryptococcus*.
- **Triazoles:**

  ▶ Fluconazole: IV, PO; Excellent bioavailability with enteral administration; penetrates the CNS; active against yeasts (unicellular fungi) but inactive against molds (fungi with hyphae).

  ▶ Itraconazole: PO; Capsules require food and an acid pH for solubilization; commercially prepared solution should be given on an empty stomach but tolerates acid pH. Useful against *Aspergillus* (allergic bronchopulmonary aspergillosis), histoplasmosis, blastomycosis.

  ▶ Voriconazole: IV, PO. Use caution with IV preparation in renal insufficiency; inhibits cytochrome P450 34A.

  ▶ Posaconazole; PO; useful for fungal prophylaxis and oropharyngeal candidiasis not responsive to fluconazole or itraconazole.

- **Echinocandins:** Often effective for refractory *Candida* and *Aspergillus*

  ▶ Caspofungin
  ▶ Micafungin
  ▶ Anidulafungin

Antiviral agents:

- Acyclovir: active against HSV and varicella zoster virus
- Gancyclovir: active against CMV and HSV

lymphoma. Children with hyperuricemia or renal insufficiency at presentation are at particularly high risk. Evidence of tumor lysis may be present prior to the initiation of the chemotherapy or after the child receives corticosteroids. See **Box 9.7.14** for a guide to monitoring for/during TLS. Preventive strategies and treatment are outlined in **Box 9.7.15**. Conditions at highest risk for TLS include:

- ALL or AML with HL (WBC > 100,000/μL)
- Leukemia with massive lymphadenopathy and/or organomegaly

- T Cell ALL
- Infant Leukemia
- Burkitt Lymphoma
- Large Cell Lymphoma

Box 9.7.13 Intracellular Molecules That Leak Into Extracellular Space and Cause TLS

Nucleotides	Purines are metabolized to xanthine and then uric acid; uric acid is poorly soluble in water and can crystallize in renal tubules causing renal injury.
Phosphorus	Malignant cells contain more phosphorus than do normal cells. Upon cell lysis phosphorus concentrations saturate renal excretion mechanisms; calcium phosphate can precipitate in renal tubules once the [Calcium in mg/dL] × [Phosphorus in mg/dL] product exceeds 70 *i.e.* "acute nephrocalcinosis".
Potasssium	Rapid increase in serum levels may result in cardiac arrhythmias and death.
Protein	Byproduct of protein metabolism is urea and uremia develops.

Box 9.7.14 TLS: Laboratory Studies and Clinical Monitoring

- CBC, calcium, phosphate, magnesium, uric acid, urea nitrogen, creatinine, lactate dehydrogenase at presentation and then every 6–12 hrs depending on risk.
- Sequential vital signs.
- Strict assessment of intake and output.
- Body weight once to twice daily.
- Cardiorespiratory monitor with multi-lead ECG as needed for hyperkalemia (*e.g.* if K > 6 mEq/L look for wide QRS and peaked T waves).
- Close clinical evaluation for signs of hypocalcemia or renal failure.

Box 9.7.15   Prevention and Treatment of TLS

Delay cytolytic therapy (if possible) until prophylactic measures can be implemented (see "hydration therapy", "urinary alkalinization", "hyperuricemia" below). Use intravenous radiologic contrast agents with caution since these might precipitate renal failure

Hydration therapy	• **Administer IV fluid: D_5 0.2% NaCl + $NaHCO_3$ 40 mEq/L at 3000 mL/m²/day** • Urine output goal: ≥100 mL/m²/hour *OR* 3 mL/kg/hr (if body weight is < 10 kg) • Urine specific gravity goal ≤ 1.010 • Diuretics may be required (furosemide or mannitol) • Recent data suggest that alkalinization may not be as safe as use of Rasburicase (see below under Hyperuricemia) in patients at high risk for severe TLS.
Urinary (see IV fluid above)	• **Urine pH goal 6.5–7.5** to aid in excretion of uric acid. Note urine pH > 7.5 may increase precipitation of $CaPO_4$ and xanthine crystals • Adjust amount of $NaHCO_3$ in IV fluid to achieve urine pH and serum [sodium] goals

Hyperkalemia (*Hyperkalemia,* 6.2)	• Moderate and asymptomatic (≥6.0 mEql/L): **sodium polystyrene sulfonate orally**
	• Severe and/or symptomatic (> 7.0 mEq/L):
	  ▸ **Calcium gluconate 100–200 mg/kg IV**
	  ▸ **D_{25} (2 ml/kg) IV + regular insulin 0.1 units/kg IV**
	  ▸ **Dialysis** may be necessary

Hyperphosphatemia (*Hyperphosphatemia* 6.2)	• **Aluminum hydroxide 50–150 mg/kg/day divided every 4–6 hrs Adults: $Al(OH)_3$ 30–40 mL 3–4 times/day** • Dialysis or continuous renal replacement therapy may be necessary
Hyperuricemia (uric acid crystals form in renal tubules and distal collecting system and are associated with oliguria)	• **Allopurinol 300 mg/m² PO divided TID**: Decreases production of uric acid by inhibiting xanthine oxidase. If possible, start 12–24 hrs before induction of cytolytic therapy <center>*OR*</center>• **Urate oxidase (Rasburicase)**: Metabolizes uric acid. Should be considered in high risk situations; contraindicated in G6PD deficiency, pregnancy, and lactation. Alkalinization is not necessary when rasburicase is given.

Box 9.7.16   Differential Diagnosis of Abdominal Masses

Neonates

Renal
- Hydronephrosis
- Multicystic dysplastic kidney
- Mesoblastic nephroma
- Polycystic kidney disease
- Wilms' tumor
- Rhabdoid tumor

Pelvic
- Ovarian cyst
- Hydrocolpos
- Hydrometrocolpos
- Gastrointestinal duplication

Infants and Children

Retroperitoneal
- Neuroblastoma
- Wilms' tumor
- Renal sarcoma
- Lymphoma

Liver
- Hepatoblastoma
- Hemangioendothelioma
- Hepatocellular carcinoma
- Hamartoma
- Embryonal sarcoma

Gastrointestinal
- Mesenteric adenopathy secondary to lymphoma
- Fecal mass
- GIST (GI stromal tumor)

Pelvic
- Rhabdomyosarcoma
- Ovarian cysts
- Ovarian malignancies
- Teratomas

Other
- Omental or mesenteric cyst
- Hepatosplenomegaly secondary to an infiltrative process
- Desmoid Tumor

Malignant Abdominal Masses. An abdominal mass in childhood may represent organomegaly, congenital anomaly, or tumor. In the newborn period abdominal masses are most commonly benign congenital anomalies. Beyond the newborn period malignancies predominate (**Box 9.7.16**).

An abdominal mass may lead to organ dysfunction through a variety of means (**Box 9.7.17**). In extreme cases, abdominal compartment syndrome may develop (*e.g.* rapidly expanding abdominal Burkitt Lymphoma). Diagnostic studies are listed in **Boxes 9.7.18 and 9.7.19**.

Box 9.7.17   Potential Consequences of an Abdominal Mass

- Gastrointestinal: Obstruction; perforation; hemorrhage; intussusception.
- Genitourinary: Obstruction; renal insufficiency or failure; hypertension due to compression of renal vasculature or catecholamine release.
- Respiratory: Compromise due to increased intra-abdominal pressure.
- Cardiovascular: Lower body venous stasis due to compression of inferior vena cava.
- Metabolic: TLS, such as in abdominal lymphoma.

Box 9.7.18   Initial Laboratory and Imaging Studies for Evaluation of an Abdominal Mass

- CBC
- Electolytes
- Liver function tests
- Uric acid and LDH
- Urinalysis

- Imaging Studies, obtained in a step-wise fashion
  ▸ Abdominal plain films
  ▸ Ultrasound
  ▸ CT Scan with oral and IV contrast (if possible)
  ▸ MRI if needed for surgical approach

Box 9.7.19   Further Diagnostic Studies in Evaluation of an Abdominal Mass

- Adrenal Tumor — Urine homovanillic acid (HVA) and urine vanillylmandelic acid (VMA)
- Ovarian Lesions — Serum beta-human chorionic gonadotropin (βhCG); Alpha- fetoprotein(AFP); CA 125
- Liver mass — βhCG and AFP

Management should be directed at relieving acute complications such as renal failure, hypertension, or bleeding. If abdominal compartment syndrome is suspected bladder pressure monitoring may be helpful, and early surgical consultation is essential. Definitive treatment will depend upon the tissue diagnosis.

Chapter 10

Trauma and Burns

Unintentional injury accounts for more than half of all childhood deaths. Trauma is responsible for more deaths and severely disabling sequelae among patients aged 1–14 yrs than all other diseases combined. Approximately 70% of pediatric trauma deaths are due to traumatic brain injury (TBI); a majority of these are motor vehicle-related. Although far less common, thoracic trauma takes second place as a cause of traumatic death in children; these are also overwhelmingly automobile-related. Abdominal injuries are more common than thoracic injuries, and are less likely to result in death. The evolution of non-operative care for splenic and hepatic trauma (approximately 2/3 of abdominal injuries) has been highly successful, with over 90% of patients successfully managed non-operatively with intensive care monitoring.

10.1 Traumatic Brain Injury

Head trauma results in approximately 50,000–100,000 pediatric hospital admissions and 7000–9000 deaths per year, with nearly 30,000 children per year left permanently disabled. Injuries may be penetrating or blunt, with acceleration–deceleration injuries resulting in contusion and/or shear injuries. The insult of TBI derives not only from the primary, immediate tissue damage resulting from the injury but also from the secondary insults of ischemia and brain swelling. Severe TBI (GCS <9) shares some of the pathophysiologic features of ischemia, with its associated failure in oxygen delivery, brain

471

Box 10.1.1   Clinical Types of Traumatic Brain Injury

- Cerebral concussion: Altered mental status; +/– loss of consciousness; normal head CT.
- Mass lesions: Epidural and subdural hematomas (see text).
- Traumatic axonal injury (TAI): Direct shearing of blood vessels at the white/gray matter interface or a delayed result of axonal biochemical injury; sometimes called diffuse axonal injury (DAI).
- Brain contusions: Focal injury at the point of impact (an object strikes the brain; *coup* injury) and at the opposite side of the brain (where the brain strikes an object; *contrecoup* injury) may occur. In acceleration/deceleration injuries, "the object" may be the inner skull surface.
- Subarachnoid hemorrhage: Shearing of the pial vessels.

---

swelling and both necrotic and programmed modes of cell death. However, unlike the management of pure asphyxial injury, intracranial pressure (ICP) monitoring and goal-directed treatment of raised ICP has improved outcome in TBI and have become accepted standards. Rapid identification of neurosurgically remediable lesions is essential. Serial brain imaging studies are important for monitoring the evolution of injuries (**Box 10.1.1**).

Key Features and Pathophysiology in Acute TBI

- **Mass lesions** (with or without associated intraparenchymal injury; *Raised Intracranial Pressure, 5.5, **Fig. 5.5.5***):

  ▶ *Epidural hematoma* (EDH): a collection of blood between the dura and inner table of the calvarium; its classic appearance on CT scan is a convex-shaped hematoma between skull and brain that does not cross boundaries defined by dural attachments to sutures. It is rarely associated with birth trauma, and more commonly associated with low velocity impacts such as falls. Most common locations in children are frontal and parieto-occipital (*usually* arterial blood, and associated with linear skull fracture in 40–80% of cases) and the posterior fossa (*usually* venous blood).

▸ *Subdural hematoma* (SDH): A collection of blood in the potential space between the dura and arachnoid membranes; its classic appearance on CT scan is a concave or crescent-shaped hematoma; a SDH can cross suture lines but is contained by dural attachments at the falx cerebri and tentorium cerebelli. SDH may occur at birth, especially if assisted by forceps or vacuum extraction; this injury is typically asymptomatic. SDH in head injured infants and children is especially frequent among patients with non-accidental head trauma, but may occur in any injury generated by lateral or rotational forces causing shearing of veins that bridge the brain surface to the dural sinuses (*usually* fronto-parietal) or less commonly, from disruption of small cortical arteries (*usually* temporo-parietal). Over-drainage of CSF (traumatic or iatrogenic) may result in traction on bridging dural vessels leading to subdural bleeding.

▸ The clinical effects of both EDH and SDH reflect the location and size of the collection. Timely neurosurgical evaluation is critical for reversal of mass effect and avoidance of morbidity and mortality.

• **Contributors to secondary parenchymal injury:**

▸ Brain swelling may occur by multiple mechanisms (**Fig. 10.1.1**). Brain cell swelling may be more mediator-dependent than "cytotoxic" (*i.e.* failure of the cell membrane to exclude salt, other osmoles, and therefore water, from the intracellular compartment) in TBI.

▸ Ischemia, either locally due to interruption of blood supply (by direct interruption or mass effect) or globally from systemic causes (*e.g.* shock).

▸ Increased cerebral blood volume or cerebral hyperemia: its importance is uncertain.

▸ Cell death may occur immediately (by necrosis) and/or by programmed cell death (PCD, apoptosis) which is cell protein regulated (*Hypoxic-Ischemic Encephalopathy, 5.3*).

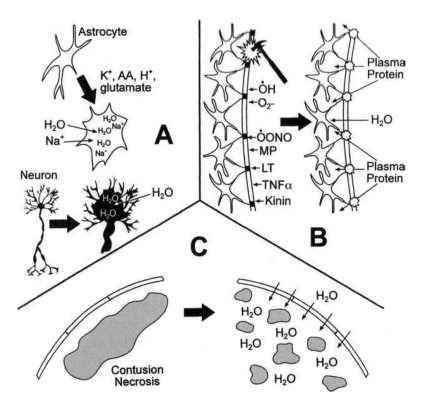

Fig. 10.1.1.   Pathophysiologic Factors in TBI. A, Mediator-driven brain cell swelling (*e.g.* glutamate, K+, acidosis and arachadonic acid-mediated astrocyte swelling). B, Leakage of intravascular contents through a damaged blood-brain barrier (tight junctions between brain capillary endothelial cells formed by astrocyte foot processes). Vascular integrity may be disrupted by direct trauma or by biochemical injury from free radicals, proteases, kinins, leukotrienes and cytokines. C, Osmotically-driven swelling in areas of contusion necrosis: necrotic tissue decomposes to constituent molecules; re-formation of an osmotic barrier around these areas leads to local edema. Redrawn with permission from Kochanek PM, Clark SB, Ruppel RA, Dixon CE, Cerebral resuscitation after traumatic brain injury and cardiopulmonary arrest in infants and children in the new millennium, in Orlowski JP (ed.), *Pediatr Clin N Amer* **48**(3):664, 2001.

Evaluation and Management Strategies. Urgent neurosurgical evaluation should be obtained for patients with focal neurologic findings, signs of raised ICP, penetrating injuries or epidural or subdural hemorrhage. Head CT scan should be obtained as soon as feasible.

- Attention to airway, breathing and circulation: Assess vital signs and monitor pulse oximetry. Hypoxemia, hypercarbia and hypotension (a late sign of shock) exacerbate secondary brain injury; these should be prevented or, if present, reversed. The presence of hypotension on admission is reported to increase mortality by nearly 60%. Signs of shock should be corrected before development of hypotension whenever possible. Prevention of these complicating disturbances should be a continuous part of on-going care.

- Do not use the nasal route for ETT's, enteric or other tubes in the presence of a possible basilar skull fracture.

- Protect the cervical spine as indicated until C-spine injury can be ruled out (*Spinal Cord Injury, 10.2*).

- Assess the neurologic status. Note pupillary reactivity, extraocular movements, brainstem reflexes, response to pain and DTR's. Identify signs of raised ICP. Patients with GCS ≤8 should be tracheally intubated.

- Optimize oxygen delivery: maintain optimal O_2 saturation (>95%) and hemoglobin (~10 gms/dL in severe TBI) and ensure an adequate mean arterial blood pressure (MAP) which is critical for maintenance of cerebral perfusion pressure (CPP) in face of an elevated ICP (CPP = MAP − ICP). The *usual* goal for CPP is 40–50 for infants and toddlers, 50–60 in children, >60–70 for adolescents and >70 for adults.

- Keep head mid-line to ensure unimpeded venous drainage from the intracranial compartment and head of bed elevated ~30° if no contraindications are present (*Spinal Cord Injury, 10.2*).

- Avoid hyper- and hypo-carbia; usual goal for $PaCO_2$ is 35–40 mmHg.

- Seizure activity increases O_2 consumption and worsens secondary injury. Treat seizure activity; identify non-convulsive status epilepticus by EEG if indicated. Empiric anticonvulsants are warranted in patients with severe TBI.

- Provide analgesia and sedation as needed; pain and anxiety may increase cerebral O_2 consumption. Avoid agents that adversely affect blood pressure. Opiates/opioids (*e.g.* morphine, fentanyl) and benzodiazepines (*e.g.* midazolam, if tolerated) are among agents frequently chosen for the pediatric age group. In patients without an ICP monitor, take care to avoid distortion of the neurologic examination by sedative drugs.

- Avoid hypo-osmolality by use of isotonic solutions (*e.g.* NaCl 0.9%) and by serial monitoring of serum sodium for evidence of antidiuretic hormone excess, cerebral salt wasting and diabetes insipidus.
- Avoid hyperglycemia: *Usual* goal for glucose in brain-injured pediatric patients is 80–150 mg/dL.
- Correct coagulopathy; severe TBI may result in disseminated intravascular coagulation. For patients with intracranial blood or an ICP monitor, the *usual* goal is an INR < 1.3 and platelets >50 K/μL.
- Control temperature: Even low-grade fever may increase ICP; fever and hyperthermia are associated with exacerbation of secondary injury and poor outcome. The role for therapeutic hypothermia is not yet defined.
- Indications for placement of an ICP monitor (*Appendix, part 2, X*):
  ▸ Abnormal head CT with GCS ≤ 8
  ▸ Anticipated increased ICP
  ▸ Inability to obtain accurate serial neurologic examinations
  ▸ Unavailability of timely neuroimaging
  ▸ Need for osmotherapy (mannitol; NaCl 3%) to treat raised ICP (*Raised Intracranial Pressure, 5.5*)
- CSF drainage (*Hydrocephalus and CSF diversion, 11.2.2*): The external ventricular drain provides accurate measurements of ICP as well as the capability of CSF removal to help relieve raised ICP.
- Barbiturate coma (*Raised ICP, 5.5*).
- Decompressive craniectomy: Surgical creation of a cranial defect (an artificial fontanel) to allow for swelling while preserving blood flow. Patient selection is individualized; reported outcomes are varied.
- Jugular venous bulb O_2 saturation ($SjvO_2$): A fiberoptic catheter with its port accurately positioned at the jugular bulb (at the skull base) permits measurement of O_2 saturation of blood as it leaves the brain (normal, 60–80%). Globally increased cerebral O_2 consumption (as seen in seizure and fever) or inadequate O_2 delivery result in a decreased $SjvO_2$ (< 50%).

- Transcranial Doppler allows for serial regional assessments of cerebral blood flow; this technique, most commonly applied to the middle cerebral artery, measures flow velocity and is limited by difficulties in obtaining adequate visualization through the bony skull, its restriction to assessment of relatively large vessels and difficulties with consistency from study to study.
- Serial images of the brain should be repeated as needed to re-assess evolving injuries. Some patients (*e.g.* those with traumatic axonal injury or hypoxic-ischemic injury) may have normal CT scans initially; any deterioration in mental status, neurologic findings or ICP should be re-evaluated. Head CT identifies surgically remediable lesions is usually easy to obtain and can be completed quickly; even unstable patients can be imaged with resuscitation in progress. Magnetic resonance imaging (MRI) offers greater detail, and a more definitive view of the posterior fossa; imaging takes much longer, and patient accessibility is limited.
- The differential diagnoses of severe TBI are listed in **Box 10.1.2**.

Post-TBI Paroxysmal Autonomic Instability with Dystonia (*PAID*; **Box 10.1.3**) occurs in up to one-third of patients with severe TBI and traumatic diffuse axonal injury (as graded by the Rancho Los Amigos Scale, level ≤ IV, **Box 10.1.4**). Episodes usually begin 5–7 days after injury, occur 1–3 times/day, last 1–10 hrs and recur for weeks to months. Dysfunction of control centers (diencephalon, periaqueductal gray substance, lateral parabrachial nucleus, rostral ventricular medulla) or connections of the diencephalon to cortical,

---

Box 10.1.2 Differential Considerations in "R/O TBI" or "R/O Head Trauma"

- Coagulopathy
- Osteogenesis imperfecta
- Benign extra-axial fluid of infancy
- Subdural collections secondary to infection
- Glutaric aciduria type I
- Rupture of arachnoid cyst with subdural bleeding

Box 10.1.3   Post-TBI Paroxysmal Autonomic Instability with Dystonia (PAID)*

PAID is defined by the presence of four or more of the following:
- Fever (> 38.3°C)
- Tachycardia
- Hypertension
- Tachypnea
- Excessive diaphoresis
- Extensor posturing or severe dystonia

---

*Rabinstein AA, Benarroch EE, *Current Treatment Options in Neurology*, 10:151–157, 2008.

Box 10.1.4   Rancho Los Amigos Scale

Level	Descriptive
I	Unresponsive; in deep sleep.
II	Generalized response: inconsistent, non-purposeful and non-specific.
III	Localized response: specific (*e.g.* turn head toward sound or focus on object; follow simple command) but inconsistent.
IV	Confused, agitated, heightened activity, disoriented; may perform automatic motor skills (sitting, reaching, walking) but not purposefully.
V	Confused and inappropriate; responsive to simple commands but agitated and confused with more complex commands; highly distracted and has difficulty learning.
VI	Confused but appropriate; performs goal directed behaviors after cuing; can remember old skills but no recent memory; emerging awareness of self and others.
VII	Purposeful and appropriate; alert, oriented; able to recall past and recent events; able to learn new activities; deficits in stress tolerance, judgment, abstract reasoning, social skills, and intellect may persist.

subcortical and brainstem loci that mediate vegetative control mechanisms may contribute to elevated blood pressure, heart rate, respiratory rate and temperature. Rigidity, seen experimentally with lesions of the midbrain, is a typical feature.

Management Principles of PAID: (1) Exclude infection and other potential causes (**Box 10.1.5**); (2) treat seizures if these are suspected; (3) treat pain as needed; (4) avoid external or internal triggers such as pain, bladder distension, manipulation of bladder catheters, repositioning; (5) ensure adequate hydration to compensate for diaphoresis; and (6) pharmacologic treatment (**Box 10.1.6**).

Box 10.1.5   Differential Diagnosis of PAID

- Neuroleptic malignant syndrome (NMS): Occurs in 1% of patients receiving dopamine receptor blockers (*e.g.* metoclopramide) or withdrawal of levodopa, carbidopa and amantidine (*Drug-Induced Toxic Hyperthermic Syndromes, 13.3*).
- Malignant hyperthermia (MH): Associated with inhalational anesthethics or depolarizing muscle relaxants (*Drug-Induced Toxic Hyperthermic Syndromes, 13.3*).
- Diencephalic seizures: Hypo- or hyperthermia and sweating are common; associated with tumors or entrapment of the 3rd ventricle, diencephalic tumors, agenesis of the corpus callosum and suprasellar arachnoid cysts; responsive to anticonvulsants.
- Autonomic dysreflexia: Occurs after spinal cord injury above T-8. Noxious stimuli below T-8 cause uncontrolled sympathetic discharge: ↑ BP, headache, flushing and sweating of upper trunk and face.
- Agitation, extensor posturing and thrashing without PAID: May occur after emergence from coma; ↑BP and ↑ temperature are not present; if purposeful movements are present during episodes of agitation, PAID is not present.
- Seizures
- Narcotic withdrawal
- Hydrocephalus (or other causes of ↑ ICP) which may trigger PAID
- Cushing response: Associated with bradycardia, irregular breathing and brainstem disruption on MRI

Box 10.1.6 Pharmacologic Treatment of PAID

- **Morphine and β-blockers** are the mainstays of treatment. These should be administered as soon as episodes of PAID begin and will need to be continued for days to weeks before tapering is possible.

  ▸ **Morphine** may abort episodes of PAID probably by analgesic action and modulation of central pathways. Monitor for interactions with benzodiazepines and barbiturates.

  ▸ **Propranolol** is highly lipophylic and penetrates the blood-brain barrier more efficiently than most other β-blockers. Use cautiously with clonidine or verapamil (may produce A-V block) or lidocaine (co-administration with propranolol may increase lidocaine levels and depress myocardial function).

- **Clonidine** is an α_2-receptor agonist with central and peripheral effects. It is most effective in mitigating hypertension and tachycardia. See warnings regarding concomitant use of propranolol and clonidine. Tricyclic antidepressants (TCA) may decrease the antihypertensive effects of clonidine. Monitor for excessive hypotension between episodes of PAID. Cyclosporine toxicity may be increased with clonidine usage. Hypertension may occur with abrupt withdrawal from clonidine.

- **Bromocryptine** is a dopamine (D_2) agonist. Its effect is modest and delayed. It is contraindicated in uncontrolled hypertension. Bromocryptine may decrease the seizure threshold and may increase levels of cyclosporine, sirolimus, and tacrolimus.

- **Baclofen** is a $GABA_B$ agonist given enterally or intrathecally. It has been effective in selective refractory cases. Baclofen IT inhibits transmission of spinal reflexes without cerebral effects; it should not be given in the presence of spinal cord injury because of possible autonomic dysreflexia. Acute baclofen withdrawal may produce a clinical syndrome compatible with PAID. Simultaneous TCA usage may produce confusion or excess hypotonia. Monitor for elevation in liver enzymes, bronchial hyper-reactivity, excess weakness or sedation.

- **Benzodiazepines** (lorezepam, midazolam and diazepam) bind to $GABA_A$ receptors and presumably act as muscle relaxants. Monitor for sedation, hypotension and respiratory depression.

(Continued)

Box 10.1.6   Pharmacologic Treatment of PAID (Continued)

- **Gabapentin** is structurally similar to GABA but it does not influence GABA receptors; its mechanism of action is unclear. It is most often used for mild dysautonomic symptoms, but may be used if other agents have failed.
- **Dantrolene** interferes with release of calcium from the sarcoplasmic reticulum and may help decrease severe dystonic posturing. Its CNS depressive effects are additive with other CNS depressants. Monitor liver enzymes before and during therapy.

Warning: Dopamine antagonists (*e.g.* chlorpromazine and haloperidol) worsen PAID and should be avoided.

10.2 Spinal Cord Injury (SCI)

SCI is uncommon among pediatric patients, who account for approximately 10% of all victims of spinal cord trauma. SCI remains a costly event for families and society. Nearly half of these patients suffer a complete cord injury, and nearly 60% of cord-injured patients are quadriplegic. Cervical spine (C-spine) injury occurs in 1–2% of pediatric blunt trauma victims, and is largely related to motor vehicle accidents. Because of its particularly devastating nature, injury of the C-spine is a focus of this discussion, but SCI in general is addressed. Early recognition of these injuries is essential for optimal outcome. If acute recovery is achieved, productive survival into the sixth to seventh decades is attainable.

Anatomic differences in children < 8 yrs as compared to adults predispose to injury of the upper cervical spinal cord by contributing to hypermobility and susceptibility to high torque forces of the C-spine:

- A relatively large head, weaker cervical musculature and greater ligamentous laxity of the C-spine.
- Anterior wedging of vertebral bodies is noted more frequently after trauma in developing children than in adults.

- Flattened facet joints, particularly from C1–C4, allow slippage of vertebral bodies across each other in the axial plane.
- Children are predisposed to fractures at the vertebral body growth plates (these centers are more susceptible to sheer) and ligamentous injuries.
- The greater elasticity of the spinal column compared with the spinal cord may result in difficult to detect injuries. SCI in children may not be associated with spine fracture in ~10–20% of patients; depending on the study, 4–66% of spinal cord injuries present without radiographic abnormality on plain films or CT scan (SCIWORA; also see **Box 10.2.1**). If a C-spine fracture is present there is a 10% chance of an additional fracture along the spine.

Mechanisms of injury and associated fractures are described in **Box 10.2.1**. The C-spine should be treated as if it were injured in all patients with known or suspected trauma; spine precautions should be in place prior to evaluation of the entire spine (**Box 10.2.2**). Typically, a cervical collar is applied and the patient is placed on a backboard until a spine injury can be ruled out. These devices provide adequate stabilization of the spine during extrication and transportation. Upon arrival to the hospital, the child should be removed from the backboard immediately to prevent skin breakdown; placing the child supine on a padded stretcher or bed provides adequate stabilization of the fractured spine.

The collar should be left in place until the child's cervical spine is evaluated and cleared from injury. Similarly, the thoracic and lumbar spine should be maintained in an aligned fashion until clearance can be obtained. The child should be "log-rolled" until thoracic and lumbar spine stability is determined. Approximately 50% of children with C-spine injury have neurologic deficits; if neurologic deficits are present, SCI should be assumed even if the radiologic evaluation is normal. Classic features are pain, muscle spasm and decreased range of motion of the spine; paresthesias or paresis may be present. The mechanism of injury is historically important and a high index of suspicion is warranted to diagnose and care for these injuries in pediatric patients (**Boxes 10.2.3–10.2.5**).

Box 10.2.1   Mechanisms of Cervical Spinal Cord Injury and Associated Fractures*

- Axial loading (vertical compression)

  Typically, a direct blow to the head along the vertical axis; compression fractures (*e.g.* C1 injury); burst fractures result from axial loading which drives the intervertebral disk into the vertebral body below; usually results in a fracture through the vertebral body. Portions of the vertebral body or the disk can herniate into the spinal cord.

- Flexion

  Most common injuries of the C-spine; rupture of posterior ligaments may be followed by injury in a posterior to anterior direction, resulting in anterior subluxation, compression (wedge fractures of the anterior vertebral body) and facet dislocation.

- Hyper-extension

  Rapid anterior to posterior force ("whiplash"). May cause compression of the posterior elements and stretch of the anterior longitudinal ligament. Atlas avulsion fracture most common; lamia and pillar fractures are also seen. Hangman's fracture involves the posterior neural arch of C1 or the pedicles of C2 from compression by the occiput.

  C2 fractures of the dens comprise three fracture types. Type I is an avulsion fracture of the tip of the dens. Type II fractures through the dens and Type III is a fracture through the base of the dens extending into the vertebral body.

- Dislocation

  Less common than other injury types; results from rotational force. May affect vascular structures; typically unstable and may require stabilization.

  Atlanto-Occipital Dissociation (AOD) is a disruption of the ligamentous attachments between the skull base and first cervical vertebra. Stretching of the spinal cord results in neurological deficit.

*Fractures of the transverse processes are usually minor and do not cause SCI. Spinal cord injury without radiographic abnormality (SCIWORA) is usually detectable by MRI.

Box 10.2.2   Evaluation of Patients with Known or Suspected Spine/Spinal Cord Injury

- Perform the Primary Survey for all trauma patients (*Appendix, part 2, VII; General Approach to the Critically Ill Child, 1.2*) and intervene as indicated (**Box 10.2.3**).
- Vital signs: Relative bradycardia with hypotension suggests neurogenic shock with an injury above T6–8; this results from unopposed vagal stimulation.
- Neurologic assessment for disability:

  ▸ GCS (*Altered Mental Status, 5.1; Box 5.1.3*)
  ▸ Assess muscle group function (*e.g.* wiggle fingers/toes). If deficits are identified, check:

    ▪ Dorsiflexion of the wrist (C6), extension of the elbow (C7), extension of the knee (L2–4) and dorsiflexion of the great toe (L5)
    ▪ Strength and drift.
    ▪ Flaccidity suggests lower motor neuron or spinal cord injury.

  ▸ Sensory: Pinprick sensation, joint proprioception; determine presence of a sensory level. Sacral sparing can indicate an incomplete spinal cord lesion. Isolated sensory deficits are the most common findings in patients with C-spine injury.
  ▸ Reflexes:

    ▪ Spontaneous respiration: Difficulties suggest a lesion at or above C4.
    ▪ Abdominal: Absence suggests injury at or above T1–12.
    ▪ Babinski: First toe dorsiflexes and fanning of toes suggests upper motor neuron lesion.
    ▪ Cremasteric: Absent with lesions at or above L1–2.
    ▪ Bulbocavernosus: Tension on a bladder catheter or pressure on the glans penis normally results in contraction of the anal sphincter. Absence confirms SCI above S2–4.
    ▪ Priapism: Results from unopposed parasympathetic stimulation; suggests a lesion of the sympathetic chain above T6–8. Usually seen in complete cord injury.
    ▪ Rectal tone: A ↓ suggests a lesion at or above S2–S4.
    ▪ Absence of deep tendon reflexes (usually lasing < 24 hrs) is classic for spinal cord injury below the level affected.

Box 10.2.3   Management of Known or Suspected Spinal Cord Injury

- Assume SCI until this is ruled out by mechanism of injury, physical examination and/or radiologic evaluation.
- Remove the patient from the backboard as soon as possible; maintain cervical immobilization with an appropriate cervical collar and logroll the patient when necessary until the spine is fully evaluated and known to be intact ("cleared;" **Box 10.2.4**).
- Emergency resuscitation:

  ▸ Avoid hypoxia, hypercarbia and hypotension.

  ▸ C-spine precautions should be taken in airway management in all instances in which C-spine injury is not ruled out (*Bag-Mask Ventilation and Tracheal Intubation, 15.2*).

  ▸ If neurogenic shock (hypotension and bradycardia due to SCI) is present, central venous and arterial access is indicated.

  ▸ Volume resuscitation with isotonic fluid should be followed by vasoactive support (dopamine or norepinephrine) when indicated to restore normal perfusion and blood pressure in the high-normal range. Phenylephrine should be used with caution because of associated bradycardia.

  ▸ Blood and blood products should be given as indicated (*Shock, 3.5*).

  ▸ Decompress the stomach (gastric tube) and the bladder (urinary catheter).

- Consider prophylaxis against deep venous thrombosis for patients >8 yrs or with an adult size body habitus

  ▸ Sequential compression devices

  ▸ Low molecular weight heparin (after timing of potential surgical intervention is determined).

  ▸ Inferior vena cava filter: If the patient has an adult habitus, placement of a temporary IVC filter may be considered. This device is typically removed when the threat of DVT is sufficiently remote or when anticoagulation is safe.

(Continued)

Box 10.2.3   Management of Known or Suspected Spinal Cord Injury (Continued)

- Steroids: There are no level 1 data to recommend their use in children.
  - ▶ High dose methylprednisolone has been used with equivocal results but remains a treatment option. If given, early administration may convey some benefit:
    - Give methylprednisolone 30 mg/kg IV over 45 mins within THREE HOURS of injury.
    - Follow by methylprednisolone 5.4 mg/kg/hr for 23 hrs.
- Maintain normothermia and avoid increased body temperature by use of antipyretics and/or cooling.
- H-2 blocker or PPI prophylaxis is recommended even if steroids are not given.
- Obtain neurosurgical or spine surgery consultation.
- Consider use of a specialty bed that provides rotational, kinetic therapy and/or a mattress suited for long-term skin-care.
- Consult rehabilitation medicine for long-term planning and goals.
- Consult physical and occupational therapy for splinting to prevent wrist and foot drop, if indicated, and for range of motion exercises.
- Address nutritional support needs.
- Provide a bowel regimen to minimize ileus, and to prevent constipation and bowel obstruction.

SCI evolves in a manner similar to traumatic brain injury; the primary injury is the direct result of traumatic forces; secondary injury due to ischemia, hypoxia, inflammation, excitotoxicity, ion disturbances and apoptosis ensues over the first 8–12 hrs following SCI. Spinal cord edema maximizes between the third and sixth day post-injury. It is this process of secondary injury which can be favorably altered by meticulous critical care.

Box 10.2.4   Approach to "Clearance" of the C-Spine and Spinal Cord Following Injury

- For patients >8 yrs using data from the National X-Radiography Use Study Group (NEXUS Trial), all the following must be present to R/O C-spine injury at the bedside:

  ▶ Normal level of consciousness and absence of drug-induced alterations in mental status.
  ▶ No painful distracting injury.
  ▶ No focal neurologic deficit.
  ▶ No tenderness of the C-spine (see below).

  For those >8 yrs, if none of the above is present, clinical clearance of the C-spine can be accomplished without radiologic study provided there are no signs or symptoms suggesting spine injury.

- For patients <8 yrs or those unable to be "cleared clinically" (as above), obtain CT scan with multiplanar reformatting capabilities of the entire C-spine. If the scan is negative and there is no evidence of neurological deficit, the collar can be removed. If the patient is comatose, has signs of neurological deficits or significant bone pain on palpation, an MRI should be obtained to assess the integrity of the spinal cord and ligamentous attachments.

- To evaluate the C-spine for tenderness/injury at the bedside in relatively low-risk patients:

  ▶ The C-collar may be removed for examination of the neck.
  ▶ Palpate the spinous processes for tenderness, muscle spasm, or deformity/"step-off".
  ▶ Ask the patient to rotate the chin slowly toward each shoulder.
  ▶ Ask the patient to touch each ear to its ipsilateral shoulder.
  ▶ Ask the patient to touch chin to chest.

  If no pain is encountered, the cervical collar may be discontinued. If pain is encountered at any step, the cervical collar should be replaced and further radiologic evaluation should proceed.

(Continued)

Box 10.2.4   Approach to "Clearance" of the C-Spine and Spinal Cord Following Injury (Continued)

• If C-spine injury is suspected, radiologic imaging should be obtained.

▸ Plain radiographs (AP, cross-table lateral and odontoid views): Include the C7–T1 junction. Overall sensitivity from infancy to adulthood for C-spine injury is ~90%. These images pose interpretation-related difficulties in children due to the greater incidence of avulsion and epiphyseal separation injuries, the normal absence of cervical lordosis and the variations in appearances such as pseudosubluxation in the pediatric age group.

▸ If three-view plain films are non-revealing, flexion and extension views may identify C-spine instability and ligamentous injury, but these require active flexion and extension (patient cooperation) with the ability to stop the maneuver if pain occurs. Passive positioning or motion beyond the point of pain may cause or worsen spinal cord injury. The practitioner should be in attendance for performance of these views.

▸ CT scan: Radiation exposure (esp. thyroid) constitutes a risk. CT should be reserved for patients who have inadequate or abnormal plain films of the C-spine or for those with normal plain films but a high clinical suspicion of C-spine injury. These images should permit reformatting in different planes for review.

▸ MRI: Modality of choice for patients with neurologic symptoms or signs and normal plain films; optimal for assessment of ligamentous injury and does not confer the risk of radiation. MRI identifies most (previously designated) instances of SCIWORA.

Box 10.2.5   Approach to "Clearance" of the Thoracic and Lumbar Spine

- Attempt clinical clearance by
  - ▶ Assessment for pain on palpation
  - ▶ Noting any external signs of injury or palpable deformity ("step-offs")
  - ▶ If the examination is normal, spine injury may be excluded clinically.
- If clinical clearance is not possible or if suspicion of spine injury is present, image the spine.
  - ▶ If the patient has already had CT scan of the chest and/or abdomen, images of the spine may be reformatted for review.
  - ▶ If CT is not available, 2-view plain films of the spine should be obtained to R/O fracture.
  - ▶ If a fracture is not identified and there are no neurologic deficits, the spine may be "cleared."
  - ▶ If suspicion of spine injury persists because of symptoms, MRI should be considered.

10.3 Thoracic Trauma

Pediatric thoracic trauma accounts for 4–25% of pediatric injuries, and results from both blunt (85%) and penetrating (15%) mechanisms. Isolated penetrating thoracic trauma in children has a 5% mortality rate. The anatomy of children differs from that of adults; some differences that contribute to pediatric morbidity and mortality associated with chest trauma include:

- A shorter, narrower, and more compressible trachea make needle cricothyroidotomy more difficult. Right mainstem intubation and accidental extubation are more likely.
- A more compliant chest wall (rib fractures are uncommon in younger children) which transmits energy to underlying structures more readily.

- A mobile mediastinum is more susceptible to the thoracic pressure changes. Diminisihed venous return may be caused by a tension pneumothorax causing obstructive shock.

Box 10.3.1   Evaluation of the Pediatric Patient with Suspected Chest Trauma

- Attention to Airway, Breathing, Circulation, Disability (neurologic status) and Environmental issues are fundamental to the primary survey (*Appendix, part 2, VII; General Approach to the Critically Ill Child, 1.2*).
- Inspect the thorax. Note specifically lacerations, bruises, penetrating wounds, flail chest (paradoxical motion of the chest wall due to fractured ribs and loss of chest wall rigidity), abdominal breathing or other signs of respiratory distress, asymmetry of chest wall motion and tracheal deviation.
- Listen for equality and adequacy of breath sounds.
- Palpate and auscultate the chest for crepitus (grating, popping or snapping sounds and sensations related to subcutaneous emphysema which may indicate rib fractures or air leak syndromes). Do not repeat palpation if pain is elicited.
- An upright (if possible) AP CXR should be obtained once the back-board is removed. If there is penetrating trauma, external wounds should be marked with radio-opaque markers to help delineate missile trajectory.
- Fracture of a first rib may be a marker for significant vascular injury.
- Chest CT is helpful in diagnosis of occult pneumothorax, mediastinal injury and in determination of missile trajectory in penetrating trauma.
- Angiography for an aortic arch injury is indicated:
  - If the chest CT scan is equivocal for a vascular injury
  - Prior to possible endovascular repair
  - When another vascular injury is suspected or identified and angiography is performed, the aorta should be evaluated as well.

Box 10.3.2   Immediately Life-threatening Thoracic Injuries

Injury	Clinical Findings	Interventions
Tension pneumothorax (PTX)	Air compresses the heart ($\downarrow$s venous return) causing jugular venous distension (JVD) and eventually cardiovascular collapse. The trachea deviates away from the side of PTX and breath sounds are $\downarrow$ on the affected side.	Needle decompression with an 18–20 G needle in the 5th intercostal space, mid-axillary line (to avoid pulmonary artery puncture in children <10 yrs); use a 14 G catheter-over-needle in the same location for the larger child. [An imaginary line drawn from the nipple posteriorly (in the transverse plane) to the mid-axillary line usually identifies the 4th intercostal space.]
Cardiac tamponade	May present with hypotension, muffled heart sounds and JVD (Beck's triad)	Pericardiocentesis or operative drainage and repair of any accompanying heart injury.
Hemothorax	Chest tube yields ≥ 15 ml/ kg blood or drainage is ≥ 2–3 ml/kg per hr for ≥ 3 hrs	Operative exploration/ intervention
Aortic injury	May diagnose with CT scan, trans-esophageal USG or aortogram.	Non-operative therapy: β blockade Operative repair: thoracotomy or endovascular stenting, depending on proper graft sizing.

Steps in evaluation of thoracic injury are outlined in **Box 10.3.1**; immediately life-threatening and potentially life-threatening chest injuries are listed in **Boxes 10.3.2 and 10.3.3**. Management is outlined in **Box 10.3.4**.

Box 10.3.3   Potentially Life-threatening Thoracic Injuries

Injury	Clinical Findings	Interventions
Pulmonary contusion*	Hypoxia, ↑work of breathing	Chest PT (rotational and/or percussive; the latter is contraindicated in certain injuries including flail chest, rib fractures); supplemental O_2 and deep breathing maneuvers, avoid fluid overload.
Small pneumothorax	Chest pain, atelectasis, hypoxia	Small bore chest tube in mid-axillary line and angle tube anteriorly; place drainage system at minus 20 cm H_2O.
Rib fractures	Uncommon but present in ~20% of cases of nonaccidental trauma.	Treat underlying injuries (*e.g.* pneumothorax or hemothorax) if present.
Traumatic asphyxia	Petechiae cephalad to nipple line (compression of thorax with a closed glottis**).	Elevate head of bed; provide supplemental O_2 (*Hypoxic-Ischemic Encephalopathy, 5.3*).
Blunt cardiac injury[†]	Although rare, dysrthymias may occur.	Consider 24 hr heart rhythm monitoring and/or USG to assess valve and wall motion dysfunction.

*Most common pediatric chest injury.
**The heart is compressed and blood flow temporarily reverses in the SVC causing capillaries to rupture (petechiae).
[†]The heart may be injured when compressed between the sternum and spine.

Box 10.3.4   Management of Thoracic Trauma

- Support airway and breathing:

  ‣ Provide supplemental O_2; early tracheal intubation should be considered; a surgical airway is rarely required.

  ‣ Strategize to prevent atelectasis and evacuate secretions; usually most effectively accomplished with tracheal intubation except with relatively minor injuries. Ventilator care should incorporate strategies to minimize barotrauma, volutrauma and oxygen toxicity (*e.g.* tidal volumes ~6 ml/kg, with aggressive use of PEEP to achieve goal FiO_2 <0.5. HFV may be indicated in severe lung injuries. Independent lung ventilation is a consideration in the older child with unilateral lung injury and severe hypoxemia.

  ‣ For non-intubated patients, incentive spirometry should be instituted as soon as possible.

  ‣ Chest tube (CT) placement is indicated when:

    ▪ Pneumothorax >10% of the volume of the hemithorax
    ▪ Subcutaneous air with evidence of rib fractures after trauma
    ▪ Hemodynamic instability with evidence of a hemothorax on CXR
    ▪ CXR with opacification of hemithorax and without evidence of lobar collapse; this is consistent with hemothorax. A large bore tube (to drain blood clot) is indicated.
    ▪ The patient is receiving positive pressure ventilation and it is felt that pneumothorax will likely increase in size with this support. Placement of a CT for an occult pneumothorax (present on CT but not visible on plain film) during PPV is controversial.

- Support the cardiovascular system. Two large bore peripheral IV's and/or central venous access should be secured. Intraosseous access may be necessary as emergently indicated.

  ‣ Pericardiocentesis should be performed if cardiac tamponade is present or strongly suspected.

  ‣ Support the circulation with isotonic fluids beginning with NaCl 0.9% 20 ml/kg, to a maximum of 50 ml/kg preferably followed by blood products (PRBC 10 ml/kg) as indicated. Monitor HR, perfusion, BP, urine output and serum lactic acid as indicators of circulatory sufficiency (*General Approach to the Critically Ill Child, 1.2*). Monitor central venous pressure as indicated.

(Continued)

Box 10.3.4   **Management of Thoracic Trauma**
(Continued)

- Pain control is necessary for comfort as well as respiratory care; painful inspiration limits chest wall movement and cough, potentially leading to atelectasis and infection. Considerations include narcotics, patient-controlled analgesia, non-steroidal anti-inflammatory agents, lidocaine patch and epidural analgesia (*Analgesia, Sedation and Neuromuscular Blockade, 13.2*).
- Chest tube care for traumatic PTX and/or hemothorax: Initially place CT's to suction; if CXR at 24 hrs reveals re-expanded lung, the CT should be placed to water seal. If repeat CXR after 6 hrs with CT under water seal does not demonstrate PTX, and if fluid out is minimal (<1–3 ml/kg/day), removal of the tube should be considered (*Thoracentesis, Chest Tube Placement and Removal, 15.4; Box 15.4.7*).

10.4 Abdominal Trauma

The abdomen is the third most commonly injured body region in children and the most common site for unrecognized injury resulting in pediatric death; the overall mortality is 8.5%. Blunt force trauma, commonly related to motor vehicle accidents results in 80% of pediatric abdominal injuries. Non-operative management has a 95% success rate in treating solid organ injuries of the pediatric abdomen.

Anatomic differences in children compared to adults impact on susceptibility to injury and resuscitation strategies. The abdominal wall in children is thinner and less muscular than adults, providing less protection from external forces.

The pediatric rib cage is more pliable and flexible which results in fewer fractures but provides less energy absorption and organ protection. Children have greater solid organ mass by proportion, which increases the likelihood of injury on impact. The liver (15%), spleen (27%), and kidney (27%) are most likely to be injured by blunt trauma. Immature peritoneal attachments are present in children, making the hollow viscera more susceptible to rapid deceleration forces or abdominal compression (*e.g.* seatbelt-related injury). Robust compensation by the cardiovascular system allows preservation of blood pressure until late in the course; hypotension is an ominous sign (*Shock, 3.5*). In addition, a child's relatively greater body surface area allows more rapid loss of heat. The approach to assessment of abdominal trauma is outlined in **Box 10.4.1**. The American Association for Surgery of Trauma (AAST) provides a CT-based organ injury grading system (www.aast.org).

Box 10.4.1   Assessment of Abdominal Trauma

- Attention to airway, breathing, circulation, neurologic status and temperature control; Evaluate for life-threatening injury and initiate resuscitation (*General Approach to the Critically Ill Child, 1.2; Appendix, part 2, VII*).
- Conduct a Secondary Survey or "head-to-toe" assessment; inspect, auscultate and palpate the abdomen; palpate flanks and back. Decompress the stomach and bladder.
- Diagnostic Peritoneal Lavage (DPL): Determines the presence of hemoperitoneum; not routinely used because small child size, large catheter size, sedation issues for children, and most blunt solid organ injuries are handled non-operatively. DPL lets the healthcare provider know only that there is hemoperitoneum, not what organ is injured.
- Obtain necessary images (see below)
- Tertiary Survey: The full survey is repeated by a different examiner in the first 24 hrs. Follow-up radiology and laboratory testing as indicated.

- **Initial laboratory tests:**

▸ Bedside glucose	▸ As indicated:
▸ CBC	▪ Type and screen or
▸ Electrolytes, Mg, Phosphorus	crossmatch
▸ Blood alcohol	▪ Lactic acid
▸ Urine toxicology screen	▪ ABG/base deficit
	▪ Urine HCG

- **Serial laboratory tests** are important to determine trends, and may be indicated at intervals from a few hours to daily for days depending on the injury: CBC, electrolytes, lactic acid, magnesium, phosphorus, liver enzymes and function tests, blood gases, lipase.

(Continued)

Box 10.4.1   Assessment of Abdominal Trauma (Continued)

- **Imaging**
  - ▶ Focused Abdominal Sonogram for Trauma (FAST) helps identify free fluid in the abdomen, pneumothorax, and pericardial effusion. Its usefulness in children is controversial. This technique can be used in children weighing >50 kg as the peritoneal, pleural and pericardial cavities are better defined in this group.
  - ▶ Plain radiographs: Useful for determination of missile trajectory in penetrating trauma when used with radio-opaque markers (*e.g.* paperclips).
  - ▶ Computed Axial Tomography (CT): Requires patient stability, usually requires both oral and IV contrast and is highly specific and sensitive. The missed injury rate in children may approach 20%, but the correlation between mortality and morbidity and missed injury rate has not been proven.

Box 10.4.2   Key Points in the Management of Pediatric Abdominal Trauma

- Secure IV access: 2 large bore PIV's or central venous access as indicated
- Arterial access for BP monitoring and blood sampling as indicated.
- Maintain gastric and bladder decompression.
- Monitor serial physical examinations and laboratory studies as outlined (**Box 10.4.1**).
- Most patients will be unable to take by mouth for at least ~48 hrs, particularly those with splenic or bowel injury. Appropriate nutritional needs should be addressed early in the course for patients expected to be "NPO" for greater than 7 days. Enteral feeding should be attempted as soon as bowel function returns as evidenced by flatus, bowel sounds, and bowel movements. Prior to starting an enteral feeding regimen if the child is NPO, an IV solution containing dextrose with appropriate electrolytes should be administered to prevent protein catabolism. Total parenteral nutrition (TPN) is reserved for the child who has contraindications for enteral feeding, *e.g.* enterocutaneous fistula, bowel obstruction, prolonged use of barbiturates.

(Continued)

Box 10.4.2   Key Points in the Management of Pediatric Abdominal Trauma (Continued)

- Consider naso- or oro-gastric decompression if vomiting is a problem; R/O intestinal obstruction. In some cases an anti-emetic (*e.g.* ondansetron) may be warranted.
- Provide DVT prophylaxis for immobile children sustaining crush injuries, amputations, or if the child has an adult body habitus.
- Bed rest is recommended for ~1 day per grade of injury (www.aast.org). *e.g.* A patient with a grade 3 liver laceration should be "on bed rest" for ~3 days.
- Care of the lungs to avoid atelectasis and/or pneumonia is extremely important. Encourage cough and deep breathing through use of incentive spirometry or other age-appropriate techniques such as bubble-blowing, pin-wheel games, *etc*.
- Address pain control. Inadequate analgesia can lead to emotional as well as respiratory complications.
- Provide peri-operative antibiotics as indicated. For abdominal surgery with minimal contamination, usually one day of second generation cephalosporin should suffice. For a patient with a ruptured viscus, anaerobic coverage (*e.g.* piperacillin-tazobactam) is typically provided for at least 24 hours.
- Address physical and occupational therapy needs.
- Provide post-splenectomy vaccines as indicated ≥14 days after emergency splenectomy (**Box 10.4.3**).

The management of pediatric abdominal trauma has evolved from mandatory exploration to cautious observation. Operative intervention for solid organ injury is based upon physiologic derangements rather than anatomical grade. However, hollow viscous injuries usually require operative intervention. These injuries account for 3% of abdominal injuries, and may be identified only as free fluid on CT scan without solid organ injury or by increasing pain on examination, abdominal distension, fever or increasing leukocytosis. The importance of serial physical examinations and good communication

Box 10.4.3   Recommended Post-Splenectomy Vaccines

Vaccine	Comments
• Pneumococcal Polysaccharide (PPSV)	PPSV 23 (contains polysaccharides from 23 serotypes) is recommended for fully immunized children ≥ 2 yrs and adults. A 7-valent conjugate pneumococcal vaccine vaccine (PCV-7) has greater immunogenicity and is recommended for patients ≥ 6 wks, incompletely immunized children 2–5 yrs and unimmunized children 5–9 yrs. Boosters are recommended.
• Haemophilus influenza (Hib; multiple conjugate vaccines available)	Children who have received a primary series of Hib vaccines and one booster dose at 12 mos. do not require further vaccination for Hib. Unimmunized children 12–59 mos or those who have received only one dose of conjugate vaccine before 12 mos should receive 2 doses of vaccine separated by 2 months. Those who received 2 doses prior to 12 mos of age should receive one additional dose. Otherwise healthy unimmunized children >59 mos should receive one dose of any conjugate vaccine. There are no recommendations for boosters, but anti-polyribosyl antibody titers can be measured and booster dosing may be considered.
• Meningococcal (MCV4, Menactra®)	Recommended for patients 2–55 yrs. Patients 2–10 yrs, and possibly older children, should be revaccinated in 3 yrs unless there is history of Guillain-Barre Syndrome.
• Influenza	Annually

• Consideration should be given to daily oral prophylaxis with penicillin or amoxicillin until 5 yrs of age, or at least 3 yrs post-splenectomy. Some authorities recommend prophylaxis until age 18 yrs or for life.

Box 10.4.4 Clinical Pathways for Patients with Abdominal Solid Organ Injury

Injury Grade	ICU Stay (days)	Hospital Stay (days)	Home-bound (weeks)	Contact Activity Restriction (weeks)
I	none	1	1	3
II	none	2	1–2	4
III	1	3	3	5
IV	1	4	3	6
V	1	5	3	8

between critical care and trauma surgery teams cannot be overstated. Key points in management of pediatric abdominal trauma are outlined in **Boxes 10.4.2–10.4.4**.

10.5 Child Abuse

Child abuse is not uncommon and clinicians who provide trauma care for children must be constantly looking for injuries or circumstances that warrant suspicion of abuse (**Boxes 10.5.1–10.5.3**). Child abuse is defined by federal legislation that provides minimum guidelines for states to incorporate into their criminal and civil statutes. Subsequently, each state has a working legal definition of child abuse and neglect. Child Protective Services (CPS) is the branch of public social services that investigates reports of child abuse and neglect in which caretakers are involved as possible perpetrators. Law enforcement is involved in many of these cases and also has primary responsibility for investigating cases in which strangers and non-caretakers are the alleged perpetrators.

All states list health care workers as mandated reporters of child maltreatment. To report a case to CPS, the provider need only have a suspicion that maltreatment or neglect has occurred, not proof. CPS is responsible for investigation when the agency believes the report meets a minimal standard of likelihood. All states mandate reporting

---

Box 10.5.1   Key Historical Issues Warranting Suspicion of Child Abuse*

- Conflicting history of accidental injury between caregivers, between caregiver and child, or over time.
- History of accidental injury clearly inconsistent with the force, energy or mechanism required to produce the observed injury.
- History of self-induced, accidental injury clearly inconsistent with the victim's developmental capabilities.
- Fatal or severe injuries attributed to a short distance (*e.g.*, household) fall.
- Specific denial of traumatic event(s) in the presence of traumatic injuries.

- Significant delay in seeking medical care despite definitive clinical signs of illness or injury.
- History of accidental injury attributed to the actions of another child whose own developmental capabilities are inadequate to have accomplished the reported actions.
- History of injury clearly inconsistent with estimated age of the injury.
- Persistently absent, unavailable, or disinterested caregiver(s).
- History or record of repetitive injuries.

---

* Modified from Hymel KP, Hall CA, Diagnosing pediatric head trauma, *Pediatric Annals*, **34**(5):358–370, 2005.

without risk of liability if the report is made without malicious intent. A medical provider can incur liability for failing to report a case of suspected child maltreatment. It is important to emphasize to parents (or other caretakers) that reporting is not an accusation, but is a legal requirement based on a current assessment.

Physical abuse is the most common type of child maltreatment seen in the PICU. Child abuse is believed to be the etiology of 10% of traumatic injuries in children < 5 yrs. Approximately 1700 children die each year from inflicted injuries and nearly 45% of those children are younger than 1 yr.

Box 10.5.2   Key Physical Findings that Raise Suspicion of Child Abuse*

- Bruises, abrasions, lacerations
  ▸ Patterned: resembling an object or paired oval (pinch marks)
  ▸ In pre-ambulatory infant
  ▸ Extensive
  ▸ Multiple ages
  ▸ Located on trunk
  ▸ Involving more than single body surface or plane
  ▸ Located in sites not overlying bony prominences
  ▸ Located in anogenital region or buttocks
  ▸ Involving ear lobes

- General physical exam
  ▸ Multiple injuries (*e.g.* fractures of different bones or skin injuries indicating multiple impact points)
  ▸ Multiple mechanisms of injury (*e.g.* fracture and burn)
  ▸ Multiple injuries at various stages of healing (*e.g.* fractures, burns, bruises)
  ▸ Signs of concurrent medical, hygienic, supervisory, or nutritional neglect

* Modified from Hymel KP, Hall CA, Diagnosing pediatric head trauma, *Pediatric Annals*, **34**(5):358–370, 2005.

Box 10.5.3   Cranial Injuries and Fractures that Raise Suspicion of Child Abuse*

Cranial Injuries:
- Clinical presentation with medically unexplained loss of consciousness, respiratory distress, apnea, persistent irritability, lethargy, hypotonia, seizures, coma, recurrent vomiting and/or poor feeding in an infant or young child.
- Retinal, subdural or subarachnoid hemorrhage in an infant or young child occurring in the absence of a specific history of a motor vehicle accident, long-distance fall, or equivalent severe accidental trauma.
- Facial/scalp soft tissue injuries in a pre-ambulatory infant involving the earlobe(s), those which are patterned (*e.g.*, slap mark) or associated with intra-oral trauma or bleeding (*e.g.*, torn frenulum, gingival laceration).
- Skull fracture(s) in pre-ambulatory infants, or that are multiple, complex or diastatic in a child with a history of a short distance (*e.g.* household) fall.

(Continued)

Box 10.5.3   Cranial Injuries and Fractures that Raise Suspicion of Child Abuse* (Continued)

- Radiological evidence of pediatric intracranial injuries of multiple ages during infancy that remain unexplained by traumatic childbirth.
- Fatal or severe pediatric head injuries occurring in the absence of specific history of motor vehicle accident, long distance fall, or equivalent severe accidental trauma.

Fractures:

- **High specificity for inflicted trauma:**
  ‣ Classic metaphyseal lesions
  ‣ Rib fractures, particularly posterior
  ‣ Scapular fractures
  ‣ Spinous process fractures
- **Common in inflicted trauma, but of low specificity:**
  ‣ Subperiosteal new bone formation
  ‣ Clavicular fractures
  ‣ Long bone shaft fractures
  ‣ Linear skull fractures

- **Moderate specificity for inflicted trauma:**
  ‣ Multiple fractures, especially if bilateral
  ‣ Fractures of different ages
  ‣ Epiphyseal separation
  ‣ Vertebral body fractures and subluxations
  ‣ Digit fractures
  ‣ Complex skull fractures

---

* Modified from Hymel KP, Hall CA, Diagnosing pediatric head trauma, *Pediatric Annals*, **34**(5):358–370, 2005.

Important factors to assess in possible abuse situations are the history, the child's developmental abilities, physical findings, and the presence of risk factors for abuse. Documentation must be carefully done and should include the elements outlined in **Box 10.5.4**.

Factors that put children at risk for physical abuse involve characteristics of both the perpetrator and the child, and are commonly exacerbated by social and environmental stressors. Perpetrators, in order of frequency, are most commonly fathers, mothers' boyfriends, babysitters (female), and mothers. Risk factors for the perpetrator

---

Box 10.5.4   Documentation of Abuse*

- **The medical record may be admitted as evidence in court.** Accurate, detailed, legible records are essential (consider dictation).
- **The record should include:**
  - ▶ Date and time of injury
  - ▶ When first noted
  - ▶ Where the injury occurred
  - ▶ Who was there and witnessed the injury
  - ▶ What led up to the injury
  - ▶ How the child and caretaker responded to the injury
  - ▶ Lapse in time before seeking care for the injury
- **Child's interview and medical history (separate interview):** Child's name, medical record number, date of birth
- **Caregiver statements (separate interview, optimally conducted by social worker):**
  - ▶ Name, relationship to child
  - ▶ Date, time statement made
  - ▶ Exact wording with quotation marks and identification of speaker
  - ▶ Behavior and mood of speaker
  - ▶ Practitioner's questions, statements, and actions
  - ▶ Witnesses to interview (names and titles of those present)
- **Physical exam findings, evidence collection; includes photographs** of all findings with child's name, record number, ruler, color scale (often done by law enforcement)

---

* Modified from Wang NE, Baz B, Physical abuse in children, *Pediatric Emergency Medicine Reports* 12(9):97–108, 2007.

include history of abuse or neglect as a child, lower level of education, young or single parenthood, and unstable social situations. A caretaker also may be more likely to perpetrate abuse when suffering from a psychiatric illness, when under the influence of drugs or alcohol, or when inexperienced or unprepared for parenthood. Other environmental risk factors include domestic violence and increased family stressors such as natural disasters.

Innate factors that put the child at greater risk for abuse include young age (80% of child fatalities occur in children <4 yrs), chronic illness and disability, speech and language disorders, learning disability, conduct disorders (*e.g.* hyperactivity), and psychological illness. Although the data are controversial, it is thought that medical conditions such as prematurity and low birth weight also may be independent risk factors of abuse later in life. Most importantly, history of previous abuse is a significant risk factor for future abuse: a physically abused child has a 35% chance of suffering further abuse and a 10% chance of dying from the abuse if it is not identified and addressed at initial presentation.

Bruises, including ecchymoses and hematomas, are the most commonly found injury in abusive trauma, accounting for up to 40% of injuries. Bruises result from direct blunt force to the skin with resulting rupture of capillaries and leakage of blood into subcutaneous tissue. Discoloration may appear immediately, or hours to days after an injury is sustained. The only evidence concerning color is that yellowish discoloration indicates that the time elapsed after injury occurred is >18–24 hrs.

Distinguishing between accidental traumatic bruises and inflicted injuries in children can be difficult, but recognizable geometric shapes from implements such as belts, whips, and hand prints are suggestive of abusive injury. Accidental bruising most often occurs over bony prominences, such as joints (elbows, knees) or pretibial areas, the forehead, and the front of the body, as a result of play. Bruising to the back of the body, inner arms or thighs, trunk, genitalia, cheeks, ears, eyes, and neck are more suspicious of abusive injury. Bruising in non-ambulatory babies is non-accidental trauma unless proven otherwise. Multiple and/or clustered bruises, especially bruises of different ages suggest repeated inflicted injuries.

Bite marks are associated with both physical and sexual abuse of children. They can appear as circular, elliptical, or arrow-shaped bruises or abrasions, and may have central clearing or associated erythema and petechiae within the bite-mark itself. Human bites tend to be more superficial than animal bites; they do not always leave individual tooth marks, and lack the tearing and deep punctures typical of animal bites. Further, adult human bite marks made by permanent teeth may be differentiated by the intercanine distance which is at least 2.5–3 cm when permanent teeth are present.

The pattern, size, contour, and color of a bite mark can be evaluated by a forensic odontologist or pathologist (or) a physician or dentist who is knowledgeable in patterns of child abuse injuries.

Blood-group substances and DNA (in epithelial cells) can be secreted in saliva and may be deposited in bites. Even if they have dried, they can be collected using the double-swab technique: (1) a sterile cotton swab moistened with distilled water is used to wipe the area in question, dried, and then placed in a specimen tube; (2) a second sterile, dry cotton swab is used to clean the same area and then is dried and placed in a specimen tube; (3) a third control sample should be obtained from an uninvolved area of the child's skin. All samples should be sent to a certified forensic laboratory for a prompt analysis. The chain of custody must be maintained on all samples submitted for forensic analysis.

Thorough documentation in the patient's chart of any suspicious bruise or bite mark is recommended, using written description, drawings, and careful photographic evidence with a color wheel and ruler.

Fractures are the second most common injury in physical abuse, and are detected in 30–50% of abused children. Any skeletal fracture may be the result of abusive trauma. Each fracture must be assessed in the context of the child's development, medical history, and history of the injury. A child's skeleton is more porous than an adult's, and is more prone to compression injuries that may result in green stick (bone bent and broken only on the convex side) and buckle fractures (one side of the bone buckles without breaking the convex side). Further, the periosteum is more prone to separation from the bone in a child, but their joint capsules and ligaments are known to be more resistant to mechanical stressors than bone and cartilage, making dislocations less likely in childhood. Finally, bone healing is more rapid in children then in adults. Spiral fractures result from rotational forces, such as twisting or torquing of the extremity. In non-ambulatory children, these are considered highly suspicious for abuse. Metaphyseal fractures also are considered to be highly suspicious for abuse. These fractures are subtle findings on radiographs, often appearing as chips or fractures from the corner of the bone known as corner or "bucket handle" fractures (**Fig. 10.5.1**).

Rib fractures account for up to 27% of all abusive skeletal injuries, and occur as a result of direct blows as well as anteroposterior compression of the chest wall, such as occurs when holding and shaking an infant. Many abusive rib fractures are posterior and adjacent to the vertebral body due to the levering of forces over the transverse process of the vertebra. To diagnose these difficult-to-detect fractures, skeletal surveys are recommended in children < 2 yrs in whom abuse is suspected (**Box 10.5.3**). Oblique views of the ribs increase detection of rib fractures. Repeat skeletal surveys in 10–14 days after the initial

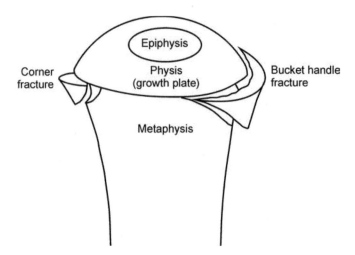

Fig. 10.5.1.   Bone Fractures Characteristic for Nonaccidental Trauma.

presentation and radionuclide bone scanning also may detect new rib fractures and subtle long bone fractures not evident on initial skeletal survey.

Central Nervous System Injury. The ability to distinguish between accidental and abusive head injury may be facilitated by an understanding of the biomechanics of brain injury. Sudden angular deceleration of the brain and cerebral vessels from violent shaking results in diffuse brain injury, with or without subdural hemorrhage, a hallmark of inflicted craniocerebral trauma ("shaken-baby syndrome" now known as "Abusive Head Trauma"). Such injuries are in contrast to those seen in low velocity injuries such as household falls, where specific contact (translational) forces are applied to the surface of the head.

CNS trauma is found in up to one-quarter of abused children. Sequelae include intracranial hemorrhage (subdural and subarachnoid), and intraparenchymal bleeding. The classic presentation linking CNS trauma to abuse are findings of (1) subdural hematoma; (2) retinal hemorrhages (65–95% of cases) and (3) skeletal fractures, including metaphyseal (**Fig. 10.5.1**) and posterior rib fractures (30–70% of cases) caused when the child is shaken violently. A minority of patients will have all three of the "classic triad". Clinical deterioration from an acute SDH (subdural hematoma) typically occurs at the time of injury without a "lucid interval". Rapid onset of morbidity and mortality from traumatic brain injury in a previously healthy child is particularly suspicious for inflicted injury. Children who have minor forms of head trauma and less ominous symptoms, such as vomiting and irritability, may not be recognized until they present later with a more serious injury.

Burns (*Burns, 10.6*), which are found in up to 20% of abused children, are frequently due to intentional injury. Burns result from contact between heat energy and skin, and may be caused by hot liquids, chemicals, contact with hot objects, flames (causing flash burns), and electricity. Children with burns suspicious for abuse need evaluation for other abusive injuries such as fractures, head trauma, and abdominal trauma.

Abdominal Trauma (*Abdominal Trauma, 10.4*). Severe abdominal injury is an uncommon but well recognized manifestation of abuse. The historian rarely includes a history of abdominal trauma. Less severe injury is under-recognized because symptoms are nonspecific and external manifestations are often lacking. Most abusive abdominal injury is caused by blunt trauma resulting in solid organ injury, perforation of hollow viscous, or shearing of mesenteric vessels. Isolated solid organ injuries are common with both accidental and inflicted injuries, however, hollow visceral injuries more commonly are associated with abuse. Recent reports of abdominal

Box 10.5.5   Potentially Useful Laboratory and Imaging Data in Suspected Child Abuse*

Study	Presentation	Examples of Co-Morbidities and Alternative Diagnoses
CBC, differential	Bleeding, bruising, pallor	Anemia, infection, thrombocytopenia, blood dyscrasias
PT, PTT, fibrinogen	Bleeding, bruising	Primary vs. secondary coagulopathies
C-reactive protein, ESR	Nonspecific	Infection, inflammatory response
Electrolytes, glucose, BUN, creatinine	Seizures, AMS dehydration	Electrolyte imbalance, hypo- or hyperglycemia, azotemia
Liver panel, lipase, amylase, stool for occult blood	Abdominal injury	Liver disease, liver dysfunction, pancreatitis
Urine (and serum) toxicology screens	Seizures, AMS	Drug ingestion (accidental vs. intentional)
Calcium, Phosphorus, 25(OH) and 1,25 (OH)$_2$ Vitamin D	Fractures	Metabolic bone disease
Skeletal survey**	Fractures; screening purposes	Metabolic bone disease; occult fractures
Radionuclide bone scan	Bone pain; screening purposes	Acute rib fractures, occult fractures, occult bone disease
CSF studies[†]	Seizures, AMS	CNS infection
Head CT; brain MRI	Any suspected head trauma	Identification of traumatic vs. non-traumatic lesions; further evaluation with brain MRI may be indicated to identify blood products and injuries not visualized on CT.

* Modified from Wang NE, Baz B, Physical abuse in children, *Pediatric Emergency Medicine Reports* 12(9):97–108, 2007.
**For children <2 yrs: AP views of humeri, forearms, hands, femurs, lower legs and feet, chest, pelvis, lateral view of axial skeleton (infants) and AP and lateral skull
[†]Head CT should be performed prior to LP if head trauma is suspected.

trauma secondary to abuse reveal that liver injuries are most common, followed by duodeno-jejunal rupture, duodenal rupture, and pancreatic, vena cava, and renal trauma. These injuries are thought to be due to compression of abdominal viscera against the vertebral column following a punch or kick. The small size of the child's abdomen predisposes to multiple organ injury. Children with severe liver or mesenteric injury often present with signs and symptoms of acute bleeding, including hemorrhagic shock. Mortality is extremely high owing to delays in presentation and magnitude of injuries. Abdominal trauma is diagnosed by physical examination, screening for elevation of LFTs, amylase, lipase, urinalysis, sonography and abdominal CT.

Differential Diagnosis. The diagnosis of accidental versus abusive injuries is crucial for the child's proper medical and social management, and may be confounded by the presence of underlying medical conditions. Whereas the past medical history often will elucidate previously diagnosed conditions, the exploration of the differential diagnosis for physical abuse should be undertaken in those cases that are unclear or suggest an alternative etiology of injury. The evaluation should include laboratory data as indicated based on the child's presentation (**Boxes 10.5.3 and 10.5.5**).

10.6 Burns

Approximately 10,000 children suffer burn injuries each year, with half occurring in the less than two year age group. Nearly 2500 children die each year as a result of burn injury, including smoke inhalation. This makes burn injury the third leading cause of accidental death in children in the United States.

Burns can result from a variety of situations; however the most common are scald, contact, flame, and chemical. Scald burns are seen primarily in the toddler population, frequently when young, newly ambulatory children are able to reach tables or countertops. Boiling water, freshly poured tea, or soups are typical liquids that come within the reach of a toddler. Contact burns result from a young child touching or grasping a hot object or appliance. Older oven doors, range tops, and curling irons are frequent culprits. Flame burns involve an older age group as compared to scald burns. In addition to house fires as the source, lighting or throwing an accelerant onto a flame source will result in a flash burn, or, worse yet, the ignition of clothing. Trash fires may contain aerosol or paint cans that can explode violently, showering bystanders with flames. More recently, the popularity of online videos demonstrating risky behaviors with fire has spawned a new type of causative agent as adolescents attempt to imitate these actions. Finally, the use or exposure to caustic chemicals can result in a significant injury.

Intentionally inflicted burns are typically seen in the younger child, between 1 and 4 yrs of age. Suspicion of an intentional burn should be raised when the history provided does not match the injury seen or the developmental age of the child. Immersion scald burns are common types of non-accidental injury with typical physical findings. Sharp lines of demarcation of burned skin are seen when a child is held in scalding water with a fixed water level. Children will often draw up their knees in an attempt to avoid the water, leaving a burn injury to the feet, buttocks, and perineum, often with an easily seen waterline. Occasionally, the soles of the feet and circular areas of the buttocks will be spared from deeper burns as these areas are pressed to the bathtub or sink and partially protected.

Injury Classification. Figure 10.6.1 shows a cross-section of the skin and the depth of injury that may occur. First degree burns are sunburn-like in nature, involve only the superficial layer of epidermis, and resolve with minimal intervention. Second degree burns are typically the result of a scald injury or a brief contact burn injury. Large, fluid-filled bullae are common and often rupture, revealing moist tissue. These burns are painful and will heal with minimal to no scarring. Third degree burns result from flame burns or prolonged immersion injury or contact. Most third degree burns will be minimally painful, if at all, and will have a dry, pale appearance. Obvious char injury of the skin is consistent with a deep third degree burn. The diagnosis of deep second degree burn is typically made after surgical debridement, and represents a level of injury between second and third degree burns. Very little is known about how to avoid the progression of these injuries to full third degree

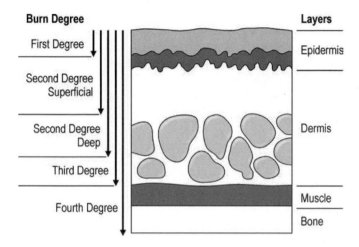

Fig. 10.6.1. Degree Burn as it Relates to Depth of Tissue Involvement.

burns. Tissue factors, inflammatory mediators, and apoptosis have all been implicated in the evolution of these burns. Continued monitoring and repeated surgical evaluations and debridement remain the optimal treatment regimen at present. Finally, fourth degree burns involve muscle, fascia or bone, and represent the most severe type of burn injury. Burns of these depths will often require amputation or significant tissue loss.

Initial Management. In all cases of burn injury, the initial priority is to stop the burning process. Removal from the source of heat, removal of clothing, and direct cooling measures are typically accomplished by first responders prior to arrival at a hospital setting. It is important to realize that a diaper may collect, retain, and continue to emit significant amounts of thermal energy and therefore should be removed. Once the burning process is halted, routine resuscitative measures by first responders or emergency room personnel should proceed. There are no definitive recommendations regarding topical therapy or use of sterile sheets; these practices are "burn-unit-dependent".

Airway. Assessment of the airway is particularly relevant for any potential smoke or inhalational injury, as well as any flash burn to the

---

Box 10.6.1   Clinical Signs of Airway Burn Injury

- Burns taking place in a closed space/environment
- Burns to the face, neck, or lips
- Singed nasal hairs
- Carbonaceous material in mouth or nares
- Darkened oral or nasal mucosa
- Stridor, hoarseness, voice change, respiratory distress

---

face. Flash burns can result in inhalation of superheated air, directly injuring the structures of the upper airway with minimal facial burns. Signs signaling airway involvement are listed (**Box 10.6.1**). With burns larger than 30% total BSA (**Fig. 10.6.2**), airway control is often recommended, given the likelihood of edema and acute lung injury. If any of these criteria are present, serious consideration should be given to securing the airway, especially if transport to a burn center is anticipated. When tracheal intubation is planned, ETTs smaller than would be chosen based on age should be available should the airway prove to be swollen. Additionally, the use of a cuffed endotracheal tube is preferred, given the high incidence of acute lung injury and ARDS in burn victims.

Fluid Requirements. Fluid resuscitation is the mainstay of burn management in the first 24 hrs. Emergency resuscitation is accomplished with Lactated Ringers solution (some experts may use 0.9% NaCl for this phase); colloid is generally avoided in the acute phase of burn resuscitation. With large burns, tissue injury gives way to massive inflammatory mediator release, capillary leak, hypermetabolism, and fluid extravasation. While there are a number of ways to estimate fluid requirements, most centers rely on the Parkland formula for initial estimation of fluid needs for patients with second and third degree burns. Based on the Parkland formula, the total fluid to be given in the first 24 hrs = 4 ml/kg × %BSA burned (**Fig. 10.6.2**), giving 1/2 over first 8 hrs, 1/2 over remaining 16 hrs. For patients < 40 kg, most experts add maintenance volume to

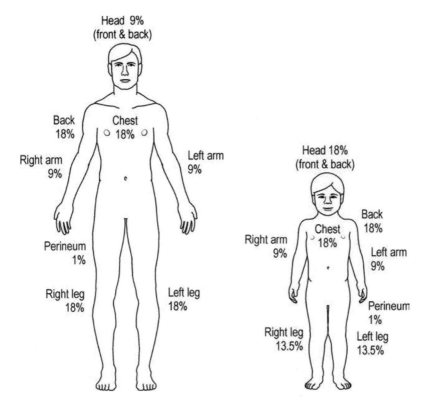

Fig. 10.6.2. Total Body Surface Area Calculator. Children have a proportionally larger cranial surface area compared to adults. These estimates can be used to estimate the surface area of a burn. Adult percentage burn guidelines are typically used for children > 6–10 yrs depending on body habitus.

this "total fluid" calculation. This regimen will be familiar to pediatricians in concept because of its similarity to resuscitation for dehydration in children. It emphasizes the enormous volume requirements a large burn will have in the first day, as a 10 kg toddler with a 50% burn will have an initial fluid rate of 250 ml/hr. Lactated Ringers solution is the most commonly chosen rehydration fluid. For smaller children, maintenance fluids containing dextrose should be added separately to the fluid regimen because of the smaller energy stores available. Patients with > 15–20% of body surface area burned or with perineal burn injury should have a urinary catheter placed for close monitoring of UOP. Hourly UOP goal of 2 ml/kg is typically used to assess adequacy of fluid resuscitation. This may appear to conflict with Pediatric Advanced Life Support (PALS) guidelines which emphasize that disturbances in end organ function are a late finding in shock. However, burned children have large amounts of circulating lactic acid, poor temperature regulation, and obvious limitations in availability of skin to assess perfusion. Thus, PALS recommendations may apply poorly to severely burned children. At the end of the day, aggressive fluid administration and close hemodynamic monitoring will provide the required volume for resuscitation.

Circulation. With circumferential burns, the likelihood of vascular compromise increases greatly. This is more commonly seen with flame and thermal burns, but can also occur with scald burns as the tissue swells. Third degree burns result in almost complete loss of skin elasticity and compliance, and, as extravasation of fluids takes place, arterial blood flow decreases. Loss of palpable or Doppler pulses in a circumferential burn is an indication for emergent escharotomy, in which the burn is incised to the subcutaneous tissue (to expose the fatty tissue) to allow for unrestricted edematous changes. Large thoracic burns may compromise lung expansion, necessitating escharotomies of the trunk. Early surgical involvement is recommended for any circumferential burn.

Pain Control. Narcotics are the mainstay of pain management for burned children; requirements are often in excess of recommended dosages. Morphine, fentanyl, and acetaminophen/codeine preparations are all appropriate choices for analgesia for an acute burn. Larger burns may have such large pain medication needs that continuous infusions and mechanical ventilation becomes necessary.

Tetanus Prophylaxis. All burns require documentation of tetanus immunization status and booster administration, if necessary. In the absence of known immunization status, tetanus immune globulin should also be given.

Infection. Unless a burn wound is grossly contaminated, prophylactic antibiotics are not recommended. Large third degree burns will likely become infected at some point during hospitalization; prophylactic antibiotic use increases the chances of selecting for resistant organisms.

Burn Centers. Because of the need for specialized care and treatment of the burned patient, burn centers have evolved as the best practice model for the care of these patients. Once the patient is stabilized, current recommendations are to transfer as soon as possible to the nearest accepting burn center. Risks of transfer are far outweighed by the improvement in outcomes reported by large burn centers. The American Burn Association has published a list of transfer guidelines for referring facilities (**Box 10.6.2**). Given these guidelines, most, if not all, pediatric patients will require notification of a regional burn center. While immediate transfer is not always necessary, especially for smaller burns, recommendations for wound management and outpatient surgery can be established. In the case of larger, more catastrophic burns, early notification while initial resuscitation is in progress can help expedite the transfer process as well as provide some helpful initial treatment recommendations.

Box 10.6.2   Burn Center Transfer Criteria

- Partial thickness burns (second degree) greater than 10% total BSA
- Burns that involve the face, hands, feet, genitals, perineum, or major joints
- Third degree burns, any size, any age group
- Electrical burns, including lightening
- Chemical burns
- Inhalation injury
- Burn injury in patients with pre-existing medical diagnoses
- Burns involving concomitant trauma in which the burn injury provides the greater risk
- Burned children in hospitals without qualified personnel or equipment for the care of children
- Burn injury in patients who will require special social, emotional, or long-term rehabilitation

Chapter 11

Peri-Operative Pediatric Surgical Critical Care

11.1 Caring for the Child Through the Hands of the Pediatric Surgeon

The pediatric general surgeon leads the care of the ill or injured child during peri-operative resuscitation, establishes the surgical diagnosis and performs procedures throughout major body compartments. A basic understanding of the surgeon's perspective for each surgical patient or candidate is essential for meaningful participation in the critical care of these children.

Pre-Operative Evaluation and Resuscitation. An accurate history determines the diagnosis in nearly 90% of cases. The patient's age, gender, race and a thorough review of the seven defining characteristics of the patient's symptom complex (**Box 11.1.1**) and signs on physical examination will narrow the surgical differential diagnosis.

Box 11.1.1 Defining Characteristics of Symptoms*

- Duration: acute vs. chronic
- Severity: grade severity from 1 (very mild) through 10 (very severe)
- Temporal pattern: constant vs. intermittent
- Location of pain: localized vs. radiating
- Associated symptoms
- Ameliorating factors
- Aggravating factors

---

* Limited by [developmental] age.

517

Patients in urgent need of surgical intervention may be admitted to the PICU for pre-operative resuscitation. This requires that the surgeon discuss the patient's current problems and provide essential orders and guidelines for patient care. The surgeon should also discuss interventions (airway care, vascular access, placement of a bladder catheter, gastric tube, *etc.*) and/or preoperative studies to assist in estimating a time frame for surgical intervention, and outline expectations so that the team is knowledgeable regarding any potential deterioration in status (*e.g.* "Notify the surgeon for....").

Box 11.1.2   Pre-Operative Resuscitation and Stabilization in the PICU

- Attention to airway and breathing. Supply oxygen and evaluate the need for tracheal intubation and/or mechanical ventilatory support as indicated.
- Resuscitate shock (*Care of the Circulation, 3; Shock, 3.5*). Evaluate the immediate and potential intra-operative need for blood products (red blood cells, plasma, platelets) and discuss this with the surgeon as indicated.
- Provide vascular access as needed/discuss with surgeon.
- Normalize the body temperature unless otherwise indicated (*e.g.* "HIE protocol in progress").
- Correct hypoglycemia and manage hyperglycemia as indicated (*Hypo- and Hyperglycemia, 6.4*)
- Provide necessary analgesia and anxiolysis as needed while ensuring respiratory and hemodynamic stability.
- Maintain *NPO* status.
- Obtain laboratory data as indicated (**Box 11.1.3**).
- Provide hydration, usually with an isotonic or nearly isotonic solution; most pediatric patients will require a dextrose-containing fluid.
- Correct lactic acidosis by correcting circulatory shock; monitor serial determinations of the serum lactate as needed.
- Identify and manage electrolyte disturbances.
- Identify renal insufficiency, hepatic insufficiency, or evidence of endocrine dysfunction.
- Establish clear communication with the surgeon/surgery team regarding changes in patient status.

Patients who are adequately resuscitated and prepared for anesthesia and surgery are better able to tolerate surgical stress (**Box 11.1.2**).

Laboratory Evaluation. Analysis of blood and body fluids may narrow the list of possible diagnoses, and assist in describing the metabolic condition to the anesthesiologist. In the otherwise healthy child undergoing routine elective surgery, when history is clear and physical findings are confirmatory, laboratory or imaging studies are not routinely necessary. However, in the critically ill or injured patient, certain laboratory data are critical (**Box 11.1.3**).

Box 11.1.3   Rationale for Pre-Operative Laboratory Data

- WBC with differential and CRP: Infection vs. malignancy
- Hemoglobin/Hematocrit: O_2 carrying capacity
- Platelet count/PT, PTT, INR: Risk for bleeding
- Electrolytes, glucose, urea nitrogen and creatinine: Metabolic imbalance, renal and endocrine function
- Lactic acid: Marker for anaerobic metabolism (shock)
- Urine: Screen for infection, hydration status, renal compromise
- Pregnancy screen (urine and/or serum) for girls ≥10 yrs
- Liver enzymes and function tests: Evidence of biliary obstruction vs. infection
- Serum markers for tumor as indicated
- Albumin/pre-albumin: Nutritional baseline and protein stores

---

Radiologic Imaging. Consultation with a pediatric radiologist is important to minimize radiation exposure and to assess need for sedation during imaging procedures. Knowledge of specific question(s) is key to choosing the appropriate imaging strategy. Ultrasound can delineate solid tissue from air or fluid filled spaces. Complex imaging (CT and MRI) with 3-D reconstruction and contrast angiography is often helpful in providing an anatomic roadmap needed in extirpative surgery such as tumor resection. Identification of non-resectable invasion into vital organs may significantly alter the operative strategy. A variety of other imaging techniques may be helpful to the surgeon: *e.g.* nuclear medicine scans for evaluation of gastric emptying and renal function, and radiolabeled tracers (MIBG; iodine-131-meta-iodobenzylguanidine) for localization of pheochromocytoma or neuro-blastomas, to describe a few.

Differential Diagnosis. The differential diagnosis will be determined by the history, physical examination, laboratory data and imaging. A pre-operative diagnosis is declared as a leading diagnosis for any operative procedure, but the surgeon prepares for the possibility of alternative and related diagnoses in order to plan the procedure (*e.g.* location of incision, open vs. minimally invasive approach, *etc.*).

Informed Consent. The surgeon provides the parent/guardian with an explanation of the child's condition, a description of the procedure to be performed, a list of the risks and benefits, possible complications, outcomes and potential alternatives. Documentation of translation for special language needs is essential. In the case of life-saving interventions when a parent or guardian is not immediately available, declaration of medical necessity with support of the risk management services is appropriate.

Anesthesia Consultation. Pre-operative anesthesia consultation is critical prior to induction of general anesthesia and requires respiratory, cardiovascular and metabolic evaluation of the patient. Emergent procedures may not allow time for correction of metabolic abnormalities or bleeding disorders, and the anesthesiologist needs to be armed with as much preoperative information as possible to support resuscitation and maintenance of critical organ function during the procedure. For elective procedures, the choice of airway, and regional or local anesthetic blocks as an adjunct or primary modality can be selected in collaboration with the surgeon as appropriate for the child.

Operative Planning. There may be additional evaluations, operating room (OR) resources and personnel that will assist the surgeon and the anesthesiologist with provision of critical care during surgery. These include:

- Pre-operative echocardiogram to evaluate cardiac performance and optimize cardiac function for surgery.

- Endoscopy as needed for evaluation of vocal cord function prior to neck dissection.
- Pulmonary function testing as needed prior to lung resections.
- Bowel preparation for GI surgeries.
- Expert nursing assistance with specialized team training.
- Surgical assistant for tissue retraction and exposure.
- Display of surgical and vascular anatomy available in the OR.
- Intra-operative equipment needs such as: C-arm fluorography, laser, Argon beam.
- Pathology considerations such as special handling of specimens.
- Availability of blood products.

Operative Procedures. The approach in the operative suite begins with an assessment by the surgeon and anesthesiologist in the *pre-operative holding area* to confirm the status of the child and ensure appropriate anesthesia and operative consents. Changes in the interval history are documented, mode of anesthesia is confirmed, surgical site marking takes place, and preoperative antibiotics and anxiolysis are provided as indicated. These are all important patient safety and quality measures that have been proven to reduce risk and improve patient outcomes. The child is moved to the OR and a "time out" are performed identifying the patient and the procedure with the entire team in the room. Intra-operative monitoring is then established as described (**Box 11.1.4**).

Box 11.1.4   Routine Intra-operative Monitoring

- ECG
- Pulse oximetry
- Capnography
- Lung compliance
- Blood pressure: non-invasive +/− invasive
- CVP as needed
- Temperature monitoring
- Train-of-four for neuromuscular blockade monitoring
- Nasogastric decompression
- Bladder drainage (Foley catheter)

The Procedure. The child is positioned for optimal placement of the incision and exposure of surgical anatomy. The steps of the procedure are reviewed with the team and succinctly summarized in fewer than 10 steps to clarify the operative plan. The OR team follows procedures similar to the aviation industry with frequent communication of the patient's condition among team members including progress toward completing the goals of the procedure. This allows coordination and allocation of resources and designation of the appropriate unit of disposition for patient recovery (*e.g.* post-anesthesia care unit vs. PICU). Indications for post-operative recovery in the PICU include children who already have respiratory failure and will not achieve extubation as a result of surgery, the need for pain management and sedation which may prohibit extubation, and the need for ongoing resuscitation.

Surgical Drains. The decision to place a surgical drain is driven by the desire to provide egress for infection, blood or body fluids, and to monitor the progress of healing of the operated organ. A variety of surgically placed tubes and their function are described (**Box 11.1.5**). It is important to learn from the surgeon the location, anticipated function and expected quality and quantity of output from each drain so that monitoring can be optimized, the surgeon can be notified of potential problems and fluid, electrolyte, protein and blood losses may be appropriately replaced. Analysis of the evacuated fluid is sometimes helpful in confirming the origin of drainage (*e.g.* high amylase content of abdominal drainage suggests a pancreatic source). Great care should be taken to ensure that tubes and drains placed in the OR remain stable in position; they are often not replaceable at the bedside. Application of restraints is often indicated for the very young or those just awakening from anesthesia.

Under specific circumstances the abdominal wall may be left open after laparotomy in order to avoid excessive abdominal compartment pressures (ACS) leading to potential visceral injuries and renal failure. Fluid shifts occurring as a result of the systemic inflammatory response syndrome (SIRS), particularly following trauma or infection may require temporary delay of abdominal wall closure. The goal in these cases is to return to the OR when the infection, inflammatory response

---

Box 11.1.5   Surgical Drains

- Penrose: soft, malleable radio-opaque hose-like drain of rubber; contains either latex or silicone. Desirable for small infants with intestinal perforation to permit drainage of fluid that may accumulate at the operative site.
- Closed suction drain with flutes or perforations connected to bulb suction (*e.g.* Hemovac®). Intraperitoneal location allows drainage of fluids and helps monitor GI anastomotic sites for leakage. A subcutaneous location promotes closure of dead space and ameliorates development of seromas/hematomas.
- Thoracostomy tubes: semi-rigid tubes placed in the pleural space to evacuate air, blood or fluid. Placed routinely after thoracotomy.
- Nasogastric, gastric and enteric tubes: These serve to decompress the GI tract and may serve as feeding access. When these tubes are placed intra-operatively special care must be taken since they may not be replaceable at bedside due to injuries, more proximal surgical sites or obstructions.
- Ureteral stents: These protect ureters during dissection by allowing identification of ureters by palpation. They also protect ureteral anastomsis from leak/stricture.
- Suprapubic and transurethral Foley catheters: These decompress the bladder and allow monitoring of urine output (renal perfusion) during resuscitation.

---

and edema resolve; fascial closure then can be achieved. Bogota bags, Gore-Tex® patch or vacuum assisted closure (V.A.C.®) devices have been applied for this purpose.

Surgical Complications

Anesthesia Considerations. The surgeon and anesthesiologist work as a team to safely perform induction of anesthesia. Securing the airway can be complicated by loss of the airway prior to intubation due to relaxation of the tongue and soft tissues. Proper chin lift to sniffing position will assist airway patency. Spontaneous breathing allows the safest access during intubation especially in the setting of mediastinal tumors. The stomach should be drained to avoid reflux and laryngospasm. Anticipation of the difficult airway (*Bag-Mask Ventilation and Tracheal Intubation, 15.2*), and recognition and management of anesthetic complications such as MH (*Drug-Induced Toxic Hyperthermic Syndromes, 13.3*) require a skilled and cohesive OR team.

Acute Operative Complications. Knowledge of the local anatomy and blood supply is essential to reduce the risk of ischemia to remaining organ systems when repairing tissue or preparing specimens for resection. Sites of gastrointestinal anastomosis should be inspected for patency and leak prior to closure. The use of the bipolar cautery can reduce the risk of thermal injury to surrounding tissues. Minimally invasive instruments such as the Harmonic Scalpel™ and vessel sealant devices (LigaSure™) have increased the efficiency of resections while reducing the risk of bleeding. The Harmonic Scalpel cuts through tissue by oscillating the working head of the device at approximately 20,000 Hz causing protein denaturation; the vessel sealant devices deliver low voltage, high amperage electrical energy to seal tissue. Intra-operative identification of nerve and vascular injuries with immediate repair allow the opportunity for optimal outcomes.

Surgical cases can be described in three major categories: **clean, clean-contaminated**, and **contaminated**. Infections are reduced by preoperative scrub of the operative field with bactericidal agents with a timed contact of at least three minutes and allowed to dry prior to incision. Cases that do not involve a preoperative infection, do not have risk for contamination of the field by the GI tract, and do not involve implantation of a foreign body (*e.g.* mesh or *Gortex*® to close a defect) do not require prophylactic antibiotics. There is no evidence to suggest that antibiotics will reduce the rate of wound infections of approximately 2% in these **clean** cases. **Clean-contaminated** cases are procedures that involve the biliary, GI, respiratory, and genitourinary tracts, or surgeries involving a minor break in sterile technique (*e.g.* gunshot wound; a breech requiring change of a sterile glove). Infection rates in these cases approximate 4%. One dose of broad spectrum antibiotics, respectful of allergies, one hour preceding the procedure is recommended as prophylaxis. **Contaminated** cases have the highest reported infection rates at 10%. These cases include traumatic contaminated wounds, perforated viscus, patients with other sources of active infection, and cases associated with a major break in sterile technique. Both a preoperative dose and a therapeutic course of antibiotics, respectful of allergies, is appropriate in these cases.

Early, rapidly progressing necrotizing soft tissue infections are important to consider in the differential diagnosis since even with aggressive therapy mortality is as high as 25–85%. This type of infection, which may occur as an operative complication or as a primary, presenting infection (necrotizing fasciitis) may demonstrate little in the way of skin manifestations but can present with high fever and result in significant deep soft tissue destruction due to microvascular thrombosis. Debridement down to bleeding tissue is required with open packed wounds and serial debridement until infection is cleared. The etiology is usually polymicrobial but *Streptococcus pyogenes* and/or *Clostridia* are isolated pathogens in 20% of cases.

Late Surgical Complications. Intra-abdominal abscess as a complication of perforated GI or GU tract may occur in up to 10% of cases and can present anywhere from 1–3 weeks post-surgery. A contained abscess can be managed by catheter drainage using interventional radiology techniques. If not contained, a leaking anastomosis may cause sepsis and a surgical approach is then needed to repair. Strictures of the bowel can occur at 4–6 weeks following necrotizing enterocolitis (8–10%), ischemic strictures can occur following blunt or penetrating trauma to the abdomen, or previous resections. Esophageal strictures following repair of atresia are asymptomatic until extremely tight and therefore contrast swallow studies are required for surveillance and early detection. Treatment of esophageal strictures with dilation over several months is generally successful. Anal strictures can usually be avoided by routine daily dilations beginning at 2 weeks following anorectal surgeries. Adhesive bowel obstruction following laparotomy represents approximately a 4% risk of occurrence throughout the child's life span, and presents as abdominal distension with vomiting.

Incisional hernias are rare in children, but occur in the setting of technical errors, nutritional deficiencies, or connective tissue disorders. Internal hernias result from mesenteric defects left open after surgeries and can cause closed loop bowel obstruction. Reoperation, reduction of hernia with sack, lysis of adhesions, and closure of the defect is required.

Metabolic/endocrinologic complications from thyroid, parathyroid, pancreas, and gastric reduction surgery require collaboration of the pediatrician and the surgeon to identify and manage over time.

Post-operative Management. Post-operatively, the surgical patient must recover a fluid deficit incurred from extravasation of blood and body fluid caused by the mechanical trauma of surgery. These losses result from excessive fluid accumulation into peritoneal and pleural spaces and the GI tract lumen, collectively referred to as the "third space." In the absence of sepsis following operation, capillary leak will abate in 24–48 hrs depending on the extent of surgery. During this phase, additional crystalloid is usually required to support the intravascular volume. Central venous monitoring may help in determination of pre-load, and monitoring of urine output helps assess appropriate end organ perfusion. Abdominal compartment syndrome (ACS) should be considered in the post-operative setting of major abdominal surgery, when preload is adequate and urine output is falling. Diagnosis can be made by the combination of physical findings, renal ultrasonography, and bladder pressure monitoring (*Abdominal Hypertension, 8.7*).

Key metabolic changes resulting from surgery are outlined (**Box 11.1.6**). In order to blunt the catabolic response to major

---

Box 11.1.6   Key Endocrine and Metabolic Responses Following Surgery

Hormone	Metabolic response
Glucagon ↑	Protein breakdown ↑↑
Catecholamine ↑	Protein balance ↓↓↓
Insulin ↓ then ↑	Glucose turnover ↓ then ↑
Cortisol ↑	Fatty acid turnover ↑

Box.11.1.7   Features of Post-operative Care

- Adequacy of airway: If tracheally intubated, consider suctioning of the airway, CXR, ABG.
- Assess circulation and resuscitate as needed.
- Review the OR record in detail for medications received, input/output data, results of intra-operative studies, *etc.*
- Note location, depth of placement (by external markings), security and output of surgically placed drains and tubes.
- Attend to analgesia and sedation needs.
- Obtain baseline laboratory studies as needed: these usually include Hb/Hct, glucose, electrolytes including Mg and phosphorus.
- Measure lactic acid if indicated.
- Discuss the anticipated duration of intubation, wound care, drain locations and expected outputs, limitations of activity and "notify for..." plans with the surgeon or surgical designee.

---

surgery, parenteral nutritional support may be required and should be targeted at meeting protein and caloric needs (See *Appendix, part 2, VI* for a guide to nutritional requirements) until resumption of enteral feeding is possible. Additional post-operative considerations are summarized (**Boxes 11.1.7 and 11.1.8**).

Surgical Outcomes. Parents, guardians and children (with appropriate developmental and emotional assessement) should be educated about the prognosis of their condition. Setting appropriate expectations will reduce the anxiety of the entire family. Providing information and access to support groups can help families and children cope with chronic conditions such as malignancy, morbid obesity, and anorectal malformations. Surgeons have moved beyond survival as an indicator of outcomes. The surgical goal is to generate a successful technical outcome that enables the child to return to an improved or baseline level of function. (See Bayne A, Kirkland P, Prepare children for surgery one stage at a time, *OR Nurse 2011*, **2**(8): 36–39, 2008).

Box 11.1.8   Additional Post-operative Considerations

- Antibiotics are continued to treat infection and to minimize the risk for infection in the setting of an open abdomen. Dressings of contaminated wounds are changed frequently, allowing debridement.
- Analgesia and sedation needs should be addressed in advance to minimize pain and anxiety.
- Discuss any limitations in positioning, sitting, standing, *etc.* and the appropriate timing for these activities with the surgeon.
- Early ambulation helps in the return of bowel function, so promoting this may be important in overall recovery.
- Incentive spirometry is helpful to avoid atelectasis after extubation. Age-appropriate equivalents such as blowing bubbles or blowing a pinwheel should be substituted.
- Surgical drains remain until dry or with minimal output. The quality of the drainage should be evaluated for possible anastomotic leak when indicated (*e.g.* bile or food draining from the peritoneal cavity).
- When tolerating a regular diet and comfortable on pain medication by mouth, the patient is discharged to home with follow up (usually at 2–4 weeks) for out-patient evaluation.
- No heavy lifting, sports or physical education is permitted until surgical follow-up and "clearance" by the surgeon.

11.2   Care Surrounding Specific Surgical Procedures

11.2.1   *Scoliosis repair overview*

Scoliosis is a spinal deformity resulting in a curvature of the spine in the coronal plain. Most cases are idiopathic in otherwise healthy adolescents but some develop as a result of a neuromuscular disorder such as cerebral palsy or muscular dystrophy. Surgery is typically recommended when the cobb angle (a measurement of the side-to-side curvature of the spine on an AP radiograph) is greater than 50 degrees. The goal of surgery is to create a spinal fusion and halt further progression of the curve. The operation utilizes spinal implants in the form of rods, screws, wires, hooks, and cables to correct the curvature and stabilize the spine which also aids in incorporation of the bone graft. Some type of bone graft is needed and traditionally harvested from the patient's iliac crest. The usual approach to the spine is through a dorsal vertical incision, but large or very stiff curves may require an additional "anterior release" performed through a thoracotomy or flank incision. Scoliosis surgeries are major procedures often requiring ≥ 3–6 hours in the operating room. It starts with an extended exposure of the spine (frequently 10–15 vertebral segments), followed by application of the instrumentation to correct the curve. Finally, the bone graft is placed over the instrumented vertebrae. Prior to placing the bone graft, a high-speed burr is used to decorticate exposed posterior (± anterior) bone, which creates a bleeding surface more conducive to the fusion process. This decortication process will result in significant ongoing bleeding from the bone for several days. Some form of deep suction drain is placed to capture this blood. Patients undergoing scoliosis surgery are monitored with sensory and motor evoked potentials during the procedure. Electrical impulses are transmitted between scalp and extremity electrodes with the hope of detecting a potentially catastrophic change in spinal cord function that could result in paralysis. Both mechanical and vascular factors can contribute to this complication, and early detection is critical. Intraoperative monitoring precludes the use of traditional gas anesthetics and paralytic agents; therefore, long acting IV sedatives are given to accomplish the surgery. This can delay extubation at the end of the procedure.

Postoperative Care:

Extubation. The decision to extubate the patient at the end of the procedure is based on several factors including core temperature, level of sedation, net fluid balance, vital signs, and medical co-morbidities. An intra-thecal injection of long acting opioid is often given at the end of the procedure to help with postoperative pain management. Some loss of respiratory drive can be expected and cautious use of supplemental analgesia is needed to avoid respiratory depression. Close attention to ventilatory drive (respiratory rate, depth and measures of oxygenation *and* ventilation) is required for the first 12–16 hrs postoperatively. Simple reliance on pulse oximetry is dangerous particularly when supplemental O_2 is given. End-tidal CO_2 monitoring is useful (*General Approach to the Critically Ill Child, 1.2*) when correlated with

PCO_2 (blood gases). Respiratory acidosis after extubation may require consideration for re-intubation. CPAP (*Non-invasive Ventilatory Support: CPAP, BLPAP, 2.8.2*) or administration of continuous naloxone may be alternative options.

Bleeding. Deeply positioned suction drains need frequent monitoring because high outputs may occur over the first 24 hrs; output is often proportional to the number of spinal levels fused. Several hundred milliliters of output per hour is not uncommon in the first few hours after the procedure. Frequent monitoring of hemoglobin (every 4–6 hrs) is essential. Hemoglobin ≤ 7.5 gms/dL is a general guideline for transfusion especially over the first 12–24 hrs postprocedure. Low hemoglobin levels can be tolerated more safely several days post-operatively. The early hours are characterized by a steady decline in circulating red cell volume. Low or borderline hemoglobin levels or signs of volume depletion (tachycardia, decreased peripheral pulses, delayed capillary refill, decreased urine output, increased serum lactic acid) may require administration of blood products rather than crystalloid. Note that blood pressure may be *increased* or normal despite marked volume depletion and that hypotension is a late sign of shock in a child. An appropriate infusion rate for transfusion of blood products is needed to replace a potentially critical deficit, recognizing that ongoing bleeding likely is taking place at the surgical site. Excessive drain output should prompt a check of the hemoglobin, platelet count, serum calcium, and coagulation profile. Disseminated intravascular coagulopathy may occur. Coagulopathy associated with bleeding should be treated aggressively.

Fluids and Electrolytes. Fluid and electrolyte balance should be monitored. Patients are at risk for increased ADH secretion; serum sodium should be monitored and measures taken to avoid resultant hyponatremia. Potassium, magnesium and phosphorus should be replaced as needed (*Electrolyte Disturbances, 6.2*).

Neurologic Checks. Scoliosis surgery has a risk of permanent neurologic impairment and paralysis. The risk is highest at the time of curve correction intra- operatively. Although very rare, some patients can lose neurologic function after the procedure, usually within the first 24 hrs. Hourly neurologic checks the night of surgery can alert the surgeon to the need for immediate action such as returning to the operating room to remove the implants.

11.2.2 *Tracheostomy*

The first report of successful pediatric tracheostomy was for relief of foreign body related airway obstruction in 1766. Historically, pediatric tracheostomy was often performed emergently for diphtheritic croup, tetanus, epiglottitis, laryngotracheobronchitis, neurologic disease and foreign bodies. With the advent of immunizations against common infectious diseases, widespread availability of endotracheal intubation, new adjuncts for tracheal intubation of the difficult airway

---

Box 11.2.1   Potential Indications for Tracheostomy in Pediatric Patients

- Upper airway obstruction caused by:
  - ▸ Subglottic stenosis, congenital or acquired (most common)
  - ▸ Congenital malformations
  - ▸ Airway malacia
  - ▸ Laryngeal cleft
  - ▸ Vocal cord palsies
  - ▸ Papillomatosis
  - ▸ Mass lesions (*e.g.* tumors, abscess)
  - ▸ Trauma
  - ▸ Burns or equivalent disorders or injuries (*e.g.* Stevens Johnson Syndrome; radiation injury; caustic ingestions)
  - ▸ Functional obstructions (*e.g.* severe obstructive sleep apnea not amenable to non-invasive assistance)
- Need for long term mechanical ventilation*
- For removal of secretions
- Inability to protect the airway (*e.g.* chronic aspiration)
- Emergent tracheostomy: Inability to intubate the trachea

---

* Pediatric patients with potentially reversible problems may tolerate endotracheal intubation for many weeks or months without need for tracheostomy.

Box 11.2.2   Key Points Regarding Tracheostomy Tubes and Post-Operative Care:

- Post-operative care is typically provided in a PICU where airway care and monitoring can be provided until the first successful TT change is completed (usually one week).
- Accidental decannulation is life-threatening. The type and size TT placed should be known by the critical care team; ALWAYS have scissors to cut tracheostomy ties and a second TT of the same size AND the two next smaller sizes at the bedside. An appropriately sized ETT may be temporarily inserted into the tracheostomy site or through the glottis in an emergency if an appropriately sized TT is unavailable.
- The TT size inscribed on the flange generally indicates the *inner* diameter of the TT; when TT replacement with a different size is necessary, the *outer* diameter (usually noted by the manufacturer on the package) of the original tube often dictates the next most appropriate size. Differences in length should also be considered.
- Attempted replacement of a TT through a freshly created tracheostomy may lead to inadvertent placement of the TT in a facial plane between the skin surface and the trachea ("false lumen"). Failure to re-enter the trachea should be recognized and rectified.
- Inspired gases should be warmed and humidified; failure to provide warm, humidified gases may result in drying of secretions, mucus plugging and TT occlusion.
- Analgesia and sedation needs should be addressed; muscle relaxation may be appropriate in selected mechanically ventilated patients.
- The presence of a TT in the trachea alters the relationship between the glottis and epiglottis such that aspiration is encouraged by incomplete glottis closure. All patients should be evaluated by a speech pathologist prior to oral feeding and for vocalization potential once stable and surgically "cleared" for advancement to oral feeding.

(*Bag-mask Ventilation and Tracheal Intubation, 15.2*) and pediatric critical care services, emergency tracheostomy is rarely required (**Box 11.2.1**). Key points regarding tracheostomies and their care and potential complications of tracheostomy are listed in (**Boxes 11.2.2 and 11.2.3**).

Outline of operative procedure as commonly performed:

- Tracheostomy is typically performed over an endotracheal tube (ETT) or percutaneously with bronchoscopic guidance.
- Patients < 12 mos: vertical skin incision.
- The strap musculature and thyroid isthmus are divided. The thymus and innominate vessels are below the level of the tracheotomy and excluded from the surgical field.
- The cricoid is elevated with a cricoid hook and the second and third tracheal rings are located.

Box 11.2.3   Complications of Tracheostomy

Early (First Week)	Intervention
• Accidental decannulation	Re-establish airway.
• TT obstruction	Bag-to-tracheostomy ventilation, suction, saline and/or bicarbonate lavage if needed; exchange TT if necessary.
• Pneumothorax	Chest tube if indicated; if small, may be monitored closely with serial CXRs.
• Pneumomediastinum	Monitor; usually self-resolves
• Bleeding	If severe, notify surgeon; check platelets, PT/PTT; support with volume/blood products.
• Stoma infection; tracheitis	Appropriate cultures and antibiotics.
• Dysphagia, aspiration, poor cough	Consult with speech pathologist; diagnostic studies (video swallow) as indicated

Late: All early complications, PLUS

• Granuloma formation	Surgical consultation for removal if obstructive.
• Suction trauma	Ensure that the suction catheter tip is not passed beyond the distal tip of the TT.
• Colonization, tracheitis, pneumonia	Appropriate cultures and antibiotics.

(Continued)

Box 11.2.3   Complications of Tracheostomy (Continued)

• Late-bleeding	If associated with suctioning, R/O airway trauma; proceed as for early-occurring bleeding; Persistent late bleeding not responsive to conservative measures may herald innominate artery erosion;* surgical re-evaluation is essential; surgical re-exploration or angiography may be required.
• Tracheomalacia	Nutrition; growth; positive pressure (CPAP).

---

* Tracheo-innominate fistula formation (usually due to erosion of the tip of a low-lying TT into the innominate artery as it crosses the antero-lateral tracheal surface) is rare but life-threatening. If hemorrhage is significant, tamponade should be attempted by insertion of a cuffed ETT through the tracheostomy with hyperinflation of the cuff at the fistulous tract. The position of the cuff would need to be manipulated to determine its optimal position. In larger patients (*e.g.* adults), after the ETT is inserted, a finger is also inserted with upward pressure on the artery until surgical help arrives. For pediatric patients with this complication, size of the trachea (and the doctor's finger) present obvious difficulties with this emergency intervention. Hence, late bleeding should be reported to the appropriate surgeon as soon as possible.

- The trachea is incised vertically at the third tracheal ring.
- Prolene suture (4.0) is passed through each divided side of the trachea ("stay sutures").
- Steri-strips are *clearly* labeled "RIGHT" and "LEFT;" these secure each respective stay suture in a loop. Gentle upward traction on these sutures allows visualization of the trachea.
- An appropriately sized tracheostomy tube (TT) is placed; once ventilation through the TT is confirmed the ETT is withdrawn.
- Clearly labeled "stay sutures" are securely taped to the skin; in event of accidental TT dislodgement, these can be useful to identify the trachea and re-insert the TT. The flange of the TT is sutured to the skin.

- Stay sutures are removed by the surgeon, usually on the 7th post-operative day, after an adequate tracheo-cutaneous fistula has been established.
- Post-procedure CXR is obtained to confirm the radiographic position of the TT in relation to the carina and to R/O pneumothorax.

Pertinent Questions to ask and/or plans to make with the surgeon:

- If this patient is accidentally decannulated and the TT cannot be replaced, will endotracheal intubation ("from above") be feasible? If not, what should be done by the bedside team and whom should be called?
- Does the tracheostomy have stay sutures?
- Is the TT sewn to the skin (usually in patients >2 yrs)?
- When will the first TT change be performed?
- If the tracheotomy is performed because of upper airway obstruction or anomaly, pre-and post-procedure photographs are indicated. Are there any endoscopic photographs available in the chart?
- Was a tracheal stent (used in laryngeal reconstruction) placed above the tracheostomy? If so, emergent intubation from above is not possible. Specifics should be discussed with the surgeon.
- Ask the surgeon to draw a picture of any altered or unusual anatomy.
- Is there an inner cannula for the TT? (These are *not* used in TT's <4.0 mm internal diameter.)

Potential benefits of tracheostomy include:

- ↓ Work of breathing
- ↓ Airway resistance
- ↓ Peak inspiratory pressure and auto-PEEP compared to conventional ventilation via an ETT
- ↑ Patient comfort
- ↑Potential for communication
- ↑Patient mobility
- Facilitates transition from ICU care

In the absence of the need for maintaining high airway pressures, uncuffed tracheostomy tubes that allow air leak around the tube are preferable to permit vocalization and minimize the effect on swallowing.

Long-term care for the patient with a tracheostomy requires:

- Caretaker education and demonstration of competency in changing the tracheostomy tube, suctioning the airway and ability to perform emergency procedures in airway care, including CPR.
- Resources for monitoring, provision of humidification, suctioning, and other adjuncts as needed be in place and evaluated by a home-visit by medical personnel before the patient with a new tracheostomy is discharged home.
- TT's are generally changed and cleaned weekly; inner cannulae are removed and cleaned daily. Half-strength hydrogen peroxide may serve as a cleanser.
- Routine change of a TT in the hospital requires preparation similar to that for tracheal intubation (*Bag-Mask Ventilation and Tracheal Intubation, 15.2*); the possibility of failed access through the tracheal stoma with the need to intubate the trachea from the mouth or nose should be considered in preparing for the procedure. Oxygen, suction, appropriately sized suction catheters, TT's (including one that is at least a half size smaller than the current size) and ties should be available, in addition to all equipment required for conventional intubation of the trachea. Proper positioning for optimal exposure of the neck is essential for a "seamless" exchange of airways.

The decision to remove a TT and allow closure of the tracheostomy (**"decannulation"**) depends on the following:

- The original reason for the tracheostomy and whether or not that need is no longer present (*e.g.* no further need for mechanical ventilatory support).
- The patient's general health.
- The ability to clear secretions.
- Bronchoscopic assessment for granulation tissue or other factors that may interfere with successful decannulation.

- Successful TT occlusion for ≥ 24 hrs; a sleep study may be warranted.
- Removal of the TT results in spontaneous closure of the tracheostomy with within hours to days.

11.2.3 *Hydrocephalus and CSF diversion*

Under normal conditions, CSF is continually produced, circulated around the brain and spinal cord and reabsorbed into the systemic circulation so as to maintain intracranial contents at a stable volume and pressure. Excessive CSF production (rare) or interference in CSF circulation and/or reabsorption result in hydrocephalus which is necessarily accompanied by an increase in intraventricular volume and pressure. Hydrocephalus should be considered the result of a pathologic condition rather than a "final diagnosis".

CSF is continuously produced by the choroid plexus within the lateral, third, and fourth ventricles and as a by-product of cerebral and spinal cord metabolism. CSF formation occurs at a rate of 0.3 ml/min in adults (approximately 400–500 ml/day), regardless of intracranial pressure (ICP) as long as the choroid plexus and the brain itself are perfused. Age, body mass, and various disease states affect the rate of CSF production. The total volume of CSF in infants is ~50 ml compared with ~150 ml in normal adults; this difference becomes negligible after 1–2 yrs of age.

The secretion of CSF (which is biochemically indistinguishable from brain extracellular fluid) by the choroid plexus is a metabolically active process involving ion pumps and enzyme systems similar to those found in the distal tubule of the kidney. Although of limited clinical usefulness, diuretics such as carbonic anhydrase inhibitors and furosemide can limit CSF production. Unlike CSF secretion, CSF reabsorption is a purely passive process driven in a linear fashion by the pressure differential between the subarachnoid space and the venous circulation, specifically, the major dural venous sinuses. The balance between CSF secretion and reabsorption helps maintain ICP within the normal range. With the exception of a tumor of the choroid plexus that causes excessive CSF secretion, the diseases that cause hydrocephalus do so by interfering with CSF reabsorption. Under these conditions, a greater ICP to dural venous sinus pressure gradient is required to reabsorb CSF into the venous circulation.

To reach the subarachnoid space and villi, CSF passes through a series of channels and pathways. Pulsations of the choroid plexus propel CSF from the lateral ventricles into the third ventricle via the foramen of Monro then into the fourth ventricle through the aqueduct of Sylvius. From the fourth ventricle (through either the lateral foramina of Luschka or the foramen of Magendie) CSF exits the ventricular system and travels around the brainstem and spinal cord and over the surface of the brain, where it is absorbed by the arachnoid villi. Alternate pathways for CSF absorption may come into play when ICP is increased. CSF may travel into the paranasal sinuses, conjunctiva, and surrounding (extra-cranial) lymphatics, as well as along the cranial or spinal nerves to be absorbed into the systemic circulation.

Hydrocephalus may be classified as congenital or acquired, communicating or non-communicating, and intra- or extra-ventricular. The description of communicating vs. non-communicating hydrocephalus may be most helpful in understanding etiology and treatment options (**Box 11.2.4**). Non-communicating hydrocephalus can result from blockage of any part of the ventricular system, obstructing the passage of CSF from one ventricle into another or from the ventricular system into the subarachnoid cisterns. This results in enlargement of the ventricular system proximal to the site of obstruction. For example, when the aqueduct of Sylvius is obstructed, the lateral and third ventricles enlarge but the fourth ventricle remains normal in size.

Communicating hydrocephalus occurs when CSF flow or absorption is blocked in the subarachnoid spaces, basilar cisterns, and the arachnoid villi. CSF may circulate freely throughout the entire ventricular system and cisterns but not be adequately absorbed; the lateral, third and fourth ventricles are enlarged. Communicating hydrocephalus may be associated with meningitis (bacterial or viral), intraventricular hemorrhage, trauma, or a congenital malformation of the subarachnoid spaces.

Box 11.2.4   Classification and Causes of Hydrocephalus

- "Non-communicating" (Intraventricular) hydrocephalus: may occur secondary to obstruction at the following sites:
  ▸ Lateral ventricle: neoplasm; ventriculitis
  ▸ Foramen of Monro: agenesis; mass; ventriculitis; hemorrhage
  ▸ Third ventricle
    ■ Anterior: mass lesions such as craniopharyngioma; glioma; sellar mass; aneurysm
    ■ Posterior: pineal neoplasm; quadrigeminal cyst; malformations of the Vein of Galen; arachnoid cyst
  ▸ Aqueduct of Sylvius: congenital stenosis (the most common cause of non-communicating obstruction; 7% of hydrocephalic males have Bickers-Adams Syndrome, X-linked); may be associated with perinatal infections; ventriculitis; hemorrhage; Vein of Galen malformation or other mass causing external compression of the aqueduct; Arnold-Chiari Malformation
  ▸ Fourth ventricle: Dandy-Walker cyst (associated with cerebellar malformations; hydrocephalus results from obstruction of foramina of Luschka and Magendie); ventriculitis; hemorrhage; Arnold-Chiari malformation
- "Communicating" (Extra-ventricular) hydrocephalus may occur secondary to any of the following:
  ▸ Obstruction in the subarachnoid space due to: hemorrhage; infection; ↑ CSF protein; mass; meningeal infiltration
  ▸ Obstruction of the basal cisterns: hemorrhage; infection; neoplastic seeding
  ▸ Lesions at the supra- and infra-tentorial junction: Arnold-Chiari malformation; achondroplasia associated with deformities of the skull base.
  ▸ Obstruction of arachnoid granulations*: trauma, hemorrhage, infection, or subdural hematoma may damage these structures and interfere with CSF drainage. Congenital hypoplasia of arachnoid granulations may occur.

* Protrusions of the arachnoid through the dura mater through which CSF enters the venous system; small granulations are also called arachnoid villi, arachnoid granulations act as one-way valves to allow CSF to leave the subarachnoid space.

"Hydrocephalus *ex vacuo*" is not true hydrocephalus. The ventricles are enlarged, but intraventricular pressure is not increased. The ventricular enlargement is secondary to atrophy of the brain parenchyma as evidenced by enlargement of the sulci and loss of brain tissue on radiologic evaluation; it is manifested over time by decreased head circumference.

Raised ICP is associated with poor functional neurologic outcomes. If raised ICP is due to hydrocephalus, the diversion of CSF to a body cavity where absorption can occur should result in normalization of ICP. Ventriculoperitoneal (VP) shunts continue to be a mainstay of treatment to reduce the amount of intracranial CSF, decrease ICP, and therefore minimize potential damage to the brain (**Fig. 11.2.2**).

Clinical Manifestations at Diagnosis. Although the signs and symptoms of hydrocephalus may vary depending on its cause, there are common clinical manifestations associated with increased CSF volume and ICP (**Box 11.2.5**). The presence or absence of an expandable cranium and the volume and compliance of cerebral tissue determine the severity of symptoms. If the accumulation of excessive CSF occurs slowly, an infant or young child may be asymptomatic until the hydrocephalus is advanced. Infants are less likely to be acutely ill because their skull and sutures can expand to accommodate increasing ventricular size, thereby mitigating an elevation in ICP.

Specific signs and symptoms of increased ICP are evident in children over 18–24 months of age with fused cranial sutures (**Box 11.2.5**). Depending on the cause of hydrocephalus and the severity of increased ICP, these symptoms can be either acute or chronic and intermittent.

Early recognition of hydrocephalus can prevent brain herniation. The frontal and periventricular areas of the brain are particularly prone to diminished perfusion as hydrocephalus progresses. Herniation syndromes (*Raised Intracranial Pressure, 5.5, Fig. 5.5.5*) can permanently damage brain parenchyma as a result of raised ICP or direct mechanical compression of the brain. Shunt evaluation and management are described in **Box 11.2.6 and Fig. 11.2.2**, (further discussion occurs in the following section).

Box 11.2.5   Signs and Symptoms of Increased ICP

Infants	Children
• ↑ Head circumference	• Headache, esp. on awakening,
• Rapid head growth	or when headache causes
• Seizures*	awakening during sleep
• Full fontanel	• Nausea
• Split cranial sutures	• Vomiting
• Dilated scalp veins	• Irritability and/or lethargy; apathy
• Developmental delay or	• Seizures*
loss of milestones	• Alterations in motor development
• Increased tone; hyperreflexia	• Spasticity; ataxia
• Macewen's sign ("cracked-	• Urinary incontinence
pot sound" heard with	• New-onset or worsening strabismus
percussion over dilated	• Electrolyte (esp. sodium) imbalance
ventricles)	• Disturbances in growth and
Late Signs:	development (due to pressure
• Lethargy	on the hypothalamus)
• Poor feeding; vomiting	• Visual disturbances (due to
• Seizures*	pressure on cranial nerves II, III
• Limitation of upward gaze	and VI)
("setting sun sign")	• Stridor
• Sixth nerve palsy	• Bradycardia
• Irregular respirations	• Papilledema (may occur late)
• Apnea	

* Seizures may occur at any point during the development of raised ICP depending on individual risk factors (see discussion below).

Radiologic Imaging. Computed tomography (CT) scans typically demonstrate increased ventricular size in hydrocephalus. Magnetic resonance imaging (MRI) is sensitive for periventricular edema (T-1 weighted images). Obstruction due to posterior fossa lesions are better visualized on MRI as compared to CT. Newer techniques to assess the flow of CSF are being refined. *Ex vacuo* hydrocephalus may be differentiated from true hydrocephalus by the presence of well-defined sulci (CT *or* MRI) and the absence of periventricular edema (MRI). Ultrasonography is most useful in the neonate when the fontanels are open; both hydrocephalus and intraventricular hemorrhage can be identified. Angiography may identify the rare vascular malformation associated with hydrocephalus.

A series of **plain films** (AP and lateral views) of the skull, neck, chest, and abdomen ("shunt series") is useful in identification of shunt discontinuity which leads to signs and symptoms of shunt malfunction. With the exception of the valve and connectors, most components are radio-opaque to allow for identification of a disconnection. On plain films, split sutures suggest hydrocephalus, a small posterior fossa suggests aqueductal stenosis, and a large posterior fossa suggests Dandy-Walker syndrome.

CSF Diversion ("CSF Shunts"). Surgical treatment for hydrocephalus is directed at restoring CSF flow by either removing the obstruction to CSF flow or creating a new CSF pathway. The latter typically involves placement of a ventricular catheter or shunt to divert CSF flow, usually to the peritoneal cavity for absorption.

Shunt Components. CSF shunts consist typically of three parts: a ventricular catheter, a valve, and a distal catheter (**Fig. 11.2.1**). The

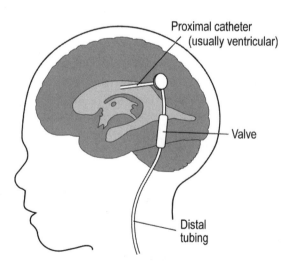

Fig. 11.2.1.   A Typical CSF Shunt Apparatus.

Box 11.2.6   Shunt Evaluation and Management

- Palpation of shunt apparatus: Type of shunt and presence of valve may be discernible by an experienced examiner.
- Note erythema, swelling, leakage of fluid, *etc.* associated with the course of the shunt.
- Patency of valve: An easily depressed valve is consistent with distal patency; rapid refill suggest proximal patency; however, sensitivity of this procedure is only 18–20% for shunt obstruction.
- Imaging:

  ▸ Shunt series: AP and lateral radiographs of the skull, neck, thorax and abdomen to identify any hardware discontinuity.

  ▸ Head CT: Comparison with prior, baseline images are critical to evaluate ventricular size. Ventriculomegaly may persist in some patients despite a functioning shunt. Conversely, some patients have shunt malfunctions and high ICP despite small or unchanged ventricles on CT. A "negative" CT scan does not rule out shunt obstruction, particularly if symptoms persist.

- Neurosurgical consultation should be obtained.
- Aspiration of fluid from the shunt should be discussed with the neurosurgeon. CSF cell count, culture, Gram stain, glucose and protein should be obtained. Once shunt obstruction has been demonstrated, the neurosurgeon plans the neurosurgical intervention. If the patient is stable, operative intervention may not occur immediately; the patient should be monitored closely (usually in a PICU) because of their potential for rapid deterioration.
- Patients should be maintained NPO; IVF should be isotonic and excessive fluid volumes should be avoided. The serum sodium should be monitored and hyponatremia should be avoided.
- Coagulopathy should be corrected.
- The usefulness of mannitol or other diuretic therapy should be discussed with the neurosurgeon.
- If the neurologic status deteriorates, airway, breathing and circulation should be appropriately resuscitated; the neurosurgeon should be notified immediately so that definitive interventions may proceed as indicated.

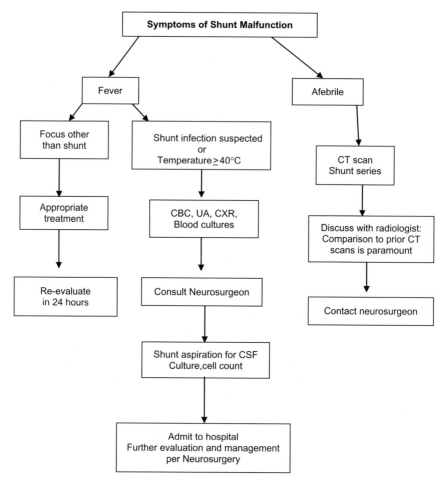

Fig. 11.2.2.   **Approach to Evaluation and Management of CSF Shunt Malfunction.**

ventricular catheter passes from the ventricle through the cortical mantle out of the skull through a burr hole to reach the external surface of the skull, where it is joined to the inlet of the valve. There are a variety of valve designs that incorporate various clever mechanical mechanisms, but the purpose of each is to prevent excessive CSF drainage. Excessive ventricular drainage can lead to postural headaches, subdural hemorrhage and chronic changes in brain compliance that promote recurrent proximal shunt failure. Most valves include a reservoir that can be punctured percutaneously with a needle for diagnostic purposes. The valve is connected to a distal catheter that carries CSF to a body site where it can be reabsorbed into the venous circulation at low pressure. Popular sites for CSF diversion are the peritoneal cavity, the pleural cavity, the gall bladder, the right atrium of the heart, and the internal jugular vein. Lumbar CSF shunts are schematically similar except that a lumbar intrathecal catheter takes the place of the ventricular catheter in communicating hydrocephalus.

Shunt Complications. The attractive feature of the CSF shunt is its nearly universal applicability in the management of hydrocephalus regardless of cause. The burden of the CSF shunt is a high rate of complications. The most common complications are described in (**Box 11.2.7**). Both retrospective and prospective studies consistently document that 30–40% of shunts fail on either a mechanical or an infectious basis in the first year after initial placement, and an additional 15% fail in the second year. The incidence of infection after shunt placement is approximately 8–12% in large series and usually occurs within the first few months post-procedure. The various types of non-infectious shunt failure occur at different intervals after shunt surgery. Obstruction of the shunt system can occur at any time after shunt placement and at any point along the shunt. The mean survival time for a VP shunt is 5 yrs; 80% of patients require shunt revision by the 10th year. The mortality from initial shunt insertion is estimated at 0.1%; mortality from shunt failure is estimated at 1–4%. Shunts in children with tumors and intraventricular hemorrhage were found to have the highest rates of complications requiring revision.

The presentation of shunt malfunction generally suggests one of three events: acute ICP elevation; chronic, insidiously progressive ICP elevation, and/or infection. The symptoms and signs of acute ICP elevation are familiar: headache, nausea, vomiting, acute papilledema, and occasionally sixth nerve palsy. Parental descriptions of distention of scalp veins or puffiness around the eyes should not be dismissed, even though the physiologic mechanisms and the findings themselves may not be obvious. Many of these findings are age related and mimic the signs of untreated hydrocephalus with raised ICP

Box 11.2.7   CSF Shunt Complications

Most Common Causes (Overall Incidence) and Key Points

- Shunt Occlusion (49%)
  ▶ May result from acute or chronic inflammation, overgrowth of the choroid plexus, accumulation of cellular debris or blood in the tubing, or secondary to distal or proximal shunt tip occlusion from ↑ in body size.

- Shunt hardware disconnections (13%)
  ▶ May occur at any section of the shunt but are esp. common at sites of mobility and with patient growth. Retained shunt fragments have been left in place if there is no evidence of infection or foreign body reaction.

- Infection (19%)
  ▶ Risk is ~8–10% per surgical procedure
  ▶ Most often a result of contamination at surgery, and most likely to present within 3–6 mos of the surgical procedure. Late infections likely have different sources.
  ▶ CSF fistulization of the surgical wound, wound dehiscence and skin breakdown over the shunt hardware account for most of the remaining infections.
  ▶ Fever is usually present; redness and swelling at surgical sites or overlying shunt tubing, drainage of pus or CSF from a surgical wound are highly suggestive; nuchal rigidity; abdominal pain and signs of peritonitis may be present if the peritoneal cavity is involved.
  ▶ Patients with epilepsy may have ↑ in seizure frequency; patients with myelomeningocele may have dysphonia, dysphagia, or disturbed respirations (underlying Chiari II malformation); progressive myelopathy may be related to underlying syringomyelia.
  ▶ *Staphylococcus epidermidis*, followed by *S. aureus*, followed by Gram-negative enteric bacteria (*Enterococcus faecalis*) and *Proprionibacterium* are the most common causative agents.

(Continued)

> **Box 11.2.7   CSF Shunt Complications (Continued)**
>
> - Other Causes of Shunt Malfunction
>   - ▸ Shunt migration: Signs and symptoms depend on shunt destination (*e.g.* GI and GU tracts, chest, cranium, umbilicus, *et al.*)
>   - ▸ Over- or under-drainage of CSF from the ventricles (*e.g.* "slit ventricle" syndrome)
>   - ▸ Mechanical malfunction of hardware
>   - ▸ Intra-abdominal infection
>   - ▸ Pseudocyst formation: Presentation with an expanding intra-abdominal mass; signs and symptoms may mimic an acute abdomen. Diagnosis may be made by USG or at laparotomy.

(**Box 11.2.5**). The diagnosis of shunt malfunction should be eliminated before ascribing symptoms to another cause (*e.g.* gastroenteritis or viral syndrome). Obstruction is associated with infection in almost one third of cases and initiation of antibiotic therapy is indicated unless shunt infection can be ruled out in a timely manner.

Early recognition of shunt obstruction and appropriate intervention are essential if morbidity and mortality related to raised ICP is to be avoided. Shunt obstruction may occur at either the proximal (ventricular) end, at the interposed valve, or at the distal end (usually in the peritoneal space). Proximal obstruction is more common than distal obstruction. The valve between the proximal and distal tubing may also become occluded with brain debris or tissue colonization.

Distal obstruction may also result from kinking of the tubing, migration, disconnections, *et al.* (**Box 11.2.7**).

Seizures. Forty-eight percent of children with VP shunts have seizures; there is a high correlation with the underlying neurologic disorder. There is insufficient direct evidence of an association between seizures and shunt surgery to warrant routine prophylaxis with antiepileptic drugs. However, seizure activity can be a presenting sign of CSF shunt malfunction, particularly in patients who are vulnerable to their occurrence (*e.g.* patients with known seizure disorders). Also, shunt malfunction may present as a first-time seizure. Various types of seizure may be observed, including generalized tonic-clonic, focal motor, simple partial, and petit mal. New seizures should prompt evaluation for a CNS infection and antiepileptic drugs should be considered. If anticonvulsant drugs are given, levels should be monitored.

Determination of functional shunt integrity may or may not be straightforward. Availability of prior head CT images is essential because comparisons of ventricular size typically allow conclusions regarding whether or not CSF is draining adequately. For example, an image of the brain while a well-functioning shunt is present or after hydrocephalus is relieved by external drainage serves as a baseline for that patient should he present with symptoms of possible shunt malfunction. At the time of malfunction, the head CT may reveal ventricular enlargement. However, changes in ventricular volume are not always apparent, particularly when brain tissue is poorly compliant or early-on in the development of symptoms. The ability to "pump the shunt," *i.e.* manually compress an externally palpable value and test its refilling capacity (its re-expansion with CSF) has been a misleading source of reassurance and is not a reliable test in the face of possible shunt malfunction.

Symptoms of shunt malfunction are often influenced by the type of shunt and its location. For example, ventriculo-atrial (VA) shunts are associated with chronic pulmonary thromboembolism and cor pulmonale. Chronic VA shunt infection (usually with coagulase negative *staphylococcus*) is uniquely associated with immune-mediated glomerulonephritis ("shunt nephritis").

Abdominal pseudocysts may develop around the peritoneal end of the VP shunt causing shunt malfunction and may become infected. Children with an infected pseudocyst may have fever, abdominal pain, anorexia, nausea, vomiting, or diarrhea; there may be abdominal guarding and unwillingness to walk. Abdominal ultrasound and CSF cultures should help differentiate between an acute abdomen and a shunt infection. Specific signs of appendicitis can be demonstrated by abdominal CT scan. A history of recent or recurrent shunt revisions also substantially increases the risk for infection.

Shunt infections (Box 11.2.5) are a common complication described in up to one third of patients. Most often, infection occurs within the first few months after surgery. There is a positive association between the frequency of infection and the number of shunt revisions, a longer operative time, the presence of a myelomeningocele, prematurity, age less than 6 months and individual surgical operators. Presentation often is insidious and may include a change in mental status, fever, irritability, malaise, or nausea. Aspiration of CSF from the shunt ("shunt tap") may reveal increased leukocyte count, elevated protein, decreased glucose and a culture positive for bacteria. Fluid should be obtained from the reservoir only after discussion with the neurosurgeon. The culture results should be emphasized because the protein, glucose and cell count may be normal despite infection. Cultures of lumbar CSF or CSF obtained directly from the ventricle are less frequently positive as compared to CSF obtained directly through the shunt. If increased ICP is suspected or present, LP is contraindicated (*Lumbar Puncture, 15.5*).

Treatment options include antibiotics with or without removal of the shunt. The highest success rate has been reported with shunt removal or shunt externalization combined with antibiotics. Ventriculitis warrants removal of the shunt, external ventricular drainage (placement of an external ventricular drain or "EVD") and IV antibiotics with or without intraventricular antibiotics (depending on the organism and the ability of the required antibiotic to penetrate the CNS). Once the CSF is sterile the shunt should be replaced. In a child who presents with infection and *a functioning shunt*, the shunt may be left in place while treatment with antibiotics proceeds. The shunt should be replaced after the CSF is sterile. However, treatment should be individualized. Initial antibiotic therapy should be broad in spectrum. Gram stain results should be incorporated into the initial antibiotic plan, but therapy should not be narrowed until final identification of the organism is available and antibiotic sensitivities are known. Commonly used IV antibiotic combinations include an anti-Staphylococcal agent (*e.g.* vancomycin or nafcillin depending on local staphylococcal sensitivities) plus a third generation cephalosporin (*e.g.* cefotaxime); an aminoglycoside should be added if history or Gram stain suggests Gram negative infection.

In an ongoing effort to find alternatives to the placement of shunt hardware, the endoscopic third ventriculostomy (ETV) has become a rewarding alternative for selected patients with obstructive hydrocephalus. The procedure involves formation of a surgical defect in the floor of the third ventricle, allowing CSF to reach the subarachnoid space and therefore, bypass obstructions caudal to the third ventricle. Its success is related to age (older patients are better candidates than younger patients) and the cause of the hydrocephalus (noninfectious causes such as a mass or aqueductal stenosis are associated with a higher success rate). Shunt placement has been avoided in up to 65–70% of "the best candidates," but operative risks are increased and mortality has been estimated at one percent (Garton HJL, Piatt JH, Hydrocephalus, *Pediatr Clin N America* **51**: 305–325, 2004).

Chapter 12

Environmental Emergencies

12.1 Snake Bites

Few circumstances invoke terror and trepidation for children, parents, and clinicians as does the snakebite. Fortunately, less than 25% of North American snakes are venomous, and pediatric snake envenomation in the United States is relatively rare and mortality is uncommon. However, compared to adults, children represent a number of unique challenges. First, children are inquisitive and lack a learned aversion to venomous snakes, placing them at risk for envenomation. Second, due to higher venom to body mass ratio, systemic signs, symptoms and mortality are more common in children. Finally, the application and dosing of the standard antivenom, frequently the mainstay of treatment, has not been well studied in the pediatric population.

North American Venomous Snakes and Snake Identification. Most venomous snakes in the United States belong to the family *Viperidae* and are known as pit vipers, identified by a sensory pit between the eye and nostril bilaterally. This family includes 18 species of rattlesnakes (*genera* Crotalus and Sistrurus) as well as the *Agkistrodon genus*, including the copperhead and cottonmouth species. The other venomous family (*Elapidae*) includes the coral snakes. Fortunately, the majority of U.S. venomous species exhibit characteristics that are easily identifiable as venomous (**Box 12.1.1**).

Although capturing a snake that has bitten a child is not recommended, families may present with the offending snake. After ensuring

---

Box 12.1.1 Venomous Snake Characteristics

- A larger head to neck ratio. (The head of a <u>non</u>-venomous snake is typically more proportional to neck size.)
- A triangular head
- Sensory pits between the eye and nostril (pit vipers)
- Elliptical pupils
- A single row of ventral plates distal to the anal plate
- Fang marks on skin versus a row of small teeth

---

that the snake is dead, it is important to differentiate venomous from non-venomous snakes.

Pharmacology of Snake Venom. Snake venom is a complex mixture of chemical constituents, primarily enzymatic proteins that exhibit both inter- and intra-species variation. The effects of venom injection include local immobilization, tissue digestion, tissue necrosis, and the additional potential of direct neurotoxicity, coagulopathy, myotoxicity and cardiotoxicity. Although there is a tendency to categorize individual species venom according to the organ or tissue most affected, venom proteins bind to multiple receptors and can affect multiple organ systems simultaneously. Damage to capillary endothelium with extravasation of fluid into the extracellular space is a common and consistent effect, particularly at the site of the bite. Significant third-spacing of volume can lead to hemoconcentration, hypovolemic shock, acute kidney injury and lactic acidosis. Fortunately, sufficient homology is observed within the venom of North American snakes to render antivenom effective across the *Viperidae* family. Distinct antivenom is necessary for coral snake bites.

Signs and Symptoms of Envenomation. Panic is a common reaction to snakebite. It is difficult but important to discern fear-induced autonomic signs from those of systemic envenomation. Accordingly, many children will exhibit tachycardia, nausea, vomiting or syncope in the early post-bite period. The earliest local sign in most pit viper envenomations is pain, and many children relate that copperhead bites are quite painful. Mojave rattlesnake bites are reportedly less painful.

- Local symptoms and signs: These include pain, paresthesia, burning, or numbness. For most North American species, the most notable local sign is edema secondary to venom-induced alterations in vascular permeability, with onset in 30–60 mins. Hemorrhagic bullae and regional lymphadenopathy may be present, with ecchymosis more common following rattlesnake bites.
- Systemic: Early signs of systemic envenomation include nausea, vomiting, and lethargy. Gustatory and perioral findings include perioral paresthesia and a metallic taste (rattlesnake). Many systemic symptoms are secondary to hypovolemia, including tachycardia, hypotension, and altered mental status. Acute kidney injury may be due to hypovolemia or myoglobinuria. Tachypnea and respiratory failure are more common following coral snake bites (neurotoxin with respiratory paralysis).
- Coagulation: Coagulopathy may manifest as thrombocytopenia, consumptive hypofibrinogenemia, and may prolong the PT/ PTT. Coagulopathy is of variable incidence and severity among species, being less common with copperhead envenomation, but having the potential for unmeasurable PT and PTT after rattlesnake envenomation.
- Although **coral snakes** do not have hypodermic fangs and have a higher incidence of dry bites, envenomation tends to be more severe than that of other North American species. The venom is primarily neurotoxic, leading to cranial nerve palsies, respiratory depression and paralysis. The onset of systemic effects may be delayed up to 12 hours, and once present, are less reversible with antivenom.

Determination of Severity of Envenomation. One of the first priorities following a reported snakebite is to determine the degree of envenomation. It is imperative to remember that 30–60% of bites are "dry", in which a clinically insignificant amount of venom is injected. An absence of local and systemic signs and symptoms and absence of coagulopathy after an observation period of 6–8 hours is consistent with a dry bite. Because the venom of most North American species has some coagulopathic effects, bloody drainage from puncture wounds is a use-

Box 12.1.2	Severity of Envenomation		
Findings	Minimal	Moderate	Severe
Local	Swelling, erythema, +/− ecchymosis confined to site of the bite*	Progression of swelling, erythema, and/or ecchymosis beyond the site of the bite	Rapid swelling or progression involving the entire extremity
Systemic	None	Non-life-threatening signs or symptoms, including nausea, vomiting, perioral paresthesia, fasciculations, metallic taste (rattlesnake)	Severe signs and symptoms, including hypotension, altered sensorium, tachycardia unrelated to pain/ anxiety, tachypnea
Coagulopathy	None	Abnormal coagulation profile without clinical bleeding	Markedly abnormal coagulation profile with clinical bleeding; PT/PTT may be unmeasurable; severe thrombocytopenia; hypofibrinogenemia

* This means that the local response does not extend proximal to the nearest joint.

ful clue to true envenomation. Although a number of classification systems exist, bites should be assessed according to severity of envenomation (**Box 12.1.2**). Of note, the severity of envenomation is predicated upon the most significant abnormality. As an example, edema confined to the region of the fang marks in combination with a mildly abnormal coagulation profile represents a moderate envenomation.

Treatment and Use of Antivenom. The treatment of snakebites is rife with myth and lore, particularly with the advent of the internet; the "do not's" of initial treatment are nearly as important as proper methods (**Box 12.1.3**).

Box 12.1.3 Treatment of Snakebites

- **Initial "Don'ts":**
  ▶ Do not lance or incise the puncture sites.
  ▶ Do not apply suction to the puncture site or apply ice.
  ▶ Do not apply a tourniquet. Tourniquets are reserved for dire circumstances in which emergency care is unavailable. The goal is to prevent venous return from the extremity to the central circulation, but it is critical that arterial flow is not impaired. If placement of a tourniquet is necessary, use a device that is wide and non-constricting, placed ~10 cm. above the bite, and under which two fingers can pass easily.

- **Initial "Do's":**
  ▶ Attempt to calm and reassure the child.
  ▶ Immediately initiate transfer to a facility that can provide definitive care.
  ▶ Expose the bite site and assess for additional bites.
  ▶ Immobilize the extremity and minimize movement and ambulation.
  ▶ Remove clothing, watches and jewelry; edema may progress rapidly.
  ▶ Mark and time the margins of edema and erythema to assist with serial examinations for progression.
  ▶ Measure and time serial determinations of extremity circumference.

- **Definitive Care:** Definitive care is directed at organ system support and administration of antivenom. Antivenom binds and neutralizes venom toxins; it is imperative to remember that attenuation and reversal of venom-induced effects on organ systems depends upon the timely administration of antivenom. For the severely envenomated child, a *horizontal* resuscitation, during which multiple interventions (*e.g.* IV access and the primary survey) proceed concurrently, is optimal.
  ▶ Support airway, breathing and circulation; give oxygen as necessary.
  ▶ Obtain pertinent history.

(Continued)

Box 12.1.3   Treatment of Snakebites (Continued)

▸ Perform a thorough examination, focusing on fang marks and local signs as well as neurologic, respiratory and cardiovascular systems.

▸ Establish IV access with a large bore catheter in a non-envenomated extremity.

▸ Measure and record extremity circumference, repeating every 30–60 mins and as needed.

▸ Mark and time the leading margin of edema or ecchymosis.

▸ If a compartment syndrome is suspected, EARLY surgical consultation is warranted. Muscle compartment pressures should be measured (pressure should be < 30 mmHg).

▸ Obtain plain X-rays of the effected extremity for retained fang (s) which may be a continued source of toxin.

▸ Obtain baseline laboratory data: electrolytes, creatine phosphokinase (esp. if compartment syndrome is suspected); platelet count, PT, PTT and fibrinogen.

▸ Do not administer antibiotics routinely.

▸ Evaluate tetanus status and immunize if the patient has received < 3 doses of toxoid, if the immunization history is unknown, or if > 5 yrs have lapsed since the last vaccine.

▸ Control pain with narcotics; avoid NSAID's if coagulopathy is present.

▸ Keep the affected extremity at the level of the heart.

▸ Administer antivenom as indicated (see text).

▸ Monitor the patient in an ICU if antivenom is administered.

▸ Treat coagulopathy with antivenom, not with blood products.

Antivenin *Crotalidae* Polyvalent (ACP, Wyeth Ayerst) was the sole antivenin available prior to the approval of *Crotalidae* Polyvalent Immune Fab (CroFab™, Protherics) by the Food and Drug Administration in 2000. ACP, which contains whole serum IgG obtained from immunized horses, utilizes venom from select North American crotalid as well as South American species. CroFab™ is an ovine product utilizing only the Fab fragment of the immunoglobulin generated from North American rattlesnakes (Eastern and Western Diamondback, Mojave) and water moccasin species. The Fab fragment binds venom toxins rendering them clinically inert, and the Fab-toxin complex is eliminated by the reticuloendothelial system. Anaphylaxis and serum sickness are less frequent than with use of ACP. Accordingly, CroFab™ has replaced ACP as the more commonly used antivenin in North America.

- **Indications:** Rigorous, evidence-based guidelines for the use of antivenom have not been developed. In general, antivenom should be considered for moderate local signs including progression of edema or ecchymosis beyond the site of the bite. Antivenom should be administered for all moderate and severe envenomations (**Box 12.1.2**).
- **Dosage:** The dosage of CroFab™ is dependent upon clinical response. Although not specifically approved for pediatric envenomation, Crofab™ is commonly used in children and adolescents, and appears to be both safe and efficacious. Initial dosing is 4–6 vials IV in a monitored setting. Response, defined as arrest of both local and systemic symptoms, is assessed over one hour. In the absence of response, the initial dose is repeated every hour until clinical response is achieved. Due to the shorter half life of the Fab product relative to venom, systemic symptoms, particularly coagulopathy, can recur. Therefore, two vials should be given every 6 hrs for three doses after clinical control is achieved (**Fig. 12.1.1**).
- **Coral snake antivenom** is distinct from that used for other North American species. Because the systemic effects of coral snake envenomation may be both delayed and less responsive to antivenom after onset, antivenom should be administered when envenomation is suspected. Five vials should be administered IV in a monitored setting. See www.FDA.gov for current status of coral snake antivenom for these envenomations.

Complications of Envenomation and Antivenom

Surgical intervention is not routinely indicated for bite wounds, particularly those resulting from North American species. However, the potential for compartment syndrome warrants vigilant surveillance.

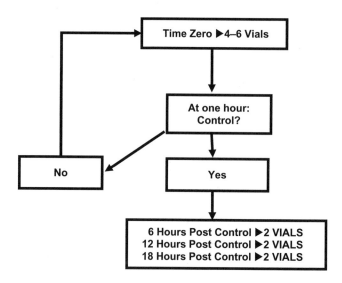

Fig. 12.1.1. Dosing Algorithm for *Crotalidae* Polyvalent Immune Fab (CroFab™).

Signs and symptoms of compartment syndrome include taut swelling of the extremity, pain with active and passive movement of the extremity, and paresthesia or hyperesthesia distal to the involved compartment. It should be noted that subtle neurologic findings may be the first sign of compartment syndrome, and ischemia with loss of pulses is a late finding. With clinical suspicion, pressure should be measured, with pressure ≥ 30 mmHg prompting surgical input. In the U.S., compartment syndrome is more commonly seen with myonecrosis associated with rattlesnake venom, although it has been reported with cottonmouth bites.

12.2 Inhalation Injury

Inhalation injury in children results from exposure to smoke from a flame source or superheated air from a fire or explosion. Though other parts of the body may be injured as well this section focuses solely on injury to the airways and lungs and the management of carbon monoxide poisoning.

Airway injury may be confined to the supraglottic airway alone or may be present below the glottis (even distal to multiple levels of bronchi). Supraglottic injury is most common in children; smaller airway caliber and turbulent flow decreases the extent of smoke and superheated air penetration. With prolonged smoke exposure or older age (*e.g.* adolescents), lower airway involvement becomes more likely and can increase morbidity and mortality. Reasons for concern for airway involvement are noted in **Box 12.2.1**.

Box 12.2.1   History, Signs and Symptoms Concerning for Airway Involvement

- Burned in enclosed space (house, car)
- Hoarseness or stridor
- Carbonaceous material in or around nose or mouth
- Respiratory distress
- Explosive or rapid ignition of accelerant into face
- Singed nasal hairs
- Burns to face, neck, lips

Inhalational injury can also cause many, if not all, of the clinical signs and symptoms associated with acute lung injury and ARDS. This effect has been found to be independently associated with inhalation injury, separate from any burn injury to the remainder of the body. Increased pulmonary vascular permeability and resultant pulmonary edema formation are seen with isolated smoke inhalation. Direct irritation of the airways leads to activation of leukocytes and humoral mediators, further propagating the inflammatory cascade. Vaporized toxins and chemicals, typically seen in workplace fires, can further injure the airways and lung parenchyma.

Airway control via endotracheal intubation is the preferred treatment for respiratory compromise following inhalational injury. With extensive fluid resuscitation often required for burn patients, early, elective intubation is favored over emergent intubation and should be accomplished before transporting from a referring institution. Since airway swelling may decrease airway caliber, smaller than anticipated sized endotracheal tubes should be immediately available at the time of intubation. The use of cuffed endotracheal tubes is preferred because progression of lung disease should be anticipated.

In pediatric patients, fiberoptic bronchoscopy is useful for airway evaluation; thermal injury to the larger airways can be documented and followed for healing, and carbonaceous smoke deposits can be washed from the airways during therapeutic bronchoscopy.

Lung protective strategies (permissive hypercapnea, lung recruitment maneuvers, low tidal volume strategies) are routinely used to treat lung injury in burned children though they have not been specifically researched in this patient population (*Mechanical Support of Ventilation, 2.8*). High frequency oscillatory ventilation, as well as volume diffusive ventilators (high frequency, time cycled, pressure ventilator) have shown specific effectiveness in burned patients.

Carbon monoxide (CO) is a colorless, odorless gas that results from the burning of combustible materials. It is the leading cause of accidental poisoning fatalities in the United States each year. Other than by fires, CO is also produced from improperly vented household appliances, kerosene or propane heaters and automobile exhaust.

CO exerts its toxic effects as a result of its high affinity for hemoglobin. CO binds reversibly to Hb but has an affinity for Hb approximately 250 times greater than oxygen. This results in a leftward shift in the oxygen-Hb dissociation curve and a decreased availability of O_2 to tissues (*Appendix, part 2, III; Oxyhemoglobin Dissociated Curve*). CO additionally binds to myoglobin, resulting in direct myocardial impairment, adding to the baseline effects of impaired O_2 delivery. Finally, CO damages neuronal cells directly via a number of cellular toxicities including inactivation of cytochrome oxidase and nitric oxide release. These CNS-specific effects help explain the prevalence of signs and symptoms even at low CO levels ($< 10\%$ of total Hb; **Box 12.2.2**).

Blood gas analysis can measure carboxylated hemoglobin in blood and is the preferred method of diagnosis. Chronic smokers may have a Co-Hb level up to 10% and infants that have residual fetal hemoglobin may have a falsely elevated Co-Hb level, but typically not higher than 10%. Children are typically more sensitive to the effects of Co-Hb because of their high metabolic rate. They may also become symptomatic

Box 12.2.2   Signs and Symptoms of Carbon Monoxide Poisoning

• Headache	• Confusion	• Depression	• Dizziness
• Agitation	• Seizures	• Lethargy	• Hallucinations
• Syncope	• Visual changes	• Impaired	• Abdominal pain
• Nausea	• Vomiting	judgment	• Shortness of
		• Chest pain	breath

at lower levels of Co-Hb exposure and may have fewer clinical signs as compared to adults. Currently, there are no recommendations for institution of treatment for children with elevated Co-Hb levels who are asymptomatic. If systemic injuries or illness preclude an adequate neurologic assessment, the level of Co-Hb must be weighed against the potential risks of treatment.

The mainstay of therapy is oxygen. CO competes with O_2 for the hemoglobin binding site; its half-life in room air is 4–5 hours versus 60–80 minutes when breathing 100% oxygen. Increasing the partial pressure of inspired oxygen through the use of a hyperbaric chamber can reduce the half-life of CO-Hb to 20 minutes. The use of hyperbaric oxygen for carbon monoxide poisoning remains controversial due to a lack of clearly demonstrated improved outcomes. While children may show greater toxicity, the long-term injury from exposure seems to be less than that for comparable adult Co-Hb levels. The goal of hyperbaric oxygen is twofold: first, to reduce circulating levels of CO-Hb acutely and second, to attenuate neuronal damage. Some centers advocate the use of hyperbaric oxygen for all significant Co-Hb exposures, even if the Co-Hb levels have normalized. An additional concern is limited access to the patient in the hyberbaric chamber during the pressurization period; emergency interventions are not possible until the decompression cycle is completed.

12.3 Drowning (Submersion Injury)

Drowning is defined as the process resulting in respiratory impairment from submersion or immersion in a liquid medium whether or not death is an outcome. Submersion accidents are one of the most common causes of cerebral hypoxic-ischemic injury in children. Death from drowning refers to any cause of death, at any time, if there is a clear chain of causality related to a submersion event. The terms near-drowning and secondary drowning, which imply an outcome of survival beyond 24 hrs after submersion, are no longer used.

Submersion accidents remain the second most common cause of injury and death in children 1–4 yrs of age. Most of these drowning deaths occur in residential pools. Infant drowning occurs most often in bathtubs and accounts for about 13% of all submersion events; some of these events may result from intentional abuse. Up to 20% of submersion injuries involve adolescents and these accidents are primarily related to water sport activities, use of illicit drugs, alcohol and risk-taking behaviors. Fewer than 5% of submersions are associated with major trauma and cervical spine injuries are rare, occurring in less than 0.5% of drowning episodes.

The initial phase of the pathophysiology of a drowning event is marked by intense fright, panic, and a struggle to maintain the airway above water. If this effort is unsuccessful, the victim submerges and voluntary breath holding occurs. Breath holding is maintained until the stimulus of air-hunger is overwhelming. Fluid is swallowed first into the stomach and then subsequently vomited and aspirated into the lungs by active inhalation. Transient laryngospasm may occur at the time of initial aspiration. As hypoxic relaxation of laryngospasm ensues, alveoli are flooded with further pulmonary aspiration. Active aspiration of fluid into the lungs occurs in at least 90% of all severe submersion events. Approximately 10% of severe submersion events are characterized by persistent laryngospasm with minimal aspiration of liquid. During this so-called "dry drowning" the lungs are spared from liquid aspiration, but hypoxia persists and leads to asphyxiation and neurogenic pulmonary edema. The final steps are cardiovascular collapse with severe bradycardia/asystole leading to onset of global cerebral hypoxic-ischemic injury (*Hypoxic Ischemic Encephalopathy, 5.3*).

The remarkable changes in blood gas values in normothermic animals during the early phases of submersion have been studied. Within moments of drowning, there is rapid onset of respiratory acidosis. There is a precipitous decline in blood oxygen tension to as low as 4 mmHg within 5 mins of the submersion event. Within 2–4 mins, there is sufficient hypoxemia to cause loss of consciousness. Carbon dioxide tension doubles by 10 minutes and the blood pH falls below 7.0. Cardiac arrest occurs within 5–10 mins of total alveolar flooding or complete airway obstruction (laryngospasm). Following cessation of brain circulation, residual oxygen stores are depleted in about 10 secs and exhaustion of high energy phosphates occurs within 5 mins. It is widely accepted that the onset of irreversible neuronal damage begins soon thereafter.

Following a submersion event, most children survive and due to initial laryngospasm they present with relatively dry lungs and little respiratory distress. Only with active aspiration of gastric contents or a complete cardiac arrest leading to passive aspiration of large amounts of fluid does the drowning victim present with significant pulmonary abnormalities. Fresh or salt water aspiration into the lungs can lead to rapid changes in the normal function of surfactant. Aspiration of fresh water dilutes and washes out surfactant, rendering alveoli unstable. Salt water, with a tonicity similar to 3% saline, generates an influx of protein rich plasma from the pulmonary capillaries, resulting in secondary surfactant dysfunction. The net physiologic effect of either type of surfactant inactivation is to create widespread areas of ventilation/perfusion (V/Q) abnormalities and intrapulmonary shunting of blood. Pulmonary aspiration may also trigger an inflammatory response in the alveolar capillary membranes and progress to acute respiratory distress syndrome (ARDS). Finally, alveolar rupture and free-air in the thorax have been observed after drowning. This may result from bronchospasm or forced expiration against bronchi that are filled with fluid or debris.

Hypoxic cardiac injury is first manifest by severe bradycardia, followed by mechanical asystole with pulseless electrical activity and eventual electrical asystole. Some drowning victims present with ventricular tachycardia or ventricular fibrillation. In the majority of submersion events in which cardiopulmonary arrest has occurred, permanent cardiac dysfunction is rare after return of spontaneous circulation (ROSC). After ROSC the cardiovascular system is often characterized by a transient state of low cardiac output associated with elevated systemic vascular resistance caused by release of endogenous catecholamines and hypothermia. These hemodynamic changes mimic those of cardiogenic shock. Increased afterload in the presence of sustained myocardial ischemia may produce cardiac failure with high ventricular end diastolic filling pressures.

Clinically significant changes in blood volume or electrolyte concentrations occur only if large volumes of aspirated fluid (11–22 ml/kg) are absorbed into the systemic circulation. Typically, drowning victims aspirate small volumes (3–4 ml/kg), causing minimal changes in electrolyte concentrations. In most reports of submersion accidents, electrolytes are measured in the normal physiologic range.

Other than immediate resuscitation, rapid onset core hypothermia is the only recognized co-morbidity associated with a reduction in hypoxic brain injury. The definition of hypothermia is a core body temperature of less than 35°C (95°F). The current record for longest cold water submersion with an intact neurological recovery is 66 mins in a two and one-half year old female with core body temperatures as low as 13.7°C (57°F). The key to hypoxic cerebral survival may be associated with cerebral hypothermia. Brain metabolism and cerebral oxygen demand are reduced by roughly 7% per degree Celsius drop in body temperature. At 30°C, cerebral metabolic rate is reduced by nearly 50% and the brain can tolerate no-blood-flow for about 20 mins. Under controlled conditions in the operating room, induction of deep hypothermia (18–25°C) can protect the brain from hypoxic injury for as long as 70–110 mins. In cold water drowning, cerebral preservation occurs naturally when the brain becomes hypothermic before asphyxial cardiac arrest. The critical factor for cerebral outcome is the rate of cerebral cooling and the overall temperature of the brain before arterial hypoxia has fallen to injurious levels.

In warm-water drowning, hypoxic and asphyxial cardiac arrest usually develops before or during cerebral cooling, which does not assure protection from anoxic brain damage. Under these conditions, the presence of a rectal temperature in the ED consistent with severe hypothermia is thought to reflect prolonged exposure to anoxia, equilibrium with ambient water temperatures, and usually correlates with extensive neurological injury. Even in warm water environments (>20°C), it is not uncommon for a child submerged for approximately 5 mins to have a core body temperature in the range of 32–34°C when removed from the water.

Management. Initial priorities of the non-cardiac arrest patient are focused on support of respiratory function. The use of BLPAP/CPAP is reserved for conscious and cooperative victims with residual pulmonary edema or atelectasis who require >50% oxygen to maintain arterial saturations greater that 93%. A functioning NG tube should be placed. If not already done, tracheal intubation of the unresponsive patient or those in severe respiratory distress should be accomplished (*Bag-Mask Ventilation and Tracheal Intubation, 15.2*). Mechanical ventilation should utilize lung protective strategies with careful adjustment of PEEP. Hyperventilation should be avoided.

The fundamental goals of treatment for all post submersion victims are to promote and maintain optimal cerebral blood flow and systemic oxygen delivery. Rapid restoration of euvolemia and vasopressor support of persistent hypotension is essential to restore oxygen delivery to the tissues and attenuate further secondary organ damage. Nearly all drowning victims require fluid resuscitation (10–20 ml/kg) using crystalloid or colloid. The fluid resuscitation must be tailored to cardiac function so as to avoid exacerbation of pulmonary edema from high cardiac filling pressures. After cardiac arrest, the cardiovascular system is typically characterized by transient myocardial dysfunction. An appreciation of the degree of post-arrest cardiogenic shock is essential to gauge the proper amount of fluid and vasotropic support. Repeated assessments of vital signs, physical findings (*e.g.* rales), urine output, measurements of blood lactic acid, venous saturation, and qualitative echocardiograms are all valuable adjuncts to guide selection and adjustments of fluid and catecholamine therapy (*Shock, 3.5*).

Hypothermia is common after drowning among children. Wet clothing should be removed and hypothermic patients should be passively or actively re-warmed. Passive techniques include drying the skin, increasing the ambient room temperature, and using blankets or other insulators to prevent heat loss. Active external warming involves use of radiant heat sources, warm packs, and forced warm air devices (e.g. Bair Hugger®). All post-arrest or comatose submersion victims whose core temperature is ≤32°C should not receive *active* warming measures. If the core temperature is <32°C, the current recommendation is to initiate passive warming to 32–34°C (i.e. mild hypothermia). The Brain Resuscitation Task Force recommends that drowning victims who remain comatose after ROSC be immediately treated with deliberate mild hypothermia (32–34°C) for 12–24 hrs. Patients treated with mild hypothermia should be endotracheally intubated and mechanically ventilated. Shivering should be prevented (e.g. with use of meperidine). Hypnotics, analgesics and neuromuscular blockade may be used as required to maintain mild hypothermia. Vigilance should be maintained for occurrence of pneumonia. At completion of induced hypothermia, passive rewarming is recommended at a rate no greater than 0.5–1.0°C per hour.

There are several other fundamental caveats of post-submersion care that are known to influence neurologic outcome. Post resuscitative hyperthermia in the post-anoxic period increases CNS metabolism by 7% per degree C and may tip the balance of cerebral oxygen supply and demand toward cerebral ischemia. Hyperthermia resulting from release of inflammatory cytokines or from overzealous efforts to re-warm the patient should be prevented. Pyrexia in drowning patients who have had cardiac arrest should be treated aggressively during the first 24–48 hrs with antipyretics and/or active cooling measures. Antipyretics (e.g. acetaminophen, aspirin and other non-steroidal anti-inflammatory drugs) work by inhibiting cyclooxygenase-mediated prostaglandin synthesis in the brain, thus lowering the hypothalamic temperature set-point. The efficacy of anti-pyretic agents is tightly linked to conditions where the brain's ability to thermoregulate is intact. Therefore, these agents are more likely to be ineffective in brain-injured patients with impaired thermoregulatory mechanisms.

Hyponatremia will intensify the potential for cerebral edema; frequently measure and control serum sodium concentration in the high normal range of 140–150 mEq/L. Permissive hypercapnia, a method of lung protection, will accelerate the potential for cerebral edema in those with potential hypoxic brain injury and should be avoided until this complication can be ruled out. Monitoring of $ETCO_2$ can alert the team to untoward increases in $PaCO_2$. Uncontrolled hyperglycemia (glucose >150 mg/dL in patients with neurologic injury) is associated with worse neurological outcomes. Similarly important is avoidance of hypoglycemia, which increases metabolic stress on recovering neurons.

Adjuvant therapies may be beneficial in the drowning victim. These may include antibiotics, diuretics and/or exogenous surfactant. Currently, there is no evidence to support use of prophylactic antibiotics following drowning. However, it is common to give broad spectrum antibiotics when aspiration of grossly contaminated water from sewers, septic tanks, hot tubs and toilets, or when massive aspiration of gastric contents has occurred. The use of loop diuretics in the ED should be reserved for submersion victims with significant respiratory distress from pulmonary edema (*e.g.* post-obstructive laryngospasm) who have stable hemodynamics and perfusion. Large clinical studies of exogenous surfactant for ARDS/ALI have not demonstrated improved outcomes, but subgroup analysis suggests aspiration-induced ARDS may benefit from its administration.

Outcome and Prognosis. In the US, nearly 71% of all submersion victims survive neurologically intact while 29% have a poor outcome, defined as death (17%) or survival in a vegetative state (12%). When cardiac arrest has occurred, the prognosis is much worse. Only 50% of these patients have ROSC and 25% survive to hospital discharge; only 6% survive neurologically intact.

Historical, clinical and laboratory variables have been unable to predict, with 100% specificity, those victims who will have a poor neurological outcome. The most dependable predictors of outcome following warm water submersions are factors that reflect the duration and extent of hypoxia and ischemia before ED arrival. Unfavorable prognostic signs are listed in **Box 12.3.1**. Despite

---

**Box 12.3.1   Unfavorable Prognostic Signs for Drowning
Patients in the Emergency Department**

- Submersion in warm (>20°C) water
- Duration of warm water submersion >25 mins
- Delayed resuscitation (>10 mins)
- Epinephrine given prior to arrival in the ED
- Pulseless on arrival to the ED
- Coma on arrival to the ED
- Fixed and dilated pupils in the ED
- Initial pH <7.10 on arrival to the ED
- Initial serum glucose >200 mg/dL
- Apnea in the ED

---

these many ominous variables, prognostic formulas are not 100% specific; therefore, the critical decision to cease treatment in the ED should be rare and always based on the conservative judgment and experience of the physician in attendance. There is growing evidence that the earliest opportunity to accurately prognosticate a vegetative outcome is 48 hrs after admission to the PICU.

12.4 Lightning Injury

Lightning is an electrical phenomenon that can cause significant morbidity and mortality among victims in its path. Lightning injuries are rare in children and research examining these injuries is limited. Identifying these injuries and primary prevention of lightning injuries are important in providing quality medical care and reducing morbidity and mortality.

Lightning is caused by multiple factors that result in a unidirectional massive impulse that can be measured in millions of volts. The physics behind lightning is extremely complex. A lightning strike is the result of electrical differences between a cloud and the earth. Discharge of the potential difference is normally prevented because air is a good insulator. When the potential difference becomes great enough, the insulation normally provided by surrounding air is disrupted, and the charge, which can be positive or negative, is dissipated as lightning. Lightning may cause injury by:

- Direct strike: lightning attaches directly to the victim; most likely to occur when a person is exposed and unable to find shelter.
- Contact injury: occurs when touching an object to which lightning attaches.
- Side flash or "splash" injury: occurs when a nearby object (tree, building, *etc.*) is struck by lightning and the current travels partly down that object before a portion "jumps" to a nearby victim. The current is seeking the path of least resistance and can jump from a primary object to a person nearby if they impose less resistance.
- Step voltage (ground current) occurs when lightning spreads radially from a point on the ground and diminishes in strength as the radius from the location of the initial strike increases. Humans offer less resistance than the earth. The normal human stride allows for a great potential difference between the legs. Therefore, current travels up one leg and down the other in the path of least resistance rather than continuing along the ground.
- Blunt injury can occur when a person is close to the concussive force of the shockwave produced as lightning strikes nearby. It can lead to a victim being thrown up to 10 yards.

Patients with lightning injuries can be categorized into three different groups depending on the severity of their injuries (**Boxes 12.4.1 and 12.4.2**). Lightning injuries are very different from generator-produced high-voltage electrical injuries, which often have a more prolonged exposure to electric current.

Assessment and Treatment of Lightning Injuries. The diagnosis of lightning injury may be difficult. Victims are often confused and amnestic to the event. Witnesses, physical findings, and history of thunderstorm are not always present. The first steps are the

Box 12.4.1   Lightning Injury Classification

Mild Injury	Moderate Injury	Severe Injury
• Patients are awake • Vital signs are stable • Possible transient hypertension • Dysesthesias in affected extremity • Confusion and amnesia (hours to days) • Temporary loss of consciousness (LOC) • Temporary deafness/blindness • Paresthesias • Muscle pain • Tympanic membrane (TM) rupture	• Temporary cardiopulmonary standstill with spontaneous recovery • Disoriented, combative or comatose • Motor paralysis (usually lower extremities) with mottled skin and decreased pulses • Seizures • 1st and 2nd degree burns • TM rupture • Prone to long-term sequelae*	• May be in cardiac arrest with ventricular standstill or fibrillation on presentation • TM rupture with hemotympanum and CSF otorrhea • Prognosis is poor because of direct lightning damage often complicated by delayed CPR with resultant anoxic brain injury.

* Sleep disorders, irritability, difficulty with fine psychomotor functions, weakness, paresthesias, post-traumatic stress disorder (PTSD).

"ABCDE's" of resuscitation: airway, breathing, circulation, disability and exposure-environment. Victims are often struck during a thunderstorm and they are frequently wet and cold. Hypothermia should be anticipated and treated appropriately. Useful laboratory and radiologic data are listed and treatment is outlined (**Boxes 12.4.3 and 12.4.4**).

Box 12.4.2   Lightning Injuries Based on Organ System

- **Cardiopulmonary injuries:** The most common cause of death in a lightning victim is ventricular standstill caused by a large direct current leading to cardiopulmonary arrest. This insult produces a depolarization of the entire myocardium resulting in ventricular standstill (asystole). An organized rhythm with contractions generally resumes in a short period of time due to the inherent automaticity of the heart. However, the respiratory arrest, caused by paralysis of the medullary respiratory center, is thought to last much longer than cardiac arrest. Unless the victim receives immediate CPR, hypoxia is thought to induce arrhythmias and perhaps secondary cardiac arrest after initial ROSC. ST segment changes consistent with ischemia are common, but may not occur until the 2nd day. The QT interval may be prolonged. Most ECG changes resolve within a few days, but some persist for months. Autopsies have confirmed myocardial infarction in children. Pulmonary edema may accompany cardiac injury; pulmonary contusion/hemorrhage may result from blunt injury or direct lung damage.

- **Neurologic injuries:** These cause the greatest number of long-term problems. Up to 72% have an initial loss of consciousness. Confusion and amnesia (usually anterograde) are almost universal with victims unable to assimilate new experiences for several days. A prolonged state of coma indicates poor prognosis. Transient "lightning paralysis" (keraunoparalysis) is specific for lightning injury. Extreme vasoconstriction occurs in one or more extremities (usually the lower extremities) and usually resolves within minutes to 1 hour. The affected extremities are cold, clammy, mottled, insensate, and pulseless. Seizures may accompany initial arrest or result from hypoxia or intracranial damage. Children are prone to delayed seizures which may present as "absence spells", blackouts and memory loss. The most devastating complications are hypoxic-ischemic encephalopathy, cerebral/cerebellar infarction, intracranial hemorrhage, spinal cord injury, and myelopathy. Direct cellular damage to the respiratory center and anterior brainstem has been shown. Survivors have persistent sleep disturbances, difficulty with fine mental and motor function, dysesthesias, headaches, mood abnormalities, emotional lability, concentration and cognitive disturbances, storm phobias, and PTSD. Delayed occurrence of pain, parethesias and headaches are common along the tract of the current passage.

(Continued)

Box 12.4.2   Lightning injuries Based on Organ System (Continued)

- **Burns:** Significant deep-tissue injury does not usually occur since the duration of exposure is just milliseconds. If the patient is in contact with a metal object a deep tissue burn can occur.

  Discrete entry and exit points are rare in lightning injury. Individuals with cranial burns are reported to be four times more likely to die than those without cranial burns. "Feathering" burns are pathognomonic of a lightning strike. This is thought to be a result of flashover current traveling on the surface of the skin rather than passing through the patient's body. It is actually not a burn, but is thought to be an inflammatory response to current passing through the skin.

- **Other problems include:** Persistent hypotension, cataracts, intense photophobia, perforated tympanic membranes (may be associated with intracranial injury), temporary vertigo, deafness and tinnitus, hemoglobinuria and myoglobinuria.

Box 12.4.3   Recommended Laboratory and Radiologic Data in Lightning Injury

- Urinalysis
- CBC
- Electrolytes, urea nitrogen and creatinine
- Glucose
- ABG as indicated
- ECG
- CK
- Troponin I and CK–MB
- Radiographs as indicated
- Cervical spine imaging (plain films, CT, MRI as indicated)
- Head CT/Brain MRI as indicated

Box 12.4.4   Management of Lightning Injuries

- Institute CPR as indicated. Prolonged CPR does not improve survival.
- Elective intubation should be achieved prior to signs of upper airway obstruction in patients with injuries to the face, mouth, and anterior neck.
- Cardiovascular therapy: Vascular spasm may make pulses difficult to palpate though central pulses are usually preserved. Hypotension should be corrected with volume (NaCl 0.9%) and vasoactive support as needed. The cause of hypotension (hypovolemia, abdominal or chest injuries, fractures, spinal shock, cardiogenic shock, or deep burns) should be identified. Cardiac monitoring and serial cardiac enzymes should be obtained if there is evidence of ischemia, complaints of chest pain, or evidence of arrhythmias. Transient hypertension is usually of short duration and requires no therapy. Arterial and CVP monitoring may be indicated.
- IVF: In normotensive and hypertensive patients, judicious fluid administration is recommended to avoid increasing the risk of cerebral edema. In hypotensive patients, volume resuscitation with an isotonic sodium salt solution is essential. A goal for urine output is 1–1.5 ml/kg/hr in children and 1.5–2 ml/kg/hr in infants.
- Treat rhabdomyolysis as indicated (*Rhabdomyolysis, 7.4*).
- Fasciotomy is rarely indicated. Intense vasospasm due to sympathetic instability is usually transient (hours).
- ICP monitoring may be indicated.
- Treat seizures with anticonvulsant drugs.
- Burns are generally superficial, and may not be apparent until hours after admission. Treat with standard therapy.
- Ophthalmologic consultation as indicated.
- Tympanic membrane rupture: Otorrhea (and/or hemotympanum) suggest basilar skull fracture and should be evaluated by head CT. Hearing loss requires ENT consultation. TM rupture usually responds to conservative management and heals spontaneously.

12.5 Hypothermia

Hypothermia is defined as a core body temperature less than 35°C. It is further categorized as mild (35–32°C), moderate (31.9–28°C) and severe (< 28°C). Core body temperature is most accurately measured in the pulmonary artery; the urinary bladder, rectum, esophagus, oral cavity, and external auditory canal have also been used. Normal body temperature is maintained by a balance of heat loss and heat gain. Peripheral thermoreceptors send afferent impulses via the lateral spinothalamic tract to the central thermostat in the hypothalamus. Differences between hypothalamic set point and core temperature initiate biologic thermoregulation. As adaptive thermoregulatory mechanisms are overwhelmed, the body is unable to adequately generate sufficient heat to maintain normothermia. In significant hypothermia, all organ systems, most importantly the CNS, cardiovascular and renal systems are affected (**Box 12.5.1**).

Hypothermia occurs when there is a decrease in heat production, increase in heat loss, impairment in thermoregulation or a combination of these factors. Most commonly, hypothermia results from exposure to a cold environment. It can also develop secondary to other causes, such as metabolic derangements, infections, endocrine CNS dysfunction, or exposure to toxins (**Box 12.5.2**).

Clinical features seen in the hypothermic patient vary with the degree of hypothermia (**Box 12.5.3**). A thorough history and physical examination should be performed to recognize these features. An electrocardiogram may show changes consistent with hypothermia (**Fig. 12.5.1**). The laboratory evaluation and management are summarized in **Boxes 12.5.3 and 12.5.4.**

Cardiac Arrest. Unresponsive hypothermic patients or those in cardiac arrest should be tracheally intubated. This permits ventilation with warm, humidified oxygen and protection from aspiration. Palpation of a pulse in severe hypothermia is difficult due to extreme bradycardia and vasoconstriction. If there is any doubt, CPR should be initiated. The treatment of markedly hypothermic patients (core temperature < 30°C) in cardiac arrest is directed at rapid active core rewarming. The hypothermic heart may be unresponsive to defibrillation, pacemaker

Box 12.5.1   Clinical Findings Based on Degree of Hypothermia

	Mild Hypothermia	Moderate Hypothermia	Severe Hypothermia
CNS	Confusion; amnesia; ataxia; ↓ cerebral metabolism	Unconsciousness; diminished gag reflex; dilated pupils	↓ or absent EEG activity; nonreactive pupils; loss of ocular reflexes
Cardio-vascular	Vasoconstriction; ↑CO; tachycardia followed by bradycardia; hypertension	Bradycardia; ↓ contractility; slowed cardiac conduction; Osborn waves (**Fig. 12.5.1**); arrhythmias	Progressive bradycardia, ↓CO and BP; ventricular arrhythmias; asystole
Respiratory	Tachypnea; bronchospasm; impaired mucosal function	Hypoventilation; V/Q mismatch; ↓VO$_2$, ↓ pulmonary compliance	Lung capillary damage; pulmonary edema; ↓ VO$_2$; apnea
Metabolic/ Renal	↑ Metabolism; ↑ VO$_2$; impaired renal concentrating ability; cold diuresis; hypovolemia; ↓ K$^+$	↓ Renal blood flow and GFR; ↓ UOP; ↑ K$^+$; ↑ glucose; lactic acidosis; loss of insulin activity	↓ Basal metabolism; lactic acidosis; renal failure
Gastro-intestinal	Nausea, vomiting, ileus	Pancreatitis; gastric ulcers	Same as moderate
Neuro-muscular	Shivering and ↑ tone, followed by muscle fatigue	Extinction of shivering; hyporeflexia; rigidity	Areflexia; rhabdomyolysis

Box 12.5.2   Predisposing Factors and Etiologies of Hypothermia

- **Decreased heat production:** hypopituitarism, hypoadrenalism, hypothyroidism, lactic acidosis, ketoacidosis, hypoglycemia, malnutrition (marasmus, kwashiorkor), extreme physical exertion, extremes of age, impaired shivering, lack of adaptation
- **Increased heat loss:** exposure to cold environment, dermatologic impairment (burns, exfoliative dermatitis), toxicologic/pharmacologic induced vasodilation or impaired vasoconstriction, iatrogenic causes: emergency delivery of newborns, infusion of cold fluid, overzealous treatment of hyperthermia
- **Impaired thermoregulation:** CNS trauma, cardiovascular accident, neuropathies, spinal cord transection, DKA, congenital intracranial anomalies, multiple sclerosis
- **Other associated conditions:** Shaken baby syndrome, sickle cell anemia, SIDS, pancreatitis, Shapiro's syndrome, sepsis, shock, systemic lupus erythematosus, uremia, severe DKA

Box 12.5.3   Laboratory Evaluation of Hypothermia

- CBC: Thrombocytopenia and leukopenia may result from bone marrow suppression or splenic sequestration. Hematocrit increases due to a decline in plasma volume.
- Electrolytes: Hypokalemia or hyperkalemia can occur. Hyperglycemia occurs acutely, but hypoglycemia can be seen in subacute or chronic states.
- Liver enzymes and function tests: Abnormal due to ↓ liver perfusion.
- Urea nitrogen and creatinine: Decreased renal function leads to ↑urea nitrogen and creatinine.
- Blood Gases: Metabolic and respiratory acidosis occurs due to ↓CO, impaired metabolism, and respiratory failure.
- Coagulation studies: Prolonged PT and PTT due to the inhibition of the enzymatic reactions of the clotting cascade *in vivo*.

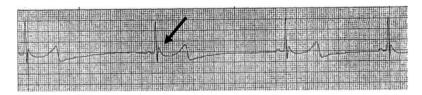

Fig 12.5.1.   Osborne Waves (at the J Point) in a Hypothermic Patient. Other changes may include prolongation of the QT_c interval.

Box 12.5.4   Management of Hypothermia

- Assess, support and monitor the airway, breathing and circulation; if central venous access is needed in moderate or severe hypothermia, take care to avoid stimulation of the heart with a guidewire or catheter since this may result in potentially life-threatening arrhythmias.
- Immobilize the cervical spine if trauma is a consideration.
- Identify and treat hypoglycemia.
- Remove the patient from the cold environment and remove any wet clothing.
- The core temperature should be measured by a "low reading" thermometer.
- Rewarming techniques based on the severity of hypothermia and the clinical situation should start immediately (see below).
- Mechanical mainpulation of patients should be minimized to avoid cardiac arrhythmias.
- Fluid resuscitation: Mildly hypothermic patients usually require only modest amounts of crystalloids. Those patients who are more significantly hypothermic are often quite dehydrated due to volume shifts and increased blood viscosity. These patients must receive adequate fluid resuscitation. Most patients require initial IV volume resuscitation with warmed crystalloid (*e.g.* NaCl 0.9%) with ongoing efforts adapted based on laboratory values and patient condition.

(Continued)

Box 12.5.4   Management of Hypothermia (Continued)

- Rewarming:
  - ▶ Passive External Rewarming: Usually effective for mild hypothermia and is only successful if thermoregulatory mechanisms are intact and patient is able to shiver.
    - ▪ Cover the head, neck and body with blankets
    - ▪ Reduce evaporative heat loss by drying the patient
  - ▶ Active External Rewarming: Usually effective for mild to moderate hypothermia; an intact circulation is required to return blood warmed in the peripheral circulation to the core circulation.
    - ▪ Apply heat directly to the body surface; use caution to avoid burns.
    - ▪ Apply warm blankets, radiant warmers, forced-heated-air devices (*e.g.* Bair Hugger®) or immerse in warm water
    - ▪ Complications include: core temperature "after-drop" and acidosis (due to return of cold blood and lactic acid to the heart and central circulation), as well as hypotension (due to venous pooling)
  - ▶ Active Internal Rewarming: Usually used in treating severe hypothermia
    - ▪ Instill heated humidified gases (40–45°C) via a tracheal tube
    - ▪ Infuse IV fluids warmed to 40–42°C
    - ▪ Lavage gastric, bladder, colon and pleural and peritoneal spaces with warmed saline (40–42°C)
    - ▪ Consider ECMO, hemodialysis and cardiopulmonary bypass when less invasive active rewarming has failed or in the presence of an unresponsive hypothermic cardiac arrest or a nonperfusing cardiac rhythm.

---

stimulation and cardiovascular drugs. If ventricular fibrillation or ventricular tachycardia is present, one defibrillation attempt is usually recommended. If the patient does not respond initially, further attempts are deferred until the core temperature rises to 30°C. Multiple doses of cardiotropic medications are usually discouraged due to potential toxicity of accumulated cardioactive drugs in the peripheral vascular bed.

These medications should be given after the core temperature rises above 30°C; however, dosing intervals should be increased. Rapidly precipitated hypothermia may provide a protective effect on the brain and other organs; physicians should use clinical judgment to decide when to cease resuscitative efforts in a victim of hypothermic arrest.

Outcomes. The overall reported patient mortality from hypothermia is 12%, however this increases to almost 40% when limited to patients with moderate-to-severe hypothermia. The presence of asphyxia or hypoxic brain injury prior to the development of hypothermia increases this risk. Neurodevelopmental and psychological disturbances have been reported in infants and newborns who have survived accidental hypothermia.

12.6 Hyperthermia

Normal body temperature varies from 36–37.5°C. Core temperature is most accurately measured in the pulmonary artery, but bladder, esophageal, rectal and tympanic sites have been used. Fever is a regulated rise in body temperature ≥ 38.3°C resulting from a cytokine-induced increase in the hypothalamic set-point. Hyperthermia is an unregulated rise in body temperature caused by an inability to eliminate heat adequately (**Box 12.6.1**). This discussion addresses heat-related illness resulting from environmental heat and/or an inability to dissipate heat. Hyperthermic syndromes related to drug exposure are discussed in *Drug-Induced Toxic Hyperthermic Syndromes, 13.3*; it is essential to review the drug exposure history and identify drug-related hyperthermia since specific therapies may be indicated.

The distinction between fever and hyperthermia can usually be made based on history. If history is unclear, the patient should be managed aggressively for heat stroke because of the high morbidity and mortality associated with this disorder. In addition, evaluation for infection should be considered and treatment for infection should be initiated so long as infection remains a possibility. Laboratory evaluation, systemic complications and management principles are outlined in **Boxes 12.6.2 through 12.6.4**.

Box 12.6.1   Fever and Hyperthermia: Definitions and Pathophysiologic Differences

- **Fever:** Interleukin 1-beta and interleukin-6 act on the anterior hypothalamus resulting in ↑ prostaglandin synthesis (esp. PGE_2), raising the temperature set-point. The body responds by shivering, increasing the metabolic rate and with peripheral vasoconstriction (to ↓ heat loss) to help achieve the new "goal" of the hypothalamus. Associated events include ↑ neutrophil activity, lymphocyte proliferation and ↓ availability of minerals (iron and zinc) needed for bacterial replication. These potential advantages may be out-weighed by the disadvantages of associated tachycardia, ↑ VO_2, ↑ CO_2 production, patient discomfort and lowering of the seizure threshold. Fever is detrimental in the presence of brain injury. Elevations in temperature due to fever generally respond to antipyretics. Environmental cooling with tepid water (~30°C) may be helpful; avoid interventions that produce shivering, which further increases body temperature.
- **Hyperthermia:** Core temperature >38°C despite normal thermoregulatory mechanisms and hypothalamic temperature set point. **Classic heat stroke** is a core temperature ≥ 40°C associated with altered mental status +/− seizures and +/− ataxia resulting from environmental heat exposure. **Exertional heat stroke** is a core temperature of ≥ 40°C associated with extreme physical exercise, usually in a hot, humid environment. Either may occur with or without impairment of heat loss (*e.g.* anhidrosis).

   The duration of hyperthermia parallels the extent of organ injury. Permanent neurologic injury occurs when core temperature exceeds 42°C (for ≥ 45 min) at which point oxidative phosphorylation is uncoupled, and multiple organ failure ensues. It is important to note that the true core temperature may be underestimated when the temperature is measured at sites other than the PA. Environmental heat stroke does not respond to antipyretics.

Box 12.6.2   Laboratory Evaluation of Severe Hyperthermia

- Bedside glucose
- Blood gases
- CBC
- PT, PTT, INR, Fibrinogen
- Serum electrolytes
- Urea nitrogen and creatinine
- Liver enzymes

- Creatine kinase
- Urinalysis
- Urine drug screen
- Chest X-Ray
- 12-lead ECG
- Echocardiogram if indicated
- Brain imaging if indicated

Box 12.6.3   Complications of Severe Hyperthermia

- Hypoglycemia
- Acute respiratory distress syndrome
- Disseminated intravascular coagulation
- Renal failure
- Hepatic failure (acute hepatic necrosis)

- Rhabdomyolysis
- Arrhythmias
- Altered mental status
- Seizures
- Cerebral edema

Box 12.6.4   Management Principles in Hyperthermia

- Attention to airway, breathing and circulation; most patients with hyperthermia have some degree of dehydration. Volume resuscitation should restore intravascular volume with care to avoid excessive hydration. Patients unresponsive to fluid resuscitation (*e.g.* 0.9% NaCl ≥60 ml/kg) should be evaluated for the need for vasoactive medications.
- Remove clothing and optimize heat loss.
- Correct hypoglycemia.
- Evaporative cooling is the most frequently recommended method of external cooling. The skin should be sprayed/misted with tepid water or saline, and a fan directed over the skin surface. A cooling blanket under the patient and ice packs applied to the groin, axillae and neck may be helpful. Sedation with benzodiazepines +/− tracheal intubation with neuromuscular blockade may be necessary to prevent shivering.

(Continued)

Box 12.6.4   Management Principles in Hyperthermia (Continued)

- Internal cooling can be attempted with gastric, bladder, and/or rectal lavage using cold saline (0.9% NaCl); these methods may be of no greater benefit than evaporative cooling. Cardiopulmonary bypass can lower the core temperature most effectively, but its availability limits its use.
- Active cooling may be stopped as the temperature approaches 38°C.
- Dantrolene has been used in selected patients who were unresponsive to traditional cooling methods.
- Antipyretics are ineffective in severe hyperthermia and may aggravate liver injury (acetaminophen) or coagulopathy (NSAIDS).
- Monitor for and treat potential complications of organ failure.

Chapter 13

Bedside Pharmacotherapy in the PICU

A basic understanding of clinical pharmacology that can be applied at the bedside is a powerful tool. A conceptual approach to this complex topic is presented to promote critical thinking and provide a basis for navigation through treatment decisions. Due to a paucity of clinical trials and the complexity of illness within the PICU population, a clinical pharmacist is an invaluable resource as a PICU team member.

13.1 Pharmacodynamics and Pharmacokinetics

Pharmacology is the study of how a medication interacts with the body. Pharmacokinetics is the discipline which describes the pathway through which a medication is absorbed, distributed, metabolized and eliminated. Clinically useful pharmacokinetic parameters are described in **Box 13.1.1.** Pharmacodynamics describes how drugs interact with the body on the molecular level to produce their effects.

Absorption. Bioavailability of medications administered by non-intravenous routes must be adequate to ensure efficacy. Adequate perfusion is necessary for adequate absorption of non-IV administered medications (IM, GI, subQ, transdermal, intranasal and endotracheal routes). Some medications may require a specific envionment to achieve adequate bioavailability. The IV route is often preferred in the PICU because it affords rapid onset, 100% bioavailability, ease of titration, and eliminates potential limitations posed by the GI tract during critical illness.

Box 13.1.1   Pharmacokinetic Concepts: Definitions

Bioavailability (*F*): Percentage of an administered dose that reaches systemic circulation.

Serum half-life (*t 1/2*): Time needed to reduce the serum drug concentration by one-half. Useful for assessing/calculating **steady state** [SS; the time at which the rate of drug administration = rate of elimination (~5 half-lives)].

Apparent volume of distribution (*Vd*): Amount of drug in the body divided by the plasma drug concentration. Useful in determining the loading dose, which is equal to *Vd* × (desired plasma concentration ÷ *F*).

Clearance (*Cl*): The ratio of the rate of drug elimination to its concentration in blood or plasma; relates to the amount of drug removed per unit of time. Useful for determining the maintenance dose.

Distribution characteristics of medications are especially important when treating disease of the CNS, urinary tract, lung or bone. Medications must reach the target site to elicit the desired therapeutic effect. Consultation with a clinical pharmacist may be helpful in optimizing therapy. Loading doses are required when the therapeutic concentration must be achieved rapidly (*e.g.* phenytoin, phenobarbital). Drug concentrations (*e.g.* aminoglycoside peaks) should be measured after the distribution phase (*e.g.* 30 min after a 30 min infusion is completed) to avoid collection of misleading data.

Metabolism serves multiple roles pharmacologically. Biotransformation reactions (primarily by the liver) often transform active drugs into less-active or inactive form(s), but conversely convert prodrugs (inactive or less-active drugs) into more active compounds. Metabolism typically results in a more polar and water soluble compound (to enhance elimination), but metabolites can also retain some pharmacologic activity. Overall, hepatic metabolism increases dramatically between six months and five years of age and declines slowly thereafter; this impacts recommended maintenance dosing of certain drugs (*e.g.* phenytoin). In addition, genetic variations in metabolic pathways among different ethnic groups and even within ethnic groups can affect drug concentrations dramatically (pharmacogenomics).

Elimination/excretion. Elimination is the process by which a drug is removed from the body. All active metabolites should be considered when addressing elimination of drug. The clinical focus should be on elimination of desired and undesired drug effects rather than "drug elimination" alone. Drug elimination primarily occurs via renal excretion and hepatic metabolism. Renal or hepatic damage or hypoperfusion can affect both pharmacokinetic and pharmacodynamic properties of a medication necessitating dosage adjustments. Clearance and half-life can be measured for many drugs (*e.g.* aminoglycosides). Creatinine clearance (Cl_{cr}) is currently the gold standard for quantifying renal function to determine the need for drug therapy modification, but changes in Cl_{cr} are often difficult to estimate in critically ill populations, necessitating the use of other more global measures of renal function, such as urine output. Small changes in a patient's serum creatinine can signify a more dramatic alteration in clinical Cl_{cr} especially in young infants.

Obese pediatric patients present unique pharmacokinetic clinical challenges. Dose and/or dosage intervals may be uncertain due to a lack of evidence-based data. Clinical pharmacists and physicians often collaborate and apply known pharmacokinetic properties of medications to optimize safe but efficacious dosing in this population. Adolescents may also present unique pharmacokinetic situations; pediatric weight based dosing (not exceeding the usual adult maximum dose) is utilized in most situations. With few exceptions, this standard practice is rarely substantiated by clinical data. Commonly used drugs dosed on ideal body weight (IBW; *Appendix, part 1*) include acyclovir, corticosteroids, nondepolarizing NMB's, digoxin and aminophylline. Aminoglycosides are dosed on actual body weight (ABW) unless the patient weighs more than 20% above IBW. In these cases, use the adjusted weight for dosing: IBW + 0.4 (ABW−IBW).

Pharmacodynamic monitoring in the critically ill child is an inexact science, largely based on observation because pediatric clinical trials are often lacking. Developmental changes, genetic heterogeneity and diverse disease states can produce multiple pharmacodynamic scenarios. The same drug in the same dose given to three different patients may yield three different effects. For example, the response to benzodiazepines can result in agitation rather than anxiolysis depending on the patient. Assessment at the bedside is essential to determine and evaluate clinically relevant pharmacodynamic effects, including the overall response to therapy.

Drug Interactions. Attention to potential drug-drug interactions is important, particularly when the following are involved: chemotherapeutic agents, warfarin, azole antifungals, antiepileptics, anti-arrhythmics, erythromycin, monoamine oxidase inhibitors (*e.g.* linezolid), sedatives, theophylline, carbamazepine, cyclosporine, levothyroxine and lithium. The prescription of each drug should prompt a series of questions for the prescriber (**Box 13.1.2**); the participation

---

Box 13.1.2　Important Questions to Ask When Prescribing a Drug

- Are the goals of the medication worthy of the associated risks? Note all warnings and contraindications.
- Will the chosen route of administration yield the desired onset of action and minimize undesired effects?
- Which is the appropriate weight (ideal, actual or adjusted; see *Appendix, part 1* for definitions) to use for drug dose calculation?
- Will the drug reach the intended site of action? Think about absorption and distribution.
- Are there any clinically relevant interactions between the drug and existing conditions or established medications?
- Has the patient been exposed to this or a similar medication in the past? If so, what was the dose given and what was the effect (*e.g.* allergic reactions)?
- Can the patient adequately eliminate the drug? Think about renal and hepatic function (*Cl*).
- If drug levels are monitored, will the reported concentration of drug be meaningful and accurate? When adjusting doses for drugs with a narrow therapeutic index (*e.g.* gentamicin) based on serum concentrations, ensure that the drug was at steady state (~5 half-lives) when assayed. Repeat drug levels when in doubt. Possible sources of error include sampling through the same catheter as that used for drug administration, improper timing of the assay and laboratory error.

of a clinical pharmacist can optimize patient safety and quality of care. With the transition to computerized prescribing, many systems contain automated databases to provide overdose and drug-drug interaction warnings at the point of order entry. Evaluation of the significance of these "alerts" may require additional pharmacy assistance since not all warning systems are reliable in the pediatric

---

Box 13.1.3 Aminoglycosides (AG): Key Concepts

- AG's demonstrate concentration-dependent killing and have a significant post-antibiotic effect. They possess excellent activity against Gram negative aerobes, with some efficacy against Gram positive organisms (*e.g.* synergistic effect with beta lactams when treating *Enterococci*).
- Dosing is based on actual body weight unless the patient weight >20% of ideal weight (see Obese Pediatric Patients, above).
- AG clearance is closely correlated with Cl_{cr}. Adjustments in dosing interval are necessary in renal insufficiency to avoid toxicity.
- AG's distribute into the extracellular fluid compartment; patients with "third-spacing", cystic fibrosis and significant burns require higher doses due to an ↑ *Vd*.
- Proper timing and correct assessment of serum concentrations are paramount. Peak concentrations should be obtained 30 mins after completion of infusion; trough concentrations should be obtained 30 mins prior to the next dose, preferably once the drug is at SS.
- Desired peak values ↑ with severity of infection. Poor drug penetration at the intended site of action also requires higher peak serum levels.
- Dosing for term neonates ≤2 wks should be based on neonatal dosing protocols.
- Risk of nephrotoxicity is ↑ when trough levels of gentamicin or tobramycin consistently exceed 2 mcg/ml (8 mcg/ml for amikacin) and/or when other nephrotoxic agents are given simultaneously. Risk of ototoxicity increases with prolonged exposure. Symptoms include dizziness, hearing loss, vertigo and tinnitus. Deafness is usually irreversible.

population. The possibility of drug interactions as a precipitant for PICU admission or as a cause for a new problem in a PICU patient should be kept in mind.

Key concepts regarding specific drugs commonly used in the PICU. Key concepts regarding the aminoglycosides, vancomycin,

---

Box 13.1.4   Vancomycin: Key Concepts

- Excellent activity against gram positive aerobes, including MRSA, and *Enterococci*.
- Use actual body weight (even in the obese) when calculating the dose.
- Some experts recommend a loading dose (25–30 mg/kg) in critically ill patients.
- Trough serum concentrations should be maintained >10 mg/L to prevent development of drug resistance and treatment failures. Trough levels 15–20 mg/L are recommended for complicated infections (pneumonia, meningitis, osteomyelitis, endocarditis) due to *S. aureus*.
- For patients who develop "red man's syndrome" with large doses, infusion times should be lengthened (*e.g.* one hour for every 10–15 mg/kg). Certain opioids (*e.g.* morphine, but not fentanyl or hydromorphone) potentiate this reaction.
- If therapy is to be continued for >48 hrs, a trough concentration is recommended prior to the 4th or 5th dose if renal function is normal. When trough levels in the 15–20 mg/L range are required, the initial therapeutic trough should be validated in 3–5 days and then weekly. For patients with unstable renal function and/or hemodynamics, more frequent monitoring of trough vancomycin levels is required to prevent ototoxicity and nephrotoxicity.
- When treating Staphylococcus with an MIC ≥1 mg/L, consultation with an infectious disease specialist and clinical pharmacist is recommended to ensure optimal treatment.
- Clinical evidence for monitoring peak levels is lacking; however, some experts recommend targeting peak levels of 30–45 mg/L when treating endocarditis or CNS infections.

Box 13.1.5   Phenytoin and Fosphenytoin: Key Concepts

- Fosphenytoin is a water-soluble prodrug of phenytoin; compared to phenytoin, it is potentially less expensive, has fewer hemodynamic side-effects, a broader compatibility profile, and a lesser risk of extravasation-related complications.
- Fosphenytoin may be given both IV and IM; there is no enteral form. Phenytoin cannot be given IM, but is available for enteral administration. Enteral absorption may be erratic in neonates because of ↓ F related to ↓ gastric acid production in this age-group. Tube feeding can result in binding of drug, reducing *F*.
- The doses of both drugs are based on ideal body weight for obese patients.
- Fosphenytoin/phenytoin: check post-load level 2 hrs after completion of fosphenytoin infusion, and one hour after phenytoin infusion. Subsequent levels are monitored as clinically indicated; SS is generally not reached until 5–7 days of therapy depending on age and dose.
- Free phenytoin levels are preferred over total levels in patients with hypoalbuminemia, patients on dialysis, or < 6 mos of age. Total levels may be falsely sub-therapeutic due to ↓ protein binding in these situations.
- To correct a total phenytoin level to an adjusted phenytoin level for hypoalbuminemia (albumin in the range of 2–3.5 gm/dL):

  Adjusted level = Measured level ÷ [(albumin × 0.25) + 0.1]

- To re-load a patient with a sub-therapeutic phenytoin level:

  Loading dose (mg) = (Desired concentration − Actual concentration in mcg/ml) × *Vd* (L)

  Where *Vd* = 1 L/kg for neonates, 0.8 L/kg for children < 1 yr and 0.7 L/kg for patients > 1 yr.

- Nystagmus may be the first sign of toxicity, first apparent during far lateral gaze, progressing to midline gaze.

phenytoin and fosphenytoin are summarized (**Boxes 13.1.2 through 13.1.5**). See the Drug Monitoring Guide in the *Appendix, part 2, XIII* for appropriate timing of peak and trough drug levels for drugs commonly used in the PICU.

Box 13.1.6   Bedside Pharmacotherapy Pearls

- Decisions based on drug levels drawn prior to *SS* can lead to inaccurate clinical decision-making which could result in adverse patient outcomes.
- The *t* 1/2 fluctuates with changes in disease state, dose, *Vd* and *Cl*.
- Hepatic clearance can be affected by ↓ hepatic blood flow, drug interactions, protein binding and hepatic injury.
- Estimated Cl_{cr} may be significantly different from the actual Cl_{cr} in critically ill patients, highlighting the need for drug monitoring. If ≥ 40% of a drug or its active metabolite is renally eliminated, renal insufficiency usually requires dose adjustment.
- Drugs which adhere to saturable (zero-order) kinetics at standard doses (*e.g.* phenytoin) should be adjusted in small increments to prevent large changes in serum concentrations.
- The clinical status should dictate the frequency of drug monitoring. If clinical deterioration occurs, the frequency of drug monitoring should increase. Adjusting therapy for improved clearance is as important as adjustments made for poor clearance.
- The risk of nephrotoxicity rises when multiple nephrotoxic agents are given (*e.g.* vancomycin, aminoglycosides, acyclovir, furosemide, and amphotericin B).
- Escalation of a continuous infusion of drug with a prolonged t 1/2 (*e.g. long term* midazolam infusion) without supplemental dosing prior to escalation of the infusion dose can result in significant accumulation. Administration of a supplemental dose followed by an ↑ in the hourly infusion dose can achieve the desired effect and avoid drug accumulation. (*E.g.* midazolam: give the amount to be received in one hour as a "*prn*" dose if hemodynamically tolerated, then increase the infusion dose.)
- Avoid morphine in the presence of asthma and hypovolemia due to histamine release and the related risk of histamine mediated bronchospasm and vasodilation. Hydromorphone and fentanyl are alternative analgesics in this setting.

(Continued)

Box 13.1.6   Bedside Pharmacotherapy Pearls (Continued)

- Midazolam is currently the most frequently chosen sedative in the PICU due to its short t 1/2 (with *intermittent* dosing) relative to other sedatives and proven safety profile. Lorazepam and midazolam have similar wake-up times in long term sedation scenarios; lorazepam is somewhat less expensive, but is not considered "first line" for continuous infusions in pediatric patients due to potential accumulation of the propylene glycol diluent.
- Ketamine can be extremely useful in asthmatics due to its bronchodilatory effects or in hemodynamically-compromised patients when a benzodiazepine/opioid combination risks hypotension. Avoid in pulmonary hypertension. Low dose midazolam can decrease the hypertensive and psychomimetic effects caused by ketamine.
- Fentanyl is the preferred analgesic in hemodynamic compromise or patients with renal insufficiency. Rapid injection may cause chest wall rigidity; give >5 mcg/kg over 5–10 min.
- Pentobarbital is a useful third-line sedative in hemodynamically stable patients but has no analgesic effects at sedative doses. It can have negative inotropic effects along with peripheral vasodilation; therefore, hypotension can occur.
- All opioids (except meperidine) may cause bradycardia via vagal stimulation. Meperidine is vagolytic and may cause tachycardia.
- Consider initiating a bowel regimen (*e.g.* docusate +/− senna) when *starting* opioid therapy if no contraindications are present.

13.2 Analgesia, Sedation and Neuromuscular Blockade

Relief from pain (analgesia) and relief from anxiety and agitation (anxiolysis and sedation) are fundamental in the delivery of pediatric critical care. Achieving these goals is important for the emotional well-being and safety of each patient and may be essential to decrease oxygen consumption, maintain optimal gas exchange, influence vasomotor responses and enhance blood flow to vital organs. Individual needs should be addressed continuously; anticipatory planning and communication among well-informed disciplines, patient and family should produce the greatest benefit with the least risk.

Pain is the sensation of discomfort resulting from localized tissue injury and/or a systemic feeling of discomfort (*e.g.* nausea). Pain is complicated by the desire to escape (and fear of inability to do so) leading to anxiety. Localized pain leads to local muscle contraction which itself becomes painful. In addition, anticipation of pain can actually cause the sensation of pain.

Peripheral nerves contain axons from primary sensory, motor and sympathetic post-ganglionic neurons. Three types of axons comprise the primary sensory afferents: A-beta (AB; not normally involved in pain perception); A-delta (Aδ; myelinated; fast) and C fibers (unmyelinated; slow). Both Aδ and C fibers supply skin and deep tissues; these fibers are capable of transmitting pain when *sensitized,* earning them the designation "afferent nociceptors". Sensitization occurs via substances released from injured tissue (*e.g.* prostaglandins, bradykinins, leukotrienes, potassium, *et al.*) which enhance the sensation of pain; under these conditions, even light touch (which ordinarily would not cause pain) can become painful. The nociceptor itself then releases chemical mediators (secondary activation) which cause vasodilatation, mast cell degranulation, serotonin release from platelets and further inflammation. Nociceptors transmit to the dorsal horn of spinal gray matter, where impulses are transmitted largely through the spinothalamic tract to the brain (thalami and cortex) resulting in both the immediate sensation of pain and the residual sensation of pain that endures after the initial painful stimulus has resolved. The ability to feel pain is present in the term newborn; the participating neurologic pain pathways are present in the fetus.

In the ICU, stimuli not typically associated with pain (*e.g.* repositioning) or stimuli inherent to common interventions (*e.g.* presence of an endotracheal tube, chest tube, tracheal suctioning *etc.*) may cause pain. Pain is further exacerbated by anxiety and fear of the unknown; it is likely that all PICU patients experience some degree of discomfort, often complicated by the inability to communicate. There

Box 13.2.1   Assessment of Pain*

- Neonate (all gestational ages): Physiologic measures (HR, RR, BP, O_2 saturations) and other indicators (posture, tone, sleep pattern, facial expressions, color and quality of cry).
- FLACC (2 mos–7 yrs): Based on facial expression, leg position, degree of activity, quality of cry and consolability. From Merkel *et al.* The FLACC: a behavioral scale for scoring postoperative pain in young children, *Pediatr Nursing* **23**:293–297, 1997.
- Wong-Baker Faces Pain Rating Scale (> 3 yrs): The child is asked to choose the face which best describes the degree of discomfort. Faces range from happy (0) to frowning with tears (using either 5 or 10 as the maximum); from Jacob E, Pain Assessment and Management in Children, in Hockenberry MJ, Wilson D (*eds.*), *Wong's Essentials of Pediatric Nursing, 8th ed.*, Mosby, St. Louis, p. 162, 2009.
- Assorted numerical scales (school-age and beyond): The patient is asked to grade his/her pain on a scale of 0–10 (with zero meaning no pain and 10, the worst pain imaginable).

*This assessment may be obscured by sedative drugs, neuromuscular blockade, CNS injury *etc.* and does not address sedation needs. Pain is typically accompanied by tachycardia, hypertension, and mydriasis. These same findings may indicate fear, anxiety, hypoxia, acidosis, shock and other conditions that potentially could worsen with administration of analgesics. A careful bedside assessment should accompany the administration of analgesics to eliminate other causes of these alterations which may require interventions other than analgesia.

are multiple tools useful for pain assessment based on developmental cues (see **Box 13.2.1** for examples). All scales are most helpful when used serially and consistently with monitoring of the result of each intervention.

Commonly used terms:

- *Tolerance*: the need for increased doses of a given drug to achieve the same physiologic effect. Tachyphylaxis refers to enzyme-mediated tolerance.

- *Incomplete cross-tolerance*: tolerance to a currently administered drug that does not extend completely to other drugs in the same class.
- *Dependence*: the need for continuation of a drug manifested by physical signs of withdrawal (**Boxes 13.2.2 and 13.2.3**).
- *Addiction*: psychological dependence driving obsessive, compulsive use of a drug (or engagement in other behavior); not a feature of drug use among the acutely critically ill.

Box 13.2.2   Signs and Symptoms of Opiate Withdrawal

- Irritability; high pitched cry; agitation
- Anxiety, fear
- Self-inflicted scratch marks on the skin due to agitation (young infants; neonates)
- Tachycardia; hypertension (mild)
- Insomnia; yawning
- Sneezing; lacrimation; rhinorrhea
- Poor feeding; disorganized suck; excessive sucking
- Nausea, vomiting, diarrhea
- ↑ Temperature; temperature instability
- Drug craving
- Hypertonicity
- Hyperacusis
- Diaphoresis; piloerection
- Myalgias, arthralgias
- Tremulousness
- Seizures

Box 13.2.3   Signs and Symptoms of Benzodiazepine Withdrawal

- Alterations in mental status, depression, anxiety, dysphoria, hallucinations, acute psychosis, personality change
- Heightened perception, hyperesthesia, parethesias, insomnia
- Dizziness, ataxia, tremor, seizures
- Tachyarrhythmia
- Palpitations
- Hypertension
- Tachypnea
- Diaphoresis
- ↓ Visual acuity
- Nausea, vomiting
- ↑ Temperature (+/−)
- Skeletal muscle spasm, myalgia

- *Neuropathic pain*: pain that originates from damaged or dysfunctional neural tissue. It is typically resistant to treatment with standard analgesics.
- *Hyperalgesia*: a pathologic, augmented response to pain that occurs after repeated painful stimuli.
- *Allodynia*: the pathologic experience of pain after stimuli that are not normally painful; it is often a feature of neuropathic pain.
- *Referred pain*: pain that has a visceral source, but is perceived at a site distant from its origin which is thought to share the same spinal sensory segment(s).

Hyperalgesia and allodynia are potential consequences of inadequately treated pain; adequate pain control avoids these complications. Tolerance and dependence are anticipated effects of the prolonged use of benzodiazepines, opiates, and other neurotropic drugs commonly used for analgesia and sedation. Incomplete cross-tolerance to opiates should be considered when one opiate analgesic is exchanged for an alternative opiate; the dose requirement for the "new" drug may be less than the anticipated "equi-analgesic" dose.

Analgesia and anxiolysis do not always require medication. Environmental comforts such as soothing company, application of warmth or cooling, lighting and temperature control, music, massage, hypnosis and other techniques can be successful in replacing or complementing pharmacologic interventions. Use of 25% sucrose either to coat a pacifier or by instillation of 1 mL in each cheek has been successful in minimizing pain for infants < 6 mos prior to painful procedures such as venipuncture.

Local anesthesia can be very effective in eliminating or decreasing pain, and minimizing the dose of systemic analgesia required to effect comfort. Some available options are described in **Box 13.2.4**.

Sedation is most commonly provided in the PICU to alleviate anxiety, control agitation and minimize movement that endangers the patient and protects the airway, vascular access and other essential devices, dressings and wounds. It may also be required to protect against undesirable muscle activity or elevations in temperature. As is

Box 13.2.4   Commonly Chosen Options for Local Anesthesia

- **Eutectic mixture of local anesthetics** (EMLA®): an emulsion of prilocaine 2.5% and lidocaine 2.5%; potentially useful at sites of anticipated skin puncture for patients of any age beginning at term. Commonly used for venipuncture, IV insertion, LP; adjunctive to SubQ infiltration with lidocaine for deeper pain as occurs with bone marrow aspirations, *etc.* Only for use on intact skin at recommended dose. Cream is applied over a small area and covered with an occlusive dressing (*e.g.* Saran™ wrap or Tegaderm™) which should be maintained for one hour prior to procedure. Contraindicated in methemoglobinemia and in patients <12 mos who are receiving drugs that may induce methemoglobin. Limitations are the one hour "wait" time and variable efficacy (particularly in dark-skinned patients). Topical lidocaine (*e.g.* L-M-X®) is an alternative; it contains benzyl alcohol and should be avoided in neonates. A lidocaine patch (*e.g.* Lidoderm®) can be applied to skin over the most painful area and provide relief from local pain such as that associated with rib fracture and post-herpetic neuralgia. The patch may remain in place for 12 hr in any 24 hr period. Toxic effects are more likely to occur when large amounts of lidocaine are applied or when a large area of skin is covered. Manufacturers' guidelines should be followed.
- **Lidocaine and tetracaine** applied topically as a patch (Synera® patch); approved for patients > 3 yrs (but has been used in younger patients); effective in 20–30 mins. Indicated for use on intact skin for vascular puncture and IV insertion. Heat generated by the activated patch helps anesthetize the skin more rapidly and causes vasodilatation which may be helpful in achieving venous access. Synera should not be applied in the MRI scanner.
- **Infiltration with Lidocaine**: Indicated for laceration repair, venous or arterial puncture, LP, bone marrow aspiration, nerve blocks *et al.*; best performed using a small needle (27 or 30 gauge) through clean, intact skin. Care should be taken to ensure that the *total* dose of lidocaine does not exceed 4.5 mg/kg over a two hour period. All sources of lidocaine (*e.g.* instillation of lidocaine in the airway during

(Continued)

Box 13.2.4   Commonly Chosen Options for Local Anesthesia (Continued)

endoscopy) should be included to calculate the dose. Aspiration (by pulling back on the syringe plunger) at each tissue level prior to lidocaine injection has been recommended to ensure that lidocaine is not injected into a blood vessel. Some have suggested that lidocaine be injected immediately into the subcutaneous tissue on skin entry to effect anesthesia since intravascular injection of small amounts (0.1–0.2 ml) while advancing the needle are inconsequential. Addition of 1 ml (= 1 mEq) 8.4% sodium bicarbonate to 9 ml of 1% lidocaine may alleviate the burning caused by instillation of lidocaine. In most patients, onset of anesthesia occurs in 2–5 mins lasting 30 mins to ~2 hrs. Epinephrine and lidocaine mixtures can minimize bleeding and systemic absorption of lidocaine, but should not be used in areas supplied by end arteries such as digits, the nose, ears and penis. Lidocaine with epinephrine can also be buffered with bicarbonate.

- **Intrathecal or epidural opiates** are particularly useful for post-operative and chronic pain when stable autonomic nervous system and neuromuscular function is desirable. The risk of rostral spread and respiratory depression is minimized with the use of continuous epidural infusion of short-acting agents such as fentanyl or sufentanyl. These techniques require anesthesia care and close monitoring.

the case with analgesics, sedatives may be given as needed (*"PRN"*), by scheduled dosing, continuous infusions or a combination of these; the smallest dose of sedative or analgesic that achieves the desired effect should be used. Decisions regarding agent(s), route and regimen require individualization of patient needs, knowledge of patient-specific limitations (*e.g.* Is the airway intubated or is the patient breathing spontaneously?) and ability to weigh risks and benefits of options in given circumstances. Advantages and disadvantages of commonly used analgesics and sedatives are described (**Boxes 13.2.5 and 13.2.6**).

Initiation of weaning of analgesics and sedation is generally undertaken when the need for these drugs is waning or no longer

Box 13.2.5   Commonly Chosen Analgesics: Key Advantages and Disadvantages

Non-opiates:

- **Acetaminophen** (PO, PR, IV): ↓ Nociception, ↓ prostaglandin synthesis in the CNS. No respiratory depression; antipyretic; effective for mild to moderate pain; may result in ↓ dosing of opiates for more severe pain. Not useful as a single agent for severe pain; Delayed onset (10–60 mins) if enterally administered.
- **Non-steroidal anti-inflammatory drugs** (NSAIDS; PO; oral suspension of ibuprofen has been given PR; Ketorolac (PO, IV IM): ↓ Prostaglandin synthesis; nonselective NSAIDS ↓ activities of both cyclooxygenase (COX) 1 and 2. No respiratory depression; anti-pyretic and anti-inflammatory; may result in ↓ requirement for opiates for more severe pain; esp. useful in treatment of visceral/bone pain. Anti-platelet activity due to inhibition of COX-1; GI ulcers and bleeding may occur. Risk of acute renal failure due to renal vasoconstriction esp. with pre-existing renal insufficiency, dehydration, hypercalcemia. May ↑ BP; multiple dosing I.M. or IV is outside product labeling for patients <16 yrs but is supported by the medical literature. Ketorolac use should be limited to ≤ 5 days.
- **Ketamine** (IM, IV): Direct action on the cerebral cortex and limbic system; NMDA receptor antagonist in the spinal cord. Potent dissociative anesthetic; amnestic. Effective for hyperalgesia and allodynia. Bronchodilatory effects (useful in asthmatics); usually preserves respiratory drive, airway tone, laryngeal reflexes and BP (useful in patients with marginal or low BP who require sedation). Causes ↑ salivation; emergence syndromes (agitation, nightmares, hallucinations) occur in up to 12% of patients within 24 hrs of administration. Severe reactions may require treatment with small doses of short-acting barbiturate or benzodiazepine.

Opiates are derived from opium poppy; **Opioids** are synthetic or semi-synthetic compounds. Both are agonists at the μ receptors is spiral cord and brain. Affinity for the μ receptor dictates the potency of the narcotic. All can cause respiratory depression and ↓ in HR and BP.

- **Morphine** (PO, SubQ, IV, IM); Preservative-free preparations available for epidural and intrathecal use. Provides rapid relief of severe pain. Causes histamine release which may lead to pruritis and bronchospasm. A primary metabolite (morphine-3-glucuronide) is excitotoxic*.

(Continued)

> **Box 13.2.5 Commonly Chosen Analgesics: Key Advantages and Disadvantages (Continued)**
>
> - **Fentanyl** (IV; transdermal patch for chronic pain in tolerant patients): Onset < 30 sec; rarely causes pruritis; well suited for continuous infusion. Rapid IV infusion may cause chest wall rigidity, *esp.* in neonates. Tolerance is common.
> - **Hydromorphone** (PO, SubQ, IV, IM): Does not cause histamine release. Metabolite (hydromorphone-3-glucuronide) is excitotoxic*.
> - **Methadone** (PO, SubQ, IV, IM): Duration > 24 hrs. Useful in narcotic weaning strategies because of its long half-life; the least dialyzable of the opiate analgesics, making it useful in patients requiring dialysis. May cause prolongation of QT_c interval.
>
> **Notes: Meperidine** is not recommended for use as an analgesic; it offers no benefits compared to morphine and the meperidine metabolite, normeperidine, is associated with dysphoria, tremors and seizures. Meperidine is useful in control of shivering; can be useful as premedication for treatment with drugs known to cause chills (*e.g.* amphotericin B) or prior to giving blood products for patients at ↑ risk for transfusion-related shivering.

*__Excitotoxicity__ may lead to seizures.

exists. For patients who have received narcotics and benzodiazepines on a regular basis (most often by continuous infusion) during a critical illness, substitution of longer-acting drugs such as methadone and diazepam or lorazepam given enterally can facilitate the weaning process and minimize the need for IV access sites, potentially enhancing patient mobility and facilitating transitional care. For example, a child whose GI tract is functional and who has received narcotic and benzodiazepine for ~7 days (*e.g.* fentanyl 2 mcg/kg/hr and midazolam 0.15 mg/kg/hr) may be appropriately weaned by instituting methadone 0.1 mg/kg/dose (0.05–0.2 mg/kg/dose, max dose 10 mg) and diazepam 0.1 mg/kg/dose (0.1–0.2 mg/kg/dose, max dose 10 mg) enterally every 6 hrs. This will allow the rapid discontinuation of the continuous IV infusions of both fentanyl (after the second dose of methadone) and midazolam (after the second dose of diazepam) if the desired level of analgesia and

Box 13.2.6   Commonly Chosen Sedative/Hypnotic Agents

Benzodiazepines: Widely used to treat anxiety and agitation; not analgesic; may be helpful in reducing the need for opiates when anxiety is a component of discomfort. All cause respiratory depression with variable effect on BP. Effects result from binding to a site on the gamma aminobutyric acid (GABA) receptor complex, where they enhance neural inhibition.

- Midazolam (PO, Intranasal, IV, IM, PR): Rapid onset (1–2 min) and brief (1–4 hrs) duration. Well suited for continuous infusion; amnesic. Potentially useful in the absence of IV access. May causes ↓ BP; avoid in hemodynamic instability.
- Lorazepam (PO, IV, IM Intranasal): Slower onset (5–15 min) and longer duration (2–6 hrs) as compared to midazolam. Not well suited for continuous infusion because of accumulation of its preservative (propylene glycol).
- Diazepam (PO, IV, PR): Onset 1–2 mins lasting 6–12 hrs; unsuitable for continuous infusion. Potentially useful in the absence of IV access. An active metabolite (desmethyldiazepam) has a half-life of 50–100 hrs; this may lead to prolonged over-sedation and toxicity in neonates and young infants (< 6 mos). In older patients, this feature may be an advantage as evidenced by the usefulness of diazepam as part of a weaning strategy from benzodiazepine dependence. IV and rectal preparations contain benzyl alcohol; exposure to large doses is associated with potential fatal toxicity ("gasping syndrome") in neonates.

Barbiturates: An alternative to benzodiazepines; also binds to GABA receptor complex to ↑ neural inhibitory activity; hyperalgesic effect. All cause respiratory depression and ↓ BP.

- Thiopental (IV, PR): Ultra-short-acting; useful for induction of anesthesia; facilitates tracheal intubation and decreases ICP.
- Pentobarbital (IV, IM): Most commonly used to induce barbiturate coma when ICP is elevated or to achieve burst-suppression in refractory status epilepticus. Long-acting; terminal half-life ~25 hrs. Obscures neurologic findings; when given continuously may take days to metabolize after discontinuation.

(Continued)

Box 13.2.6   Commonly Chosen Sedative/Hypnotic Agents (Continued)

Dexmedetomidine (IV): a more specific α-2 adrenergic agonist than clonidine. Binds to sites in the periphery, spinal cord and brain; sedative and analgesic effects; treats shivering; attenuates ↑ HR, ↑ BP and delirium associated with ketamine; minimal effects on respiration; may ↓ requirement for opiates. Limited data in critically ill children; currently, manufacturer recommends use < 24 hrs. Rapid IV administration produces reflex bradycardia and hypertension; ↓ HR and ↑ BP may occur independently of each other with continuous infusion.

Chloral Hydrate (PO, PR): Hypnotic; useful for intermittent dosing in patients tolerant to high doses of benzodiazepine. Mechanism of action not known. Causes respiratory depression; active metabolites (trichloroethanol; trichloroacetic acid) with long half-lives (>10 hrs); not recommended for use in neonates, for continuous sedation in the ICU or for procedural sedation.

Propofol (IV): Potent anesthetic/sedative; onset is rapid (within 30 sec) and duration is brief (3–10 mins depending on dose); well-suited for procedural sedation by skilled providers. Respiratory depression and hypotension are common complications, particularly if dosing needs are over-estimated. Results in greenish discoloration of urine. Not for continuous infusion "in PICU patients" per product labeling. Prolonged infusions in children have been associated with metabolic acidosis and death. Contraindicated if egg or soy allergy is present (controversial).

sedation have been achieved. The staggering of administered doses so that the patient receives alternately methadone or diazepam every three hours may be helpful. Appropriate doses of methadone and diazepam should be identified based on clinical effects, and should be adjusted as needed.

Rapid discontinuation of analgesics and/or sedatives may result in an abstinence syndrome (**Boxes 13.2.2 and 13.2.3**) especially in patients who have required opiate analgesia and/or benzodiazepines for > 4–7 days. A gradual reduction in dose can effect pain-free awakening from pharmacologic sleep. Weaning schedules should be individualized depending on dose and duration of drug administration. A minimum reduction in dose of approximately 10–15% per day is usually well tolerated. For patients who require both analgesics and sedatives, provision of analgesia beyond the period of sedative discontinuation may be needed to avoid allowing the patient to awaken in pain.

Treatment of iatrogenic withdrawal in the PICU typically requires supportive care and re-introduction of an analgesic and/or sedative agent, *e.g.* a benzodiazepine. Clonidine (a centrally acting alpha-2 adrenergic agonist) is an effective agent in treating or avoiding narcotic withdrawal. Signs and symptoms of drug withdrawal may be indistinguishable from infection; the latter should be considered in the differential diagnosis.

Use of reversal agents (naloxone for narcotics; flumazenil for benzodiazepines) may precipitate pain, agitation and withdrawal symptoms if the antagonized drug has been given for a prolonged period. The half-life of naloxone is brief; a continuous infusion may be required in narcotic overdose. Flumazenil is used primarily to reverse the effect of benzodiazepines after general anesthesia and may be useful to reverse paradoxical excitation produced by midazolam in some patients. Both naloxone and flumazenil should be available when narcotics and/or benzodiazepines are used for procedural sedation.

Patient-controlled analgesia (PCA) may be suitable for patients > 5 yrs who are developmentally and physically able to press a button in response to a need for pain medication. Selected patients < 5 yrs may be candidates, particularly if they are experienced in associating pain relief with medication (*e.g.* the chronically ill). PCA is most often used to deliver opiate analgesia (*e.g.* morphine); a programmable pump allows self-delivery of small doses several minutes apart (*e.g.* 5–10 mins) with a pre-determined hourly maximum dose, beyond which the pump will not deliver additional drug. A low dose "basal" infusion of drug may or may not be infused along with self-administered "bolus" doses; the basal dose contributes to the hourly maximum dose. The total amount of drug delivered is retrievable and the numbers of attempts made to self-deliver analgesia are recorded; these data can be used to evaluate patient need and/or ability to use this modality. The inclusion of a basal dose has been associated in some series with an increase in adverse events such as respiratory depression, without significant improvements in pain control when compared to PCA without basal dosing. PCA by proxy (care-giver or family member presses the PCA button to deliver analgesia) has gained attention, both for its efficacy as well as concerns for an increase in adverse events. Whatever approach is chosen, it is important that dosing regimens be individualized, and continuous cardiorespiratory and Pox monitoring be supervised by staff with a mastery of pediatric assessment skills and resuscitation.

Neuromuscular blockers (NMB) are used in the ICU to eliminate (or in some cases, minimize) the activity of skeletal muscle in order to accomplish certain interventions in which movement or certain reflexes may be detrimental, improve patient-ventilator synchrony, optimize gas exchange, and/or pulmonary blood flow, minimize barotrauma, lower raised ICP, decrease O_2 consumption, and suppress movements that interfere with care. Neuromuscular blockade provides *no* analgesia or alteration in mental status and it is imperative that adequate pain relief and sedation be instituted *before and provided during* NMB use.

NMBs are structurally similar to acetylcholine (ACh) and are divided between depolarizing and non-depolarizing NMBs. Depolarizing agents (*e.g.* succinylcholine) bind to cholinergic receptors on the motor end-plate causing an initial muscle depolarization followed by blockade of depolarization. Stimulation of the nicotinic acetylcholine receptor is thought to be associated with muscle fasciculations (not typically seen in young children) and an increase in ICP, intraocular pressure, intragastric pressure and possibly muscle pain. Re-depolarization does not occur because calcium does not re-accumulate in the sarcoplasmic reticulum until the depolarizing agent leaves the receptor. Its normal fate is hydrolysis by pseudocholinesterase. Nondepolarizing NMBs competitively inhibit acetylcholine at the motor endplate by binding to the receptor and rendering it non-functional or by obstructing ion channels so that an electrical potential cannot be generated. Characteristics of commonly used NMBs are described in **Box 13.2.7**.

It is essential that the airway is deemed accessible prior to administration of NMB for tracheal intubation and that the airway remains safely secured when NMB is required for mechanically ventilated

---

Box 13.2.7   Neuromuscular Blocking Agents

Depolarizing Agents: Acetylcholine receptor agonists (ARA)

• **Succinylcholine** is used primarily to facilitate tracheal intubation or treat laryngospasm. Frequently chosen for rapid onset (< 1 min) and brief duration (7–8 mins) of paralysis, making it well suited for rapid sequence intubation. Spontaneous respirations resume within an average of 9 mins (a major advantage if tracheal intubation has failed). Serum K^+ ↑s by 0.5–1 mEq/L limiting its use in patients with hyperkalemia. May cause malignant hyperthermia (MH). Untoward effects associated with initial depolarization during tracheal intubation may be blunted by giving a "defasiculating dose" (~10% of the paralyzing dose) of a non-depolarizing agent. Contraindications to use of succinylcholine: > 24–48 hrs *after* acute thermal injury (↑↑ risk of hyperkalemia); personal or family history of MH; ≥ 7 days post-crush injury or denervation; progressive neuromuscular disease of any cause. Masseter muscle rigidity preventing laryngoscopy after succinylcholine may herald MH. No reversal agent(s) for any effects of ARA are available.

Nondepolarizing Agents: Competitive antagonists at the acetylcholine receptor. The onset of action is slower and duration is longer among these agents as compared to succinylcholine; they do not cause MH or hyperkalemia. Hypokalemia and hypocalcemia potentiate neuromuscular blockade with non-depolarizing agents. Non-depolarizing agents are divided into the benzylisoquinolones and the aminosteroids based on structure. Reversal of nondepolarizing agents occurs with their metabolism, redistribution from receptor-binding and/or cholinesterase inhibition (*e.g.* neostigmine; bradycardia and asystole are potential effects from neostigmine).

(Continued)

Box 13.2.7   Neuromuscular Blocking Agents (Continued)

Examples of Benzylisoquinolones:

- Mivicurium: Onset 1–3 mins; duration is brief (9–20 mins); the only paralytic in its class that is metabolized by pseudocholinesterase. ↑ risk of histamine-associated ↓ BP with higher doses.
- Cisatracurium: Onset 1.5–2 mins; intermediate duration;* preferred for continuous paralysis over vecuronium when ↑ risk of myopathy exists (*e.g.* patients requiring continuous muscle paralysis *and* systemic steroid therapy. Myopathy will not be apparent until chemical paralysis is discontinued.) Minimal risk of histamine-associated hypotension.

Examples of Aminosteroids:

- Rocuronium: Onset 1–1.5 mins; intermediate duration;* no significant hemodynamic effects.
- Vecuronium: Onset 1.5–3 mins; intermediate duration*; no significant hemodynamic effects.
- Pancuronium: Onset 1–3 mins; long acting;** ↑ HR and ↑ BP; arrhythmias in predisposed patients. ↑ arrhythmias when given with tricyclic antidepressants and halothane.

*Intermediate duration, 25–60 mins.
**Long acting, 90–100 mins.

patients. NMB can be given intermittently *PRN* or by continuous infusion. Advantages of intermittent dosing include avoidance of post-paresis myopathy which can result in flaccid areflexic tetraplegia, prolonged ventilator dependency and ICU stay. In addition, the advantages of preserving the cough reflex may favorably affect airway clearance. However, for patients who require continuous pharmacologic paralysis, the smallest dose required to produce adequate muscle relaxation should be used. The degree of competitive neuromuscular blockade (CNMB) should be monitored by testing the response to peripheral nerve stimulation using the "Train-of-four" method. Two electrodes are placed approximately 2 cm apart over a peripheral nerve (usually the ulnar, facial or posterior tibial nerves). Four small electrical impulses are delivered; the associated muscle responds with a twitch corresponding to the percentage of receptor sites blocked by the NMB. Current is delivered in milliamps (mAmp) beginning at 20 and progressively increasing to a maximum of 80 mAmp. The desired degree of blockade (85–90% blockade) correlates with 1–2 twitches, which is usually achievable with a stimulus in the 20–50 mAmp. range when NMB dose is optimal. The absence of a twitch response indicates that all receptors are blocked and that CNMB is excessive. A four twitch response indicates that <75% of receptors are blocked, which *may* be inadequate for the clinical circumstance. The required depth of blockade should be individualized; monitoring of the degree of blockade should be frequent (every 30–60 mins) until the desired level of blockade is achieved and stable. The monitoring can be less frequent (per PICU protocol) thereafter.

The degree of analgesia and sedation should be monitored continuously during administration of NMB. Currently, the physical examination (pupillary size, HR, BP, the hemodynaminc response to stimulation) are the mainstay of monitoring in the ICU. Bispectral index monitoring (BIS) was designed for intra-operative use to help ensure that general anesthesia is present throughout the procedure; BIS monitoring may be used in the PICU to supplement physical examination for monitoring of the depth of sedation. BIS monitoring relies on EEG data to generate a numeric correlate with the degree of sedation and potential for recall in patients >1 yr. BIS monitoring electrodes are applied to the forehead; numeric results range from 0 (no EEG activity) to 100 (fully awake). Values in the 40–60 range are consistent with deep sedation and low probability of recall. Unreliable values may result from artifact, sensor malposition, and electrical interference. BIS values should be used in conjunction with clinical findings in bedside decision making.

13.2.1 *Procedural sedation*

Procedural sedation is a drug-induced alteration of consciousness provided specifically to facilitate accomplishment of a necessary procedure. Depending on the nature of the procedure, analgesia may be required also. As an increasing number of non-operative interventions have become available and pediatric imaging more widely utilized, the need for procedure-related motion control and analgesia has also increased. This need has resulted in the sedation of pediatric patients outside the "safety net" of the operating room and PICU. Recognition of the hazards of pediatric sedation in areas where personnel, equipment and patient access are limited, different or unavailable underscores the need for preparation and the ability to reconstruct the "PICU environment" wherever pediatric sedation is to occur. Practice Guidelines for Sedation and Analgesia by Non-Anesthesiologists (*Anesthesiology* **96**:1004–1017, 2002) and Guidelines for Monitoring and Management of Pediatric Patients During and After Sedation for Diagnostic and Therapeutic Procedures (*Pediatrics* **118**:2587–2602, 2006) provide consensus recommendations for the conduct of pediatric sedation. This section summarizes the essential elements involved in pediatric sedation for referring and participating providers. Key definitions and points are outlined (**Box 13.2.8**).

The goals of pediatric sedation as they relate to the spontaneously breathing patient are to ensure the patient's safety and welfare, alleviate anxiety, treat discomfort and pain, minimize psychological trauma, maximize amnesia when appropriate, and recover the patient to his/her pre-procedure status. Pre-procedure teaching (for patients developmentally ≥ 3 yrs and parents) may decrease the need for sedation in some patients. Non-pharmacologic methods of calming (*e.g.* distraction; coaching) should be used whenever possible to replace and/or complement the use of drugs.

Safe and successful pediatric sedation requires intensive focus on patient eligibility for sedation without tracheal intubation, development of a safe pharmacologic strategy and preparation for adverse events. Sedation results in a potential continuum of alterations in consciousness. Despite identification of an intended level of sedation, the sedationist and sedation team must be ready and able to manage the effects and complications of deeper levels of sedation, including unintended general anesthesia. This requires expertise in airway care and intensive monitoring with the ability to recognize

---

Box 13.2.8   Definitions of Varying Degrees of Sedation

- **Minimal sedation:** anxiolysis; the patient responds normally to commands; cognitive function may be impaired. Cardiorespiratory function is preserved.
- **Moderate sedation:** drug-induced depression during which the patient responds cognitively to commands by verbal cue with/without mild stimulation such as light touch. Reflex withdrawal does not qualify as a cognitive response. For infants, the response must reflect purpose or cognition. Cardiorespiratory function is preserved; however, the procedure itself (*e.g.* upper GI endoscopy or bronchoscopy) may lead to airway obstruction requiring intervention.
- **Deep sedation:** drug-induced depression from which the patient is not easily aroused, but is still able to respond purposefully after repeated verbal and/or noxious stimuli (*e.g.* No response to calling his/her name or light touch, but withdraws and pushes away the examiner's hand when a digit is pinched; may or may not say "Ouch!") Respiratory function may be impaired; cardiovascular function is usually maintained.
- **General anesthesia (GA):** drug-induced loss of consciousness from which the patient is unarousable. Airway patency is endangered, respiratory function is often impaired and cardiovascular function may be impaired.

---

and maintain desirable effects and avoid and/or reverse undesirable effects. The essence of the pre-sedation evaluation is summarized (**Box 13.2.9**).

The physician/practitioner and team (sedationist and at least one skilled assistant to monitor the patient) providing sedation should be knowledgeable about pharmacologic alternatives and be able to select appropriate agents based on the patient and planned procedure; reversal agents (naloxone, flumazenil) should be available, although their use may be limited. For patients requiring moderate-deep sedation, vascular access is appropriate. It is recommended that the person performing the procedure not be involved

---

Box 13.2.9 Key Elements of the Pre-Sedation Evaluation

- **History:** Complete, with special attention to allergies, current medications, prior sedation and/or GA experiences, personal or family history of MH, and recent intake (**Box 13.2.10**). History of snoring respirations, obstructive sleep apnea, trismus, C-spine instability or limitations in extension, drooling, recent or current URI, copious airway secretions are among the relative contraindications to sedation of a spontaneously breathing patient.
- **Physical Examination:** Focused on evaluation of the airway (*Bag-Mask Ventilation and Tracheal Intubation, 15.2; Fig. 15.2.5*), cardiopulmonary status, determination of airway accessibility and maintenance, and potential reversibility of hemodynamic instability. (*E.g.* Patients with "kissing tonsils" may have further obstruction once sedated.) Patients reliant on left-to-right shunts may develop ↓ pulmonary blood flow and ↓ Pox saturations if systemic pressures fall during sedation.
- **Laboratory/Radiologic/Other Studies:** Results of recent laboratory data (*e.g.* hemoglobin, platelet count, acid-base status, electrolytes), X-rays (*e.g.* CXR, relevant CT scans), sleep study data, EEG's, *etc.* should be reviewed; these may be relevant in weighing the risks of sedation.
- **Review of Prior Records of Sedation/GA:** Note drug exposures and any adverse events.
- Assign an American Society of Anesthesiology (**ASA**) **Classification** score (**Box 13.2.11**).
- **Discussion** of risks, benefits, and alternatives to sedation without planned intubation with the guardian(s) and patient (if developmentally appropriate); signed permission for sedation should be obtained.

---

in providing sedation. All necessary equipment for emergency airway care and resuscitation should be immediately available. The HR, BP, RR, Pox saturations and $ETCO_2$ should be monitored continuously and recorded at least every 5 min with checks of peripheral perfusion for patients deeply sedated. If BP cuff inflation results in overstimulation, this measurement may be performed less frequently in favor of checks of peripheral perfusion and the

Box 13.2.10   Minimum Fasting Period for Sedation without Tracheal Intubation*

Substance Ingested**	Minimum Pre-Sedation Fast (Hours)
Clear Liquids	2
Human milk	4
Infant formula; non-human milk	6
Light meal (*e.g.* "toast and clear liquids"); fatty meals may prolong gastric emptying and a longer fast may be desirable	6

* Practice Guidelines for Preoperative Fasting and the Use of Pharmacologic Agents to Reduce the Risk of Pulmonary Aspiration: Application to Healthy Patients Undergoing Elective Procedures (*Anesthesiology* 90: 896–905, 1999).

** For patients at ↑ risk of GE reflux/aspiration, modifications of these timeframes may be warranted.

Box 13.2.11   American Society of Anesthesiologists (ASA) Classification

Class	Definition
I	Healthy with no underlying medical problems
II	Mild systemic disease that does not interfere with daily activities (*e.g.* occasional asthma)
III	Severe systemic illness that interferes with daily activities (*e.g.* a child with cystic fibrosis whose activities are curtailed by dyspnea)
IV	Serious Systemic illness that is a continual ongoing threat to life (*e.g.* a patient requiring vasoactive and ventilatory support)
V	Life-threatening disease with instability; patient may die without the intended procedure.

aforementioned measures. The neurologic status is monitored throughout the procedure and post-procedure period until fully recovered (*i.e.* until he/she is at or very close to the pre-procedure respiratory, cardiac and neurologic state. Use of a scale (*e.g.* the Aldrete Score, a scale of 0–10 describing activity, respiration, circulation, level of consciousness, and O_2 saturation, with 10 as the normal fully awake patient) can provide an objective measure of the progress of sedation and recovery.

The majority of sedation-related adverse events resulting in neurologic injury or death are associated with poor patient selection, inadequate monitoring, inadequate rescue, medication errors and/or inadequate recovery. Sedations performed by individuals who frequently sedate patients are less likely to be associated with adverse outcomes. Complications are associated with "any drug, in any dose by any route"; it is not "safer" to give an oral sedative than an IV sedative. Polypharmacy and drugs with long half-lives (*e.g.* chloral hydrate) should be avoided, since these are associated with an increased risk of poor outcome.

13.3 Drug-Induced Toxic Hyperthermic Syndromes

Thermoregulation is a process of balancing heat gain and heat loss. Endogenous heat produced through basal metabolism (controlled by hormones and sympathetic stimulation) and muscle activity is normally lost through the skin via radiation (60%), evaporation (25%), convection (15%) and conduction (3%). The hypothalamus normally regulates body temperature within a tight range. When the environmental temperature exceeds body temperature, the balance shifts in favor of heat gain by the body (*Hyperthermia, 12.6*). Hyperthermia occurs when heat production increases and/or heat loss is impaired and the hypothalamus can no longer adequately control body temperature. The difference between the more common pyrogen-mediated fever and hyperthermia may not be immediately apparent; however, the distinction can usually be made based on history and physical examination. It is critical to distinguish the two since hyperthermia itself is life-threatening and frequently does not respond to antipyretics. There are five recognized syndromes of drug-induced hyperthermia.

Malignant Hyperthermia (MH) is a genetic biochemical muscle disorder characterized by dysfunctional calcium channels; calcium flows into the cell and increases ATP production which results in muscle contraction, accelerated muscle metabolism and uncoupling of oxidative phosphorylation. Common triggers include inhalational anesthetics (*esp.* halothane, enflurane, isoflurane) and succinylcholine. Some congenital muscle disorders increase the risk of developing MH. Children are especially susceptible to MH because of higher basal metabolic rates and less well developed metabolic controls. The classic triad of MH is hyperthermia, muscle rigidity and metabolic acidosis. Clinical findings and treatment of MH are outlined (**Boxes 13.3.1 and 13.3.2**).

Neuroleptic Malignant Syndrome (NMS) occurs in 0.01–0.02% of patients treated with antipsychotic drugs but has a mortality rate of 10%. In classical form there are four key elements: muscle rigidity, pyrexia, altered consciousness, and autonomic disturbances (diaphoresis, tachycardia, labile blood pressure, hypersalivation). If two of the four criteria are present the diagnosis should be considered. NMS is caused by blockade of dopaminergic neurons in the CNS. Although 16% of cases develop within the first 24 hrs of treatment with an

Box 13.3.1 Clinical Findings in Malignant Hyperthermia (MH)		
Early	Late	Terminal
• Tachycardia • Tachypnea • Muscle rigidity (often first seen in masseter muscles) • Ventricular dysrhythmias • Hypercarbia	• Hyperthermia • Sweating • Skin mottling • Mydriasis • ↑ Creatine kinase (CK) • Myoglobinuria • Metabolic and respiratory acidosis • Hyperkalemia	• DIC • Liver failure • Bowel ischemia • Congestive heart failure • Arrhythmias • Pulmonary edema • Neurologic injury

---

Box 13.3.2   Treatment of Malignant Hyperthermia

- Discontinue inciting agents.
- Hyperventilate with 100% oxygen.
- Administer dantrolene 2.5 mg/kg IV every 5 min as needed to block calcium release from the sarcoplasmic reticulum.
- Cooling measures for elevation of core temperature: Cooling blankets, ice packs, ice water submersion, cool water mist and fans. Goal for temperature 38–39°C. Use benzodiazepines and/or muscle paralysis to prevent shivering. Antipyretics are ineffective.
- Ensure adequate volume replacement, avoid dehydration and promote diuresis to protect kidneys; in addition to volume administration, mannitol or furosemide may be helpful.
- Use lidocaine for ventricular arrhythmias.
- Treat metabolic acidosis with sodium bicarbonate.
- Treat hyperkalemia with calcium, insulin and glucose as indicated (*Electrolyte Disturbances, 6.2, Box 6.2.10*).
- Monitor vital signs, ABG's, potassium, bicarbonate and CK serially.
- Continued monitoring in the ICU for 24 hrs after resolution of MH is warranted since MH may recur.
- The "MH Hotline" provides a valuable resource for assistance with diagnosis and care by experienced Anesthesiology staff. They can be contacted at 800-644-9737 in the USA and Canada and 011-303-389-1647 outside North America.

---

antipsychotic drug, onset may be delayed for ~30 days. Mean recovery time after discontinuation of the offending drug is 7–10 days with nearly all recovering within 30 days. The typical drugs and conditions associated with NMS, differential diagnosis, therapies and complications are listed (**Boxes 13.3.3 through 13.3.6**).

Serotonin syndrome (SS). Serotonin is synthesized in the brain from the amino acid tryptophan. Serotonin affects mood, sleep and pain perception in the CNS. Peripherally, serotonin has its predominant effect on muscles and nerves.

Serotonin does not cross the blood brain barrier. SS is the result of overstimulation of $5HT_{1A}$ (and possibly $5HT_z$) receptors in brainstem

Box 13.3.3   Typical Drugs and Pathologic Conditions Associated with Neuroleptic Malignant Syndrome (NMS)

Neuroleptics	Antiemetics	Pathologic Conditions
• Aripiprazole	• Domperidone	• Acute catatonia
• Chlorpromazine	• Droperidol	• Extreme agitation
• Clozapine	• Metoclopromide	• High doses of antipsychotics
• Fluphenazine	• Prochlorperazine	• Rapid escalation of antipsychotics
• Haloperidol	• Promethazine	
• Olanzapine		• Parenteral antipsychotics
• Paliperidone		• Other psychotropic drugs
• Perphenazine		• Substance abuse
• Quetiapine		• Neurologic disease
• Risperidone		• Acute medical illness
• Thioridazine		• Trauma
• Ziprasidone		• Surgery
		• Possibly dehydration

Box 13.3.4   Differential Diagnosis of NMS*

- Infectious: Meningitis/encephalitis/brain abscess; post-infectious encephalomyelitis (ADEM); sepsis
- Psychiatric: Idiopathic malignant catatonia; nonconvulsive status epilepticus; benign extrapyramidal side effects; structural lesions of midbrain; delirium
- Toxic: Amphetamines/hallucinogens; serotonin syndrome; anticholinergic agents; salicylates; withdrawal from dopamine agonists/sedatives
- Endocrine: Thyrotoxicosis; pheochromocytoma
- Environmental: Heat injury
- Metabolic: Malignant hyperthermia

* Adapted from Strawn JR, Keck PE, Caroff SN, Neuroleptic Malignant Syndrome, *Am J Psychiatry* **164**: 870–876, 2007.

Box 13.3.5 Management of Neuroleptic Malignant Syndrome (NMS)*

Clinical Presentation	Supportive Care	Specific Therapies
• Rigidity, tremor		Anticholiergic agent
• Rigidity, muteness, stupor	Change or ↓ antipsychotic	Lorazepam
• Rigidity (mild), catatonia or confusion, T ≤ 38°C	Discontinue antipsychotics; initiate cooling for ↑ temperature; eliminate risk factors: exhaustion and dehydration, ↑ environmental temperature, high dose/ high potency parenteral antipsychotics	Lorezepam
• Rigidity (moderate), catatonia or confusion, T 38–40°C		Lorazepam, bromocriptine or amantidine; consider electroconvulsive therapy (ECT; rarely used but may be considered in extreme cases)
• Rigidity (severe) or coma, catatonia, T ≥ 40°C		Dantrolene, bromocriptine or amantidine; consider ECT

*Adapted from Strawn JR, Keck PE, Caroff SN. Neuroleptic Malignant Syndrome, *Am J Psychiatry* **164**: 870–876, 2007.

Box 13.3.6 Complications of Neuroleptic Malignant Syndrome (NMS)

- Dehydration
- Myocardial infarction
- Electrolyte imbalance
- Cardiomyopathy
- Rhabdomyolysis (acute renal failure)
- Deep venous thrombosis
- Cardiac arrhythmias or arrest
- Pulmonary embolism

- Chest wall rigidity
- Aspiration pneumonia
- Seizures
- Disseminated intravascular coagulation
- Hepatic failure
- Sepsis
- Death

Box 13.3.7	Radomski Criteria for Serotonin (5-HT) Syndrome*		
Characteristic	Major Symptoms	Minor Symptoms	Diagnostic Considerations
Cognitive and Behavioral	• Confusion • Elevated mood • Coma/ semi-coma	• Agitation • Insomnia	• Metabolic cause • Sepsis • Thyroid storm • Toxic: *e.g.* lithium, cocaine, SSRI's (see **Box 13.3.8**) MAOI's salicylates, ecstacy, TCA's anticholinergics • Neuroleptic malignant syndrome
Autonomic	• Fever • Diaphoresis	• Tachycardia • Flushing • Tachypnea • Dyspnea • Diarrhea • Hypertension • Hypotension	
Neuromuscular	• Hyperreflexia • Myoclonus • Tremors/ shivering • Rigidity	• Incoordination • Akathasia • Mydriasis	

*Diagnosis requires at least 5 major symptoms or 3 major plus 2 minor symptoms. Adapted from Radomski JW, Dursun SM, Revelry MA, Kutcher SP. An exploratory approach to the serotonin syndrome: an update of clinical phenomenology and revised diagnostic criteria. *Med Hypotheses* **55**: 218–224, 2000.

nuclei. The diagnosis of SS is clinical (**Box 13.3.7**) and requires identification of a causative serotonergic agent as well as exclusion of other diagnoses. Some serotonin reuptake inhibitors have a long half life (*e.g.* fluoxetine); if such drugs are discontinued and a second serotonergic agent is introduced, SS may result from additive effects. Drugs can cause SS by several mechanisms (**Box 13.3.8**); treatment is outlined in **Box 13.3.9**. Most patients improve within 24 hrs after having been admitted though in 40% some symptoms persist longer. A major

Box 13.3.8   Mechanisms and Drugs Leading to Serotonin Syndrome

↑ 5HT formation	L-tryptophan
↑ Serotonin release	NMDA (ecstasy), cocaine, amphetamine, fenfluramine, phenteramine
↓ 5HT metabolism	Monamine oxidase inhibitors, isocarboxazid, phenelzine, tranyl-cypromine, selegiline, moclobemide, linezolid
Serotonin receptor direct agonists	LSD, buspirone, almotriptan, eletriptan, frovatriptan, naratriptan, rizatriptan, sumatriptan, zolmitriptan, dihydroergotamine
↓ Serotonin reuptake	Citalopram, escitalopram, fluvoxamine, fluoxetine, paroxetine, sertraline, nefazadone, trazadone, venlafaxine, amitriptyline, clomipramine, cocaine, imipramine, tramadol, dextromethorphan, meperidine, amphetamine
Nonspecific	Lithium, St. John's Wart, electroconvulsive therapy

Box 13.3.9   Management of Serotonin Syndrome

- Discontinue all serotonergic medications.
- Treat seizures, rigidity, myoclonus and agitation with benzodiazepines. If benzodiazepines fail to reduce muscular rigidity, treat with cyproheptadine ($5HT_{1A}$ receptor antagonist). If this treatment fails, proceed with tracheal intubation and paralysis using a nondepolarizing muscular blocking agent.
- Longer term anticonvulsant drug therapy should include barbiturates.
- Treat hyperthermia with external cooling.

difference between NMS and SS is that SS tends to develop within minutes to hours of exposure to the offending agent, and is more likely to present with myoclonus and hyperreflexia than rigidity.

Anticholinergic poisoning (ACP). Anticholinergic drugs competitively compete with acetylcholine for binding to cholinergic receptors with acetylcholine and cause hyperthermia by stimulation of both central and peripheral muscarinic blockade. Central cholinergic blockade causes agitation, seizures, and coma. Peripheral cholinergic blockade interferes with cutaneous heat loss by impairing sweat production. Hyperthermia results from increased heat production and decreased heat loss. The classic description of anticholinergic poisoning is characterized: "red as a beet" (vasodilatation attempts to compensate for decreased sweat production), "dry as a bone" (sweat glands do not produce sweat), "hot as a hare" (hyperthermia), "blind as a bat" (nonreactive mydriasis results in blurry vision), "mad as a hatter" (delirium, hallucinations), "full as a flask" (the detrusor muscle and uretheral sphincter are under muscarinic control and urination is prevented). Commonly ingested substances that cause ACP are listed (**Box 13.3.10**). The

---

Box 13.3.10   Commonly Ingested Substances That Cause Anticholinergic Poisoning (ACP)

- Antihistamines
- Cold medications
- Tricyclic antidepressants
- Scopolamine
- Sleep aids

- Tainted street drugs (*e.g.* heroin "cut with scopolamine")
- Jimson weed
- Atropine
- Deadly nightshade

---

differential diagnosis includes any ingestion/exposure/condition that produces an alteration in mental status (*Altered Mental Status, 5.1*), tachycardia, urinary retention or seizure. Management of ACP is outlined (**Box 13.3.11**).

Sympathomimetic poisoning (SP). The mechanism of hyperthermia in SP involves both central and peripheral disturbances in thermoregulation. Centrally, dopamine, norepinephrine and serotonin concentrations are elevated. Peripherally, vasoconstriction, increased muscle activity (agitation, seizures, rigidity) and increased heat production resulting from increased hepatic metabolism contribute to hyperthermia. Development of life-threatening hyperthermia is idiosyncratic. Common causes include cocaine, amphetamine,

Box 13.3.11   Management of Anticholinergic Poisoning (ACP)

Indication	Treatment	Considerations
Prolonged QRS or QTc	Sodium bicarbonate IV	Usual goal arterial pH = 7.5 to 7.55 (monitor QRS duration during administration)
Agitation and seizures	Benzodiazepines	Avoid phenothiazines and butyrophenones which are anticholinergics
	Physostigmine*	Monitor for bradyarrhythmia; atropine should be available
Hyperthermia	Evaporative cooling	For moderate to severe poisoning

*Used in patients who manifest both peripheral symptoms and moderate agitation/delirium due to ACP; *not* to be given in conditions other than pure ACP (e.g. avoid in TCA poisoning).

methamphetamine and derivatives, caffeine, theophylline, over-the-counter decongestants such as phenylpropanolamine, ephedrine, and pseudoephedrine. In cocaine and amphetamine intoxication, mortality is directly related to the degree of temperature elevation. Common signs, complications and therapies are listed (**Boxes 13.3.12 and 13.3.13**).

Drug withdrawal syndrome. Ethanol increases CNS inhibitory output via its effects on gamma aminobutyric acid (GABA; a major inhibitory neurotransmitter) and inhibits excitatory tone by attenuating the effects of excitatory transmitters such as glutamate *et al.* When acutely deprived of ethanol following chronic ethanol exposure, excitatory transmission predominates and withdrawal symptoms are manifested (**Box 13.3.14**).

The usual treatment includes benzodiazepines for withdrawal symptoms. Benzodiazepines increase the frequency of GABA chloride channel opening; barbiturates increase duration of channel opening and propofol may open chloride channels in the absence of GABA

Box 13.3.12   Common Signs of Sympathomimetic Poisoning (SP)

- Delusions
- Paranoia
- ↑ BP
- ↑ or ↓ HR
- ↑ Temperature
- Diaphoresis
- Piloerection

- Mydriasis
- Hyperreflexia
- In severe poisoning:
  - ➢ Seizures
  - ➢ ↓ BP
  - ➢ Dysrrhythmias

Box 13.3.13   Management of Complications of Sympathomimetic Poisoning

Complication	Treatment
Pulmonary edema	Positive pressure ventilation
Ventricular dysrrhythmias	For the first few hours post-ingestion use a non-sodium channel blocker (*e.g.* esmolol if the dysrhythmia is NOT hemodynamically significant and amiodarone if the dysrhythmia IS hemodynamically significant). After the first 2 hrs post-ingestion, lidocaine or procainamide may be given to treat ventricular arrhythmias.
Hypertension	Benzodiazepines, nitroprusside
Chest pain	Benzodiazepines, nitroglycerin (continuous infusion)
Seizures	Benzodiazepines, barbiturates
Metabolic acidosis	Consider $NaHCO_3$ IV
Rhabdomyolysis	Vigorous hydration to achieve UOP >1–2 ml/kg/hr
Hyperthermia	Diazepam, ice packs, +/− acetaminophen; dantrolene for persistent severe temperature elevation.
Hypoglycemia*	Glucose (continuous infusion)

* Hyperthermia can prevent gluconeogenesis.

Box 13.3.14   Symptoms of Ethanol Withdrawal

- Anxiety; Insomnia
- Tremulousness
- Headache
- Diaphoresis
- Alcoholic Hallucinosis (normal vital signs)

- Gastrointestinal upset
- Palpitations
- Seizures
- Delirium tremens (hallucinations, agitation, disorientation, tachycardia, hypertension, ↑ temperature) beginning 48–96 hrs after the last ingestion of alcohol.

---

stimulus. The Clinical Institute of Withdrawal Assessment for Alcohol Scale measures severity of withdrawal and can help guide IV versus oral therapy. Sustained use of opiates, benzodiazepines and the shorter acting SSRIs (*e.g.* paroxetine, venlafaxine) is associated with a withdrawal syndrome if discontinued suddenly.

Drugs that Uncouple Oxidative Phosphorylation (UCOP). Normally the transport of electrons in mitochondria is "coupled" to the formation of ATP from ADP and phosphate. The most common cause of UCOP in children is salicylate ingestion, although ingestion of less common toxins should be noted (**Box 13.3.15**). Manifestations and treatment of salicylate intoxication are listed (**Boxes 13.3.16 and 13.3.17**).

Box 13.3.15   Drugs that Uncouple Oxidative Phosphorylation

- Salicylates: aspirin and non-aspirin salicylate compounds; oil of wintergreen is notorious for its high salicylate content.
- Nitrophenols: dinitrophenols (herbicides), trinitrophenols (explosives, reagents used to Gram stain and to check for creatinine), pentachlorophenol (wood preservative).
- Ioxynyl containing herbicides

Box 13.3.16   Manifestations of Salicylate Intoxication

- Respiratory: Hyperpnea; respiratory alkalosis (early); tachypnea, noncardiogenic pulmonary edema; respiratory acidosis (late, grave prognosis).
- Neurologic: Tinnitus/altered hearing; altered mental status; convulsions; cerebral edema.
- Hyperthermia
- Metabolic: Acidosis, hypo/hypernatremia, hypokalemia; hypoglycemia, hyperglycemia, ketonemia, ketonuria, hypoglycorrhachia.
- Gastrointestinal: Vomiting, hemorrhagic gastritis, decreased motility, pylorospasm; abnormal liver enzymes.
- Dehydration caused by vomiting and ↑ perspiration (caused by ↑ temperature).
- Renal: Renal tubular damage, proteinuria; salt and water retention; hypouricemia.
- Coagulation abnormalities: hypoprothrombinemia; inhibition of Factors V, VII, and X; platelet dysfunction.

Box 13.3.17   Treatment of Salicylate Intoxication

- Correct fluid, glucose and electrolyte imbalances; central venous or pulmonary artery pressure monitoring may be required if noncardiogenic pulmonary edema or renal failure is present.
- Alkaline diuresis should be initiated: $NaHCO_3$ 1–2 mEq/kg followed by $NaHCO_3$ 130 mEq/L of D_5W to infuse at 1.5–2 times the maintenance rate. Urine pH should be maintained at 7.5–8.0.
- Consider administration of multidose activated charcoal.
- Hemodialysis should be considered in child with serum salicylate concentration 35–50 mg/dL and metabolic acidosis. Hemodialysis or hemoperfusion should be initiated for serum concentration >60 mg/dL in a child.

Chapter 14

Poisonings

14.1 Principles of Diagnosis and Decontamination

The diagnosis and management of the poisoned patient can be a challenging task, particularly when the toxin is not clearly identified by history. Physical findings and diagnostic tests may provide critical clues, but in some cases the diagnosis and optimal management pathway remain a challenge. Consultation with a medical toxicologist is advisable and always available from regional poison control centers, accessible nationwide throughout the United States by telephone (1-800-222-1222).

A thorough **history** is essential; for infants and young children, this typically requires information gathering from witnesses or those at the scene of the ingestion or exposure. Older patients may withhold information for a variety of reasons. The mental status of the patient may also contribute to confusion or concealment of portions of the history. Key historical information to be obtained is listed in **Box 14.1.1**. All potential sources of information should be sought when indicated: this includes family members, any witnesses at the scene or anyone with knowledge of possible exposures (*e.g.* friends, teachers, care providers, emergency medical and law enforcement personnel, pharmacists and other health care providers).

Any substance can be potentially dangerous in a large enough dose. However, there are certain ingestions (**Box 14.1.2**) that may be harmful, or even lethal, even in small amounts (*e.g.* one pill or a teaspoon), especially when the patient is a small child. Some

623

Box 14.1.1   Key Historical Information

- Identify toxin
  - ▶ Prescription medication(s)   ▶ Plants
  - ▶ Over the counter drug(s)   ▶ Herbal medications
  - ▶ Illegal drugs   ▶ Chemicals (*e.g.* solvents, caustics, hydrocarbons)
- Time line: When did the ingestion or exposure occur?
- Amount: How much was ingested or what was the nature of the exposure (*e.g.* splash of chemical in the eyes)?
- Accidental vs. intentional?
- Substance abuse?

Box 14.1.2   Potentially Dangerous Ingestions Even in Small Amounts

Pesticides/Herbicides
Carbamates
Organophosphates
Diquat
Paraquat
Lindane
Hydrocarbons
Toxic Alcohols
Ethylene glycol
Methanol
Topical Preparations
Benzocaine
Camphor
Eucalyptus oil
Oil of wintergreen
(methyl salicylate)

Caustic Chemicals
Selenious acid
Hydrofluoric acid
Imidazolines (eye drops and nasal sprays)
Naphazoline
Oxymetazoline
Tetrahydrozoline
Xylometazoline
Prescription Medications
Antimalarials
Clonidine
Calcium channel antagonists
Cyclic antidepressants
Lomotil (atropine/diphenoxylate)
Opiates*/opioids**
Sulfonylureas

* Naturally occurring drugs derived from the poppy plant.
** Drugs that bind to opium receptors in the brain.

ingestion-related complications are associated with a high morbidity and mortality risk. Depressed mental status, especially when accompanied by vomiting, may lead to aspiration pneumonitis and respiratory failure. Rhabdomyolysis may occur in association with prolonged seizure activity.

Some patterns of **physical findings** may suggest a particular category of ingestion. These collections of findings are often referred to as toxic syndromes or *toxidromes* (**Box 14.1.3**). If more than one toxin is involved, the pattern of symptoms is less likely to resemble a classic toxidrome.

If particular medications are known to be available, **serum levels** of these drugs may be obtained, particularly if symptoms correspond with its toxicity. In an unknown or suicidal ingestion, a broader

Box 14.1.3	Frequent Clinical Findings of Selected Toxic Syndromes (Toxidromes)			
Findings	Opioids/ Opioids*	Cholinergic*	Anticholinergics*	Sympatho-mimetics*
Mental status	Depressed	Depressed	Confused or Somnolent	Agitation
HR	NS (↓)	↓ (↑)	↑	↑
BP	NS (↓)	NS	↑	↑
Respiration	↓	NS (↑)	NS	NS
T	NS (↓)	NS	↑	↑
Pupils	Miosis	Miosis	Mydriasis	Mydriasis
Mucous-membranes	NS	↑Salivation ↑Lacrimation	Dry	NS
Skin	NS	Diaphoretic	Flushed	Diaphoretic
Bowel sounds	NS (↓)	↑	↓	NS (↑)
Urination	NS	↑	Retention	NS

↑, increased; ↓, decreased; NS, non-specific; ( ), less commonly

* *E.g.* Opioids: fentanyl, methadone; opiates: morphine; Cholinergics: organophosphates; Anticholinergics: diphenhydramine, amitriptyline; Sympathomimetics: cocaine, phencyclidine.

Box 14.1.4   Key Laboratory Tests for Specific Indications

- **CXR**: Aspiration pneumonitis
- **ABG**: Acid–base disturbance (respiratory or metabolic)
- **Co-oximetry**: Carbon monoxide poisoning or methemoglobinemia
- **Compare measured osmolality with calculation of osmolar gap**: Toxic alcohols
- **CK**: Rhabdomyolysis
- **BUN and creatinine**: Kidney toxin (*e.g.* ethylene glycol)
- **Liver enzymes and function tests**: Liver toxin (*e.g.* acetaminophen)
- **Specific drugs levels** in plasma or serum: *e.g.* Lithium, iron, carbamazepine, phenobarbital, digoxin, acetaminophen, salicylate

---

diagnostic evaluation may be considered both in an attempt to identify particular toxins (*e.g.* acetaminophen) or specific findings that may change management (*e.g.* wide QRS interval on ECG). Though not an exhaustive list, certain **diagnostic testing** is suggested, particularly in the latter, more uncertain clinical scenario. Some recommended tests are discussed briefly in **Box 14.1.4** and more extensively below.

Acetaminophen level (serum) should be obtained on *all* patients suspected of intentional overdose. Acetaminophen is widely available, has a non-specific initial clinical presentation and is readily treated by early administration of *N*-acetylcysteine ("NAC").

Salicylate level (serum). Although salicylate toxicity often causes clinical findings (*e.g.* tachypnea, tinnitus) and laboratory abnormalities (*e.g.* metabolic acidosis) these may not be evident on presentation. A salicylate level is easily obtained and may direct subsequent therapy (*e.g.* sodium bicarbonate infusion or hemodialysis).

Serum electrolytes and glucose. Profound hypoglycemia may suggest exposure to insulin or sulfonylureas. A metabolic acidosis with an elevated anion gap (AG > 16; *Appendix part 2, V*) may suggest exposure to a toxin or alternative diagnosis as noted in **Box 14.1.5**.

Electrocardiogram (ECG): An ECG may demonstrate characteristic findings that may help indicate a particular toxin (**Box 14.1.6**).

Box 14.1.5   Differential Diagnosis for Metabolic Acidosis with an Elevated Anion Gap Acidosis ("MUD PILES")

- Methanol
- Uremia
- Diabetic ketoacidosis (also starvation ketoacidosis and alcoholic ketoacidosis)
- Paraldehyde, Phenformin
- Iron, Isonazid, Ibuprofen, Inhalants (carbon monoxide, cyanide, hydrogen sulfide), Inborn errors of metabolism
- Lactic acidosis
- Ethylene glycol
- Salicylates

Box 14.1.6   Electrocardiographic Findings for Selected Toxins

- Tachycardia
  - ▶ Amphetamines
  - ▶ Anticholinergics
  - ▶ Cocaine
  - ▶ Theophylline
- Bradycardia
  - ▶ β-blockers
  - ▶ Calcium-channel antagonists
  - ▶ Clonidine
  - ▶ Digoxin

- Prolonged QTc interval
  - ▶ Antipsychotics
  - ▶ Cyclic antidepressants
  - ▶ Citalopram
- Prolonged QRS interval
  - ▶ Cocaine
  - ▶ Cyclic antidepressants
  - ▶ Propranolol
  - ▶ Chloroquine
  - ▶ Diphenhydramine
  - ▶ Propoxyphene
  - ▶ Type I antidysrhythmics (*e.g.* quinidine)

Urine toxicology screens: The urine toxicology screen available at most healthcare facilities is an immunoassay that detects a limited number of drugs of abuse, typically some opiates/opioids, benzodiazepines, barbiturates, cocaine, and amphetamines (exact components will vary). Diagnostic pitfalls exist for immunoassay

---

Box 14.1.7   Pitfalls of Urine Toxicology Screens (Immunoassays)

- Drug classes and specific substances detected may vary between individual tests and no test will screen for all possible substances.
- False-negative results may occur if a substance is present below the level of detection of the assay.
- Not all members of a drug class may be tested (opiate screens may not detect fentanyl or methadone).
- Positive results only indicate presence of a substance and not toxicity (qualitative result not quantitative).
- False-positive results due to the presence of other substances may occur (*e.g.* dextromethorphan may cause a positive reaction for phencyclidine).
- Positive results may not mean acute toxicity (*e.g.* cannabinoid metabolites may persist for weeks).
- If there are medico-legal implications, positive immunoassay results should be followed with confirmation testing (generally gas chromatography/mass spectrometry) in order to identify the specific agent.

---

screens (**Box 14.1.7**). More "comprehensive" urine toxicology screens (generally utilizing other chromatographic techniques) are also available, but still cannot detect all toxins and results are often delayed. Acute management rarely is altered by these results. The clinical status of the patient should always be the primary guide to management.

Gastrointestinal decontamination (GID) has long been considered a mainstay in the treatment of the poisoned patient. Clear clinical evidence supporting the routine use of any form of gastrointestinal decontamination has not been demonstrated. Furthermore, each method of GID carries with it certain limitations and risks. Careful consideration of these risks should be balanced with any potential benefit before attempting to utilize GID. Consultation with a medical toxicologist either at your healthcare facility or regional poison control center is strongly encouraged.

Activated charcoal (AC) is generally considered the mainstay of GID. Possessing a large relative surface area and a high absorptive capacity, AC is administered enterally with the hope of binding toxins in the GI tract before they can reach the bloodstream. Although AC is often regarded as a "universal antidote" by some, its use is not without risk and should be avoided in some circumstances (**Box 14.1.8**). It has not been shown to change clinical outcomes when used routinely. For most ingestions, the therapeutic window

---

Box 14.1.8   Activated Charcoal (AC): Key Points

- The ideal dose of AC is not known, but many recommend 1 gm/kg enterally (max. 100 gm).
- If an NG tube is used, its position must be confirmed (by radiograph) prior to instillation of charcoal.
- For most ingestions, any efficacy of AC likely decreases >1 hr post-ingestion.
- AC carries the risk for the following complications:
  ‣ Pulmonary aspiration
  ‣ Adverse GI effects including: nausea, vomiting, diarrhea, pain, and constipation
  ‣ Corneal abrasions if splashed in the eye
- AC is contraindicated in any patient with:
  ‣ Current or potential loss of consciousness or airway compromise without establishment of definitive airway (*i.e.* tracheal intubation)
  ‣ Compromised functional integrity of the GI tract (*e.g.* ileus, bowel obstruction, GI perforation, ischemic bowel)
- AC does readily adsorb the following substances and therefore is not recommended for the following ingestions:
  ‣ Metals (*e.g.* iron and lithium)
  ‣ Toxic alcohols (*e.g.* ethylene glycol and methanol)
- AC is contraindicated in hydrocarbon ingestion due to concern for vomiting and aspiration.
- AC is contraindicated in caustic ingestions (*i.e.* alkali and acids) as it will not prevent gastrointestinal damage and will obscure subsequent endoscopic evaluation.

for administration of AC is within 1 hr after ingestion. There may be exceptions when delayed gastric emptying is a factor and AC given after this time period may be helpful (*e.g.* salicylates). Although routine administration of AC is not recommended, stronger consideration should be given when a particularly toxic ingestion has no other effective therapy and no contraindication exists.

Gastric Lavage (GL). The goal of GL is to remove toxins from the stomach before they can be absorbed by using a large bore gastric tube and serial aliquots of normal saline. In the past this was most commonly performed to extract whole pills or fragments. Concerns regarding potential complications and lack of evidence that GL changes clinical outcomes have contributed to a general decline in its use. There are no uniformly agreed upon indications; it should be considered only in the most dire and life-threatening of circumstances. A summary of the key points regarding GL is listed (**Box 14.1.9**).

Whole bowel irrigation (WBI) is the administration of large volumes of polyethylene glycol electrolyte solution ("PEG-ES" or GoLYTLEY®) in an attempt to evacuate toxins more quickly from the gastrointestinal tract and reduce absorption. These large volumes of PEG-ES may be given orally or via an NG tube as many patients will not tolerate taking the required doses by mouth. It is sometimes advocated in instances where AC is not effective (*e.g.* iron poisoning) or under other specific circumstances (*e.g.* ingestion of sustained release). As with other forms of GID, there is no conclusive evidence that WBI changes clinical outcomes and adverse events are a concern with its use. This technique is summarized in **Box 14.1.10**.

Box 14.1.9   Gastric Lavage (GL): Key Points

- GL should be considered only within 1 hour of ingestion.
- Intubation is performed before GL in any patient with current or potential loss of consciousness or airway compromise.
- A large orogastric tube, usually 36–40 F, is placed. For small children a tube of at least 24 F can be utilized. Nasogastric tubes should be considered for removal of non-caustic liquid toxins only.
- The left lateral decubitus position with the head ~20° below the feet affords the potential benfits of raising the position of the pylorus (and therefore slowing gastric emptying) and lowering the risk of aspiration, regardless of whether or not an endotracheal tube is in place.
- Though the total volume of fluid for GL is debated, 1–2 L (10 ml/kg aliquots) in a small child and 2–4 L (200–300 ml aliquots) in an adolescent are generally used. Normal saline is preferred, but some use water in adolescents. Each aliquot is withdrawn in an attempt to remove toxic matter. This is repeated until the fluid withdrawn is clear.
- GL carries the risk for multiple complications:
  ▸ Pulmonary aspiration
  ▸ Gastrointestinal perforation (mechanical injury)
  ▸ Hyponatremia (with water used as lavage fluid)
  ▸ Hypernatremia (with normal saline as lavage fluid)
  ▸ Hypothermia (lavage fluid not sufficiently warmed)
- GL is contraindicated in the management of:
  ▸ Caustic ingestions (↑ concern for GI perforation)
  ▸ Hydrocarbon ingestions (↑ risk of pulmonary aspiration)
- GL is contraindicated in any patient with:
  ▸ Current or potential loss of consciousness or airway compromise without establishment of a definitive airway (*i.e.* tracheal intubation).
  ▸ Increased risk of GI bleed or perforation (*e.g.* recent surgery).

Box 14.1.10   Whole Bowel Irrigation (WBI): Key Points

- Polyethylene glycol electrolyte solution (PEG-ES) is given in doses based on age:
  9 mos –6 yrs: 500 ml/hr
  6–12 yrs: 1000 ml/hr
  Adolescents: 1500–2000 ml/hr
- If PEG-ES is refused by mouth, it may be administered via NG tube. It is advised that the patient be placed in an upright position while slowly advancing the fluid rate. The risk of aspiration should not be underestimated if this route is chosen.
- PEG-ES is continually administered until rectal effluent is clear.
- Many advocate considering WBI for the following overdoses or poisoning scenarios:
  ‣ Iron
  ‣ Lithium
  ‣ Sustained-release drug preparations
  ‣ Ingested medicinal patches
  ‣ Ingested packages of drugs of abuse (*i.e.* narcotic body packing)
- WBI risks include:
  ‣ Pulmonary aspiration
  ‣ Adverse GI effects including: nausea, vomiting, abdominal cramping and bloating.
- WBI is contraindicated in any patient with:
  ‣ Current or potential loss of consciousness or airway compromise without establishment of definitive airway (*i.e.* tracheal intubation).
  ‣ Intractable vomiting
  ‣ Compromised functional integrity of the GI tract (*e.g.* ileus, bowel obstruction, GI perforation, ischemic bowel)

14.2 Common Ingestions

Supportive care, with appropriate attention to airway, breathing and circulation is the cornerstone of medical toxicology and its importance cannot be over-emphasized. However, there are times when supportive care may not be sufficient and specific therapies or antidotes may be indicated. These examples of commonly ingested substances were chosen because they have a high potential for morbidity and mortality, frequently require prolonged observation, and often require antidotal therapy which may not be immediately familiar to the bedside clinician.

Acetaminophen [N-acetyl-p-aminophenol (APAP)] is used in many prescribed and over the counter medications as both an analgesic and an antipyretic. It is considered a safe medication at normal therapeutic doses. The maximum therapeutic APAP dose is 10 to 15 mg/kg per dose for children (75 mg/kg/day) or 1 g per dose four times a day at four-hour intervals for adults. Acute overdose is considered an amount over 7.5–15 g/dose in an adult or 150 mg/kg in a child.

APAP is well absorbed from the GI tract. It reaches its plasma peak level in 4 hours. The majority of APAP is conjugated with hepatic sulfate or glucuronide, and excreted in urine. About 5% of APAP is oxidized by the cytochrome P450 (CYP2E1) system and forms the toxic metabolite, N-acetyl-p-benzoquinone imine (NAPQI.) With ingestion of a therapeutic dose, NAPQI is conjugated with glutathione and excreted in urine. With overdose, endogenous glutathione is insufficient to detoxify NAPQI, which leads to hepatocyte injury. A majority of APAP exposures do not result in toxicity; however, the American Association of Poison Control Centers reported 5 deaths in patients

---

Box 14.2.1   Stages of Acetaminophen (APAP) Toxicity

Stages (Post-ingestion)	Clinical Manifestations
I (24 hrs)	Asymptomatic or GI symptoms (nausea, vomiting in the first 12 hrs). Liver enzymes are normal during this phase.
II (24–36 hrs)	Liver enzymes begin to rise and patients may complain of abdominal pain.
III (72–96 hrs)	Liver enzymes peak; fulminant hepatic failure with coagulopathy and encephalopathy may develop.
IV (next days–weeks)	If the patient survives, liver enzymes and function normalize.

Box 14.2.2   Management of Acetaminophen (APAP) Overdose or Suspected Overdose

- Obtain serum APAP level at least 4 hrs after ingestion.
- For acute single overdoses, the Rumack-Matthew nomogram can be used to assess the possibility of developing hepatotoxicity if the time of ingestion is known and the patient presents within 24 hrs of the ingestion.
- If the serum APAP concentration is less than the possible toxicity line the healthy patient will not develop serious hepatotoxicity and does not require antidote therapy.
- N-acetylcysteine (NAC; the precursor of glutathione) is the antidote for APAP poisoning. It should be given to patients who have a "possible hepatotoxic" level of APAP on the nomogram or to those who have already developed hepatotoxicity from APAP ingestion. (There are data that support administration of NAC no matter how late post-ingestion the patient presents. NAC is also routinely given in cases of undifferentiated liver failure.)
  - ▸ Oral: Loading dose: 140 mg/kg followed by 70 mg/kg every 4 hrs for 17 doses.
  - ▸ IV: Several protocols exist. The "21 hour protocol." A loading dose of 150 mg/kg over 1 hr followed by 50 mg/kg over 4 hrs and then 100 mg/kg over 16 hrs.
- Liver enzymes and APAP concentrations should be measured at the completion of NAC therapy. NAC should be continued if there is evidence of ongoing liver injury or if APAP is still detectable. Although an abbreviated (24 hr) course of NAC may be feasible in selected asymptomatic patients with normal liver enzymes and function, this approach is controversial and should be individualized.

<20 yrs of age in 2008. The assessment and management of APAP overdose are summarized in **Boxes 14.2.1 and 14.2.2**.

Nearly all patients who receive NAC within 8 hrs of APAP ingestion do well. Those who present later are at risk of fulminant liver failure but should still be treated with NAC. The Kings' College Hospital Criteria are predicative of mortality without liver transplant, and are used to predict the need for liver transplant: arterial blood pH < 7.30 and/or serum creatinine > 3.39 mg/dL after resuscitation; PT > 100 sec, INR > 6.5; grade III or IV hepatic encephalopathy.

Cardiovascular toxins can be divided into three groups including sodium channel blockers, antihypertensives, and cardiac glycosides. Sodium channel blockers (SCB) include tricyclic antidepressants, many antimalarial medications, type I anti-dysrhythmia medications, and local anesthetics. The antihypertensives include beta-blockers, calcium channel blockers, angiotensin converting enzyme inhibitors or receptor blockers, and others. Among the antihypertensives, the beta-blockers (BB) and calcium channel blockers (CCB) have the greatest potential to cause morbidity and mortality. The most common cardiac glycoside exposure is pharmaceutical digoxin, but many plants including foxglove, lily of the valley, oleander, and red squill contain cardiac glycosides with similar potential for toxicity.

SCB's slow the influx of sodium during Phase 0 of the cardiac action potential causing widening of the QRS complex. This increases the risk of ventricular dysrhythmias and hypotension. Seizures and altered sensorium are also common, probably due to interference with neuronal sodium channels.

BB's and CCB's work by blocking either β-adrenergic receptors or calcium channels; both classes of medications can cause cardiogenic shock. The cardiac conduction system can be interrupted resulting in bradycardia and heart block including complete AV dissociation. Cardiac contractility is also adversely affected further reducing cardiac output. Many of these medications also cause peripheral vascular smooth muscle dilation resulting in hypotension.

Cardiac glycosides inhibit the Na-K membrane pump in both myocytes and the cardiac conduction system. Interference in the conduction system, typically at the AV node, can result in bradycardia, heart block, and junctional escape rhythms. The effect on myocytes usually causes cardiac irritability resulting in premature ventricular contractions, predisposing to ventricular dysrhythmias. Assessment and management of cardiovascular toxin ingestion are summarized in **Box 14.2.3**.

Disposition. Symptomatic patients or those with a potentially serious exposure require admission to a monitored setting capable of caring for a critically ill child. Extended release CCB's present the added challenge of delayed toxicity (12–18 hrs). Most authors

Box 14.2.3   Assessment and Management of Commonly Ingested Cardiovascular Toxins

- Assess and stabilize airway, breathing and circulation (*General Approach to the Critically Ill Child, 1.2*).
- Obtain a 12-lead ECG as soon as possible.
- Gastrointestinal decontamination (*Principles of Diagnosis and Decontamination, 14.1*) should be considered especially in symptomatic patients because of the great potential for morbidity and mortality.
- Meticulous supportive care is the mainstay of therapy.
- Fluid resuscitation with crystalloid should proceed for shock in the normal manner with 20 ml/kg boluses.
- A trial of atropine for symptomatic bradycardia is indicated, but may not be effective on the poisoned heart.
- Vasoactive medications may be useful for fluid-unresponsive shock (except in the case of digoxin toxicity, which requires treatment with digoxin-immune-Fab).
- Attemps at transvenous pacing in the setting of cardiac glycoside poisoning may lead to dysrhythmias induced by the pacer itself because of an already irritable myocardium.
- **Specific Antidotes for Symptomatic Patients:** Note that patients poisoned with any of the cardiovascular toxins are frequently critically ill. Consultation with a regional poison center or toxicologist is encouraged.
  - ▸ **Calcium:** Trial administration is recommended for hypotension in CCB poisoning; may be helpful in BB poisoning. Avoid in cardiac glycoside poisoning. Calcium gluconate 10% (0.6 ml/kg; max 30 mls) given over 10–15 min is preferred over CaCl if given peripherally. If a positive clinical response is achieved, calcium gluconate 10% 1.5 ml/kg/hr may be given. Repeat doses of 0.6 ml/kg is reasonable while a continuous infusion is prepared. Serum ionized calcium should be monitored at least hourly with some advocating a goal of twice normal concentrations.
  - ▸ **Digoxin-specific antibodies (Digoxin Immune Fab):** Highly effective for cardiac glycoside exposures negating the need for other therapies. Indicated in symptomatic acute or chronic cardiac glycoside ingestions and for asymptomatic acute ingestions with serum $K+ > 5$ mEq/L. The empiric dose for acute ingestions is 5–10 vials IV over 30 min.

(Continued)

> **Box 14.2.3   Assessment and Management of Commonly
> Ingested Cardiovascular Toxins (Continued)**
>
> ▶ **Glucagon:** Effective for both CCB and BB poisoning. It is thought to ↑intracellular cAMP and ↑HR and BP. The main adverse effect is vomiting. A suggested dose is 50–150 mcg/kg IV. This dose can be repeated every 3–5 mins. A continuous infusion can be given if intermittent dosing is helpful, with the effective "bolus" dose given as an hourly infusion.
>
> ▶ **Insulin:** A growing body of evidence supports the use of high dose insulin therapy for both CCB and BB poisoning. The mechanism is unclear but animal studies and case series continue to show benefit for this treatment. The typical initial loading dose of insulin is 0.5–1 Unit/kg IV followed by an infusion of 0.5–1 Unit/kg/hr. Serum glucose monitoring (every 15–30 mins until stabilization is achieved, and then at least hourly) and dextrose supplementation as needed to maintain euglycemia are essential.
>
> ▶ **Intralipid** IV has been advocated for severe CCB or BB poisoning.
>
> ▶ **Sodium bicarbonate:** The treatment of choice for SCB poisoning with a QRS duration > 100 msec. Initial dose: sodium bicarbonate 8.4% 1–2 mEq/kg IV. Repeat every 5–10 mins with the goals of narrowing the QRS complex and controlling ventricular dysrhythmias. Once goals are met, a continuous infusion can be started to maintain blood pH of 7.50–7.55. Repeated dosing may be required if QRS widening of dysrhythmias recur. Serum sodium should be monitored and hypernatremia should be avoided.

recommend admission for 24 hrs after CCB exposure. Most other cardiac toxins should manifest symptoms within 6 hrs and patients should and observed at least that long.

Anti-diabetic agents. There are several classes of oral hypo-glycemic medications available including sulfonylureas, meglitinides, biguanides (*e.g.* metformin), glitazones, and alpha-glucosidase inhibitors. Of these, only the sulfonylureas and the meglitinides commonly induce hypoglycemia. Although metformin is not usually associated with hypoglycemia, lactic acidosis may result and can be fatal.

Sulfonylureas and meglitinides interfere with hormonal feedback in the pancreatic beta cell resulting in increased secretion of endogenous insulin. The major difference between the two classes is the duration of action. Sulfonylureas have very long half lives and have active metabolites which can result in prolonged and recurrent episodes of hypoglycemia. For reasons not entirely understood,

---

Box 14.2.4   Assessment and Management of Oral Anti-Diabetic Agent Ingestion

- Rule out hypoglycemia as a cause in all cases of altered mental status and/or seizures.
- If symptoms are mild, oral glucose should be provided. More commonly, dextrose IV is required (*Hypo- and Hyperglycemia, 6.4; Box 6.4.4*).
- If IV access is delayed, glucagon 0.025 mg/kg (max 1 mg) Im can be given pending IV access.
- Once stabilized, the patient should be given oral calories.
- Because of the long $t_{1/2}$ of the sulfonylureas hypoglycemia may recur for hours to days and continuous dextrose infusion may be needed.
- Octreotide is a somatostatin analog which decreases insulin secretion from the pancreas. Its use has been recommended in cases of recurrent hypoglycemia. Optimal dosing has not been established. Most authors recommend 2–5 mcg/kg up to the adult dose of 75 mcg given subQ every 6 hrs. Octreotide has been used primarily in sulfonylurea toxicity but the mechanism of action suggests that octreotide should be helpful for meglitinide toxicity as well.
- The asymptomatic patient potentially exposed to even one pill of a sulfonylurea should be admitted to monitor blood sugar because delayed hypoglycemia is common and has been reported to occur up to 24 hrs after initial exposure with the majority showing toxicity within 8–12 hrs. The shorter half lives of the meglitinides suggest less potential for delayed toxicity, but due to the limited data, prolonged observation is warranted in these exposures as well. Symptomatic patients, regardless of the offending agent, should be admitted for 24 hrs and until euglycemic for several hours.

sulfonylureas are known to cause delayed toxicity, especially in children, with hypoglycemia occurring as long as 18–24 hrs after exposure. The meglitinides have short half lives and may not cause such a prolonged risk of hypoglycemia. The assessment and management of oral hypoglycemic agent ingestion is summarized in **Box 14.2.4**.

Opiates (naturally-occurring) and **opioids** (semi-synthetic or synthetic) are medications that, when given in therapeutic doses cause analgesia by agonizing a variety of receptors (*mu*1, *mu*2, kappa), but predominantly via the *mu* (μ) receptors in the central and peripheral nervous systems. The terms *opiate* and *opioid* are sometimes used interchangeably. When considered as a group they can be administered IV, IM, *PO*, transdermally, or intra-nasally. There is a wide variety of these analgesics with a wide range of half-lives and potencies, ranging from ultra-short acting, highly potent opioids (*e.g.* sufentanyl), to long acting, moderate potency opioids (*e.g.* extended release oral morphine). Buprenorphine is available as an oral medication with both *mu* agonist and antagonist properties and a long half life. This medication is changing opioid addiction management, as it can be taken on an out-patient basis. Unfortunately, this results in household access to these medications, resulting in profound opioid intoxication and substantial morbidity among children.

While these medications can be highly effective analgesics when administered in therapeutic doses, they can also cause substantial morbidity and mortality when given or taken in overdose. The opioid toxidrome is classically described as miosis, bradypnea, hypotension, mental status depression and hypoxemia, possibly with respiratory arrest. It is important to recognize, however, that some synthetic opioids, such as meperidine, propoxyphene and fentanyl may not cause miosis, perhaps obscuring the toxidrome. Besides mental status and respiratory depression, non-cardiogenic pulmonary edema has also been associated with opioid administration and intoxication. Some suggest that naloxone administration may cause or predispose to non-cardiogenis pulmonary edema. However, this complication occurred before naloxone was in use, suggesting that the mechanism is unclear.

A few opioids are cardiotoxic and may cause ECG abnormalities. Propoxyphene has SCB effects, which may cause QRS widening and ventricular dysrhythmias. Dextromethorphan, a common over-the-counter cold remedy is an opioid derivative which may cause hallucinations and a toxidrome resembling phencyclidine intoxication; it may also cause a false-positive result for phencyclidine on routine urine drug screens. The assessment and management of opioid toxicity is summarized in **Box 14.2.5**.

"**Toxic alcohols**" refers to alcohols that are not intended for ingestion. The most common toxic alcohols are methanol, ethylene glycol and isopropanol. Methanol is commonly found in windshield washer fluid. Ethylene glycol is found in engine coolant ("antifreeze"). Isopropanol is used as rubbing alcohol. Many of these solutions contain high concentrations of toxic alcohols making even small ingestions potentially dangerous.

All alcohols are rapidly absorbed after ingestion. Toxic alcohols may be absorbed through many routes, including skin. Alcohol dehydrogenase and aldehyde dehydrogenase catalyze toxic alcohols into toxic metabolites that cause organ impairment. Methanol is metabolized to formaldehyde then formic acid, which is directly toxic to the optic nerve and can cause visual impairment ranging from blurred vision to irreversible blindness. Ethylene glycol is metabolized into glycoaldehyde, glycolic acid, glycoxylic acid, then into oxalic acid. The resulting oxalic acid crystals can cause renal failure by precipitation in renal tubules. These crystals are found also in heart, myocardium and other tissues. Oxalic acid can precipitate with calcium and lead to hypocalcemia, QT prolongation and dysrhythmias. Isopropanol is oxidized to acetone by alcohol dehydrogenase and may cause sedation but does not cause severe or permanent injury. Because of their acidic metabolites, methanol and ethylene glycol can produce an anion gap metabolic acidosis which can be severe. Since isopropanol is not metabolized into an acid, it does not cause metabolic acidosis, but ketonemia is common because of its metabolism to acetone. Symptoms range from confusion to coma, as with ethanol. Assessment and management of toxic alcohol ingestion is summarized in **Box 14.2.6**.

Box 14.2.5   Assessment and Management of Opioid Toxicity

- Assess and stabilize airway, breathing and circulation (*General Approach to the Critically Ill Child, 1.2*).
- An asymptomatic patient who presents after ingesting an oral opioid should be monitored with continuous heart rate and pulse oximetry monitoring.
- Naloxone is the most readily available reversal agent for opioid intoxication; Naloxone 0.1 mg/kg IV (max dose 2 mg) will reverse respiratory depression in most cases; higher doses may be required depending on the potency of the opiate/opioid. If the initial dose of naloxone fails, the dose can be doubled every 3–5 mins until the desired effect is achieved. If there is no response after 10 mg, the diagnosis should be reconsidered. The IM, subQ and ET routes yield more delayed effects. Use of naloxone by mucosal atomizer (intranasally) is emerging.
- In chronic opioid dependency, the goal of therapy should be to restore spontaneous respirations while avoiding signs and symptoms of withdrawal (namely vomiting, diarrhea, piloerection and diaphoresis); may consider smaller naloxone doses.
- Duration of action of naloxone is ~45 mins. Naloxone by continuous infusion should be considered if relapse occurs after initial naloxone administration. The starting dose is usually one-half the effective dose infused over one hour, titrating to the desired effect. Patients with persistent opioid intoxication should be closely inspected for patches (*e.g.* a transdermal fentanyl patch). Alternatively, ingestion of an extended release form of an oral opioid may require prolonged treatment.
- Check acetaminophen levels on all patients after presentation, as many products containing opioids are combined with acetaminophen.
- Patients who have ingested extended release tablets or transdermal patches may need prolonged observation as well as whole bowel irrigation to expedite drug transport time through the gastrointestinal tract and minimize systemic absorption.
- Some urine drug screens detect only heroin (opioid), morphine and codeine (opiates); other screens may detect additional dugs in this family. Because of high rates of false negative results, treatment should not be delayed pending a urine drug screen when opioid intoxication remains a clinical suspicion.

Box 14.2.6   Assessment and Management of Toxic Alcohol Ingestion

- Assess and stabilize airway, breathing and circulation (*General Approach to the Critically Ill Child, 1.2*); fluid resuscitation is often required.
- GI decontamination is rarely indicated because of the rapid absorption of alcohol from the gut.
- Measurement of toxic alcohol levels by gas chromatography is confirmatory for suspected toxic alcohol ingestion. Methanol and ethylene glycol levels >25 mg/dL are considered toxic. This test is usually performed in a reference laboratory and the result might not be available for several hours to days. Surrogate markers such as the osmolar gap, urine fluorescence, and calcium oxalate crystals in the urine, can be helpful but should not be relied upon to exclude ingestion. Treatment should not be withheld while awaiting results of confirmatory testing.
- The osmolar gap (difference between calculated osmolarity and measured osmolality; *Dehydration, 6.1; Box 6.1.2*) has been used to assess the possibility of toxic alcohol ingestion, but has several limitations. Individuals' baseline osmolar gap can vary widely, making interpretation difficult. Both methanol and ethylene glycol are metabolized to non-osmotically active metabolites. Therefore, the osmolar gap decreases over time and could be normal in late presenters.
- Calcium oxalate mono- and di-hydrate crystals can be seen in urine sediment after ethylene glycol poisoning but are nonspecific and a late finding. Fluorescence of urine with an ultraviolet light might be helpful in the setting of ethylene glycol poisoning because of the additive fluorescein in antifreeze but this is an unreliable finding.
- Monitor serum electrolytes, renal function, and acid-base balance.
- Methanol and ethylene glycol ingestions are in the differential diagnosis for anion gap metabolic acidosis of unknown etiology; metabolic acidosis from either of these alcohols can be life threatening independent of the toxic metabolites.

(Continued)

> **Box 14.2.6   Assessment and Management of Toxic Alcohol Ingestion (Continued)**
>
> - Fomepizole is a competitive antagonist of alcohol dehydrogenase and can prevent further formation of toxic metabolites from either methanol or ethylene glycol. Fomepizole (15 mg/kg IV followed by 10 mg/kg every 12 hrs) is indicated for confirmed or suspected methanol or ethylene glycol ingestion. The dose should be adjusted if the patient is undergoing hemodialysis as fomepizole is also readily dialyzable. Ethanol infusions are also effective at blocking alcohol dehydrogenase, but should only be considered when fomepizole is unavailable because they are considerably more difficult to use, especially in the pediatric patient.
> - Fomepizole is not indicated for isopropanol poisoning since its metabolite does not cause toxicity.
> - Hemodialysis is the definitive treatment for toxic alcohol poisoning. Indications include: refractory metabolic acidosis, end-organ toxicity, and renal failure. Methanol levels >25 mg/dL and ethylene glycol levels >50 mg/dL are also indications for hemodialysis. Isopropanol and ethanol are dialyzable but dialysis is rarely if ever indicated. The end point of hemodialysis is improvement of acidosis and the lowering of methanol and ethylene glycol levels to nontoxic levels.
> - While not a replacement for fomepizole and dialysis, folate can help prevent the accumulation of formic acid in methanol poisoning.
> - Thiamine and pyridoxine may prevent accumulation of toxic metabolites from ethylene glycol.
> - Isopropanol ingestions cause CNS depression but do not generally cause serious end organ toxicity, and usually improve with supportive care alone.

14.3 Terrorism Agents

The emergence of the Internet has allowed access to a wealth of information on terrorism agents. This chapter reviews the more commonly reported agents utilized by terrorists.

Cyanide consists of one atom of carbon bound to one atom of nitrogen by three molecular bonds. Inorganic cyanides (also known as cyanide salts) contain cyanide in the anion form. Cyanide salts react readily with water to form hydrogen cyanide. Hydrogen cyanide is a colorless gas at standard temperature and pressure. Cyanogen gas and cyanogen chloride are also potential terrorist agents.

The absorption of cyanide can occur via any of several routes (inhalation, ingestion, dermal, parenteral) depending on the type of cyanide compound. Rapid diffusion through the lungs followed by direct distribution to target organs accounts for the rapid lethality associated with hydrogen cyanide inhalation. Cyanide is an inhibitor of multiple enzymes in the human body (*e.g.* mitochondrial enzymes). Despite sufficient cellular oxygen delivery, the mitochondria cannot utilize oxygen or generate adenosine triphosphate (ATP). Unincorporated hydrogen ions accumulate and lactate rises.

No reliable pathognomonic clinical effect is associated with acute cyanide poisoning. The time to onset of clinical effects depends on the dose and route of exposure as well as the type of cyanide-containing compound. Such effects can occur within seconds of inhalation of hydrogen cyanide or several minutes following ingestion of an inorganic cyanide salt. Clinical manifestations may reflect rapid dysfunction of oxygen-sensitive organs, with central nervous and cardiovascular findings predominating. CNS toxicity includes headache, lightheadedness, anxiety, restlessness, agitation, confusion, lethargy, seizures, and coma. Cardiac toxicity includes bradycardia, tachycardia, atrial fibrillation, and ventricular dysrhythmias. The terminal events, however, are consistently bradycardia and hypotension.

Because of the associated nonspecific signs and symptoms and the delay in laboratory cyanide confirmation, clinicians must rely on routine laboratory studies to raise suspicion of cyanide poisoning. The triad of laboratory findings suggestive of cyanide poisoning include: (1) a narrow arterial–venous oxygen difference; (2) an anion gap metabolic acidosis; (3) an elevated lactic acid concentration in blood. Blood cyanide determination can confirm toxicity but may take days before results are available.

Because cyanide poisoning is rare, it is easy to overlook the diagnosis unless there is an obvious history of exposure. Thus, the most critical step in treatment is considering the diagnosis in high-risk situations and initiating empiric therapy with 100% oxygen, hydroxocobalamin, and thiosulfate. Hydroxocobalamin is a hemoglobin-like molecule (with cobalt instead of iron at its core) that binds to cyanide with such affinity that it can pull cyanide out of the mitochondria and restart the activity of the electron transport chain. Hydroxocobalamin is supplied in 250 ml vials; each vial contains 2.5 mg of hydroxocobalamin to be diluted in 100 ml of 0.9% NaCl. Hydroxocobalamin (5 g IV in adults and 70 mg/kg in children) is infused over 15 mins. The dose can be repeated in a serious poisoning. This antidote should be used in combination with sodium thiosulfate, which enhances the conversion of cyanide to thiocyanate which is renally excreted. Sodium thiosulfate should be given after hydroxocobalamin as an IV dose of 50 ml of a 25% solution in adults (12.5 g of sodium thiosulfate). The pediatric dose is 1.65 ml/kg of the 25% solution given over 10 mins. Hydroxocobalamin should not be infused through the same site or at the same time as sodium thiosulfate since thiosulfate inactivates hydroxocobalamin.

Nerve Agents are organophosphates and have chemical structures similar to the more familiar organophosphate pesticides such as malathion. There are a number of nerve agents that have been manufactured, including tabun, soman, sarin, cyclosarin, VX and the Russia V-type agent designated VR. These agents are among the most potent toxins known to mankind.

Acetylcholine (ACh) is a neurotransmitter found throughout the nervous system, including the CNS, the autonomic nervous system, and at the skeletal muscle motor end-plate (**Fig. 14.3.1**). ACh acts in both the CNS and peripheral nervous system by binding to and activating muscarinic and nicotinic cholinergic receptors. The enzyme, acetylcholinesterase (AChE), terminates the activity of ACh within the synaptic cleft. Nerve agents act by binding the AChE active site, rendering the enzyme incapable of inactivating ACh. As a result, ACh accumulates in the synapse and excessive stimulation occurs. Over time, a portion of the bound nerve agent is cleaved producing a stable, covalent bond between the nerve agent and AChE. This process is called *aging*. Before aging occurs, AChE reactivators such as pralidoxime chloride, can remove the nerve agent and restore enzyme function. However, once this aged covalent bond forms,

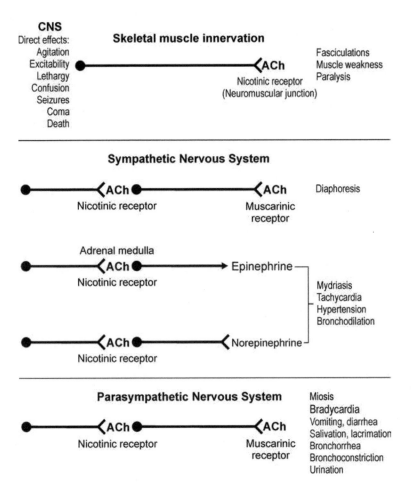

Fig. 14.3.1. Clinical Effects Seen in Nerve Agent Poisoning Caused by Excess of Acetylcholine in the Central, Autonomic, and Peripheral Nervous Systems. M, muscarinic; N, nicotinic; NE, norepinephrine.

AChE cannot be reactivated and activity is not restored until new enzyme is synthesized.

The onset, severity, and clinical effects of nerve agent poisoning vary widely. The two most prevalent routes of exposure are via dermal droplet contact and gas inhalation or absorption. Both the dose of nerve agent and the route of exposure are factors in determining clinical effects (**Boxes 14.3.1 and 14.3.2**).

Box 14.3.1 Comparison Effects of Nerve Agent Exposure: Dermal vs. Vapor

Amount of Exposure	Dermal	Vapor
Minimal	Diaphoresis and muscle fasciculations at the site of exposure	Miosis, conjunctival injection, dim vision, rhinorrhea, mild wheezing and dyspnea
Moderate	Worsening of above signs, plus: generalized muscarinic signs (may lack or have less severe eye and respiratory signs); generalized muscular weakness.	Worsening of above signs, plus: dyspnea more pronounced, ↑ing bronchorrhea and salivation, ↑ing generalized muscarinic signs, generalized muscular weakness.
Severe	Above signs plus: coma, convulsions, paralysis, apnea	Above signs plus: coma, convulsions, paralysis, apnea

Box 14.3.2 Acetylcholinesterase Inhibitor Clinical Effects ("DUMBBELS")

Diarrhea	Defecation, nausea/vomiting, salivation, abdominal cramps.
Urination	Contraction of detrusor muscle, contraction of bladder and relaxation of trigone and sphincter muscles.
Miosis	Contraction of ciliary muscles and blurred vision results.
Bradycardia	Direct cholinergic effects on heart or nicotinic effects on autonomic ganglia.
Broncho-constriction	And bronchorrhea (causing increased airway resistance) along with CNS respiratory depression and neuromuscular failure can result in respiratory failure.
Excitation	Fasciculations from nicotinic receptor stimulation at muscle end plate with muscle weakness and subsequent paralysis. Sympathomimetic effects (*e.g.* tachycardia) may also be seen due to ganglion stimulation.
Lacrimation	Lacrimal gland stimulation.
Sweating	Sweat glands are innervated by muscarinic receptors.

The clinical laboratory can measure neither serum or urine concentrations of nerve agents or their metabolites nor the concentration of AChE in synapses. Instead, the nervous system's AChE activity is approximated by measuring plasma cholinesterase (sometimes called "pseudo-cholinesterase") and erythrocyte (or RBC) cholinesterase activity to aid in or confirm diagnosis. Depression of RBC cholinesterase typically provides a more accurate reflection of the severity of toxicity, but is often less readily available than plasma cholinesterase.

Lifesaving treatment of severe nerve agent poisoning should initially focus on a patent airway, adequate ventilation and aggressive atropine administration. Succinylcholine should be avoided because it is metabolized by AChE. Copious secretions and bronchoconstriction may complicate invasive airway intervention. Aggressive atropine use decreases secretions and airway resistance. Electrographic seizures may occur in the absence of motor activity making EEG monitoring essential.

Atropine is the initial drug of choice in the symptomatic nerve agent victim. Atropine acts as a muscarinic receptor antagonist and blocks neuroeffector sites on smooth muscle, cardiac muscle, secretory gland cells, peripheral ganglia, and in the central nervous system. Intravenous, IM or ET routes are useful for administration. The dose varies with the severity of exposure and route of administration. Tachycardia is an effect of nerve agent poisoning and is not a contraindication to atropine administration. Reduction of respiratory secretions and resolution of bronchoconstriction are the therapeutic end points used to determine the appropriate dose of atropine. If bag assisted ventilation is difficult or secretions continue, then the atropine dose must be increased. Atropine has no effect on the nicotinic receptors and therefore has no effect on muscle weakness, fasciculations, tremors or paralysis. Atropine may help abort seizures. Miosis is not a useful clinical sign to guide treatment with atropine. Repeated atropine dosing based on miosis may lead to an anticholinergic syndrome. The only recommended indication for ophthalmic instillation of a mydriatic/cycloplegic agent is to relieve intractable eye pain due to ciliary spasm.

Pralidoxime chloride (2-PAMCL, Protopam Chloride) reactivates AChE by exerting a nucleophilic attack on the phosphorus of AChE resulting in an oxime-phosphate bond that splits from the AChE leaving the regenerated enzyme. This reactivation is clinically most apparent at nicotinic skeletal neuromuscular junctions, with less activity at muscarinic sites. Pralidoxime must therefore be administered concurrently with adequate atropine doses. In addition, the process of aging will prevent pralidoxime from regenerating the AChE active site and, as a result, is ineffective after aging has occurred. Therefore, the sooner the administration of pralidoxime, the greater the clinical effect. The recommended initial dose of pralidoxime is 1.0 g for adults or 15–25 mg/kg for children by intravenous route. Slow administration over 15–30 mins has been advocated to minimize side effects, including hypertension, headache, blurred vision, epigastric discomfort, nausea, and vomiting.

Effective and rapid management of nerve agent-induced seizures is critical. Benzodiazepines are effective in treating nerve agent-induced seizures. Midazolam is more potent and rapidly acting as an anticonvulsant than diazepam both via parenteral and intranasal routes. Because of its high water solubility, midazolam can be safely injected intramuscularly with very rapid absorption. Phenytoin, fosphenytoin, carbamazepine, valproic acid, felbamate, lamotrigine, magnesium sulfate, pentobarbital, phenobarbital and ketamine have no therapeutic anticonvulsant effectiveness for nerve agent-induced seizures. In animal models, successful control of seizure activity, regardless of the pharmacologic agents utilized, was predictive of survival of the lethal effects of nerve agent exposure, a more rapid behavioral recovery, and greater protection from neuropathology. Numerous epidemiologic studies have shown that the duration of human seizures correlates with outcome, with longer seizures being more refractory to treatment and associated with cognitive decline. It is therefore prudent to expeditiously and aggressively treat nerve agent induced seizures.

Saxitoxin (STX) is a potent toxin that is formed by dinoflagellates that cause a phenomenon known as a red tide. Marine life (mollusks, crabs, and fish) may feed on these and bio-accumulate the dinoflagellates toxins. Humans may inadvertently consume intoxicated seafood. Governments reportedly began experimenting with STX in the 1950s. The U.S. Department of Health and Human Services and the U.S. Department of Agriculture published final rules that set forth the requirements for possession, use, and transfer of select agents and toxins.

STX is water soluble, heat stable and is unaffected by cooking. STX is a specific high-affinity blocking ligand of voltage-dependent sodium channels, similar to tetrodotoxin. This binding inhibits sodium flux through these ion channels rendering excitable tissues such as nerves and muscle nonfunctional. Following oral exposure, STX causes prominent paresthesias, often beginning circumorally and spreading to the limbs. This can then progress to paralysis with retention of reflexes. Cranial nerve dysfunction, hypersalivation, diaphoresis, respiratory failure, hypertension, and hypotension have all been reported. STX toxicity is nearly indistinguishable from tetrodotoxin toxicity. There is no known antidote for STX toxicity. The majority of patients will recover if they receive adequate and timely supportive care.

Sodium monofluoroacetate (SMFA; also known as "1080") exists in synthetic form (CAS No. 62-74-8) as a white powder similar in appearance to flour or powdered sugar. It is odorless, tasteless, and readily dissolves into water. When present in natural water sources, it degrades within 7 days due to its metabolism by microorganisms within those environments. The only reported distinguishing characteristic is that it has a weak vinegar taste when mixed with water. It is heat stable; it does not decompose until temperatures approach 200°C (392°F). It is well absorbed from the gastrointestinal tract, the respiratory tract, open wounds, mucous membranes, and ocular exposure. The majority of human exposures reported in the medical literature have been through ingestion. Toxicity has been reported to be the same whether it is administered orally, subcutaneously, intramuscularly, or intravenously. Dusts containing SMFA are effectively toxic by inhalation.

The toxicologic mechanism of SMFA involves disruption of cellular energy production, resulting in multisystem organ failure. The parent compound, fluoroacetate, has very low cellular toxicity. Once ingested and absorbed, however, enzymatic reactions within cells

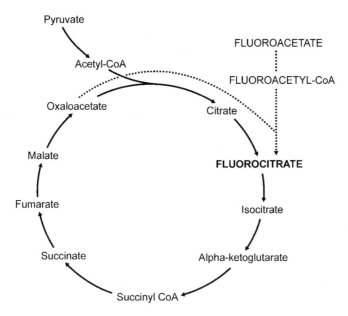

Fig. 14.3.2.   The Krebs Cycle. The effect of fluorocitrate [a product of the toxin sodium monofluoroacetate (SMFA or 1080)] on cell metabolism is shown. Fluorocitrate blocks conversion of citrate to isocitrate, disrupting glycolysis.

convert fluoroacetate to fluoroacetyl-CoA which in turn is converted to fluorocitrate, which inactivates aconitase (the enzyme necessary to metabolize citrate to isocitrate (**Fig. 14.3.2**). This results in interruption of the energy-producing Krebs cycle and the buildup of citrate. Fluorocitrate also inhibits transport of citrate into and out of mitochondria, further contributing to the buildup of citrate. Elevated citrate levels disrupt energy production via glycolysis by inhibiting the enzyme phosphofructokinase. Elevated citrate levels may also cause life-threatening hypocalcemia.

Clinical signs and symptoms associated with SMFA poisoning are nonspecific. SMFA poisoning is characterized by a latent period of 30 mins to 3 hrs following the administration of the compound by any route. Delayed onset of symptoms, however, has been reported up to 20 hours after exposure in the pediatric population. Even massive doses do not elicit immediate responses, although the latent period may be reduced.

In a retrospective study of 38 human cases of SMFA poisoning, the most frequent symptom was noted to be nausea and/or vomiting (74%). ECG changes were quite variable, ranging from mild nonspecific ST and T-wave abnormalities (72%), to ventricular tachycardia and asystole. The most common electrolyte abnormalities were hypocalcemia (42%) and hypokalemia (65%). Seven of the 38 patients died in this series (18%). Discriminate analysis identified hypotension, increased serum creatinine, and decreased blood pH as the most important predictors of mortality, with sensitivity of 86% and specificity of 96%.

There is no specific antidote for SMFA toxicity, and therapy is primarily focused on supportive care. A number of different treatments have been explored for SMFA toxicity. Because SMFA induces hypocalcemia, calcium supplementation through administration of either calcium gluconate or calcium chloride has been shown to be of benefit.

Chapter 15

Procedures, Indications and Complications

15.1 Enteric Tube (EnT) Placement

EnTs are indicated for decompression, drainage and/or irrigation of the stomach or bowel, or to provide access for instillation of feeding or medications. EnTs are most commonly inserted nasally or orally into the stomach (NGT, OGT) or into the duodenum (NDT, ODT) or jejunum (NJT, OJT). Alternatively the tube can be inserted through the abdominal wall into the stomach (gastrostomy) or jejunum (jejunostomy). A gastrojejunal tube (GJT) permits both gastric and jejunal access. Occasionally, a rectal tube is placed in the rectum. Nasal polyethylene and polyvinylchloride tubes lose flexibility and need replacement every 3 to 4 days. Polyurethane and silicone tubes remain flexible and can remain in place for longer periods. In critically ill adults, ND feeding may help achieve nutritional goals earlier, and decrease the rate of vomiting and incidence of ventilator associated pneumonia as compared to NG feeding; data for pediatric patients are lacking. Measurements for placement of nasal EnTs as well as con-traindications/complications are shown (**Boxes 15.1.1 and 15.1.2**).

NGT range in size from 10–14 French for the infant/child and 14–18 French for adults. Radiographic visualization of the position of the tube is the gold standard for verification of placement of the distal tip in the stomach. An NG "sump tube" is used to drain fluid from the stomach while venting air; the blue pigtail should be kept above the level of fluid in the stomach to prevent gastric contents from leaking back through the vent lumen. Air flow should be

Box 15.1.1　Placement of Nasal Enteric Tubes

Type	Insertion Length Determined by Surface Measurements	Appearance on Anterior–Posterior Abdominal X-Ray
NGT*	Distance from tip of the nose to the earlobe, then to the xiphoid process	Tip of NGT and all ports in stomach
NDT*	As for NGT plus distance from the xiphoid to the midaxillary line (transpyloric tube)	NDT should course horizontally to the right crossing the vertebral column (first portion of duodenum), course caudally (second portion of duodenum) and then may redirect horizontally and to the left (third portion of duodenum).
NJT*	As for NGT plus chest diameter measurement (transpyloric tube)	NJT should follow course of NDT but the NJT ascends the fourth portion of duodenum in left upper quadrant and passes the ligament of Treitz

*Secure the nasal portion of the tube to the cheek (not the forehead) to avoid nasal injury from traction on greater nasal alar cartilage and overlying skin.

To promote advancement of an EnT from the NG to the ND/J position, instill 5–10 mL of air while in the NG position before advancing through the pylorus. Position the child right side down for ~2 hrs. before obtaining an AP abdominal Xray to verify the transpyloric position. If repeated difficulty is encountered in placement of a transpyloric tube, fluoroscopic guided placement may be needed. Difficulty in placement of a transpyloric tube may occur with severe scoliosis or anatomic anomalies.

audible from the vent pigtail when intermittent suction (IS) is applied. If air flow is obstructed by the presence of fluid in the vent port, flush the vent port with air. Intermittent suction should be set at minus 80 cm H_2O for a sump tube and $\leq$ minus 20 cm H_2O for a simple single lumen NGT. Any EnT to be used for instillation of a substance (except a rectal tube/enema) should have its position confirmed by X-ray before instillation is attempted.

Box 15.1.2   Contraindications and Complications of Enteric Tubes

Contraindications	Complications
• Head trauma with anterior fossa skull fracture (nasally inserted tube may cross cribiform plate); orally inserted tubes may be used.	• Rhinorrhea; accidental tracheal intubation may lead to hypoxia, cyanosis, respiratory arrest
• Esophageal strictures or varices	• Epistaxis, skin erosion, sinusitis, otitis media
• Alkali ingestion	• Esophageal-tracheal fistula
• Unprotected airway with potential for vomiting and aspiration	• Nasal irritation
• Suspected cervical spine injury with potential for coughing/gagging	• Aspiration of formula if feeding is attempted orally or creation of esophageal sphincter incompetence

---

A gastrostomy tube (GT) is placed through the abdominal wall midway along the greater curvarture of the stomach using a urinary (Foley®) catheter, wing–tip, or mushroom catheter. It can be placed in an "open" fashion (surgically from the outer abdominal wall) or endoscopically (percutaneous endoscopic gastrostomy, "PEG"). The skin-level device (SLD) is a GT with its outer extent near the skin surface. Either a MIC–KEY® or Bard® can be placed at the time of open surgery or can replace the PEG (8 weeks after creation of the gastrostomy). Connecting tubing may be attached to the SLD during feedings to allow for greater mobility. If the skin surrounding a gastrostomy site is wet, red and irritated, antacid should be applied topically to the site; the device may need to be replaced if the retention balloon leaks. A thin, single layer of gauze between SLD and skin surface may be used to absorb formula leakage at the stoma site. Avoid "packing" the site since this may cause upward tension against the gastric wall leading to mucosal ischemia. Leakage may indicate tube displacement and the need for surgical consultation. Anytime a GT is displaced from the abdominal wall, immediately (gently) attempt to replace it with a similar GT or with a temporary Foley® catheter (of the same size or smaller) to preserve the GT tract in the abdominal wall. "Tissue growth" surrounding the exit site may indicate granulation tissue versus herniating gastric mucosa; a surgical consultant can help make the distinction. A gastrojejunostomy tube can be placed with fluoroscopic guidance in cases of severe gastroesophageal reflux if Nissen fundoplication is undesirable (*Gastroesophageal Reflux Disease, 8.4*).

Rectal tubes (RT) may be inserted to provide a fecal incontinence collector, to measure the volume of liquid stool or to prevent excoriation to the skin. A 10–12 French Malecot catheter is used in children and 22–26 French in adults. The RT is advanced into the rectum 2–4 inches in children and 4–5 inches in adults. Digitally palpate the rectum for obstruction before inserting a RT. The RT is attached to a urinary catheter bag. Remove and clean the catheter at 24 hrs intervals. Avoid placement of a RT in immunocompromised children, if rectal bleeding is present, if the patient is anticoagulated or coagulopathic, if bowel disease is present or if there has been recent rectal surgery. Enemas may be performed through RTs (*Constipation in the PICU, 8.2*).

15.2   Bag-Mask Ventilation (BMV) and Tracheal Intubation

Skillfully delivered BMV can be as effective as tracheal intubation for rescue breathing in the pre-tracheal intubation period (**Boxes 15.2.1, 15.2.2 and 15.2.3**); it should be instituted whenever urgent respiratory support is required in the absence of an established airway. Early recognition of the difficult-to-access airway (see below) is critical to planning airway interventions. Equipment for airway support includes:

- O_2 source, suction instruments (both rigid and flexible) and either a self-inflating or flow-inflating bag device.
- Self-inflating resuscitation bags are more easily used by all levels of rescuers than flow-inflating ("anesthesia") bags. Use a bag with ≥450–500 mL volume for term neonates, infants and children. The oxygen source should provide O_2 10–15 L/min for a pediatric-sized bag and 15 L/min for an adult-sized bag.

Box 15.2.1   Bag-Valve Mask Ventilation: Key Steps

- Correct positioning of the head (atlanto-occipital joint) and neck relative to the torso is essential to prevent functional obstruction of the airway (**Fig. 15.2.1**). Hyperextension of the head may "kink" the upper airway of an infant or small child because of their relatively large occiput. The nose and mouth should face the ceiling. The external auditory canal should be anterior to the shoulders.

- If cervical spine injury is suspected, maintain manual in-line neck immobilization. Jaw-thrust (**Fig. 15.2.2**) should be used to open the airway, *not* head tilt (**Fig. 15.2.3**).

- Clear the airway of debris.

- Single airway manager: The mask is held over the nose and mouth with thumb and index finger while the 3rd, 4th and 5th fingers lift the jaw along the mandible ("C" and "E" configurations, respectively that generates a complete air seal between face and mask; **Fig. 15.2.4**). Squeeze the bag with the other hand.
  Two airway managers (preferred): The mask is held in place by one rescuer using one hand on either side of the face (two "C's"); the fingers provide a bilateral jaw thrust (two "E's"), lifting the face into the mask so that a complete air seal is generated between the two surfaces.

- Second or third rescuer: Apply gentle cricoid pressure to help prevent gastric inflation/reflux of gastric contents until an endotracheal tube (ETT) is confirmed to be in the trachea. An oro- or naso-gastric (OG or NG) tube is connected to continuous suction is also helpful.

- Ensure a complete seal between face and mask

- Disable the pop-off valve and use a PEEP device on the bag when appropriate.

- Chest wall movement is the required endpoint.

- ECG and Pox monitoring should be continuous throughout the process of tracheal intubation. An audible tone reflecting Pox readings is helpful.

Box 15.2.2   Troubleshooting Problems with BMV

Failure to ventilate (absent chest wall movement):
- The most common problems are obstruction caused by the tongue and malposition of the head and neck (**Fig. 15.2.1**). Rapid "trial and error" of alternative positions (+/− an oral or NP airway) usually solves the problem.
- Check face-to-mask seal.
- Depress the pop-off valve; squeeze the bag sufficiently to deliver a tidal volume that will move the chest adequately.
- Ensure abdominal decompression by placing NG or OG tube.
- Ensure that cricoid pressure is not excessive; this may cause airway obstruction.
- R/O Pneumothorax
- R/O Equipment failure
- R/O Foreign body

Failure to oxygenate (adequate chest wall movement with oxygen desaturation):
- Check integrity of connections to O_2 source and oxygen flow supply
- Add PEEP by use of a PEEP valve.
- Too rapid a respiratory rate will result in insufficient time for alveolar inflation and may lead to air-trapping and pneumothorax, particularly when small airway obstruction is present. Initiate ventilation with a gradual inspiration and i:e ratio of at least 1:2 to 1:3. Trial and error to control inspiratory and expiratory times may solve the problem.

- An O_2 reservoir should be attached to minimize entrainment of room air when the bag spontaneously re-inflates; this generates an FiO_2 of 60–95%.
- Self-inflating bags limit peak inspiratory pressure to 35–45 cm H_2O through a pop-off valve. It is often necessary to disable the pop-off valve when airway resistance is high or lung compliance is low; this is the case for most pediatric patients with respiratory failure and lung disease. Familiarity with the equipment in your facility and PICU is essential.

Box 15.2.3   Key Points in Rapid Sequence Intubation (RSI; the six P's)

- Preparation: Identify anatomic, pathophysiologic, allergic, hereditary and historical factors that may pose difficulties to tracheal intubation and make alternative plans. Assign team roles.
- Preoxygenate with BMV (**Box 15.2.1**) for patients with inadequate respiratory effort and a non-rebreathing mask for spontaneously breathing patients.
- Pre-treatment drugs are not routinely used in pediatric patients. Considerations include:
  Atropine: overcomes the ↑ in vagal response to laryngoscopy, esp. in patients < 1 yr and in those who will receive succinylcholine (SCh). Atropine masks the bradycardia related to hypoxemia associated with unsuccessful intubation.
  Lidocaine: minimizes the ↑ in ICP associated with intubation; not needed if thiopental, etomidate or non-depolarizing muscle relaxant is used; Lidocaine may ↓ bronchospasm.
  Opiates/opioids: may be useful in conjunction with sedation immediately proximate to assisted ventilation or intubation.
- Sedation and Paralysis: The goal of sedation is loss of consciousness; consider gastric decompression or a Sellick maneuver once sedation is adequate; this is followed by a paralytic (SCh, a depolarizing agent or a non-depolarizing agent such as rapacuronium, rocuronium, vecuronium).
- Confirm placement and protect ETT security. Release cricoid pressure only after ETT placement is confirmed.

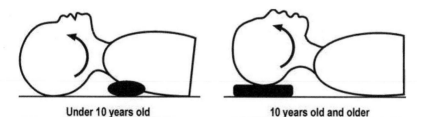

Under 10 years old   10 years old and older

Fig. 15.2.1.   Head and Neck Positions Useful in Opening the Airway.

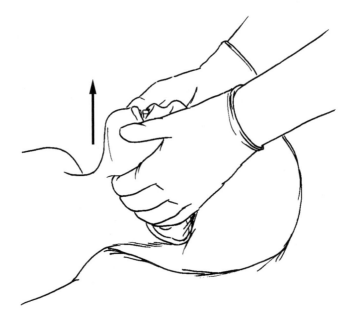

Fig. 15.2.2.   Jaw Thrust.

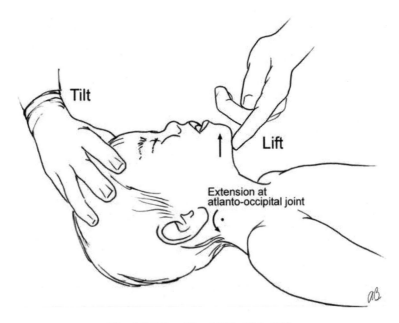

Fig. 15.2.3.   Head Tilt-Chin Lift.

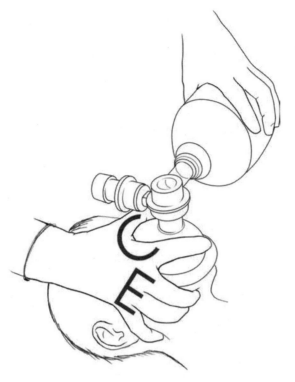

Fig. 15.2.4.   Bag-Mask Ventilation.

• Use the smallest facemask that encircles the nose and mouth, but excludes the chin and does not touch the eyes.
• Airway adjuncts [oral or nasopharyngeal (NP) airways] may facilitate BMV.

An **oral airway** is useful in the unconscious patient to help lift the tongue and anterior pharyngeal tissues away from the posterior pharynx. This assists in establishing airway patency and is helpful in BMV when the unconscious child has upper airway obstruction from these tissues. The correct size is chosen by externally matching the flange of the oral airway with the corner of the mouth; the tip of the oral airway should extend just to the angle of the mandible. Insertion is accomplished with the help of a tongue depressor or laryngoscope blade which is used to push the tongue downward (to the floor of the mouth). If not correctly positioned, the oral airway itself, or further displacement of the tongue posteriorly can worsen airway obstruction. In addition, the presence of an oral airway in an awake patient can cause gagging, vomiting and lead to aspiration.

A **NP airway** may also be helpful (*Other Aids to Support Oxygenation and Ventilation, 2.9*), particularly in the awake patient. However, the oral airway is more likely to be effective in creating airway patency for the purposes of BMV provided the patient is unconscious.

- Airways should be kept clear of secretions. The importance of suctioning the upper airway to achieve optimal airway patency cannot be overemphasized.

Tracheal intubation provides long-term airway stability, permits control of oxygenation and ventilation, allows for evacuation of secretions and analgesia and/or sedation as needed. Indications include:

- Actual or impending respiratory arrest.
- Respiratory insufficiency despite non-invasive support.
- Inability to swallow.
- Inability to clear secretions.
- Anticipated respiratory deterioration (*e.g.* severe trauma, burns, smoke inhalation).
- Prolonged transports with respiratory, hemodynamic and/or neurologic instability.
- GCS < 8.
- The need for interventions which are unsafe without airway protection (*e.g.* whole bowel irrigation in a patient with depressed level of consciousness).

Equipment for tracheal intubation. All equipment needed for BMV plus:

- Endotracheal tubes (ETT): The size is defined by the internal diameter (ID) of the tube. The appropriate size may be determined based on the patient's length (*Appendix, part 1*, Broselow tape) or based on age for patients <12 yrs:

    ▶ Uncuffed ETT: (age in years ÷ 4) + 4

▶ Cuffed (low pressure, high volume cuff) ETT: (age in years ÷ 4) + 3

For patients >12 yrs: size 6–10 mm. The ID of the tube approximates the width of the nail of the 5th finger.

- ETT's one-half and one size smaller and one-half size larger should be readily available
- Stylet, (appropriate size for ETT chosen): This is inserted in the ETT to provide rigidity. The tip of the stylet should terminate within the ETT tip, and not protrude beyond it.
- Laryngoscope: Either the large (adult) or more slender (pediatric) handle may be used. The blade may be straight (*e.g.* Miller blade) which lifts the epiglottis directly or curved (*e.g.* MacIntosh) which is positioned in the vallecula, indirectly lifting the epiglottis as the mandible is elevated anteriorly. The length of the blade should approximate the distance from frontal incisors to the mandibular angle. The straight blade is more commonly used in infants because of their relatively large and floppy epiglottis.
- End tidal CO_2 detector (colorimetric, qualitative) or capnography should be used to confirm that the ETT is in the trachea (*General Approach to the Critically Ill, Child, 1.2*). An esophageal detector device may be used in patients >20 kg to confirm tracheal placement in low to no perfusion states.
- Suction catheters of appropriate size to help clear the lower airways via the ETT after tracheal intubation.
- Avoid environmental contamination of the ETT, stylet and suction catheter before introducing these devices into the airway.

Tracheal intubation of the non-comatose patient with intact cough and gag reflexes or the patient with a full stomach generally requires that sedation and pharmacologic paralysis be provided (**Box 15.2.4**). Deeply comatose or arrested patients and the newly born generally do not require this approach. Rapid sequence intubation (RSI) employs rapidly acting medications which produce intubation-ready conditions once consciousness is lost, with the goal of eliminating the need for BMV (and the attendant risk of aspiration). Since O_2 consumption in an infant or child is 2–3 times that of an adult, BMV after loss of consciousness may still be required,

Box 15.2.4   Drugs Commonly Used To Facilitate Tracheal Intubation

Sedative Drugs	Advantages	Disadvantages	Absolute or Relative Contraindications
Midazolam	Amnestic	↓ BP; myocardial depression	Shock; ↓ cardiac function
Ketamine	↑ HR, ↑BP (↑catecholamine); bronchodilator	↑ HR, ↑ BP; may ↑ ICP, but may be useful in ↑ICP with hypotension*; epileptogenic	Hypertension; ↑ ICP; thyrotoxicosis, CHF; psychoses; conditions in which hypertension is hazardous
Propofol	Amnestic; rapid onset and short-acting; anticonvulsant	↓BP; myocardial depression	Egg or soy allergy; Avoid in hemo-dynamic instability
Etomidate	Potent sedative with usually minimal hemodynamic effect	Adrenal suppression that may last ≥24 hrs; eye movements; dystonia; myoclonus in 32%	Adrenal insufficiency; septic shock; if given during septic shock, consider treatment with dexamethasone
Thiopental	Short-acting; ↓ ICP; anticonvulsant	↓ BP; myocardial depression	Acute intermittent porphyrias; RAD due to histamine; ↓ BP
Paralytics			
Succinylcholine (SCh)**	Rapid onset (30–60 sec); brief duration (4–6 min)	Hyperkalemia; bradycardia; malignant hyperthermia; may lead to ↑ ICP and ↑ intraocular pressure	Hyperkalemia; motor neuron lesions; muscle injury ≥2–3 days duration; muscle atrophy; myopathies; eye injury; known ↓ pseudocholinesterase; potentially inaccessible airway
Rocuronium†	Rapid onset (30–60 sec)		
Vecuronium†	Onset 1–3 mins. faster onset at ↑ doses (e.g. 0.3 mg/kg)	Duration 30–40 minutes	Potentially inaccessible airway

* Etomidate may be a viable alternative.
** Depolarizing muscle relaxant.
† Nondepolarizing agent.

particularly if more than one attempt at laryngoscopy is needed. Cricoid pressure (Sellick maneuver) and gastric decompression is important in minimizing the risk of aspiration of gastric contents. The use of respiratory depressants and/or paralysis may be hazardous in patients with potentially difficult-to access airways; alternative planning with airway experts is indicated.

The main distinctions between the pediatric versus adult airway are a relatively larger tongue and epiglottis, greater tonsillar and adenoidal tissue, a more superior and anterior larynx, and smaller airways offering greater resistance to flow. The signals of a **difficult-to-access airway** include:

- Signs of upper airway obstruction (*Upper Airway Obstruction, 2.2*).
- Craniofacial anomalies or facial/oral trauma.
- Micrognathia, macroglossia, glossoptosis or "kissing" tonsils.
- Trismus or inabiltity to visualize the posterior limits of the soft palate, uvula and tonsillar pillars (**Fig. 15.2.5**)
- Cervical spine injury or cervical anomalies that decrease range of motion.
- Morbid obesity.

Tracheal intubation: Preparation and proper positioning (**Fig. 15.2.1**) are essential to success. If cervical spine instability is

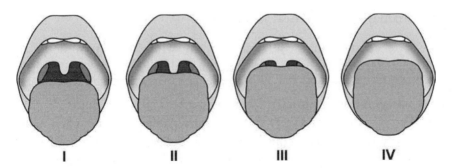

| I | II | III | IV |

Fig. 15.2.5. Mallampati Scoring helps predict a difficult tracheal intubation in an adult; it has been applied to children and adolescents who are cooperative in voluntary mouth-opening. A grade I–II view is consistent with an accessible larynx; grades III–IV are predictive of difficult laryngoscopy in an adult. However, normal infants will often demonstrate grades II–IV with spontaneous opening.

suspected, manual in-line traction should be applied to prevent neck movement and a **jaw thrust** (**Fig. 15.2.2**) not head-tilt/chin lift (**Fig. 15.2.3**), is used to access the airway.

- The laryngoscope is held in the left hand, placed into the right side of the mouth and displaces the tongue to the left as it is moved toward the hypopharynx. The blade is lifted away from the intubator to expose the larynx. Do not use the palate or upper incisors as a lever; this obscures the view and can cause injury to these structures.
- A straight blade is used to lift the epiglottis and tissue anterior to it; the tip of a curved blade sits in the vallecula; the mandible is lifted upward (forward), elevating the epiglottis. If the epiglottis is not visualized, the blade may be inserted into the esophagus and withdrawn until the epiglottis is visualized at the tongue base.
- Apply cricoid pressure if the glottis and vocal cords are not immediately identified. Moving the cricoid "up and to the right" may be helpful. The ETT should be passed through the vocal cords without force. Remove the stylet. The ETT should be inserted to a depth (cm) of approximately $3 \times ID$ (mm) of the tube.
- Bag-to-ETT ventilation should be given; a cuffed ETT may require inflation at this time. An inflation pressure $<20\,cm\,H_2O$ is recommended.

Confirmation of tracheal intubation:

- The chest should rise symmetrically with PPV. Asymmetry of chest wall movement may indicate malposition of the ETT in a mainstem bronchus (usually the right), pneumothorax or severe unilateral or asymmetric lung disease.
- A colorimetric $ETCO_2$ detector turns yellow (yes!) when CO_2 exceeds 15 mmHg, consistent with a successful tracheal intubation. In the presence of circulatory arrest and failure to perfuse the lungs, $ETCO_2$ will not be detected. Capnogaphy should reveal the $ETCO_2$ waveform (*General Approach to the Critically Ill Child, 1.2*).
- Breath sounds should be audible over both hemithoraces in the mid-axillary line. While breath sounds may be audible over the left

upper quadrant as well, especially in small infants, they should be much louder over the lung fields.

- Confirm the ETT distance above the mainstem carina by CXR.
- Decompress the stomach (*Enteric Tube Placement, 15.1*); and identify the position of the EnT on CXR; suction the airway as needed.
- If tracheal intubation is not successful, remove the ETT and repeat the effort beginning with BMV. Understanding the reason for failure will increase the chances of correcting the problem.
- Once intubation is confirmed, **secure the ETT**. This can be accomplished by painting the skin with tincture of benzoin and use of adhesive tape or with use of commercially available ETT holders. Analgesia and sedation should be provided, with muscle relaxation if needed, to ensure airway safety.

Alternatives to direct laryngoscopy for ETT placement include the Glidescope®, use of a lighted stylet, and bronchoscopically guided tracheal intubation. Skilled use of the laryngeal mask airway (LMA) may provide temporary airway control. The **Combitube®** may be useful in patients greater than 4 feet tall. **Needle cricothyrotomy** is a last resort to oxygenate during upper airway obstruction. It is safer than surgical cricothyrotomy and can be attempted for any aged patient. Ventilation is difficult to achieve, but this bridge to oxygenation could be life-saving. The head is extended and the cricothyroid membrane is identified. This membrane may be as small as 1 mm in an infant. A 20 or 22 g needle attached to a syringe is directed through the membrane in a caudal direction. If air is aspirated, remove the small bore needle and repeat the procedure using a larger bore (12–14 g) catheter over needle. If air is aspirated, thread the catheter into the airway. The adapter of a 3 mm ETT may be attached to the catheter hub. This may allow bag-assisted oxygenation, spontaneous breathing or high frequency jet ventilation. Pediatric cricothyrotomy kits are commercially available.

15.3 Vascular Access

Obtaining and maintaining appropriate vascular access requires anticipatory planning, knowledge of the ramifications of available

Box 15.3.1   Indications for Central Venous Access and Catheter Options

Indications:

- Administration of medications not deliverable or potentially hazardous if given peripherally (*e.g.* hypertonic medications, solutions, calcium, *etc.*)
- CVP monitoring
- Inability to obtain or maintain secure peripheral access in a patient who requires IV therapy
- To permit frequent sampling of venous blood when alternatives are impractical.
- For long-term IV therapies.

Catheter Options (Catheter-life expectancy)

- Polyethylene or polyurethane catheter: Inserted percutaneously at a central site; usually placed at the bedside; most commonly chosen option in critical illness. (Days to weeks)
- Silastic central catheter [*e.g.* Broviac or Hickman catheter]: Inserted surgically at a central site; a portion of the catheter courses subcutaneously after exiting the vessel and before exiting the skin *i.e.* "tunneled". A Dacron cuff surrounds a subcutaneous portion of the catheter and helps form a barrier against migration of organisms along the catheter tract; it also helps to anchor the catheter. (Months)
- Central port [*e.g.* Mediport, Port-A-Cath, Infuse-A-Port]: Inserted surgically at a central site; has a subcutaneous reservoir accessible by a percutaneous needle; also has a tunneled portion; not dislodged by activity; lowest infection rate. (Months to years).
- Peripherally Inserted Central Catheter [PICC]: Inserted percutaneously in a peripheral vein and terminates in a central vein; most often accessed via basilic or cephalic veins; may require ultrasound or fluoroscopic guidance for placement. (Days, weeks or months)
- Central venous cutdown: Multiple site options; generally a last resort; may be obviated by interventional radiologic techniques.

options, proper equipment, skilled personnel and optimization of conditions that will promote success. Most pediatric patients are well served with peripheral venous access (PIV). When critical illness or special needs are introduced, central venous access becomes essential. The decision to place a central venous catheter (CVC) and identification of the most suitable type is often as important as the ability to perform the procedure (**Boxes 15.3.1 and 15.3.2**).

Box 15.3.2	Advantages and Disadvantages of CVC Placement Sites in Children	
Site (vein)	**Advantages**	**Disadvantages**
Femoral*	Usually easily accessible even in the awake infant/ child. Allows head-up position throughout procedure; compressible vessels in event of bleeding. CVP measurement correlates well with intrathoracic measurement.	May be difficult to maintain sterility of the site over time, although no documented ↑ in infection rates compared to other sites in the pediatric population. Possible ↑ risk for catheter-related clot in patients at risk.
Subclavian (SC)	Usually easily maintainable site; can measure CVP close to the RA	↑ Risk of pneumothorax during insertion; vessels not compressible in event of bleeding; placement requires strict motion control.
Internal Jugular (IJ)	Can measure CVP close to RA; ↓ risk of pneumothorax compared to SC site	May be difficult to maintain in the short neck of an infant; risk of thoracic duct injury on the left and carotid arteries bilaterally. Placement requires strict motion control.

* Interventions at the femoral site permit continued activity at the head and neck during resuscitation.

Percutaneously placed central catheters are inserted using Seldinger technique or a modified version of this procedure (**Boxes 15.3.3, 15.3.4 and 15.3.5**). General contraindications to CVC placement at a given location include significant trauma, lesion

---

Box 15.3.3   Seldinger Technique and Immediate After-Care for Vascular Access*

- Under **sterile conditions**, the targeted vessel is accessed with a thin-walled straight needle
- Once blood is aspirated with unimpaired flow, the syringe is disconnected from the needle without dislodging the needle from the vessel.
- A guidewire is threaded through the needle into the vessel. The course of the wire should offer no resistance. Do not force a wire into a vessel.
- Withdraw the needle without dislodging the wire.
- Make a tiny cut in the skin at the point of wire entry; use a dilator (tapered at its distal tip) to create a pathway from skin surface into the receiving vessel to allow for catheter passage.
- Remove the dilator without dislodging the wire; be prepared to put pressure on the site until the vascular catheter is threaded over the guidewire. The catheter should be prepared for insertion by flushing all ports and tubing with saline or heparinized saline (1:10,000 unit solution).
- Remove the guidewire. Avoid exposing an uncapped/unclamped catheter hub to room air because of the danger of air embolus.
- Confirm blood return and ability to flush all ports of the catheter without resistance.
- The catheter should be secured with sutures or an alternative means, sometimes provided by the manufacturer. A sterile occlusive dressing that is waterproof but permeable to water and air (*e.g.* Tegaderm™) should be applied.
- Catheter position should be confirmed by X-ray.

---

* Seldinger technique can be modified for arterial access; *e.g.* when used to access a radial artery, vessel dilatation is neither required nor recommended.

Box 15.3.4   Site-Specific CVC Insertion Guidelines

Femoral vein: lies medial and parallel to the artery in the inguinal region, midway between the anterior superior iliac crest and symphysis pubis. The patient is positioned with the pelvis elevated so that the inguinal crease is flattened. The femoral vein is accessed ~0.5–1 cm below the inguinal crease in a direction parallel to the femoral artery and aiming toward the umbilicus. Post insertion X-ray (cross table lateral) should demonstrate the catheter tip to lie *anterior* to the vertebral column.

Subclavian vein: lies beneath the proximal half of the clavicle. Optimally the patient lies in Trendelenburg with a towel roll (vertically) under the thoracic spine, allowing the shoulders to "fall back". The vessel is approached from slightly caudal to the junction of the middle and medial thirds of the clavicle, keeping the needle along the inferior surface of the clavicle, in a horizontal plane with the thorax, aiming toward the sternal notch. Post-insertion X ray should demonstrate the catheter tip in the proximal third of the SVC just cranial to the right atrium (tip is at or above the level of the mainstem carina).

Internal Jugular vein: lies just anterior and lateral to the carotid artery within a triangle formed by the two bellies of the sternocleidomastoid muscle and the clavicle.

Medial (central) approach: the needle enters at the triangle's apex, lateral to the carotid pulse, at ~45° and is aimed at the ipsilateral nipple. The IJ vein is usually accessed at a depth of ~1–2 cm.

Posterior approach: the needle enters at the lateral border of the posterior belly of the sternocleiodomastoid muscle, at the junction of the middle and lower thirds (near the intersection of the external jugular vein with the posterior belly) at ~30–45°, aiming toward the sternal notch.

Post-insertion X-ray shows the catheter tip in the IJ or innominate vein, or SVC at or above the level of the carina. Ultrasound guided placement may increase safety of insertion, depending on provider skill. If IJ or SC been access is attempted, a CXR should be obtained regardless of whether or not catheter placement was successful.

Box 15.3.5   Suggested Age and Weight-Appropriate Sizes for CVC*

Neonates (<8 kg)	3.0 F	5–8 cm
<12 mos (5–15 kg)	3.0–4.0 F	5–12 cm
1–7 yrs (10–30 kg)	4.0–5.0 F	5–15 cm
≥8 yrs (≥25 kgs)	5.0–8.0 F	≥8 cm

---

* The length chosen depends on the thickness of the subcutaneous tissue, the intended location of the tip and the insertion site chosen.

Box 15.3.6   CVC Complications

Intra-procedural

- Vascular injury/perforation
- Hemorrhage; arterial puncture
- Arrhythmia caused by intracardiac guidewire or catheter
- Pneumothorax (SC, IJ)
- Cardiac tamponade
- Hemothorax (SC, IJ)
- Foreign body (*e.g.* guidewire) embolization
- Air embolus, esp. with intrathoracic access in spontaneously breathing patients. Risk decreases with Trendelenburg positioning.
- Catheter malposition: SC, left < right; IJ, right < left; femoral, right possibly < left
- Defective equipment with resultant injury

Post-procedural

- Infection; sepsis; septic shock
- Thrombosis
- Leg swelling (femoral CVC)
- Pulmonary embolus
- Superior vena cava syndrome (SC, IJ)
- Intracardiac thrombosis
- Vascular injury/perforation
- Hemorrhage
- Arrhythmia caused by migration of catheter to intracardiac position
- Catheter migration with leakage of infusate in subcutaneous, intrapleural (hydrothorax) or extra-peritoneal spaces
- Defective catheter

---

or infection at or near the insertion site, and pre-existing thrombosis or injury involving the vessel. "Semi-elective" or elective long-time access should be placed when systemic infection (risk of bacteremia) is unlikely. Complications are listed (**Box 15.3.6**).

CVC-Related Blood Stream Infections (CRBSI; Box 15.3.7). The National Nosocomial Surveillance Report in 2003 revealed 6.6 CRBSI/1000 catheter days or 3–7% of CVC's placed in PICU populations. Each CRBSI costs $34,000 –$56,000 and increases

---

Box 15.3.7   Definitions: Colonization vs. Catheter Related Blood Stream Infection (CRBSI)

Colonization denotes isolation of an organism from blood or catheter segment culture that is not isolated from peripheral blood. A **CRBSI** is a primary BSI in a patient with a CVC with at least one positive blood culture obtained from a peripheral site* and at least one of the following:

- Positive growth from the CVC blood culture ≥2 hrs before the peripheral blood culture becomes positive for "the same organism" *i.e.* the organisms share the same identity and antibiotic sensitivity pattern. ** This "time-to-positivity" technique is simple when automated culture detector devices are used. These devices identify positive cultures every 15 mins.
- Simultaneously drawn quantitative blood cultures with ≥5:1 (CVC: peripheral) ratio of the same (biogram identical) organisms. This quantitative technique is expensive, labor-intensive and not typically performed in clinical laboratories.
- Isolation of > 15 colony forming units from a catheter segment with isolation of the same organism with an identical biogram from peripheral blood.

---

* Note that blood cultures should first be drawn from peripheral blood then from the CVL in question in close proximity of each other (time-wise). Blood from other vascular devices (*e.g.* arterial catheters) should also be cultured to determine the extent of involvement.

** DNA testing may reveal "the same" biogram identical organisms to be genetically different.

the PICU stay by 14.6 days. CRBSI is the likely cause of a primary blood stream infection (BSI) in a patient who had a CVC within 48 hrs before the development of the BSI *and* the isolated organism did not originate from another site. Risk factors are summarized (**Box 15.3.8**); common offending organisms are listed (**Box 15.3.9**).

Box 15.3.8   Risk Factors for Development of CVC Infections

- Break in sterile technique; insertion without maximum barrier precautions
- Skill of operator placing the CVC; repeated attempts (which may reflect severity of illness) ↑s risk
- Prolonged presence of CVC
- Skin or hub colonization
- ↑ Number of lumens in the catheter may ↑ infection risk
- Emergency placement
- Knowledge, skill and availability of CVC maintenance staff
- Local infection of skin, tunnel site or port pocket
- Frequency of accessing/ manipulations
- Infusion of TPN
- Extremes of patient age
- Use of CVC in out-patient settings other than home
- Antibiotic use
- Unrelated bacteremia/ fungemia; endocarditis

- Shock
- Mechanical ventilation
- Immunocompromised host
- Vascular thrombosis
- Continuous renal replacement therapy
- Site: adults: SC site poses lower risk than IJ site; IJ poses lower risk than femoral site. Pediatric patients: no documented difference in risk among these sites.
- PICC's have a lower risk than any of the centrally-inserted CVC's; this may be due to the patient population (usually less sick).
- Tunneled catheters have a lower risk (1–2 per 1000 catheter days) than non-tunneled catheters. Subcutaneous infusion ports have a lower risk than tunneled catheters.
- Polyvinyl chloride and polyethylene catheters ↑ risk as compared to Teflon-coated, polyurethane or silicone elastomere catheters

Box 15.3.9   Common Organisms Causing CRBSI

- Coagulase negative *Staphylococci* are the most common cause of both CRBSI and contaminated blood cultures. Eighty percent were successfully treated with vancomycin for 10–14 days if the catheter was left in place. If the catheter can be removed, 5 days of therapy is sufficient.
- *S. aureus* CRBSI is associated with metastatic infection and catheter removal is optimal. If surgically implanted without other access options, or if thrombocytopenia is a problem, the CVC may be left in place and systemic treatment should be supplemented with "antibiotic lock" (antibiotic + anticoagulant, to fill catheter lumen and allowed to dwell; vancomycin and heparin or minocycline and EDTA in 25% ethanol are options).
- Gram negative bacillary infections often originate from the urinary tract, lung or abdomen (including translocation of gut bacteria). CVC removal with systemic treatment for 10–14 days is recommended.
- *Candida spp.* requires CVC removal and antifungal therapy for 14 days after the last positive blood culture. CVC retention for >72 hrs is associated with ↓ response to antifungal agents and ↑ morbidity and mortality.
- Emerging agents include: vancomycin-resistant enterococcus (VRE), MRSA, and multidrug-resistant gram negative bacilli and fungi.

Pathophysiology of CRBSI:

- Bacteria migrate from skin or other sources of external contamination (*e.g.* hands) into the insertion site along a fibrin sheath (biofilm). Biofilm envelops the *outer* surface of the catheter in its tract from the skin to the vessel within 24 hrs of placement and is thought to play an important role in promoting colonization. Deposition of biofilm can also occur *inside* the catheter.
- Contamination of the *inside* of the catheter ("hub contamination") usually occurs ≥ one week after CVC placement.
- Infusion of contaminated substances can also lead to CRBSI

- Bacteria may infect a CVC from a site in the body distant from the CVC via the blood stream.
- Catheter-related thrombosis significantly increases infection risk.

Prevention of CRBSI involves meticulous technique in placement and care, circumvention of risk factors when possible plus use of antibiotic (*e.g.* minocycline/rifampin) impregnated catheters. Antiseptic catheters (*e.g.* those coated with chlorhexidine/sulfadiazine silver) decrease catheter colonization but are not proven to decrease CRBSI. Skin preparation with chlorhexidine (approved for patients >2 mos) is superior to provodone iodine. The dressing should be occlusive and changed at least weekly or sooner if loose, damp or visibly soiled. Gauze and transparent dressings offer equal protection against infection. If the site is oozing, a sterile gauze dressing is preferable. Application of polymicrobial ointment at the entry site promotes growth of resistant bacteria and *Candida*. Erythema or pus at the insertion site is highly predictive of CRBSI and removal of the CVC should be considered. Scheduled replacement of CVC's has not been shown to prevent CRBSI and change of CVC's over a guidewire may increase the risk of CRBSI. If TPN or blood products are infused, IV tubing should be changed daily and needless hubs should be changed every 12 hrs. Connection sites should be maintained in sterile fashion and cleansed with isopropyl alcohol before reattachment.

CVC-Related Thrombosis (CVC-RT). Sixty percent of pediatric thrombotic disease is related to a CVC. Pathogenesis of thrombosis involves Virchow's triad: (1) endothelial damage from a CVC, sepsis, trauma or medication; (2) venous stasis from decreased mobility, leukostasis, *etc.* and (3) a hypercoaguable state as may occur with inherited thrombophilia or acquired disease (*e.g.* inflammatory states). In our practice, severe dehydration is a well recognized risk factor. The true incidence is not known since most CVC-RT's are asymptomatic but may be as high as 50% of all CVC's placed; the significance of clinically silent clots is not known.

Within about 2 weeks, nearly all CVC's become surrounded by a fibrinous sheath. Its encroachment on the catheter tip may result in inability to aspirate blood from the catheter but continued ability to

Box 15.3.10   Risk Factors for Development of CVC-Related Thrombosis (CVC-RT)

- CRBSI
- Critical illness associated with ↑ production of thrombin and DIC
- Low body weight
- Newborn age-group
- ALL and use of L-asparaginase
- Infusion of TPN
- Protein-depleted states that lead to depletion of Protein S, Protein C and anti-thrombin
- Primary thrombophilia
- Hemophilia with Factor VIII therapy
- Number of vascular access attempts
- Large bore catheters in small vessels
- External catheters as compared to subcutaneous ports
- Polyvinyl chloride or polyethylene catheters are more thrombogenic than polyurethane or silicone elastomere catheters.
- Site-related: Femoral > SC > brachial > IJ

infuse through it. Local treatment of the catheter with alteplase may reverse the obstruction. Whether or not these obstructions or fibrin sleeves herald or influence the development of CVC-RT is not known. Risk factors for development of CVC-RT, signs and symptoms and complications are listed (**Boxes 15.3.10, 15.3.11 and 15.3.12**). The time from placement to development of thrombosis is ≥2 days. Morbidity and mortality among children from CVC-RT are reported by the Canadian Registry of Venous Thromboembolic Complications to be 6.5–9.4% and 2.2%, respectively.

Diagnosis of CVC-RT requires a high index of suspicion. Venography is the "gold standard" for identification of thrombosis. Lower extremity deep venous thrombosis (DVT) is typically diagnosed by ultrasonography (USG), but CT or MRI venography may be required to visualize deep pelvic or abdominal veins. USG cannot visualize the SC or brachiocephalic veins or SVC in their entirety; however, it is the study of choice for IJ thrombus detection. Cardiac USG can detect intracardiac clot and thrombus in the proximal vena cavae.

Box 15.3.11   Clinical Signs and Symptoms Suggestive of CVC-RT

- Loss of CVC patency
- Swelling, discoloration and discomfort near or distal to the catheter site
- Superior vena cava (SVC) syndrome (swelling of the face, neck; headache; hydrocephalus)
- Pulmonary embolism

- Thrombocytopenia
- Leukocytosis
- Fever
- Chylothorax or chylopericardium (due to inability of the thoracic duct to empty into the central venous circulation)

Box 15.3.12   Complications of CVC-RT*

- Loss of IV access and the associated impact on therapy
- Post-thrombotic syndrome: chronic pain, swelling, fatigue and/or ulceration of the affected extremity; development of collateral vessels (varicose veins)

- ↑ Risk of CRBSI/sepsis
- SVC syndrome (SC, IJ, SVC catheters)
- Pulmonary embolism
- Recurrent thromboses
- Renal compromise (femoral catheters)
- Subcutaneous fibrosis

---

* The incidence of long-term sequelae (years after catheter removal) is not known.

Prevention: CVC-RT may be avoidable by use of heparin-bound CVC's and use of sequential compression devices on the lower extremities when femoral catheters are placed in adults. Their use in children is limited by available sizes. Elastic stockings may lead to venous stasis because of constricting proximal bands. Prophylactic anticoagulation does not appear to decrease the incidence of CVC-RT. Since most CVC-RT's are not symptomatic, their incidental discovery presents treatment-related questions;

Box 15.3.13   Therapy for CVC-RT

- Catheter removal is optimal. In extreme circumstances when this is not possible, treatment with low molecular weight heparin (LMWH) or warfarin may be effective; anticoagulation for 3 months followed by prophylaxis until the catheter can be removed is recommended.
- LMWH (Enoxaparin) or unfractionated heparin should be initiated in the absence of contraindications to anticoagulation.

Therapeutic goals: **LMWH**: anti-factor Xa (called by the misnomer "heparin level" in some clinical laboratories) 0.5–1.0 U/ml
Unfractionated heparin: anti-factor Xa 0.3–0.7 U/ml or aPTT 60–85 secs.

- Warfarin should be started after goal heparinization is achieved; heparin is continued until the goal INR (2.0–3.0) is maintained for 2 consecutive days. Duration of therapy (usually 3–6 mos, but sometimes longer) is determined in conjunction with the hematologist based on risk factors.
- For children with a first CVC-RT anticoagulated for 3 months and in whom the offending catheter could not be removed, continued treatment with warfarin (goal INR 1.5–1.8) or LMWH (anti-factor Xa levels 0.1–0.3) should be considered until the catheter is removed.
- Thrombolytic agents should be considered in consultation with a hematologist in the setting of right heart failure, hemodynamic instability or limb-threatening thromboembolic (VTE) disease.
- Temporary vena cava filters should be considered in older patients if VTE occurs despite therapeutic anticoagulation and in the presence of ↑ risk.

---

prophylactic therapy to minimize the risk of clot growth should be considered if the CVC cannot be removed. Treatment of CVC-RT is described (**Box 15.3.13**).

Indwelling Arterial Catheters (IAC) are usually placed when any of the following are indicated:

- Continuous blood pressure monitoring.

- Frequent ABG, lactate, or ammonia determinations.
- Frequent blood sampling not readily obtainable from other sources; eliminates potential contamination of samples from substances infusing through venous catheters.

Vessel selection should be individualized. Extremities compromised by trauma or ischemia should be avoided; sites with collateral blood supply should be chosen over sites without collateral blood supply. If collateral circulation is not present, the benefits of arterial access should out-weigh the risks of limb loss. Potential sites, catheter sizes, advantages and disadvantages are itemized in **Box 15.3.14**. To check for collateral flow through the superficial palmar arch, perform a modified Allen Test: Elevate the hand above the chest and compress the radial and ulnar arteries. Lower the hand to chest level and release the vessel *not* intended for cannulation. Color should return to the hand; if it remains pale, collateral circulation is not present ("positive Allen test"). Guidelines for radial artery catheterization and complications of IACs are described in **Boxes 15.3.14 and 15.3.15**.

Complications from IACs include bleeding, hematomas, catheter-related infection, accidental tubing disconnection resulting in hemorrhage, thrombosis, accidental infusion of medication or IVF intra-arterially and arterial occlusion. Placement of an IAC should be avoided during severe coagulopathy if possible. Sterile technique during placement and catheter care are essential, although the risk of IAC infection is much less as compared to CVCs. Patients with IAC's should be monitored closely, with appropriately set BP alarms that alert the team to loss of tubing integrity. Use the smallest length and diameter catheter appropriate to cannulate the desired vessel; this will hopefully minimize the risk of catheter-related thrombosis (**Box 15.3.14**). Any indication of loss of perfusion distal to the catheter site should prompt immediate assessment and catheter removal. Blanching of the skin at or above the catheter site that does not refill within a few seconds should be assessed for the need for catheter removal.

Box 15.3.14 Indwelling Arterial Catheters: Site Options, Suggested Catheter Sizing, Advantages and Disadvantages

Artery	Catheter Sizes* Infants	Children and Adolescents	Advantages, Disadvantages And Comments
Radial, Ulnar	24 g or 2.5 F	22 g or 2.5 F	Usually accessible and easy to immobilize; collateral circulation can be checked using the modified Allen test (see text above); low incidence of ischemic complications reported with cannulation of the radial artery.
Posterior tibial, Dorsalis pedis			Collateral flow through the lateral plantar artery (a branch of the posterior tibial artery) can be checked by compression of the dorsalis pedis artery and pinching the great toe; color to the toe should return when pressure is released.
Axillary	22–20 g or 2.5–3.0 F	20–18 g or 3.0–4.0 F	Collateral circulation is present via the thyrocervical trunk and subscapular artery.
Femoral			Frequently chosen site when central BP monitoring is required or peripheral sites are lacking. No collateral arterial circulation.

*g, gauge; F, French. The access needle should be smaller than the catheter placed. Catheters larger and/or longer than those noted above may be required in large for age or obese patients.

Box 15.3.15   Guidelines for Radial Artery Catheter Placement

- The wrist should be secured so that the access site is protected from untoward movement. Use of a cushioned board that extends both distal and proximal to the access site is helpful. The wrist should be slightly dorsiflexed and **digits should be readily visible**.
- Sterile technique; a catheter-over-needle or Seldinger technique may be used.
- The radial artery is accessed where the pulse is most readily palpable, between the distal radius and the flexor carpi radialis tendon. The vessel should be approached ~1–3 mm distal to the pulse, aiming for the pulse at ~30–45°.
- If a catheter-over-needle device is used, the catheter can be threaded over the needle once arterial blood return is evident; modified Seldinger technique may be used (**Box 15.3.3**).
- The catheter should be secured with sutures or taped appropriately to minimize the risk of catheter displacement and hemorrhage.

15.4 Thoracentesis, Chest Tube Insertion and Chest Tube Removal

Gas (pneumothorax) or fluid collections in the pleural space may require removal, particularly if they are significant in volume, increasing in size, causing symptoms or if sampling is needed for diagnostic purposes ("diagnostic thoracentesis;" DT). When evacuation of the pleural space for relief of symptoms is required "therapeutic thoracentesis" (TT) or chest tube insertion (CTI) may be indicated. Usual indications, relative contraindications, procedural guidelines and complications for drainage of the pleural space are detailed (**Boxes 15.4.1 through 15.4.6**). See *Thoracic Trauma, 10.3, Box 10.3.2* for needle decompression of tension pneumothorax. **Figure 15.4.1** illustrates the physiology of drainage of the pleural space. Guidelines for CT removal are provided (**Box 15.4.7**).

Box 15.4.1   Common Indications and Relative Contraindications for Diagnostic Thoracentesis (DT)

Indications:

- Fever with pleural fluid collection over 1 cm thickness between lung and chest wall.
- A unilateral pleural effusion or bilateral effusions of different sizes
- Features "atypical" for congestive heart failure (CHF): normal sized heart on CXR, normal heart on cardiac ultrasound, normal B-type natriuretic peptide levels, effusion that does not improve with therapy for CHF.
- Pleurisy
- A larger than expected alveolar-arterial (A-a) oxygen gradient.

Relative Contraindications:

- Bleeding diathesis: PT or PTT > normal, platelet count < 25,000/mm^3
- Serum creatinine > 6 mg/dL
- Small volume of pleural fluid (see above)
- Skin infection at point of needle insertion.

Special precaution should be taken for patients receiving positive pressure ventilation. Ultrasound guidance should be used to avoid creating a pneumothorax.

15.4.2   Performance of Thoracentesis

- Sedation and analgesia may be required. Local anesthesia alone may be sufficient for some patients.
- Place patient in upright sitting position for non-loculated, "free-flowing" effusions.
- Identify fluid collection (preferably by ultrasound insonation) above the ninth rib posteriorly, midway between the spine and posterior axillary line
- Sterilize the skin and infiltrate skin with 1% lidocaine; advance the needle toward the adjacent rib and "walk" the needle over the superior aspect of the rib. Intermittently withdraw syringe plunger before injection of lidocaine to avoid intravascular injection.

(Continued)

15.4.2   Performance of Thoracentesis (Continued)

- Attach a 30–50 mL syringe to a 22-gauge 1½" needle and advance through anesthetized tissue while applying continuous negative pressure.
- Add 1 mL of heparin 1:1000 to a 50 mL syringe to prevent clotting of bloody or proteinaceous fluid withdrawn.
- A post-procedure CXR should be obtained.

Box 15.4.3   Complications of Thoracentesis

- Pain at site
- Bleeding
- Pneumothorax

- Empyema
- Soft tissue infection
- Spleen or liver puncture

- Reaction to anesthetic
- Vasovagal event
- Seeding of needle tract with tumor

Box 15.4.4   Indications and Relative Contraindications for CT Insertion (CTI)

Indications:

- Pneumothorax (if large, symptomatic or progressive)
- Pneumothorax during mechanical ventilation
- Complicated parapneumonic effusion or empyema
- Chemical pleurodesis for pleural effusions

- Penetrating chest trauma
- Hemothorax
- Bronchopleural fistula
- Chylothorax
- Bronchopleural fistula
- Recurrent symptomatic malignant effusion

Relative Contraindications:

- Bleeding diathesis (same as for thoracentesis)
- Pleural adhesions from prior infection (CT guidance is recommended)
- Pleurodesis
- Lung transplant

Box 15.4.5 Chest Tube Insertion (CTI): Procedure

- Sedation may be required.
- Insertion (skin incision) site: usually in the anterior axillary or mid-axillary line at the 4th or 5th intercostal space (ICS)
- After sterile preparation and draping, give 1% lidocaine for local anesthesia (*Analgesia, Sedation and Neuromuscular Blockade, 13.2*). Lidocaine is infiltrated into the periosteum of ribs above and below the intercostal insertion site.
- A 2 cm incision is made parallel to the ICS, one ICS inferior to the ICS that will be penetrated.
- Advance a Kelly clamp in the closed position through the incision site and cephalad over the superior aspect of the rib and through the parietal pleura; open the Kelly clamp to spread the muscles and enlarge the opening in the parietal pleura.
- Insert a finger into the pleural space to assure there are no adhesions between the lung and pleural surface; only lyse *small* adhesions.
- Use a Silastic CT with radio-opaque strip and gaps that mark drainage ports; a larger bore CT is typically necessary for large air leaks or viscous/loculated effusions. Longer CTs are made for adults; shorter tubes are used for children.
- Clamp the distal CT with the Kelly clamp and introduce the tube into the pleural space; direct the CT apically for pneumothorax or inferiorly and posteriorly for pleural fluid; then release the tube and observe for condensation in the lumen with breathing or fluid drainage. Insure that proximal port on the side of the CT is in pleural space.
- Close the skin with mattress or interrupted sutures and tie one of the sutures to the CT to anchor it; cover with gauze or petroleum gauze; secure with tape.
- Connect the CT to the drainage system (**Fig. 15.4.1**) and set "pressure-regulating bottle" to −10 to −20 cm H_2O. Check for "air-leak" (air stream entering pleural tube) by checking for "bubbling" in the "water-sealed bottle"
- Obtain CXR; proximal port should be at least 2 cm into the pleural space from rib margin.

(Continued)

Box 15.4.5   Chest Tube Insertion (CTI): Procedure (Continued)

The Seldinger technique (*See Vascular Access, 15.3*) can be used to place an 8.5 French Fuhrman "pigtail" (multiperforated polyurethane) catheter in the pleural space for small air leaks or drainage of pleural fluid (transudate). Preparation and site selection for the CT should be similar to that used for the conventional CT however no skin incision is used prior to introducer needle placement. After local anesthesia, an introducer needle is inserted into the pleural space, aspirating for air or fluid. The guide wire is introduced and needle withdrawn. A dilator is passed over the wire and then the dilator is withdrawn. The pigtail catheter is passed over the guidewire and secured. (Note: variations on this catheter and insertion procedures exist; correct insertion procedures may differ from that which has been described.)

Box 15.4.6   Complications of Chest Tube Insertion (CTI)

- Recurrent pneumothorax
- Empyema
- Lung perforation
- Diaphragm perforation
- Subcutaneous placement
- Perforation of right ventricle (RV) or right atrium
- Cardiogenic shock from compression of RV
- Perforation of abdominal organs
- Mediastinal perforation; contralateral hemothorax or pneumothorax
- Intercostal artery bleeding
- Infection at entry site
- Re-expansion pulmonary edema

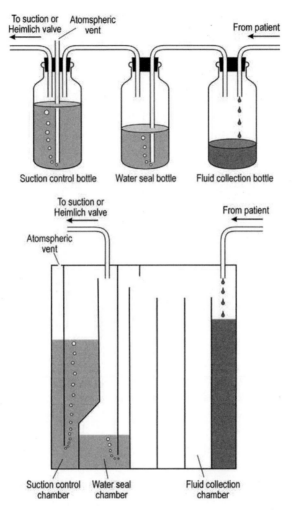

Fig. 15.4.1. **The Negative Pressure Wet-Dry Chest Tube Drainage Unit** (**"Pleur Evac"**) is used to remove air and/or fluid from the pleural space. The "pressure-regulating chamber" applies negative pressure to the CT in cm of water equal to the depth in cm that the atmospheric vent is submerged in water. The "water-seal chamber" is designed to monitor air leak from the patient; if air leak occurs then bubbles will appear (as demonstrated in the "water-seal bottle" in the figure). Also if the patient inhales and extreme negative pressure is transmitted to the "fluid collection chamber" water will ascend the submerged tube to prevent air from entering the chest. "Tidaling" (movement of water up and down in the submerged "water seal chamber" tube with each breath) occurs until the lung is completely re-inflated or if the circuit tubing becomes kinked, occluded or broken.

Box 15.4.7   Guidelines for Chest Tube Removal

- The timing of CT removal depends upon the reason for its insertion.
- If placed for pneumothorax, the absence of an air leak (absence of bubbling in the water-seal chamber) and re-expansion of the affected lung should be documented prior to CT removal. Typically, if suction was required to evacuate the pneumothorax, a trial of underwater seal without suction for 12–24 hrs is recommended. During this time, the water sealed chamber is checked frequently for evidence of air-leak (bubbling). Air leak should not be inducible by cough or positive airway pressure. A CXR obtained 12–24 hrs after the last observed air-leak should be obtained to confirm the absence of pneumothorax.
- If the patient requires positive pressure assistance (*e.g.* mechanical ventilation), some prefer to leave the CT in place until the patient is breathing spontaneously.
- If placed for drainage of pleural fluid, the volume drained in a 24 hrs period should be minimal (*e.g.* <1–3 mL/kg/day) and the CXR should be consistent with evacuation of the fluid.
- CT removal:
  - ▶ Assemble necessary equipment, including suture removal scissors or blade, additional suture material to close the CT site hole if necessary, petroleum-based gauze (if desired), dry gauze and elasticized or other sturdy tape.
  - ▶ The goal is CT removal and avoidance of entrainment of room air in to the pleural space.
  - ▶ The preferred phase of respiration during which the CT is removed varies among practicing physicians. In general, spontaneously breathing patients should have the CT removed quickly at end-inspiration. If the patient is able to cooperate, a forced Valsalva maneuver is desirable. If the patient is receiving positive pressure breaths (*e.g.* mechanical ventilation) the CT should be pulled at end-expiration.

(Continued)

Box 15.4.7   Guidelines for Chest Tube Removal (Continued)

▶ The chest wound should be *quickly* covered with an occlusive (air impregnable) dressing. If sufficiently large, the wound may require suture closure. Some operators secure CT's with a purse string suture that can be pulled tightly after CT removal to effect closure of the defect.

• The patient should be monitored and a CXR obtained if there is any suspicion of reaccumulation of pneumothorax or fluid. If the patient remains asymptomatic a CXR should be obtained 12–24 hrs after CT removal to confirm stability.

15.5 Lumbar Puncture (LP)

The risks and benefits of accessing CSF in a given patient should be weighed case-by-case in the critically ill. Inability to obtain CSF in a timely fashion should never delay administration of antibiotics when CNS infection is suspected (*Meningitis and Encephalitis, 5.4*). The indications, contraindications, procedure and complications are described (**Boxes 15.5.1, 15.5.2, 15.5.3 and 15.5.4**).

Box 15.5.1   Indications for Lumbar Puncture

• Suspected CNS infection
• Suspected subarachnoid hemorrhage when CT is not diagnostic
• For evaluation of CNS diseases such as post-infectious syndromes (*e.g.* ADEM), Guillain-Barre Syndrome, normal-pressure hydrocephalus, CNS malignancy, *et al.*
• Evaluation of inborn error of metabolism
• Administration of intrathecal medication
• Instillation of contrast material
• Treatment of raised ICP associated with *Pseudotumor cerebri*

Box 15.5.2   Contraindications to Lumbar Puncture and Special Considerations

- **Infection of the overlying skin site.** Significant trauma or other lesion (*e.g. hemangioma*) in this area may also be prohibitive or impose limitations on performance of the procedure.
- **Raised ICP:** These patients are at risk for brain herniation when a pressure differential is created between the spinal canal and intracranial fossa. Patients with risk factors for ↑ ICP should have a head CT prior to LP to assist in identification of ↑ ICP. This includes patients with altered mental status, focal neurologic signs, seizures, papilledema, craniosomatic disproportion, ventriculo-peritoneal (or alternative) shunt* and patients at high risk for brain abscess (*e.g.* those with right- to- left shunts or swollen eyes/forehead consistent with sinusitis).
- **Coagulopathy:** Platelet count < 50,000 and/or INR >1.4. There are no specific guidelines regarding abnormal PTT; significant prolongations of PTT should probably be corrected prior to LP. If the cause of coagulopathy is unknown, hematologic consultation should be sought to help identify the etiology and make recommendations regarding optimal correction of the disturbance for LP. When the risk of bleeding is high despite attempts at correction and LP cannot be postponed, fluroscopically guided LP may be considered.
- **Spinal deformities:** Identification of abnormalities in the lumbosacral area may warrant a fluoroscopically guided LP.
- **Respiratory or hemodynamic instability:** Patients with these instabilities may deteriorate in the knee-chest/flexed position.

*Neurosurgical consultation should be considered prior to LP for any patient with CNS shunt.

Box 15.5.3   Lumbar Puncture: Preparation and Performance

- Critically ill patients should be monitored by ECG, Pox and for respiratory distress or insufficiency throughout the procedure. Assure they are stable in the chosen position:
  - ▸ Lateral recumbent, knee chest; the back should be at 90° with a firm surface.
  - ▸ Sitting; the infant is supported in an upright knee-chest position. A child may sit at the edge of a bed and lean over a cushion, with elbows on knees.

(Continued)

Box 15.5.3 Lumbar Puncture: Preparation and Performance (Continued)

- An imaginary line connecting the iliac crests intersects the L-4 vertebra. The L3-4 and L4-5 interspaces can be accessed for CSF since the spinal cord terminates above this region in all age groups. For older children and adults, the L2-3 interspace may be used since the spinal cord ends at the inferior border of L1 by adulthood.
- Use sterile technique throughout the procedure. Preparation of the skin with provodone iodine (*not* chlorhexidine) should be used because contact with the meninges is anticipated.
- Local anesthesia should be used whenever possible. A surface (skin) anesthetic (*e.g.* Lidocaine and prilocaine) if time permits *plus* subcutaneous instillation of Lidocaine with a 25g needle are optimal. A mixture of Lidocaine 1% plus sodium bicarbonate 8.4% in a ratio of 9:1 minimizes burning on injection of lidocaine. Before injection of subcutaneous tissue, withdraw the syringe plunger to ensure that Lidocaine is not injected into the spinal canal or into a blood vessel. Young infants may benefit from oral sucrose on a pacifier provided there are no contraindications.
- Motion control is essential; some patients may require sedation.
- A 22g (2.5 inch for infants; 3.5 inch for children and adolescents) is introduced into the pre-identified interspace at the midline with the bevel of the needle upward (recumbent) or sideways (sitting). The needle is advanced slowly, aiming at the umbilicus. A "pop" may be felt as the needle traverses the dura. The stylet is removed intermittently to check for CSF flow.
- Opening pressure (OP) is measured with a manometer attached to the needle hub. A short connecting tubing with stopcock facilitates the attachment of the manometer to the spinal needle. Traditionally, legs and neck are extended for an accurate reading in the lateral recumbent position. If the patient is mechanically ventilated, $PaCO_2$ should be in the normal range.
  Normal OP = 50–200 mmH$_2$O; with flexion, readings of 100–280 mmH$_2$O are reported.
- After removal of an appropriate volume of CSF, the styleted needle is withdrawn and a clean dressing is applied.

Box 15.5.4   Complications of LP

- Brain herniation: Usually occurs within 12 hrs of LP in patients who had pre-existing ↑ ICP.
- Infection: Usually occurs when the puncture site is infected.
- Spinal epidural and/or subdural hematoma: Usually occurs in patients with uncorrected coagulopathy. Patients with back pain and neurologic compromise after an LP require emergent evaluation to R/O spinal hematoma.
- Epidermoid tumor: Possibly caused by introduction of epidermoid tissue into the spinal canal via a needle without a stylet or a poorly fitted stylet; may not be recognized for years after LP.
- Post LP headache: More common in adults than children; bed rest does not appear helpful. Adults in whom the spinal needle was withdrawn with the stylet in place had a ↓ in incidence of post-LP headache compared to those whose needles were withdrawn without a stylet.

Potential problems encountered during LP include:

- Patient deterioration: Abort the procedure; proceed with empiric therapy when indicated.
- "Hitting bone" with the needle: Ensure optimal positioning; redirect the needle; use a clean needle each time the skin is pierced.
- Bloody spinal fluid: Compare RBC counts in the first and last tubes; do not assume a "traumatic LP;" blood may reflect subarachnoid hemorrhage.
- Poor CSF flow: gently rotate the needle to reposition the bevel; re-insert the stylet and advance the needle ~1mm; if these fail, try withdrawing the needle by ~1mm from its original position.

15.6   Urinary Bladder Associated Procedures

Need for access to the urinary bladder in the PICU is frequent. Indwelling urinary catheters (UC) allow for continuous monitoring of urine output, timed urine collection and patient comfort. Invasive single pass urine drainage with a transurethral bladder catheter (TUBC) is often used to obtain urine for analysis and culture or to relieve a distended bladder which might be related to medication side effects or neurological disorders (*e.g.* spinal cord injury). Most UCs are made of siliconized rubber. Sizes ≥6 French (F) have a second lumen allowing inflation of a "retention balloon" at the UC tip. UC sizes should be individualized. General sizing estimates are 5F for the newborn, 6 F for infants, 8F for toddlers and children, and 12F for adolescents. Some UCs have a 3rd (infusion) port for continuous bladder irrigation (*e.g.* to wash out blood or infuse antibiotic). Passage of a UC can introduce bacteria into the urinary tract either along the surface of the catheter (biofilm) or through the UC lumen. Insertion technique must be performed under sterile conditions (**Box 15.6.1**); the operator should wear sterile latex-free gloves.

Box 15.6.1 Insertion of Transurethral Bladder Catheter

Boys:	Girls:
• With child in supine and frog-legged position retract foreskin exposing urethral meatus (reposition foreskin over the glans after procedure to avoid paraphimosis).	• With child in supine and frog-legged position retract the labia majora; use a cotton swab to retract redundant tissue from urethral orifice
• Hold penis perpendicular to lower abdomen; swab glans with podione-iodine	• Swab urethral orifice with podione-iodine from front to back
• Resistance to UC passage may be met at base of penis at external bladder sphincter; continue to try to advance UC with gentle pressure.*	• *Insert UC until urine is visualized in UC then inflate retention balloon if no resistance is encountered.

Remove the indwelling UC as soon as possible; UTI's are directly associated with duration of catheterization. Urine may be sampled with a needled syringe from a "collection port" diaphragm on the UC drainage tube after clamping the drainage tubing. Routine changing of UCs or drainage systems has not been shown to decrease the incidence of infection.

Lack of urine output in a patient with an indwelling bladder catheter should prompt evaluation of the catheter for obstruction. This may occur because of debris or blood clot in the catheter lumen, or may be due to compression or kinking of the catheter. The catheter should be inspected and the abdomen should be palpated for a distended bladder. Use of a bedside bladder scanner (ultrasound) may also help in identification of failure to adequately drain the bladder. Marked bladder distention from an obstructed urinary catheter may result in "new-onset hypertension" which resolves after bladder distention is relieved.

Suprapubic bladder aspiration (SPA) is best performed after identifying a distended bladder with bedside ultrasound with the ingant supine and in frog-legged position. Using sterile technique with sterile preparation 1 to 2 cm above the pubic symphysis, a 22 gauge needle attached to a 5 mL syringe is advanced cephalad (approximately 20°) while applying suction to the syringe. Gentle pressure may be applied to the base of the penis (boys) or the external meatus (girls) to avoid spontaneous urination. Urine sampled by SPA is the gold standard for diagnosis of urinary tract infection. Complications of SPA include hematuria (rarely gross) and anterior abdominal wall abscess (rarely).

Appendix

Part 1

Abbreviations, Definitions and Formulae

1 mmHg	$= 1.36$ cm H_2O
AA	Aplastic anemia; amino acids
A–a gradient	The difference between alveolar (A) and arterial (a) oxygen: $P_AO_2 - P_a O_2$; see Respiratory Physiology (*Appendix, part 2, III*)
ACCM	American College of Critical Care Medicine
ACCP	American College of Chest Physicians
ACE	Angiotensin converting enzyme
Acidemia	Subnormal blood pH
Acidosis	A decrease in total carbon dioxide buffering capacity without a change in blood pH. Often used clinically without regard to blood pH changes
ACS	Acute chest syndrome; Abdominal compartment syndrome
ADEM	Acute disseminated encephalomyelitis
AFP	Alpha-fetoprotein
AG	Anion gap; Measured cations – measured anions; See *Appendix, part 2*, V
AJDO$_2$	Arterial-jugular venous difference in O_2 content
AKI	Acute kidney injury
A–L	Indwelling arterial catheter ("a-line")

ALT	Alanine aminotransferase
ALTE	Apparent life-threatening event
Alveolar gas Equation	See Respiratory Physiology Supplement, *Appendix part 2, III*
ALL	Acute lymphocytic leukemia
AML	Acute myelogenous leukemia
ANC	Absolute neutrophil count
ANA	Anti-nuclear antibody
AOD	Atlanto-occipital dislocation
AOI	Apnea of infancy
AP	Anterior–posterior; an "AP X-ray" describes an image obtained by directing x-rays from a source anterior to the imaged part onto a detector placed posterior to the imaged part.
APCC	Activated prothrombin complex concentrate
aPTT	Activated partial thromboplastin time
Apt test	Test used to distinguish blood of maternal origin (adult hemoglobin) from blood originating from the newborn; swallowed maternal blood may be vomited or passed in the stools of a newborn, usually on the 2nd or 3rd day of life. Fetal hemoglobin is alkali resistant whereas maternal blood converts to hematin (brownish) on addition of alkali. Tested blood should be red, not tarry.
APV	Adaptive pressure ventilation
ARDS	Acute (or adult) respiratory distress syndrome
ARF	Acute respiratory failure; acute renal failure
ASM	Acid sphingomyelinase
ASO	Anti-streptolysin O; arterial switch operation
AST	Aspartate aminotransferase
ATN	Acute tubular necrosis
AV or av; AVSD	Atrioventricular; atrioventricular septal defect
AVM	Arterio-venous malformation
AVPU	Quick assessment tool for mental status: Alert; Responsive to voice; responsive to pain; Unresponsive.
BAL	Bronchoalveolar lavage

BAS	Balloon atrial septostomy
BB	Beta-blocker
BD	Base deficit; brain death
B-HCG	Beta-human chorionic gonadotropin
BIG IV;	Botulism immune globulin; see *Appendix,*
Baby BIG	*part 2, XII*
Bioavailability (*F*)	Percentage of an administered dose that reaches the central circulation.
BIS®	Bispectral index brain monitoring
Bladder capacity	Age in years + 2 = bladder capacity in number of ounces; adult bladder capacity is ~500 mL.
BLPAP	Bilevel positive airway pressure
BMI	Body mass index; equal to body weight (kg) ÷ [height (meters) squared]
BMR	Basal metabolic rate

Body weight

Actual (ABW)	Measured weight; should be obtained without clothing, linen, equipment, *etc.*

$$\textit{Ideal}\ (\text{IBW; kgs})\quad \text{For } 1-18\,\text{yrs} = \frac{[\text{height}\,(\text{cm}^2)\times1.65]}{1000}$$

Alternatively the 50th percentile of weight for the patient's height is a useful approximation of IBW; differs from lean body weight in that the latter is devoid of *all* fat.

Adjusted	IBW + 0.4 (ABW–IBW)
BPD	Bronchopulmonary dysplasia
BSA	Body surface area = square root of [height (cm) × weight (kg) ÷ 3600]
C.	*Chlamydophila (formerly, Chlamydia)*
CA125	cancer antigen 125; tumor marker
CaO$_2$	Content of oxygen in arterial blood. See *Appendix, part 2, IV*
CAUTI	Catheter-associated urinary tract infection
CBC	Complete blood count
CBF	Cerebral Blood Flow; Normal = 50–75 mL/100 g brain tissue

CF	Cystic fibrosis
cGMP	Cyclic guanosine monophosphate
CHD	Congenital heart disease
CHF	Congestive heart failure; more broadly, termed heart failure; also, Chronic hepatic failure
CI	Cardiac index; See *Appendix, part 2, IV*
C/I or c/i	Contraindicated
CLD/CLDI	Chronic lung disease/chronic lung disease in infants
Clearance (*Cl*)	The ratio of the rate of drug elimination to its concentration in blood or plasma; *Bedside Pharmacotherapy, 13.1.*
Cl_{cr}; Clcr	Creatinine clearance; See Fluid, Electrolyte, Renal and Acid-Base Calculations *Appendix, Part 2, V.*
CML	Chronic myelogenous leukemia
CMV	Conventional mechanical ventilation; continuous mandatory ventilation; Cytomegalovirus
CNMB	Continuous neuromuscular blocker (-ade)
CNS	Central nervous system
CO	Cardiac output; Chapter 3; *Appendix, part 2, IV*
Coronary perfusion pressure	Equal to MAP minus RA pressure
CPAP	Continuous positive airway pressure
CPF	Cough peak flow
CPP	Cerebral perfusion pressure; equal to MAP–ICP
CPR	Cardiopulmonary resuscitation; an attempt to restore spontaneous, effective ventilation and circulation
CPS	Child protective services
CRRT	Continuous renal replacement therapy
C-RT	Catheter-related thrombosis
CRT	Capillary refill time; Normal < 2 sec.
CSF	Cerebrospinal fluid; Normal volume is 50 mls in infants and ~150 mls in adults.

CT	Chest tube; Computerized tomography or CAT scan
CV	Cardiovascular
CVL	Central venous catheter ("central venous line")
CVP	Central venous pressure
CWM	Chest wall movement
CXR	Plain chest radiograph; Chest X-Ray
DA_1	Dopaminergic
DAI	Diffuse axonal injury
DBP	Diastolic blood pressure; the minimum blood pressure measured during cardiac relaxation (filling); may vary depending on the site and mode of measurement.
DDAVP	Desmopressin acetate; 1-deamino-8-D-argenine vasopressin
Dead space ventilation	See Respiratory Physiology Supplement, *Appendix III*
d-dimer	A fragment of fibrin in plasma; increased in disseminated intravascular coagulation, deep vein thrombosis and acute myocardial infarction.
DI	Diabetes insipidus
DIC	Disseminated intravascular coagulation
DNR *or* DNAR	"Do Not Resuscitate" *or* "Do Not Attempt Resuscitation;" An advanced directive NOT attempt to restore spontaneous, effective ventilation and perfusion. In clinical practice, this directive is typically defined in detail regarding appropriate and desired *vs.* inappropriate and undesired interventions which are individualized on a case-by-case basis.
DO_2	Delivery of Oxygen; *Appendix, part 2, IV.*
DPL	Diagnostic peritoneal lavage
DRI	Daily recommended intake
DTR	Deep tendon reflex(es)
Dyne	One dyne is the force that accelerates a one gram mass at the rate of one cm/second per second.

ECG	Electrocardiogram; also "EKG"
ECHO	Echocardiogram; cardiac ultrasonography
ECLS (ECMO)	Extracorporeal Life Support (also, extracorporeal membrane oxygenation)
EDH	Epidural hematoma
EDV	End diastolic volume
EFAD	Essential fatty acid deficiency
EGD	Esophagogastroduodenoscopy
ELISA	Enzyme-linked immunosorbant assay
ELT	Euglobulin lysis time: Citrated plasma is treated to precipitate the euglobulin fraction which contains inactivated clotting factors, plasminogen, tissue plasminogen activator (t-PA). When euglobulin fraction is resuspended, the addition of thrombin causes clotting. The time required for lysis of the clot by plasmin is the ELT (Normal = 90–240 mins). The ELT is prolonged in DIC but shortened in primary fibrinolysis (normal breakdown of clot).
EPAP	Expiratory positive airway pressure
ERK	Extracellular signal regulating kinase
ERV	Expiratory reserve volume
esp.	Especially
ESR	Erythrocyte sedimentation rate; a non-specific measure of inflammation
ET	Endotracheal; endothelin
ETCO$_2$	End tidal carbon dioxide
e-time	Expiratory time (time required to accomplish expiration)
ETT	Endotracheal tube
ETV	Endoscopic third ventriculostomy
EVD	External ventricular drain
Extra–axial	A collection or lesion inside the skull or spinal canal that does not arise from the CNS itself. *E.g.*, the meninges, subdural, epidural and subarachnoid blood are all considered "extra-axial".

"FAST"	Focused abdominal sonography for trauma; used in adults to R/O massive hemorrhage in the setting of trauma with shock.
FDP	Fibrin degradation products
Fig.	Figure
FFP	Fresh frozen plasma
Fr or F or FR	"French;" sizing based on diameter: 1 Fr = 0.33 mm.
FRC	Functional residual capacity
G or g	Gauge
G6PD	Glucose-6-Phosphate dehydrogenase
Gasping syndrome	Metabolic acidosis, respiratory distress, gasping respirations, seizures, cardiovascular collapse; typically occurs in neonates exposed to large amounts of benzyl alcohol, a metabolite of sodium benzoate/benzoic acid, a preservative used in certain drugs. Potentially lethal.
GCS	Glasgow Coma Scale or Score (*Altered Mental Status, 5.1*)
GER/GERD	Gastroesophageal reflux/gastroesophageal reflux disease
GFR	Glomerular filtration rate
GI	Gastrointestinal
GIR	Glucose infusion rate (mg/kg/min)
GIST	GI stromal tumor
GL	Gastric lavage
GU	Genitourinary
Hb	Hemoglobin
Hct	Hematocrit
Heimlich maneuver	Subdiaphragmatic abdominal thrusts delivered in an attempt to dislodge an obstructive foreign body from the upper airway; designed to increase intrathoracic pressure, generating an artificial cough. *Not* recommended for infants <1 yr because of potential damage to a relatively unprotected liver.
HF	Heart failure

HFNC	High flow nasal cannula
HIE	Hypoxic ischemic encephalopathy
HIV	Human immunodeficiency virus
HL	Hyperleukocytosis (WBC > 100,000/μL)
HTN	Hypertension
HOB	Head of bed
HPA	Hypothalamic-pituitary axis
HR	Heart rate; beats/min
HSV	Herpes simplex virus
HUS	Hemolytic uremic syndrome
HVA	Homovanillic acid
HZ	Hertz; cycles/second
IAP	Intra-abdominal pressure
IBD	Inflammatory bowel disease
IC	Indirect calorimetry
iCa	Ionized calcium
ICP	Intracranial pressure; normal: 5–10 mmHg (7–14 cm H_2O)
IEM	Inborn error of metabolism
I:E or i:e ratio	Ratio of inspiratory time to expiratory time
IJ	Internal jugular
IM	Intramuscular
Impedance Pneumography	A bioimpedance recording that measures respirations indirectly through electrodes on the chest wall; respiratory volume and rate are measured through the relationship between respiratory depth and thoracic impedance change.
iNO	Inhaled Nitric Oxide
IPPB	Intermittent positive pressure breathing
IPV	Intrapulmonary percussive ventilation
IO	Intraosseous (-ly)
i-time	Inspiratory time (time required to accomplish inspiration)
ITP	Intrathoracic pressure; Idiopathic thrombocytopenic purpura
IU	International units

IV	Intravenous (ly)
IVFE	Intravenous fat emulsion(s)
IVIG	Intravenous immune globulin
JCAHO	Joint Commission for the Accreditation of Health Care Organizations; currently, "The Joint Commission;" sets national standards for the delivery of health care.
JET	Junctional ectopic tachycardia
JNK	c-Jun NH_2-terminal kinase
K	Thousand; also the chemical symbol for potassium
KD	Kawasaki Disease
LBW	Low birth weight
LDH	Lactate dehydrogenase
Lean body mass	The body mass minus all fat. At chemical maturity (≥ 3 yrs), water accounts for ~70% of lean body mass and ~60% of ideal body weight.
LFT's	Liver function tests; these include bilirubin, total protein, albumin, vitamin K (reflected in PT/INR) ammonia, *etc.* "LFT's" are often equated with liver enzymes, which are not tests of liver function.
LGI	Lower gastrointestinal
LP	Lumbar puncture
LV	Left ventricle
LVH	Left ventricular hypertrophy
M.	*Mycobacterium; Mycobacteria*
MAP	Mean arterial blood pressure; equal to diastolic pressure + 1/3(systolic - diastolic)
MCFP	Mean circulatory filling pressure
MDS	Myelodysplastic syndromes
MEP	Maximal expiratory pressure
Met-Hb	Met-hemoglobin; results from oxidation of normal hemoglobin (Fe^{++}) to the ferric (Fe^{+++}) state.
MH	Malignant hyperthermia; MH Hotline: 1-800-644-9737 in the USA and Canada, and 001-303-389-1647 outside North America.

MI	Myocardial infarction
MIBG	Iodine-131-metaiodobenzylguanidine
MIC	Minimum inhibitory concentration; qualitative or quantitative determination of antimicrobial susceptibility of a specific microbe. The usual goal is selection of antibiotic therapy that will achieve a peak level 2–4 times the MIC at the site of infection. A level 10 times the MIC is usually chosen for urinary tract infections.
Minute ventilation	Tidal volume × respiratory rate; the volume of gas (mLs) exchanged in one minute.
MIP	Maximum inspiratory pressure
Mixed venous blood gas	Blood gas determination from pulmonary artery blood; when this is unavailable, blood from a source close to the right atrium has been substituted.
Mixing study	Differentiates factor deficiency from presence of an inhibitor. The patient's plasma is mixed 1:1 with normal pooled plasma, and the abnormal clotting study is repeated. If the test is normal with the "help" of pooled plasma, then a factor deficiency is most likely. If the test remains abnormal, an inhibitor is the likely cause of the coagulopathy. For example in hemophilia, mixing normal plasma with patient plasma results in correction of the coagulopathy.
mPaw	Mean airway pressure
MRA; MRV	Magnetic resonance arteriography; magnetic resonance venography
MRI:	Magnetic resonance imaging; See *Appendix, part 2, XV*
N/A	Not applicable
ND	Nasoduodenal; a route chosen to bypass the stomach (*e.g.* for feeding in cases of severe gastroesophageal reflux)

NEC	Necrotizing enterocolitis
NG	Nasogastric
NHLBI	National Heart, Lung and Blood Institute (branch of the National Institute of Health)
NICU	Neonatal Intensive Care Unit; see Standards in Levels of Neonatal Care, *Paediatr Child Health* **11(5)**: 303–306, 2006.
Levels 1, 2, 3	*Level 1*: Provides normal newborn nursery care; further subdivision includes level 1 nurseries that provide phototherapy (1a) and those that include infants with a corrected age >34 weeks or weight >1800 g, or have a mild illness or those convalescing from intensive care (1b). Level 1b nurseries also have the ability to initiate and maintain IV therapies, tube feedings and O_2 therapy. *Level 2a*; Special Care Newborn Nursery; include care for infants with a corrected age ≥32 weeks or weight >1500 g who are moderately ill. *Level 2b* nurseries provide mechanical ventilation for brief periods (<24 hrs) or CPAP; some implement and care for CVC's, including umbilical catheters. *Level 3*: Cares for neonates of all ages and weights. Level 3b nurseries would include availability of surgical interventions but would not include ECMO, hemofiltration and hemodialysis, congenital heart surgery requiring cardiopulmonary bypass. Level 3c nurseries offer the latter services.
NIRS	Near infra-red spectroscopy
NIV	Non-invasive ventilation
NiVNP	Non-invasive ventilation, negative pressure
NJ	Naso-jejunal
NMB	Neuromuscular blocker (-ade)

NMDA	N-methyl-D-aspartate
NMS	Neuroleptic malignant syndrome
NO	Nitric oxide
NPO	*Nones per os*; nothing by mouth
NPPV	Non-invasive positive pressure ventilation
NSAID	Non-steroidal anti-inflammatory drug
Off–label drug use	The use or prescription of a drug for reason(s) other than those approved by the Food and Drug Administration (FDA) Center for Drug Evaluation and Research. The FDA regulates the ability of a manufacturer to promote a drug for a given indication based on clinical trial data; however, the FDA may not regulate the ability to use or prescribe a drug for an indication not included in the "labeling".
OI	Oxygenation index: $[mPaw \times FiO_2 \times 100] \div PaO_2$
OSA/OSAS	Obstructive sleep apnea/OSA Syndrome
Osmolality	The number of osmoles or milliosmoles per kilogram water (solvent), measured by an osmometer based on freezing point or vapor pressure. The laboratory is able to measure osmolality, *not* osmolarity.
Osmolarity	The number of osmoles or milliosmoles per liter of solution. This value can be calculated from the measured osmoles.
PA	Pulmonary artery
PA Catheter	Pulmonary artery catheter; Swan–Ganz Catheter®
PAI	Plasminogen activator inhibitor
PAID	Paroxysmal autonomic instability with dystonia
PAT	Pain Assessment Tools (NICU, *etc*)
Paw	Airway pressure
PAWP	Pulmonary artery wedge pressure
PC	Pressure controlled (ventilation)
PCD	Programmed cell death; apoptosis
PCP	*Pneumocystis carinii* pneumonia (agent renamed *Pneumocystis jiroveci*)

PEEP	Positive end-expiratory pressure
PEFR	Peak expiratory flow rate
PEG	Percutaneous endoscopic (endoscopically-placed) gastrostomy
PEP	Positive expiratory pressure
PF	Peak flow
PGE_1/PGE-1	Prostaglandin E-1
PGI_2	Prostaglindin I-2 or prostacyclin
PHT, PHTN	Pulmonary hypertension
PICU	Pediatric Intensive Care Unit; see standards in *Guidelines and Levels of Care for Pediatric Intensive Care Units*, Pediatrics, **114**: 1144–1125, 2004.
Levels 1, 2	*Level 1:* Capable of providing definitive care and a multidisciplinary approach for a broad range of pediatric critical illness with the exclusion of premature newborns. These PICU's will have a full complement of pediatric subspecialists (including pediatric intensivists and the fulltime availability of a pediatric surgeon). *Level 2:* Generally care for less critically patients and differ from level 1 units in that a full spectrum of subspecialists is not mandatory; however, the same standards in quality of care are applied to both level 1 and level 2 units. Well-established communication should be constructed between level 2 and level 1 PICU's to facilitate appropriate referrals.
PIP	Peak inspiratory pressure; PIP = inspiratory pressure (or ΔP) + PEEP
PMI	Point of maximal impulse
PN	Parenteral nutrition
PO	*per os*; by mouth
Pox	Pulse oximeter (-try)
PPE	Parapneumonic effusion

PPI	Proton-pump inhibitor
PPV	Positive pressure ventilation
PRBC	Packed red blood cells
PRES	Posterior reversible encephalopathy syndrome
PRISM score	PRISM III; Pediatric Risk of Mortality Index; a predictor of mortality for children hospitalized in PICUs of various sizes developed in 1996. The equation is scored using the most abnormal values of variable sets for the first 12 hrs and the second 12 hrs of the PICU stay. Variable sets are 1] cardiovascular and neurologic vital signs 2] acid/base blood gases 3] chemistry tests 4] hematology tests 5] other factors. The first four "physiologic variables" are subdivided into 26 ranges and there are eight "other factors" that are also added into the final score. Higher total PRISM scores are associated with higher risk of mortality.
PRN	*Pro re nata*; as needed
PRVC	Pressure-regulated volume control (ventilation)
PSG	Polysomnogram; polysomnography
PT	Prothrombin time; physiotherapy (*e.g.* chest PT)
PTSD	Post-traumatic stress disorder
PTT, aPTT	Partial thromboplastin time, activated partial thromboplastin time
PVR	Pulmonary vascular resistance
PVS	Persistent vegetative state
QTc prolongation	The corrected QT interval equals [the measured QT interval] ÷ [the square root of the immediately prior R–R interval]. Normal values are: 1) 0.440 sec is the 97th percentile at 3–4 days of age 2) ≤ 0.45 sec in infants < 6 mos 3) ≤ 0.44 sec in children and adults

R	Resistance; mathematically described as the change in pressure between two points divided by flow.
RA	Right atrium (-atrial)
RAD	Reactive airway disease
RANCHO	Rancho Los Amigos Scale; a grading system for post-TBI patients that assists with evaluation of rehabilitation potential.
RBC	Red blood cells
RMSF	Rocky mountain spotted fever
R/O, r/o	Rule out
ROSC	Return of spontaneous circulation
RQ	Respiratory quotient; CO_2 eliminated/O_2 consumed
RR	Respiratory rate; breaths/min
rSO_2	Regional O_2 saturation; measured by near infra-red spectroscopy (NIRS)
RSV	Respiratory syncytial virus
RV	Right ventricle
RVH	Right ventricular hypertrophy
S.	*Streptococcus; Staphylococcus*
SBP	Systolic blood pressure; maximal arterial pressure during contraction of the left ventricle; may vary depending on the site and mode of measurement (*e.g.* A-L vs. cuff).
SCC	Spinal cord compression
SCCM	Society of Critical Care Medicine
SCD	Sickle cell disease
Scr	Serum creatinine
S_CVO_2	Central venous oxygen saturation
SDH	Subdural hematoma
SIRS	Systemic Inflammatory Response Syndrome
SjO_2; $SjvO_2$	Jugular venous oxygen saturation
SLA	Soluble liver antigen
SMS	Superior mediastinal syndrome
SNP	Sodium nitroprusside

Solute	A substance dissolved in a solvent.
Solvent	A substance, usually a liquid, in which other substances dissolve.
Spp.	Species
SS	Steady state; reached in approximately five half-lives of a given drug; Serotonin syndrome
STEC	Shiga-like toxin-producing *E. coli*
STX	Shiga-like toxin
SubQ	Subcutaneous (-ly)
SUN	Serum urea nitrogen; traditionally called BUN (a misnomer since urea nitrogen is no longer measured in blood, but in serum)
SVCS	Superior vena cava syndrome
SvO_2; $ScvO_2$	Venous O_2 saturation; usually refers to venous saturation from pulmonary arterial blood; blood from a central source close to the right atrium has been substituted when PA blood cannot be obtained.
SVR	Systemic vascular resistance
SWI	Stroke work index; See *Appendix, part 2, IV*
$T_{1/2}$	Half-life; also $t_{1/2}$
T	Temperature
T&A	Tonsilloadenoidectomy
TAI	Traumatic axonal injury
TAPVC (R)	Total anomalous pulmonary venous connection (return)
TBI	Traumatic brain injury
TCA	Tracheal cross-sectional area; tricyclic antidepressant; tricarboxylic acid cycle
$t\,CO_2$	Measured total carbon dioxide; includes carbon dioxide as H_2CO_3 plus HCO_3^- plus CO_2.
TCT	Total clotting time
TEE	Total energy expenditure; transesophageal echocardiogram
TGA	Transposition of the Great Arteries
Ti	Inspiratory time
TIA	Transient ischemic attack

TID	*Tres in diem*; three times per day
TLS	Tumor lysis syndrome; thoraco-lumbar-sacral spine
Tmp	Transmural pressure; the pressure difference between two sides of a wall; the pressure inside a tube minus the pressure outside the tube.
TMP-SMX	Trimethoprim and sulfamethoxazole
TOF	Tetralogy of Fallot
Train-of-four	Peripheral nerve stimulation to help assess the degree of neuromuscular blockade (*Analgesia, Sedation and Neuromuscular Blockade, 13.2*).
TRALI	Transfusion-related acute lung injury
Trauma Center	The Committee on Trauma Verification Program facilitates the process by which the American College of Surgeons deems that a given center is capable of and permitted to perform as a trauma center based on the document: *Resources for Optimal Care of the Injured Patient.*
Levels I through IV	*Level I*: A tertiary care, regional resource trauma center which should be accessible to all those who require its resources. Every aspect of acute care through the rehabilitation process is available. *Level II*: Provides initial definitive care; may not be able to provide the comprehensive care accessible in a level 1 facility. *Level III*: Provides prompt assessment and emergency care, including emergency surgery, and stabilization for transport as indicated. *Level IV*: Provides advanced trauma life support in remote areas until appropriate patient transfer can be accomplished.
TT	Tracheostomy tube
TV	Tidal volume
TXA	Thromboxane
UAO	Upper airway obstruction

UGI	Upper gastointestinal
UOP	Urine output
USG	Ultrasonography; ultrasound examination
VAP	Ventilator-associated pneumonia
VBG	Venous blood gas
VC	Vital capacity; Volume controlled (ventilation)
Vd	Volume of distribution; equal to the amount of drug in the body ÷ the drug concentration in plasma
VF *or* V-fib.	Ventricular fibrillation
VIP-oma	Vasoactive intestinal peptide-producing tumor
VMA	Vanillylmandelic acid
VO$_2$	Oxygen consumption; *Appendix, part 2, IV*
VP/VA shunts	Ventriculoperitoneal/ventriculo-atrial CSF diversion; refers to the procedure or the hardware used.
VT *or* V Tach.	Ventricular tachycardia
V/Q	Ventilation to perfusion ratio
Wall stress	A measure of tension; when applied to the heart, wall stress = (Pressure within the ventricle × Radius of the ventricle) ÷ 2 Also known as the La place equation.
WSACS	World Society on Abdominal Compartment Syndrome

Part 2

I. Normal Vital Signs

Normal Heart Rates (BMP) for Infants, Children and Adolescents

Age	Heart Rate (mean)	Age	Heart Rate (mean)
0–7 days	95–160 (125)	4–5 yr	65–135 (110)
1–3 wk	105–180 (145)	6–8 yr	60–130 (100)
1–6 mo	110–180 (145)	9–11 yr	60–100 (85)
6–12 mo	110–170 (135)	12–16 yr	60–110 (85)
1–3 yr	90–150 (120)	>16 yr	60–100 (80)

Normal Respiratory Rates (RR/min) for Infants, Children and Adolescents

Age	Respiratory Rate
Infant (birth to 1 yr)	30–60
1–3 yr	24–40
3–6 yr	22–34
6–12 yr	18–30
12–18 yr	12–16

Minimum (Low Normal) Systolic Blood Pressures (mmHg) Based on Age

Age	Minimum Systolic BP
Infant (birth to 1 yr)	60
1–3 yr	> 70
3–6 yr	> 75
6–12 yr	> 80
12–18 yr	> 90

Upper Limits of Normal* for Blood Pressure in Boys and Girls < 12 mos of Age*

Age	Systolic		Diastolic	
	Boys	Girls	Boys	Girls
1st week	87	76	68	68
Months				
1	101	98	65	65
2	106	101	63	64
3	106	104	63	64
4	106	105	63	65
5	105	106	65	65
6	105	106	66	66
7	105	106	67	66
8	105	106	68	66
9	105	106	68	67
10	105	106	69	67
11	105	105	69	67
12	105	105	69	67

* Report of the Second Task Force on Blood Pressure Control in Children — 1987. *Pediatrics* 79(1):1987.

Blood Pressure Levels for Boys by Age and Height Percentile

Age (Yr)	BP %ile	Systolic BP (mmHg) Percentile of height							Diastolic BP (mmHg) Percentile of height						
		5th	10th	25th	50th	75th	90th	95th	5th	10th	25th	50th	75th	90th	95th
1	50th	80	81	83	85	87	88	89	34	35	36	37	38	39	39
	90th	94	95	97	99	100	102	103	49	50	51	52	53	53	54
	95th	98	99	101	103	104	106	106	54	54	55	56	57	58	58
	99th	105	106	108	110	112	113	114	61	62	63	64	65	66	66
2	50th	84	85	87	88	90	92	92	39	40	41	42	43	44	44
	90th	97	99	100	102	104	105	106	54	55	56	57	58	58	59
	95th	101	102	104	106	108	109	110	59	59	60	61	62	63	63
	99th	109	110	111	113	115	117	117	66	67	68	69	70	71	71
3	50th	86	87	89	91	93	94	95	44	44	45	46	47	48	48
	90th	100	101	103	105	107	108	109	59	59	60	61	62	63	63
	95th	104	105	107	109	110	112	113	63	63	64	65	66	67	67
	99th	111	112	114	116	118	119	120	71	71	72	73	74	75	75
4	50th	88	89	91	93	95	96	97	47	48	49	50	51	51	52
	90th	102	103	105	107	109	110	111	62	63	64	65	66	66	67
	95th	106	107	109	111	112	114	115	66	67	68	69	70	71	71
	99th	113	114	116	118	120	121	122	74	75	76	77	78	78	79
5	50th	90	91	93	95	96	98	98	50	51	52	53	54	55	55
	90th	104	105	106	108	110	111	112	65	66	67	68	69	69	70
	95th	108	109	110	112	114	115	116	69	70	71	72	73	74	74
	99th	115	116	118	120	121	123	123	77	78	79	80	81	81	82
6	50th	91	92	94	96	98	99	100	53	53	54	55	56	57	57
	90th	105	106	108	10	111	113	113	68	68	69	70	71	72	72
	95th	109	110	112	114	115	117	117	72	72	73	74	75	76	76
	99th	116	117	119	121	123	124	125	80	80	81	82	83	84	84
7	50th	92	94	95	97	99	100	101	55	55	56	57	58	59	59
	90th	106	107	109	111	113	114	115	70	70	71	72	73	74	74
	95th	110	111	113	115	117	118	119	74	74	75	76	77	78	78
	99th	117	118	120	122	124	125	126	82	82	83	84	85	86	86
8	50th	94	95	97	99	100	102	102	56	57	58	59	60	60	61
	90th	107	109	110	112	114	115	116	71	72	72	73	74	75	76
	95th	111	112	114	116	118	119	120	75	76	77	78	79	79	80
	99th	119	120	122	123	125	127	127	83	84	85	86	87	87	88
9	50th	95	96	98	100	102	103	104	57	58	59	60	61	61	62
	90th	109	110	112	114	115	117	118	72	73	74	75	76	76	77
	95th	113	114	116	118	119	121	121	76	77	78	79	80	81	81
	99th	120	121	123	125	127	128	129	84	85	86	87	88	88	89
10	50th	97	98	100	102	103	105	106	58	59	60	61	6	62	63
	90th	111	112	114	115	117	119	119	73	73	74	75	76	77	78
	95th	115	116	117	119	121	122	123	77	78	79	80	81	81	82
	99th	112	123	125	127	128	130	130	85	86	86	88	88	89	90

(Continued)

(Continued)

Age (Yr)	BP %ile	Systolic BP (mmHg) Percentile of height							Diastolic BP (mmHg) Percentile of height						
		5th	10th	25th	50th	75th	90th	95th	5th	10th	25th	50th	75th	90th	95th
11	50th	99	100	102	104	105	107	107	59	59	60	61	62	63	63
	90th	113	114	115	117	119	120	121	74	74	75	76	77	78	78
	95th	117	118	119	121	123	124	125	78	78	79	80	81	82	82
	99th	124	125	127	129	130	132	132	86	86	87	88	89	90	90
12	50th	101	102	104	106	108	109	110	59	60	61	62	63	63	64
	90th	115	116	118	120	121	123	123	74	75	75	76	77	78	79
	95th	119	120	122	123	125	127	127	78	79	80	81	82	82	83
	99th	126	127	129	131	133	134	135	86	87	88	89	90	90	91
13	50th	104	105	106	108	110	111	112	60	60	61	62	63	64	64
	90th	117	118	120	122	124	125	126	75	75	76	77	78	79	79
	95th	121	122	124	126	128	129	130	79	79	80	81	82	83	83
	99th	128	130	131	133	135	136	137	87	87	88	89	90	91	91
14	50th	106	107	109	111	113	114	115	60	61	62	63	64	65	65
	90th	120	121	123	125	126	128	128	75	76	77	78	79	79	80
	95th	124	125	127	128	130	132	132	80	80	81	82	83	84	84
	99th	131	132	134	136	138	139	140	87	88	89	90	91	92	92
15	50th	109	110	112	113	115	117	117	61	62	63	64	65	66	66
	90th	122	124	125	127	129	130	131	76	77	78	79	80	80	81
	95th	126	127	129	131	133	134	135	81	81	82	83	84	85	85
	99th	134	135	136	138	140	142	142	88	89	90	91	92	93	93
16	50th	111	112	114	116	118	119	120	63	63	64	65	66	67	67
	90th	125	126	128	130	131	133	134	78	78	79	80	81	82	82
	95th	129	130	132	134	135	137	138	82	83	83	84	85	86	87
	99th	136	137	139	141	143	144	145	90	90	91	92	93	94	94
17	50th	114	115	116	118	120	121	122	65	66	66	67	68	69	70
	90th	127	128	130	132	134	135	136	80	80	81	82	83	84	84
	95th	131	132	134	136	138	139	140	84	85	86	87	87	88	89
	99th	139	140	141	143	145	146	147	92	93	93	94	95	96	97

* The 90th percentile is 1.28 SD, 95th percentile is 1.645 SD, and the 99th percentile is 2.326 SD over the mean.

Blood Pressure Levels for Girls by Age and Height Percentile

Age (Yr)	BP %ile	Systolic BP (mmHg)							Diastolic BP (mmHg)						
		Percentile of height							Percentile of height						
		5th	10th	25th	50th	75th	90th	95th	5th	10th	25th	50th	75th	90th	95th
1	50th	83	84	85	86	88	89	90	38	39	39	40	41	41	42
	90th	97	97	98	100	101	102	103	52	53	53	54	55	55	56
	95th	100	101	102	104	105	106	107	56	57	57	58	59	59	60
	99th	108	108	109	111	112	113	114	64	64	65	65	66	67	67
2	50th	85	85	87	88	89	91	91	43	44	44	45	46	46	47
	90th	98	99	100	101	103	104	105	57	58	58	59	60	61	61
	95th	102	103	104	105	107	108	109	61	62	62	63	64	65	65
	99th	109	110	111	112	114	115	116	69	69	70	70	71	72	72
3	50th	86	87	88	89	91	92	93	47	48	48	49	50	50	51
	90th	100	100	102	103	104	106	106	61	62	62	63	64	64	65
	95th	104	104	105	107	108	109	110	65	66	66	67	68	68	69
	99th	111	111	113	114	115	116	117	73	73	74	74	75	76	76
4	50th	88	88	90	91	92	94	94	50	50	51	52	52	53	54
	90th	101	102	103	104	106	107	108	64	64	65	66	67	67	68
	95th	105	106	107	108	110	111	112	68	68	69	70	71	71	72
	99th	112	113	114	115	117	118	119	76	76	76	77	78	79	79
5	50th	89	90	91	93	94	95	96	52	53	53	54	55	55	56
	90th	103	103	105	106	107	109	109	66	67	67	68	69	69	70
	95th	107	107	108	110	111	112	113	70	71	71	72	73	73	74
	99th	114	114	116	117	118	120	120	78	78	79	79	80	81	81
6	50th	91	92	93	94	96	97	98	54	54	55	56	56	57	58
	90th	104	105	106	108	109	110	111	68	68	69	70	70	71	72
	95th	108	109	110	111	113	114	115	72	72	73	74	74	75	76
	99th	115	116	117	119	120	121	122	80	80	80	81	82	83	83
7	50th	93	93	95	96	97	99	99	55	56	56	57	58	58	59
	90th	106	107	108	109	111	112	113	69	70	70	71	72	72	73
	95th	110	111	112	113	115	116	116	73	74	74	75	76	76	77
	99th	117	118	119	120	122	123	124	81	81	82	82	83	84	84
8	50th	95	95	96	98	99	100	101	57	57	57	58	59	60	60
	90th	108	109	110	111	113	114	114	71	71	71	72	73	74	74
	95th	112	112	114	115	116	118	118	75	75	75	76	77	78	78
	99th	119	120	121	122	123	125	125	82	82	83	83	84	85	86
9	50th	96	97	98	100	101	102	103	58	58	58	59	60	61	61
	90th	110	110	112	113	114	116	116	72	72	72	73	74	75	75
	95th	114	114	115	117	118	119	120	76	76	76	77	78	79	79
	99th	121	121	123	124	125	127	127	83	83	84	84	85	86	87
10	50th	98	99	100	102	103	104	105	59	59	59	60	61	62	62
	90th	112	112	114	115	116	118	118	73	73	73	74	75	76	76
	95th	116	116	117	119	120	121	122	77	77	77	78	79	80	80
	99th	123	123	125	126	127	129	129	84	84	85	86	86	87	88

(Continued)

(Continued)

Age (Yr)	BP %ile	Systolic BP (mmHg)							Diastolic BP (mmHg)						
		Percentile of height							Percentile of height						
		5th	10th	25th	50th	75th	90th	95th	5th	10th	25th	50th	75th	90th	95th
11	50th	100	101	102	103	105	106	107	60	60	60	61	62	63	63
	90th	114	114	116	117	118	119	120	74	74	74	75	76	77	77
	95th	118	118	119	121	122	123	124	78	78	78	79	80	81	81
	99th	125	125	126	128	129	130	131	85	85	86	87	87	88	89
12	50th	102	103	104	105	107	108	109	61	61	61	62	63	64	64
	90th	116	116	117	119	120	121	122	75	75	75	76	77	78	78
	95th	119	120	121	123	124	125	126	79	79	79	80	81	82	82
	99th	127	127	128	130	131	132	133	86	86	87	88	88	89	90
13	50th	104	105	106	107	109	110	110	62	62	62	63	64	65	65
	90th	117	118	119	121	122	123	124	76	76	76	77	78	79	79
	95th	121	122	123	124	126	127	128	80	80	80	81	82	83	83
	99th	128	129	130	132	133	134	135	87	87	88	89	89	90	91
14	50th	106	106	107	109	110	111	112	63	63	63	64	65	66	66
	90th	119	120	121	122	124	125	125	77	77	77	78	79	80	80
	95th	123	123	125	126	127	129	129	81	81	81	82	83	84	84
	99th	130	131	132	133	135	136	136	88	88	89	90	90	91	92
15	50th	107	108	109	110	111	113	113	64	64	64	65	66	67	67
	90th	120	121	122	123	125	126	127	78	78	78	79	80	81	81
	95th	124	125	126	127	129	130	131	82	82	82	83	84	85	85
	99th	131	132	133	134	136	137	138	89	89	90	91	91	92	93
16	50th	108	108	110	111	112	114	114	64	64	65	66	66	67	68
	90th	121	122	123	124	129	127	128	78	78	79	80	81	81	82
	95th	125	126	127	128	130	131	132	82	82	83	84	85	85	86
	99th	132	133	134	135	137	139	139	90	90	90	91	92	93	93
17	50th	108	109	110	111	113	114	115	64	65	65	66	67	67	68
	90th	122	122	123	125	126	127	128	78	79	79	80	81	81	82
	95th	125	126	127	129	130	131	132	82	83	83	84	85	85	86
	99th	133	133	134	136	137	138	139	90	90	91	91	92	93	93

* The 90th percentile is 1.28 SD, 95th percentile is 1.645 SD, and the 99th percentile is 2.326 SD over the mean.

Fourth Report on the Diagnosis, Evaluation, and Treatment of High Blood Pressure in Children and Adolescents. May 2004.

II. Conversion Formulae and Calculation of Body Surface Area

A. Convert degrees Celsius (C°) to degrees Fahrenheit (F°):
(9/5 × C°) + 32
B. Convert degrees Fahrenheit (F°) to degrees Celsius (C°):
(F° −32) × 5/9
C. Convert inches to centimeters (cm): multiply by 2.54
D. Convert pounds to kilograms (kg): divide by 2.2
E. Calculation of Body Surface Area (BSA)

Surface area (m²) = the square root of [(height (cm)
× weight (kg)) ÷ 3600]

Estimations of Body Surface Area (m²) Based on Weight (kg)					
Weight	BSA	Weight	BSA	Weight	BSA
2	0.12	9	0.40	40	1.32
3	0.2	10	0.44	45	1.43
4	0.23	15	0.62	50	1.53
5	0.25	20	0.79	55	1.62
6	0.29	25	0.93	60	1.70
7	0.33	30	1.07	65	1.78
8	0.36	35	1.2	70	1.84

III. Respiratory Physiology: Equations and Abbreviations

The **Laplace Equation** states that the pressure inside a bubble exceeds the pressure outside the bubble. Stated mathematically

Pressure inside a bubble = 2 × bubble surface tension
÷ radius of the bubble.

Note: Surfactant alters the properties predicted for a bubble by lowering the surface tension of the alveolar lining as its radius decreases. As the radius of the "bubble" (actually, an isolated completely spherical alveolus) decreases, surfactant prevents the pressure inside the bubble from increasing. Rather, the pressure inside the bubble remains relatively constant. In other words, surface tension on the inside of the alveolus decreases, protecting it from complete collapse.

Minute Ventilation (**MV**)
    = Tidal volume (**TV**) × Respiratory rate (**RR**), *or*
    = Alveolar Ventilation + Dead Space Ventilation

Physiologic or Total Dead Space (TDS):

$$TDS \text{ (anatomic + alveolar)} = (PaCO_2 - P_{ETCO2}) \div PaCO_2$$

Note: Dead space accounts for ~40% of the TV in a term infant; this decreases to ~ 33% by 15 yrs. of age.

Functional Residual Capacity (FRC) = ERV + RV
  ERV = Expiratory Reserve Volume = volume that can be forcibly
          exhaled after tidal volume is exhaled.
  RV = Residual Volume = volume that cannot be exhaled
          after ERV is exhaled.

Vital Capacity (VC) = Volume inhaled from maximal exhalation to maximal inhalation.

Total Lung Capacity (TLC) = all of the air in the lung at maximal inspiration (including RV).

Closing Capacity (CC) = volume of the lung at which dependent airways begin to close; in normal young subjects CC is equal to ~10% of VC and begins to increase with small airway disease.

Compliance (C) = $\Delta V/\Delta P$ or the change in lung volume per unit change in pressure.

Pressure is plotted on the X axis and volume on the Y axis. A lung with greater compliance has a steeper slope ($\Delta V/\Delta P$). Compliance measured at zero air flow is "static compliance" whereas compliance measured at peak inspiratory pressure is "dynamic compliance".

Static compliance $= \Delta V \div$ (plateau pressure $-$ PEEP)
Dynamic compliance $= \Delta V \div$ (PIP $-$ PEEP)

Resistance (R) $= \Delta P \div (\Delta V \div \Delta T)$ where T = Time
Resistance is the pressure difference that drives a specific flow of gas or liquid.

Poiseuille's equation: $\Delta P = [(\Delta V \div \Delta T)\ 8\eta l] \div \pi r^4$ where η is viscosity, l is length of tube, and r is radius of the tube. Poiseuille's equation predicts a pressure drop that produces laminar flow.

Time Constant (TC): Relates resistance and compliance.
TC (sec) = R (cm H_2O/L/sec) $\times$ C (L/cm H_2O).

One TC equals the time needed for a lung segment to reach 63% of filling or emptying volume; approximately 98% of filling or emptying occurs in 5 TCs. Depending on the breathing frequency, a lung unit with a large TC does not complete filling before exhalation begins and thus is poorly ventilated. Faster RR causes poorer ventilation of these long TC units.

Alveolar Gas Equation describes the partial pressure of oxygen in the alveolus (P_AO_2) which equals

$$P_{inspiratory}\ O_2 - (PaCO_2 \div Respiratory\ Quotient)$$

Calculation of $P_{inspiratory}\ O_2$: This is determined by the total barometric pressure (usually ~760 mmHg) from which the partial pressure of water (47 mmHg) is subtracted. When breathing room air, 21% of total pressure is oxygen; therefore 0.21 (760–47) = $P_{inspiratory}$ $O_2 = 150$ mmHg. When breathing at rest the usual $PaCO_2$ is 40 mmHg and the RQ is 0.8. Therefore $(PaCO_2 \div RQ) = 40 \div 0.8$ or 50 mmHg Therefore: $P_AO_2 = 150$ mmHg $- 50$ mmHg $= 100$ mmHg.

"A–a Gradient" is the difference between the partial pressure of oxygen in the alveolus and the partial pressure of oxygen in arterial blood, so:

A–a Gradient = P_AO_2 – PaO_2 *or* {[FiO_2 (760–47)] – ($PaCO_2$ ÷ 0.8)]} minus PaO_2

Normal A–a gradient for FiO_2 0.21: < 9 mmHg; for FiO_2 1.0: < 34 mmHg

O_2 Content of arterial or venous blood (CaO_2 or CvO_2) calculates the ml of oxygen bound per gram of hemoglobin plus mls of oxygen dissolved in plasma at 760 mmHg (1 atmosphere pressure).

$$CaO_2 = (SaO_2 ÷ 100) × [Hb × constant] + 0.0031 × PaO_2.$$
where the constant ranges from 1.34–1.39, We will use 1.36.

For example, the oxygen content of 1 dL of arterial blood with Hb of 8 gms/dL and 95% saturated Hb using a constant of 1.36 and a PaO_2 of 80 mmHg is equal to:

$$CaO_2 = (95/100) × (8 × 1.36) + (00031 × 80) = 10.59 \text{ mL}$$
of O2/dL of blood.

The oxygen content of venous blood (CvO_2) can be calculated similarly by substituting the oxygen saturation in venous blood (SvO_2) and venous PO_2 (optimally measured from the pulmonary artery but values obtained from central venous blood may be substituted).

V/Q Mismatching: Both ventilation and perfusion increase progressively as one moves lower down in an upright lung. The rate of increase, however, differs so that ventilation increases more slowly, and perfusion increases more rapidly as we move lower down the in lung. This results in apical lung which is relatively under-perfused compared to its degree of ventilation (V/Q >1) and basal lung regions which are somewhat under-ventilated in relation to perfusion (V/Q <1).

The concept of V/Q mismatch includes use of another concept called **"venous admixture."** This is a theoretical or calculated amount of mixed venous blood (blood from the pulmonary artery) that would need to be added to pulmonary end capillary blood (blood in which the

PaO_2 is equal to alveolar O_2 *i.e.*, P_AO_2) to produce the observed drop in PaO_2 between pulmonary end-capillary blood and the actual (measured) arterial PaO_2. Total cardiac output (**CO or Qt**) equals shunted blood flow (**Qs**) and pulmonary capillary blood flow. The ratio of Qs/Qt is important because it affects the ability of the lung to increase PaO_2. At a Qs/Qt of 0% there will be a linear increase in PaO_2 with increased FiO_2. If Qs/Qt is > 50%, then further increasing FiO_2 will have no effect on PaO_2. Shunt can be calculated as follows:

Intrapulmonary shunt = Qs/Qt

Qs/Qt = (Cpulmonary capillary O_2 – CaO_2)
÷ (Cpulmonary capillary O_2 – CvO_2)

Where **Cpulmonary capillary O_2 = P_AO_2 (see above); CaO_2 = O_2** content of arterial blood; **CvO_2** = oxygen content of mixed venous blood. Normal Qs/Qt is < 5%.

Fick Equation: VO_2 = CO (CaO_2 – CvO_2) where VO_2 is oxygen consumption, CO is cardiac output and CaO_2 and CvO_2 are the contents of oxygen in arterial and venous blood, respectively.

If CO falls with a constant VO_2 then CvO_2 will fall. For this reason, monitoring of mixed venous O_2 saturation is helpful in assessing the balance between O_2 delivery and consumption.

Oxygen Extraction Ratio (OER) = (CaO_2 – CvO_2) ÷ CaO_2

Note: A normal OER is 0.25; the OER increases when O_2 delivery is inadequate to meet demands.

Oxy-hemoglobin dissociation curve for hemoglobin A. The P50 of hemoglobin A is the PaO_2 at which hemoglobin is 50% saturated with oxygen (PaO_2 27 mmHg). If the curve is shifted leftward, the affinity of hemoglobin A for oxygen is increased, *i.e.* hemoglobin remains 50% saturated at a lower PaO_2, leaving less oxygen available for tissues. If conditions favor a rightward shift, the affinity of hemoglobin for oxygen decreases, *i.e.* at a PaO_2 of 27 mmHg, hemoglobin is only 30% saturated, leaving 70% available for tissues, as opposed to the 60% saturation of hemoglobin with the same PaO_2 under

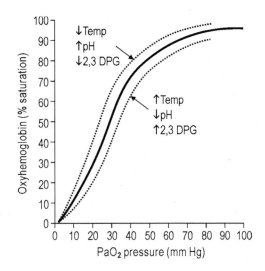

conditions favoring a leftward shift of the curve. The mnemonic "**CADET**, face right" suggests ↑CO_2, **A**cid, **D**PG (diphosphoglylcerate), **E**xercise and **T**emperature shift the oxyhemoblobin curve to the right.

	Right Shift	Left Shift
Temperature	High	Low
2,3-DPG	High	Low
P(CO_2)	High	Low
P(CO)	Low	High
pH (Bohr effect)	Acidosis	Alkalosis
Hb type	Adult Hb	Fetal Hb

IV. Hemodynamic and O_2 Delivery Equations
(*Determinants of Cardiac Output and O_2 Delivery, 3.1*)

Measure or Derived Value (Abbreviation)	Formula	Usual Normal Range	Units of Measure
Content of O_2 in	(Hb × 1.34* × SaO_2) + (PaO_2 × 0.0031)	17–20	ml/100 ml blood
Content of O_2 in venous blood (usually, mixed venous blood)	(Hb × 1.34* × SvO_2) + (PvO_2 × 0.0031)	12–15	ml/100 ml blood
A–V O_2 Difference	CaO_2 – CvO_2	3.5–5.5	ml/dL
Cardiac output (CO *or* Qt)	Stroke volume (SV in L) × Heart Rate (HR in beats/min.)		L/min
Cardiac index (CI)	CO ÷ BSA (in m^2)	3.5–5.5	$L/min/m^2$
O_2 Delivery (DO_2)	CaO_2 × CI × 10	400–600	$ml/min/m^2$
O_2 Consumption (VO_2)	(CaO_2 – CvO_2) × CI × 10	120–200	$ml/min/m^2$
SV index (SVI)	SV/m^2	30–60	ml/m^2
Systemic Vascular Resistance Index (SVRI)	[(MAP – *CVP*) ÷ CI] × 79.9	800–1600 (15–20)	$dyne\text{-}sec/cm^5/m^2$ (Wood's units)**
Pulmonary Vascular Resistance Index (PVRI)	[(MPAP – PCWP) ÷ CI] × 79.9	80–240 (<3)	$dyne\text{-}sec/cm^5/m^2$ (Wood's units)**
Left Ventricular Stroke Work Index (LVSWI)	SI × (MAP – PCWP) × 0.0136	50–62 (Adult)	$g\text{-}m/m^2$
Right Ventricular Stroke Work Index (RVSWI)	SI × (MPAP – CVP) × 0.0136	5.1–6.9	$g\text{-}m/m^2$

* Note that values 1.33–1.39 have been used.
** To calculate SVRI/PVRI in Wood's units, divide $dyne\text{-}sec/cm^5/m^2$ by 79.9.
Shortening fraction = (LV end-diastolic dimension – LV end systolic dimension) ÷ LV end-diastolic dimension; Normal range is 0.28 to 0.40.
Ejection Fraction = [(LV end-diastolic volume – LV end-systolic volume) ÷ LV end-diastolic volume] × 100; Normal range is 54% to 75%.

Ejection fraction provides a more accurate reflection of global LV function as compared to the shortening fraction. Cardiac mechanics change with age as manifested by an increase in afterload and a decrease in systolic function and contractility during normal growth and development. The most rapid changes occur between 1 and 4 years of age. Echocardiographically obtained data should be interpreted by the pediatric cardiologist. (Colan SD, Parness IA, Spevak PJ, Sanders SP, Developmental modulation of myocardial mechanincs: age- and growth-related alterations in afterload and contractility, *Pediatric Cardiology* 19(3): 619–629, 1992.)

V. Fluid, Electrolyte, Renal and Acid–Base Calculations

A. Anion Gap (mEq/L) = $[Na^+ + K^+] - [Cl^- + HCO_3^-]$; Normal: usually <16; variations exist among different laboratories since AG is calculated from other values which are measured.

Causes of an Abnormal Anion Gap

Decreased Anion Gap
- ↑ Un–measured cations: ↑Ca^{++}; ↑Mg^{++}; Lithium; TRIS buffer; hypergammaglobulinemia
- ↓ Un–measured anions: Metabolic acidosis; hypoalbuminemia
- Laboratory Error

Increased Anion Gap
- ↑ Un–measured anions: ↑lactate; ↑ketones (anions); ↑acetate; ↑sulfate; ↑phosphate; alkalemia; metabolic alkalosis with dehydration; nitrates; penicillins; methanol; ethylene glycol; salicylate; *d*–lactic acidosis *et al.*
- ↓ Un–measured cations: ↓Ca^{++}; ↓Mg^{++}
- Laboratory error

B. Creatinine clearance (Cl_{cr}) = [height or length (cm) × k] ÷ serum creatinine (mg/dL)

Age	k value*
LBW to ≤ 1yr	0.33
Full term to ≤1 yr	0.45
2–12 yrs	0.55
13–21 yrs female	0.55
13–21 yrs male	0.70

* From: Schwartz GJ, Brion LP, Spitzer A, The use of plasma creatinine concentration for estimating glomerular filtration rate in infants, children and adolescents, *Pediatr Clin N Am* **34:** 571–590, 1967.

C. Electrolyte Content of Body Fluids (mEq/L)

Fluid Source	Sodium	Potassium	Chloride
Gastric	20–80	5–20	100–150
Pancreatic	120–160	5–15	20–90
Small Intestine	100–140	5–15	90–130
Bile	120–140	5–15	80–120
Ileum	45–135	3–15	20–115
Diarrheal stool	10–90	10–80	10–110
CSF	148	3	120

D. Fractional Excretion (FE) of any substance *or* Y" = [Urine Y ÷ Plasma Y] ÷ [Urine creatinine ÷ Plasma creatinine] × 100

Fractional Excretion: Normal Values and Interpretations

FE Sodium

<1%	Consistent with a pre-renal cause (hypovolemia, CHF, renal artery stenosis, contrast induced nephropathy, *etc.*)
>2%	Consistent with an intrinsic renal cause (acute tubular necrosis, acute interstitial nephritis, glomerulonephritis, *etc.*)
>4%	Consistent with a post-renal cause (bladder stone, bilateral ureteral obstruction, *etc.*)

FE Magnesium	Normal: <3%
FE Phosphorus	Normal: 5–20%; In the presence of hypophosphatemia, a FE Phosphorus >5% is consistent with renal phosphorus wasting.

E. Calculated Osmolarity in mOsm/L solution = 2[Na (meq/L)] + [SUN (mg/dL) ÷ 2.8] + [glucose (mg/dL) ÷ 18]

Calculated osmolarity approximates measured osmolality by +/− 10 mOsm/kg H_2O unless additional (unmeasured) osmoles (*e.g.* alcohol, mannitol) are present. If additional unmeasured osmoles are present then the calculated osmolarity will exceed measured osmolality by >10 mOsm/kg.

F. *Predicted Sodium* Concentration in the Presence of Hyperglycemia = {[(Measured glucose (mg/dL) −100) ÷ 100] × 1.6} + Measured Na^+ (mEq/L)

In other words, for every 100 mg/dL increase in glucose above 100 mg/dL, the measured sodium is decreased by 1.6 mEq/L. This *predicted* value for sodium is the more commonly applied "correction" for artifactual hyponatremia in the presence of hyperglycemia.

G. Helpful Acid–Base Computations

- For any acute 10 mmHg decrease in $PaCO_2$ from 40 mmHg, blood pH will increase by 0.08 units (and vice versa).
- **To calculate the approximate base deficit (or excess):**
  - ▶ Calculate the predicted pH based on the measured $PaCO_2$.
  - ▶ Actual pH minus predicted pH = Δ pH.
  - ▶ Multiply Δ pH by 67 to determine the base deficit (a negative number) or base excess (a positive number) in mEq/L.
  - ▶ The total body bicarbonate deficit can be estimated by :

  Calculated base deficit (mEq/L) × 0.3 × ideal body weight.

Usually, only 25% of the calculated total bicarbonate deficit should be given to initiate correction of the base deficit. This dose usually approximates 1 mEq/kg of $NaHCO_3$. This should be given IV over 30–60 mins.

VI. Nutritional Requirements

Dietary Reference Intakes (DRIs): Estimated Energy Requirements (EERs)

Category Infants & Children (months)	Estimated Energy Requirements (kilocalories)
0–3	$(89 \times \text{weight [kg]} - 100) + 175$
4–6	$(89 \times \text{weight [kg]} - 100) + 56$
7–12	$(89 \times \text{weight [kg]} - 100) + 22$
13–35	$(89 \times \text{weight [kg]} - 100) + 20$
Males (yrs)	
3–8	$88.5 - 61.9 \times \text{age [yr]} + \text{PA} \times (26.7 \times \text{weight [kg]} + 903 \times \text{height [m]}) + 20$
9–18	$88.5 - 61.9 \times \text{age [yr]} + \text{PA} \times (26.7 \times \text{weight [kg]} + 903 \times \text{height [m]}) + 25$
≥ 19	$662 - 9.53 \times \text{age [yr]} + \text{PA} \times (15.91 \times \text{weight [kg]} + 539.6 \times \text{height [m]})$
Females (yrs)	
3–8	$135.3 - 30.8 \times \text{age [yr]} + \text{PA} \times (10.0 \times \text{weight [kg]} + 934 \times \text{height [m]}) + 20$
9–18	$135.3 - 30.8 \times \text{age [yr]} + \text{PA} \times (10.0 \times \text{weight [kg]} + 934 \times \text{height [m]}) + 25$
≥ 19	$354 - 6.91 \times \text{age [yr]} + \text{PA} \times (9.36 \times \text{weight [kg]} + 726 \times \text{height [m]})$

PA, Physical activity: PA = 1.0 for inactive, sedentary patients; PA = 1.13 for low level activity and PA = 1.26 for active patients.

Schofield Equations for Calculating Basal Metabolic Rate in Children

Male (yrs)	Resting Energy Expenditure (REE) in kcal/day
0–3	$0.167W + 15.174H - 617.6$
3–10	$19.59W + 1.303H + 414.9$
10–18	$16.25W + 1.372H + 515.5$
>18	$15.057W + 1.004H + 705.8$

Female (yrs)	
0–3	$16.252W + 10.232H - 413.5$
3–10	$16.969W + 1.618H + 371.2$
10–18	$8.365W + 4.65H + 200$
>18 yr	$13.623W + 23.8W + 98.2$

H = height (cm); W = weight (kg)
Adapted from Schofield W, Predicting basal metabolic rate, new standards and review of previous work, *Human Nutrition Clinical Nutrition* **39c Supp 1**, 5–41, 1985.

Assessment of Basal Metabolic Energy Requirements in Hospitalized Pediatric Patients*

	Kcal/day			Kcal/day	
Body Wt (kg)	Male	Female	Body Wt (kg)	Male	Female
3.0	120	144	16.0	750	747
4.0	191	191	17.0	780	775
5.0	270	274	18.0	810	802
6.0	330	336	19.0	840	827
7.0	390	395	20.0	870	852
8.0	445	448	22.0	910	898
9.0	495	496	24.0	980	942
10.0	545	541	26.0	1,070	984
11.0	590	582	28.0	1,100	1,025
12.0	625	620	30.0	1,140	1,063
13.0	665	655	32.0	1,190	1,101
14.0	700	687	34.0	1,230	1,137
15.0	725	718			

(Continued)

Assessment of Basal Metabolic Energy Requirements in Hospitalized Pediatric Patients* (Continued)

Body Wt (kg)	Kcal/day Male	Kcal/day Female	Body Wt (kg)	Kcal/day Male	Kcal/day Female
36.0	1,270	1,173	62.0	1,660	1,572
38.0	1,305	1,207	64.0	1,690	1,599
40.0	1,340	1,241	66.0	1,725	1,626
42.0	1,370	1,274	68.0	1,765	1,653
44.0	1,400	1,306	70.0	1,785	1,679
46.0	1,430	1,338	72.0	1,815	1,705
48.0	1,460	1,369	74.0	1,845	1,731
50.0	1,485	1,399	76.0	1,870	1,756
52.0	1,505	1,429	78.0	1,900	1,781
54.0	1,555	1,458	80.0	1,935	1,805
56.0	1,580	1,487	82.0	1,970	1,830
58.0	1,600	1,516	84.0	2,000	1,855
60.0	1,630	1,544			

"Stress Factor" Adjustments for Estimating Caloric Needs in Sick Pediatric Patients: * Multiply Basal Metabolic Requirements by Stress Factor Based on Severity of Illness

Clinical Condition	Stress Factor
Starvation	0.9
Fever	12% per degree >37C
Cardiac failure	1.15–1.25
Major surgery	1.20–1.30
Sepsis	1.40–1.50
Catch-up growth	1.5–2.0
Burns	1.5–2.0

Schofield W, Predicting basal metabolic rate, new standards and review of previous work, Human Clinical Nutrition, **39c Supp 1**, 5–41, 1985.

Example: 18-month-old, 12 kg boy admitted with sepsis and respiratory distress; tracheally intubated and heavily sedated. Basal metabolic demands: 625 kcal/day. Estimated energy requirement = Stress factor of 1.4 × 625 = 875 kcal/day. Note: Recommended dietary allowance for a normal healthy 18 mos. old is 102 kcal/kg/day or 1,224 kcal/day, which is almost 40% more than estimated requirement during critical illness.

VII. Trauma Evaluation: Summary

Primary Survey	
	Potential Interventions
Airway and Cervical Spine Control	Jaw thrust; suction; finger sweep if foreign body is visible; C–spine immobilization; artifical airway as indicated; apply cervical collar.
Breathing	Provide supplemental O_2; assist ventilation (tracheal intubation) as needed; evacuate tension pneumothorax or hemothorax; assist ventilation with flail chest.
Circulation and Control of Bleeding	Control external bleeding; Place 2 large bore PIV's; Obtain blood samples (*e.g.* CBC, PT/PTT/INR, electrolytes, type and cross-match as indicated). Perform CPR and begin advanced life-support measures as indicated. Examine the back (log roll if spine injury has not been ruled out).
Disability (AVPU)	Maintain alignment of the spine; avoid hyperventilation unless otherwise indicated.
Exposure and Environmental Control	Remove clothing/prevent heat loss with use of warm blankets, over-bed warmers, warmed blood products/IV fluids, *etc.* Avoid over-warming!
Secondary Survey	
Measure Vital Signs	Apply monitors including Pox; insert NG/OG if not already placed prior to tracheal intubation; decompress the bladder.
Assess Pain	Provide appropriate analgesia.
Head-to-toe assessment	Complete the history and physical examination, including allergies, immunization status, chronic medications, recent illnesses, menstrual history as indicated, and family history. Identify legal guardian(s). Intervene and document appropriately.
Consultations	Obtain as appropriate if not already sought during primary survey.

VIII. Decision Tree for Management of Threatening Behavior

Threatening or aggressive behavior in the pediatric patient should be evaluated so as to exclude organic causes that may require specific medical therapy (*Altered Mental Status, 5.1*). Threatening behavior not attributed to an organic cause, or illness-associated behavior that requires symptomatic intervention to facilitate management and help ensure safety may require pharmacologic intervention. The following decision tree, developed by the professional staff at Children's Hospital of The King's Daughters, is a guide to pharmacologic management of threatening behavior. Prescribers should individualize management based on patient need and response to interventions. With permission from: Chicella M, Dozier P, Fine B, Mason J, Ramirez D, Zaritsky A.

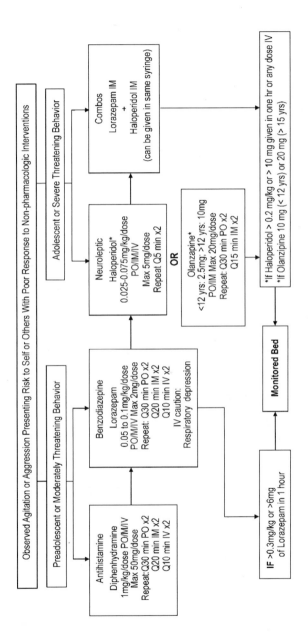

IX. A. Initial Metabolic Approach to the Encephalopathic Infant

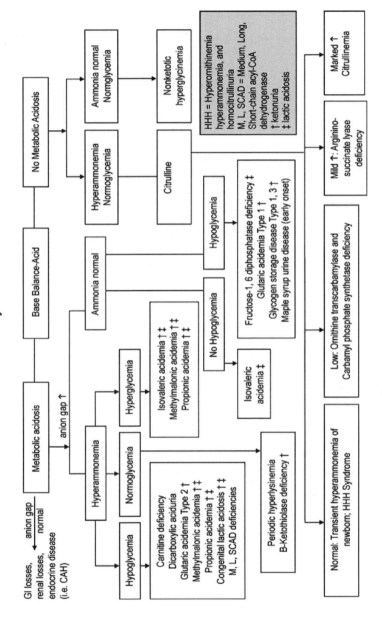

IX. B. Classification of Inborn Errors by Initial Biochemical Profile

X. A. ICP Management Decision Tree Part 1

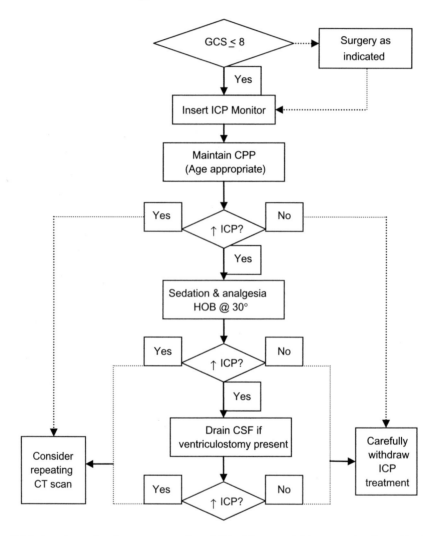

Critical pathway for the treatment of established intracranial hypertension in pediatric traumatic brain injury. From Adelson PD, Bratton SL, Carney RM *et al.* Guidelines for the acute medical management of severe traumatic brain injury in infants, children and adolescents, *Pediatr Crit Care Med* **4(3)**: S66–67, 2003.

X. B. ICP Management Decision Tree Part 2

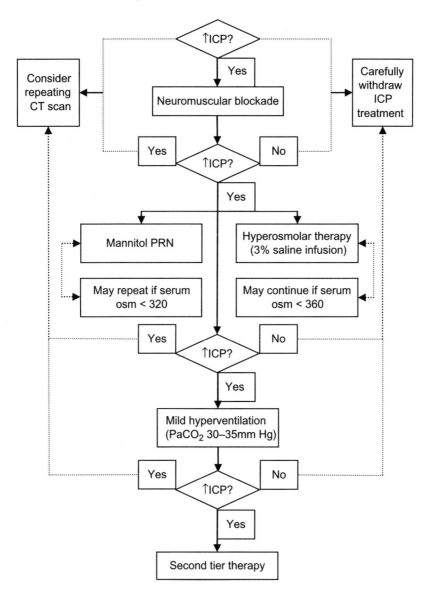

X. C. ICP Management Decision Tree Part 3

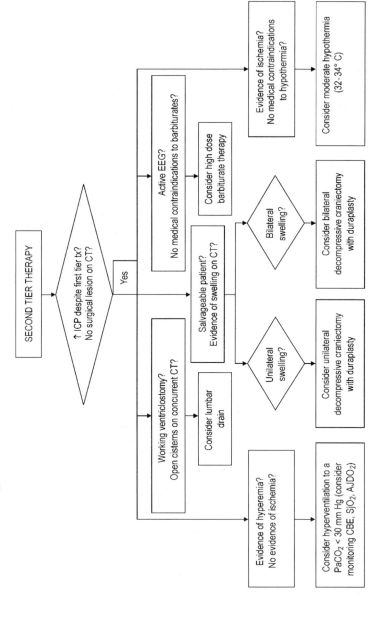

XI. Empiric Antibiotic Treatment for Sepsis/Septic Shock Based on Suspected Source of Sepsis

	Lungs	Abdomen	Skin/Soft Tissue	Urine	CNS
<3 mos	Group B *Strep.* L. monocytogenes E. coli; S. aureus Syphilis C. trachomatis RSV, influenza adenovirus, HSV, CMV VZV, enterovirus	E. coli, Enterobacter cloacae, Enterococcus sp. Bacteroides fragilis Other Gram-negative enteric bacilli	S. aureus Group B *Strep.* S. pyogenes	E. coli Group B *Strep.* Enterococcus, Klebsiella, Enterobacter Proteus Candida sp.	Group B *Strep.* L monocytogenes E. coli H. influenza N. meningitides
Empiric Antibiotic therapy	Ampicillin + Gentamicin OR ampicillin + Cefotaxime	Cefepime OR Cefotaxime + Gentamicin +/- (Clindamycin or Metronidazole) OR Piperacillin/tazobactam + gentamicin OR Meropenem	Cefotaxime + (Nafcillin or Vancomycin)	Ampicillin + Gentamicin OR Ampicillin + Cefotaxime	Ampicillin + Gentamicin OR Ampicillin + Cefotaxime

(Continued)

XI. Empiric Antibiotic Treatment for Sepsis/Septic Shock Based on Suspected Source of Sepsis (Continued)

	Lungs	Abdomen	Skin/Soft Tissue	Urine	CNS
3 mos to 5 yrs	*S. pneumoniae* *H. influenza* Group A *Strep.*, RSV influenza, adenovirus parainfluenza, *Pneumocystis jiroveci* *M. tuberculosis*	*E. coli* *Enterobacter cloacae* *Enterococcus sp.* *Bacteroides fragilis* Other Gram-negative enterics bacilli.	*S. aureus* Group A *Strep.* *Clostridium sp.*	*E. coli* *K. pneumonia* *Proteus* *Enterobacter cloacae*	*S. pneumoniae* *H. influenza* *N. meningitides*
Empiric Antibiotic Therapy	Ceftriaxone **OR** Cetotaxime +/– (Vancomycin or Linezolid if MRSA is suspected)	Cefepime **OR** Cefotaxime + Gentamicin +/– (Clindamycin or Metronidazole) **OR** Pipercillin/tazobactam + Gentamicin **OR** Meropenem	Nafcillin **OR** Cefazolin **OR** Clindamycin **OR** (Vancomycin or Linezolid if MRSA is suspected)	Ampicillin + Gentamicin **OR** Ampicillin + Cefotaxime	Vancomycin + (Ceftriaxone or Cefotaxime)

(Continued)

XI. Empiric Antibiotic Treatment for Sepsis/Septic Shock Based on Suspected Source of Sepsis (Continued)

	Lungs	Abdomen	Skin/Soft Tissue	Urine	CNS
5 yrs Adolescents	*S. pneumoniae* Group A Strep. *Mycoplasma pneumoniae* *Chlamydia pneumoniae* *M. tuberculosis*	*E. coli* *Enterococcus sp.* *B. fragilis* *Pseudomonas sp.*	*S. aureus* Group A Strep. *Clostridium sp.*	*E. coli* *Enterococcus sp.* *Staphylococcus saprophyticus*	*S. pneumoniae* *Neisseria meningitidis*
Empiric Antibiotic Therapy	Ceftriaxone **OR** Cefotaxime +/− Macrolide +/− (Vancomycin or Linezolid if MRSA is suspected)	Meropenem **OR** Imipenem **OR** Piperacillin-tazobactam	Nafcillin **OR** Cefazolin **OR** Clindamycin **OR** Vancomycin + Cefotaxime if Gram negative organisms are present on Gram stain	Ceftriaxone **OR** Cefotaxime	Vancomycin + (Ceftriaxone **OR** Cefotaxime)

XII. Therapy in Complex Infections and Supplemental Therapies in the Immunocompromised Host

Antibiotic considerations in the **immunocompromised host >6 weeks of age** with **no obvious infectious focus** (*e.g.* **fever and neutropenia**): Consider disease from Gram negative bacilli (*e.g.* from the gi tract); staphylococci and streptococci; yeast and fungi, esp. aspergillus.
Empiric therapy would include:

- [Cefepime or meropenem or piperacillin-tazobactam] AND tobramycin (amikacin or gentamicin may be alternative aminoglycosides).

- Add Vancomycin if patient has received high dose cytarabine chemotherapy, has mucositis, cellulitis, a vascular catheter, known colonization with MRSA/MSSA, or intra-abdominal or peri-rectal infection or Coagulase negative *Staphylococcus* is a concern.

- Add Metronidazole if colitis, peri-rectal lesion, typhilitis or other deep anaerobic infection is suspected.

- **If lungs are a focus,** consider community acquired organisms, *Pseudomonas,* or nosocomial Gram negative bacilli, *S. aureus,* fungi (esp. *Aspergillus*), AFB, *P. jiroveci* ("PCP"), and viral agents. Sampling by brochoalveolar Lavage (BAL) is recommended. **Empiric therapy would include:**

  ▸ Cefepime or meropenem or piperacillin-tazobactam AND vancomycin or linezolid if MRSA is a possibility.

  ▸ If pnemonitis is diffuse, add trimethoprim-sulfamethoxazole AND a macrolide (azithromycin or clarithromycin).

- For **CNS disease,** lumbar puncture prior to antibiotic therapy is optimal; however, lumbar puncture should not unduly delay administration of antibiotics. Unstable patients should receive antibiotics empirically and CSF should be obtained when the clinical circumstances permit (*Lumbar Puncture, 15.5).* Possible offending agents include *S. pnemoniae, N. meningitidis,* Gram negative organisms (esp. in the presence of a CSF shunt, foreign body or post-surgery), fungi (*Cryptococcus*), parasites

(toxoplasmosis) and viruses (arbovirus, CMV, EBV, enterovirus).
Empiric therapy would include:

▶ Cefotaxime or ceftriaxone or cefepime or meropenem PLUS vancomycin, esp. if post operative or if hardware is present.

▶ If fungal or viral CNS infection is suspected, pre-treatment LP is mandatory to guide anti-fungal or anti-viral therapy.

Considerations in Treatment of Fungal and Viral infections:
- **Antifungal agents:**

  ▶ **Amphoteracin B Liposome:** Often employed as first line agent for presumed fungal infections in the febrile neutropenic patient; effective against *Candida, Aspergillus* and *Cryptococcus.*

  ▶ **Triazoles:**
    - Fluconazole: IV, PO; excellent bioavailability with enteral administration; penetrates the CNS; active against yeasts but inactive against molds.
    - Itraconazole: PO; Capsules require food and an acid pH for solubilization; commercially prepared solution should be given on an empty stomach but tolerates acid pH. Useful against *Aspergillus* (Allergic bronchopulmonary aspergillosis), histoplasmosis, blastomycosis.
    - Voriconazole: IV, PO. Use caution with IV preparation in renal insufficiency; inhibits cytochrome P450 34A.
    - Posaconazole; PO; useful for fungal prophylaxis and oropharyngeal candidiasis not responsive to fluconazole or itraconazole.

  ▶ **Echinocandins:** Often effective for refractory *Candida* and *Aspergillus*
    - Caspofungin
    - Micafungin
    - Anidulafungin

- **Antiviral agents:**

  ▶ Acyclovir: For treatment of herpesvirus infections and varicella

  ▶ Gancyclovir: For treatment of CMV

Adjunctive Therapy in Complex Acute Infections:

- **Intravenous Immune Globulin (IVIG):** May be useful in necrotizing skin and/or soft tissue infections, Guillain-Barre Syndrome (1 gram/kg on two consecutive days), toxic shock syndrome (1 gram/kg) or as adductive therapy in agammaglobulinemia or hypogammaglobulinemia (low IgG for age).
- **Clindamycin:** added in severe staphylococcal or streptococcal infections to inhibit toxin production.
- **Specific immunoglobulin preparations:**
  - ▸ **CMV immune globulin** can be given with gancyclovir in treatment of CMV disease
  - ▸ **Botulism immune globulin (BIG-IV or "Baby BIG").** Indicated for patients <1 yr with infant botulism caused by toxin type A or B. This product and instructions for sampling and shipment of specimens can be obtained from the California Department of Health (510-231-7600 or www.infantbotulism. org). **Antitoxin for suspected foodborne or wound-related cases** (non-infant botulism) can be obtained from state health departments or the Centers for Disease Control.

- **Empiric antifungal therapy:** Consider in any patient with continued fevers without identified source after 4–7 days.
- **Granulocyte transfusion**: Use is limited in pediatrics by paucity of studies indicating clear benefit. Studies which may have an impact on children are underway (NHLBI) in nuetropenic adults. WBC transfusions carry a major risk of transfusion-related acute lung injury (TRALI).
- Use of **Granulocyte Colony Stimulation Factor (GCSF)** has been added to the therapy of febrile neutropenic cancer patients to hasten recovery of granulocytes following chemotherapy. No controlled, randomized trials have been conducted with GCSF for this purpose. There was no improvement in outcome (organ dysfunction, duration of mechanical ventilation, death) among non-neutropenic patients with SIRS or septic shock when GCSF was given as adjunctive therapy.

XIII. Therapeutic Dose Monitoring Table for Medications Commonly Used in the PICU

Medication	Therapeutic Range P, Peak; T, Trough (mcg/mL)	Toxic Range (mcg/mL)	Monitoring* (Timing of serum levels)
Amikacin	P: 20–30 T: 4–8	P: >30 T: >8	P: 30 min after 30 min infusion, 15 min after 1 hr infusion, 60 min after IM.
Gentamicin	P: 4–12 ** T: ≤1	P: n/a T: >2	P: 30 min after 30 min infusion, 15 min after 1 hr infusion, 60 min after IM.
Tobramycin	P: 4–12 ** T: ≤1	P: n/a T: >2	P: 30 min after 30 min infusion, 15 min after 1 hr infusion, 60 min after IM dose
Carbamazepine	T: 4–12 T: 4–8 (if other enzyme inducers are present)***	T: >12	P levels not clinically useful.
Digoxin	T: 0.8–2	T: >2	T immediately prior to next dose (at least 6 hrs after the prior IV dose).
Phenobarbital	T: 15–40 (T ≥70 may be required for refractory status epilepticus or cerebral salvage)	T: >40 T ≥80 (potentially lethal)	T immediately prior to next dose (must be at least 2 hrs after the prior dose). (Continued)

XIII. Therapeutic Dose Monitoring Table for Medications Commonly Used in the PICU (Continued)

Medication	Therapeutic Range P, Peak; T, Trough (mcg/mL)	Toxic Range (mcg/mL)	Monitoring* (Timing of serum levels)
Phenytoin or Fosphenyoin	$T_{(Total)}$ 10–20 $T_{(Free)}$: 1–2	T: > 20	T immediately prior to next dose P: 1 hr (for phenytoin) or 2 hrs (for fosphenytoin) after IV infusion is complete); at least 4 hrs after IM dosing.
Aminophylline or Theophylline	P: 10–20 (asthma) P: 7–12 (apnea of prematurity)	P: > 20	30 min after 30 min infusion (bolus dosing) 12–24 hrs after initiation of continuous infusion.
Valproic Acid (anticonvulsant)	T: 50–120	T: >100–150	T immediately prior to next dose
Vancomycin	P: 25–40 T: 10–20	T: > 20	P: 1 hr after infusion is complete T: ≤ 30 min before next dose

*Peak and trough concentrations are usually obtained after SS is achieved. Peak levels of anticonvulsants may be required before achieving SS, esp. if seizures are on-going. Trough levels are typically obtained within 30 mins prior to the next dose.

**Goal peak for uncomplicated uti, Gram positive endocarditis and synergy with B–lactams is 3–5 mcg/mL; for Gram negative bacteremia and other severe Gram negative infections, goal peak is 6–8 mcg/mL; for Gram negative pneumonia or acute life-threatening Gram negative infection, goal peak is 8–12 mcg/mL.

***Due to increase in unmeasured active epoxide metabolite.

XIV. Neonatal Hyperbilirubinemia

Indirect hyperbilirubinemia in the neonate is occasionally seen in the PICU when the progression of jaundice after discharge from the nursery is unexpectedly severe, or when neonatal jaundice presents as an incidental event in a PICU patient with other problems (*e.g.* congenital heart disease). Recognition, appropriate evaluation and timely intervention are essential to minimize the risk of acute bilirubin encephalopathy (kernicterus). Management guidelines are outlined in "Management of Hyperbilirubinemia in the Newborn Infant 35 or More Weeks of Gestation" by the Subcommittee on Hyperbilirubinemia, American Academy of Pediatrics (*Pediatrics*, **114(1)**: 297–316, 2004).

XV. MRI Terminology

Image contrast. The differences in signal intensity (reflected by the gray scale from white to black) that vary among pixels depending on the chemical properties of the tissues comprising the pixel.

Pulse Sequence. A repetitive, ordered combination of magnetic field perturbations (creating a precise linear spatial variation or "gradient" in the strength of the magnetic field), radiofrequency (RF) wave transmissions (often called "RF pulses"), and RF wave signal acquisitions (called "echos") used to create images of a given contrast.

Spin echo. A type of pulse sequence that creates the MRI signal by applying repeated RF pulses and acquiring repeated echos.

Inversion recovery "IR". A type of pulse sequence that creates MRI signal by first applying a special RF pulse that inverts the directional magnetization of protons and later applies a spin echo sequence to form the images. Varying the time between the inversion pulse and the application of the spin echo sequence allows for eliminating signal from certain types of tissue.

T1-weighted image. An image contrast that is usually created using a spin echo pulse sequence in which fluid is dark, fat is bright, brain white matter is bright and gray matter is gray. T1 is a measure of the time it takes for the protons in a tissue to recover their directional magnetization after having been disrupted by an RF pulse.

T2-weighted image. An image contrast that is usually created using a special type of spin echo pulse sequence (call a "fast spin echo" or "FSE") in which fluid and fat are bright, brain gray matter is light gray and white matter is dark. T2 is a measure of the time it takes for protons in a tissue to lose their magnetization by transferring energy to the surrounding protons.

"FLAIR". Fluid Attenuated Inversion Recovery. An image contrast in which an IR sequence is used to eliminate high signal from water or most simple fluids. The FLAIR sequence allows high signal associated with pathology or edema to be more conspicuous relative to physiologic fluid.

"STIR". Short Tau Inversion Recovery. An image contrast in which an IR sequence is used to eliminate signal from fat.

Index